Nursing Leadership
A Concise Encyclopedia

Second Edition

HARRIET R. FELDMAN, PhD, RN, FAAN, is professor and Interim Provost and Executive Vice President for Academic Affairs at Pace University (2010 to the present) and was dean of the Lienhard School of Nursing at Pace University (1993–2010) and interim dean of the School of Education (2006–2010). Dr. Feldman was an editor of two nursing journals: *Scholarly Inquiry for Nursing Practice: An International Journal* and *Nursing Leadership Forum.* Three of her books have received American Journal of Nursing Book of the Year Awards: 2001 (*Nurses in the Political Arena: The Public Face of Nursing,* coauthored by Dr. Sandra B. Lewenson), 2005 (*Educating Nurses for Leadership,* coedited by Dr. Martha J. Greenberg), and 2007 (*Teaching and Learning Evidence-Based Practice: A Guide for Educators,* coedited by Dr. Rona F. Levin). Other books include *Strategies for Nursing Leadership* (2001), *The Nursing Shortage: Strategies for Recruitment and Retention in Clinical Practice and Education* (2003), and *Nursing Leadership: A Concise Encyclopedia* (2008). She has more than 80 refereed publications to her credit. Dr. Feldman was chair and member of the Board of Commissioners of the Commission on Collegiate Nursing Education (2003–2010), a Fellow of the American Academy of Nursing, and a Fellow of the New York Academy of Medicine.

G. RUMAY ALEXANDER, EdD, RN, is clinical professor and director of the Office of Multicultural Affairs at the University of North Carolina at Chapel Hill School of Nursing. A frequently sought-after lecturer and consultant, Dr. Alexander is recognized nationally and internationally as an expert in diversity and inclusion management. She has been featured in three National Student Nurses' Association award-winning videos. Dr. Alexander has received numerous invitations to present nationally and internationally, consulted with 90 hospitals, and consulted on HRSA- and NIH-funded grants, and 20 nursing programs including Bournemouth University in England. She has authored four books and eight book chapters and has participated on numerous expert panels, advisory committees, and professional bodies such as Sigma Theta Tau's International Nursing Alliance, the landmarked Workforce Commission of the American Hospital Association, which produced "In Our Hands," the Robert Wood Johnson Foundation, and the National Quality Forum's Steering Committee for the first ever national voluntary consensus standards for nursing-sensitive care. She is the 2010 recipient of the American Organization of Nurse Executives' Prism Award, which recognizes, at a national level, leadership in the scholarship and science of diversity.

MARTHA J. GREENBERG, PhD, RN, is associate professor at the Lienhard School of Nursing of the College of Health Professions at Pace University in Pleasantville, New York. She has served in leadership roles as chairperson of the 4-year baccalaureate nursing program from 1995 to 2000 and again from 2007 to the present. She has received a VA Nursing Academy grant, one of 15 such grants in the United States. Dr. Greenberg is the coeditor of *Educating Nurses for Leadership,* which received a 2005 American Journal of Nursing Book of the Year Award. She maintains a clinical practice in medical-surgical nursing and serves on a variety of community boards and task forces in Westchester County, New York. Her areas of research interest are humor and complementary health and healing practices.

MARILYN JAFFE-RUIZ, EdD, RN, is professor emeritus of nursing at the Lienhard School of Nursing in the College of Health Professions, Pace University, New York, NY. Her areas of specialization include leadership, education, psychiatric mental health nursing, cultural competence, and siblings and families of the intellectually disabled. Dr. Jaffe-Ruiz served as Pace University's chief academic officer with the title of Provost and Executive Vice President for Academic Affairs from 1998 to 2003. Formerly, she was Vice Provost and, before that, dean of the Lienhard School of Nursing at Pace, a position that she held for 7 years. Dr. Jaffe-Ruiz has held faculty positions at Pace University and Columbia University. In 2001, Dr. Jaffe-Ruiz was inducted into the Teachers College Nursing Hall of Fame and made an honorary member of the Golden Key International Honor Society at Pace University. In 2006, she received the Dr. Martin Luther King Social Justice Award, and in 2002, she received the Diversity Leadership Award at Pace University. She received the Anne Krauss Volunteer of the Year Award from the New York City Chapter of the Association for the Help of Retarded Children in May 2007.

ANGELA BARRON MCBRIDE, PHD, RN, FAAN, is Distinguished Professor-University Dean Emerita at Indiana University School of Nursing. She is on the board of Indiana University Health, the largest hospital network in Indiana, and chairs the board's Committee on Quality and Patient Safety. Known for her contributions to women's mental health, she served as president of Sigma Theta Tau International (1987–1989) during the building of their International Center for Nursing Scholarship, and of the American Academy of Nursing (1993–1995). Elected in 1995 to the Institute of Medicine, Dr. McBride was named a "Living Legend" by the American Academy of Nursing in 2006. Passing on her leadership savvy, she designs the annual leadership conference of the John A. Hartford Foundation's Building Academic Geriatric Nursing Capacity Program, chairs the national advisory committee for the Robert Wood Johnson Foundation's Nurse Faculty Scholar Program, and authored *The Growth and Development of Nurse Leaders* (Springer, 2011).

MARGARET L. MCCLURE, EDD, RN, FAAN, is a professor at New York University, where she holds appointments in both the College of Nursing and the School of Medicine. For almost 20 years, she was the chief nursing officer at New York University Medical Center, where she also served as chief operating officer and hospital administrator. She has held office in several professional organizations, including the presidency of the American Organization of Nurse Executives and the American Academy of Nursing. A prolific writer and lecturer, Dr. McClure is internationally recognized as a nursing leader. Her best known contribution to the literature is *Magnet Hospitals: Attraction and Retention of Professional Nurses*, which she coauthored under the auspices of the American Academy of Nursing. In 2002, she completed a compilation of all the work that has been done regarding this subject, titled *Magnet Hospitals Revisited*. In 2007, she was named a "Living Legend" by the American Academy of Nursing.

THOMAS D. SMITH, MS, RN, DNP, NEA-BC, is chief nursing officer and senior vice president at Maimonides Medical Center in Brooklyn, New York. Dr. Smith's prior positions include chief nursing officer at Cambridge Health Alliance in Cambridge, Massachusetts, and senior vice president for nursing at the Mount Sinai Hospital in New York City, the first full-service hospital in Manhattan to receive the Magnet Award for nursing excellence. He currently serves as senior clinical advisor at the Hartford Institute for Geriatric Nursing at New York University College of Nursing. Dr. Smith is the recipient of numerous awards, including the Grace E. Davidson Award for contributions to the education of nursing students at New York University College of Nursing, the Anne Kibrick Award for excellence in nursing leadership from the University of Massachusetts, Boston, and the Dean's Legacy Award from the Frances Payne Bolton School of Nursing at Case Western Reserve University. He has served on the Board of Commissioners of the Commission on Collegiate Nursing Education and is active in the American Organization of Nurse Executives. Dr. Smith's research interests and publications focus on the nurse–patient relationship, care of the older adult, and the organization and improvement of patient care delivery.

Nursing Leadership
A Concise Encyclopedia

Second Edition

Editor-in-Chief

Harriet R. Feldman, PhD, RN, FAAN

Associate Editors

G. Rumay Alexander, EdD, RN

Martha J. Greenberg, PhD, RN

Marilyn Jaffe-Ruiz, EdD, RN, FAAN

Angela Barron McBride, PdD, RN, FAAN

Margaret L. McClure, EdD, RN, FAAN

Thomas D. Smith, MS, RN, DNP, NEA-BC

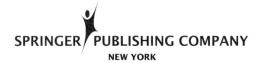

SPRINGER PUBLISHING COMPANY

NEW YORK

Springer Publishing Company, LLC
11 West 42nd Street
New York, NY 10036
www.springerpub.com

Acquisitions Editor: Allan Graubard
Production Editor: Lindsay Claire
Composition: Newgen Imaging

ISBN: 978–0-8261–2176-9
E-book ISBN: 978–0-8261–2177-6

11 12 13 / 5 4 3 2 1

The author and the publisher of this Work have made every effort to use sources believed to be reliable to provide information that is accurate and compatible with the standards generally accepted at the time of publication. The author and publisher shall not be liable for any special, consequential, or exemplary damages resulting, in whole or in part, from the readers' use of, or reliance on, the information contained in this book. The publisher has no responsibility for the persistence or accuracy of URLs for external or third-party Internet Web sites referred to in this publication and does not guarantee that any content on such Web sites is, or will remain, accurate or appropriate.

Library of Congress Cataloging-in-Publication Data

Nursing leadership : a concise encyclopedia / Harriet R. Feldman ...
[et al.], editors. — 2nd ed.
      p. ; cm.
 Includes bibliographical references and index.
 ISBN 978-0-8261-2176-9 — ISBN 978-0-8261-2177-6 (e-Book)
 I. Feldman, Harriet R.
 [DNLM: 1. Leadership—Encyclopedias—English. 2. Nursing,
Supervisory—Encyclopedias—English. 3. Nurse
Administrators—Encyclopedias—English. WY 13]
 610.7303—dc23   2011042085

Special discounts on bulk quantities of our books are available to corporations, professional associations, pharmaceutical companies, health care organizations, and other qualifying groups.

If you are interested in a custom book, including chapters from more than one of our titles, we can provide that service as well.

For details, please contact:
Special Sales Department, Springer Publishing Company, LLC
11 West 42nd Street, 15th Floor, New York, NY 10036-8002
Phone: 877-687-7476 or 212-431-4370; Fax: 212-941-7842
Email: sales@springerpub.com

Printed in the United States of America by Hamilton Printing.

Leadership skills develop over a lifetime, through the many relationships we nurture and the many people we meet along the way. There are significant people in my life who gave me their love and support so that I could get to the place where I am in my leadership journey.

To my parents, Florence and Mickey Martin, whose faith and unconditional love guided me toward success;

To my dear husband, Ron Feldman, who challenged me to realize more than I ever dreamed and always pushed me toward the next great challenge—you were my best fan;

To my children and grandchildren, you have kept me on track and cheered me on with your faith and love—you light up my life!;

To my past mentors, many of who through the years were leaders in their own right, for gently showing me the way so I could grow as a professional and a person of integrity;

My associate editors have established themselves over time as nursing leaders because of a special skill each possesses for making things happen. I could not have completed this work without their steadfast guidance and commitment. Thank you!

Harriet

CONTENTS

PREFACE

Nursing Leadership: A Concise Encyclopedia grew out of our long-standing and enduring commitment to describe and define the concept and field of nursing leadership. I believe that this encyclopedia presents an important reference to provide students, faculty, nurse managers, executives, and others with a concise resource for information about the range of knowledge and roles encompassed by the term *nursing leadership*. New entries in the second edition also reflect the changing needs of our time. Our latest thematic listing of entries in 10 distinct categories, along with the alphabetical listing, will help the reader conceptualize and access content. These categories are as follows: Characteristics of Leaders; Health Care Delivery Standards and Health Policy; Informatics and Technology; Leadership in Practice, Education, and Research; Major Leaders; Management and Executive Skills; Organizational Leadership; Professional Standards; Quality Outcomes; and Theories and Models. The section on historical nursing leaders has been revised and set apart to emphasize the important roles these individuals played in health care and organized nursing.

The associate editors and I hope that you will use the practical skills and references of each entry to further develop your understanding of what leaders and aspiring leaders need to know to be successful. Along with the six associate editors—Drs. G. Rumay Alexander, Angela Barron McBride, Martha J. Greenberg, Marilyn Jaffe-Ruiz, Margaret L. McClure, and Thomas D. Smith—there were numerous individuals who, because of their expertise, contributed by writing one or more entries. Hence, we have the benefit of many years of experience and the expertise of scores of nursing leaders. Assembling this wonderful group of leaders is part of the story. The remaining credit goes to the staff at Springer Publishing Company, with whom I have been associated for more than 25 years, and especially Allan Graubard, whose insights and reminders provided great support to the publication.

The leaders who have crossed our paths teach us important lessons about the art and science of leadership, for example, working effectively in groups, persuading others, communicating and advancing one's vision, dealing with naysayers, and celebrating success. Through them, we have reinforced values, learned to solve dilemmas, think and feel differently, and developed new attitudes and behaviors consistent with our leadership roles. I am confident that the many topics and resources of this encyclopedia will enhance your leadership skills and opportunities to be successful.

Harriet R. Feldman, PhD, RN, FAAN
Editor-in-Chief

CONTRIBUTORS

Linda H. Aiken, PhD, RN, FAAN
Claire M. Fagin Leadership Professor of
  Nursing
Professor of Sociology
Director, Center for Health Outcomes and
  Policy Research
University of Pennsylvania School of Nursing
Philadelphia, PA
  Failure to Rescue

G. Rumay Alexander, EdD, RN
Clinical Professor and Director of the Office
  of Multicultural Affairs
University of North Carolina at Chapel Hill
School of Nursing
Chapel Hill, NC
  Affirmative Action
  Cultural Diversity
  Employee Resource Groups
  Epigenetics
  Meaningful Use Rule
  National Coalition of Ethnic Minority
    Nurse Associations

**Anne W. Alexandrov PhD, RN, CCRN,
  FAAN**
University of Alabama
School of Nursing
Birmingham, AL
  Outcomes Management

**Patricia G. Archbold, DNSc, RN, FAAN,
  FGSA**
Consulting Program Administrator
Building Academic Geriatric Nursing Capacity
American Academy of Nursing
Washington, DC
  Hartford Geriatric Nursing Initiative (HGNI)

Karen A. Ballard, MA, RN, FAAN
Adjunct Faculty
PACE University and New York
  University
Nursing Consultant
New York, NY
  Advocacy
  Collective Bargaining and Unions
  Credentialing
  Employee Safety
  Health Care Reform
  Licensure

Geraldine Bednash, PhD, RN, FAAN
Chief Executive Officer and Executive
  Director
American Association of Colleges of
  Nursing
Washington, DC
  Doctor of Nursing Practice

Rachel Behrendt, DNP, RN, AOCNS
Senior Director, MAGNET Program and
  Staff Development
Thomas Jefferson University Hospitals
Philadelphia, PA
  Externships

Lazelle E. Benefield, PhD, RN, FAAN
Dean and Parry Endowed Professor
Director, Donald W. Reynolds Center of
  Geriatric Nursing Excellence
College of Nursing, University of Oklahoma
  Health Sciences Center
Oklahoma City, OK
  Aging in Place

Diane M. Billings, EdD, RN, FAAN
Chancellor's Professor Emeritus
Indiana University School of Nursing
Indianapolis, IN
Distance Education in Nursing

Marie Boltz, PhD, RN, GNP-BC
New York University College of Nursing
Associate Director for Practice
Hartford Institute for Geriatric Nursing and
Assistant Professor
New York, NY
Nurses Improving Care for Healthsystem
Elders (NICHE)

Susan Bowar-Ferres, PhD, RN, NEA-BC
Adjunct Professor of Nursing
College of Nursing
New York University Professor of Nursing &
Nursing Administration
School of Medicine
NYU Board Member
Nurses Educational Funds, Inc.
New York, NY
Leadership in Practice Settings

Susan A. Boyer, RN, MEd, FAHCEP
Executive Director
Vermont Nurses In Partnership, Inc.
Windsor, VT
Preceptorship: Pathway to Safe Practice and
Clinical Reasoning

Carrie Bright, IOM, CAE
Executive Director
American Midwifery Certification Board,
Inc.
Linthicum, MD
American Midwifery Certification Board

Ingrid E. Brodin, RN, BS, MS
Cambridge Health Alliance
Cambridge, MA
Rapid Response Teams

Jo Ann Brooks, PhD, RN, FAAN, FCCP
Vice President System Quality and Safety
Indiana University Health
Indianapolis, IN
Continuous Quality Improvement
Sentinel Events

Marion E. Broome, PhD, RN, FAAN
Indiana University School of Nursing
Indianapolis, IN
Conflict of Interest in Research
Editing and Reviewing

Billye J. Brown, EdD, RN(R), FAAN
Professor Emeritus
University of Texas at Austin
School of Nursing
Manchaca, TX
Executive Search

Mary C. Brucker, CNM, PhD, FACNM
Accreditation Commission for Midwifery
Education, Chair
Silver Spring, MD
Accreditation Commission for Midwifery
Education

Peter I. Buerhaus, PhD, RN, FAAN
Valere Potter Professor of Nursing
Director Center for Interdisciplinary Health
Workforce Studies
Institute for Medicine and Public Health
Vanderbilt University Medical Center
Nashville, TN
Nursing Shortage in the United States

Jennifer Butlin, EdD
Executive Director
Commission on Collegiate Nursing
Education
Washington, DC
Commission on Collegiate Nursing
Education

Jacquelyn Campbell, PhD, RN
Anna D. Wolf Chair
Johns Hopkins University School of Nursing
Baltimore, MD
*Robert Wood Johnson Foundation Nurse
Faculty Scholars Program*

Elizabeth Capezuti, PhD, RN, FAAN
Associate Professor
New York University College of Nursing
Co-director
Hartford Institute for Geriatric Nursing
New York, NY
*Nurses Improving Care for Healthsystem
Elders (NICHE)*

**Laura Caramanica RN, PhD, CENP, PhD,
FACHE**
Vice President/Chief Nursing Officer
WellStar Kennestone Hospital
Marietta, GA
*Pay-for-Performance and Value-Based
Purchasing*

Shirley S. Chater, PhD, RN
Chair, National Advisory Committee
Robert Wood Johnson Foundation
Executive Nurse Fellows Program
President Emerita
Texas Woman's University
Denton-Dallas-Houston, TX
Former Commissioner, U.S. Social Security
Administration (1993–1998)
*Professional Presence
Robert Wood Johnson Foundation
Executive Nurse Fellows Program*

Jeannie P. Cimiotti, DNSc, RN
Associate Professor
Executive Director, New Jersey
Collaborating Center for Nursing
Rutgers University College of Nursing
Newark, NJ
Failure to Rescue

Sean P. Clarke, PhD, RN, FAAN
RBC Financial Group Chair in
Cardiovascular Nursing Research
Associate Professor
Lawrence S. Bloomburg Faculty of Nursing
University of Toronto
Peter Munk Cardiac Centre, University
Health Network
Toronto, Onterio, Canada
Failure to Rescue

Brenda L. Cleary, PhD, RN, FAAN
National Advisory Committees of RWJF-
funded New Graduate RN Project
Oregon Consortium and Western Governors
University MAP-RN Initiative
Center to Champion Nursing in America

Vicki S. Conn, PhD, RN, FAAN
Associate Dean and Potter Brinton Professor
Editor, *Western Journal of Nursing Research*
University of Missouri School of Nursing
Columbia, MO
Writing for Publication

Christine Coughlin, EdD, RN
Associate Professor
Adelphi University
Garden City, NY
*Employee Performance Appraisal
Teamwork*

Marilyn Cox, MSN, RN, NEA-BC
Senior Vice President of Nursing
Riley Hospital for Children
Indiana University Health
Indianapolis, IN
Transforming Care at the Bedside

Linda Cronenwett, PhD, RN, FAAN
Beerstecher-Blackwell Term Professor
School of Nursing
University of North Carolina
Chapel Hill, NC
Quality and Safety Education for Nurses

Judi DeBlasio, RN, MSN
Associate Professor
Undergraduate Clinical Placement and
   Recruitment Coordinator
Pace University
College of Health Professions
Lienhard School of Nursing
Pleasantville, NY
   Student Recruitment

Connie White Delaney, PhD, RN, FAAN
Professor and Dean
School of Nursing
University of Minnesota
Minneapolis, MN
   Leveraging

Darlene Del Prato, PhD, RN
Associate Professor and Chair Department
   of Nursing and Health Professions
Coordinator
MS Nursing Education program
SUNY Institute of Technology
Utica, NY
   Academic Mobbing
   Horizontal Violence

Joanne Disch, PhD, RN, FAAN
Clinical Professor and Director
Katharine J. Densford International
   Center for Nursing
Leadership Chair
Population Health & Systems
   Co-operative Unit
Katherine R. and C. Walton Lillehei Chair in
   Nursing Leadership
University of Minnesota School of Nursing
Minneapolis, MN
   Advanced Practice Registered Nurses
   Chairing Key Organizational Committees
   Raise the Voice!

Marianne Ditomassi, RN, DNP, MBA
Executive Director
Patient Care Services and Magnet Program
   Director
Massachusetts General Hospital
Boston, MA
   Nurse Satisfaction in the Professional
      Practice Environment
   Professional Practice Model

Jane Dolan
   Student Recruitment

Gloria F. Donnelly, Ph.D., RN, FAAN
Dean and Professor
College of Nursing and Health
   Professions
Drexel University
Philadelphia, PA
   Faculty Retention
   Managing Finances in Nursing Programs
   Student Retention

**Karen Drenkard, PhD, RN, NEA-BC,
   FAAN**
Executive Director
American Nurses Credentialing Center
Silver Spring, MD
   Transformational Leadership

Patricia R. Ebright, PhD, RN
Indiana University
School of Nursing
Indianapolis, IN
   Patient Safety

David N. Ekstrom
Associate Professor and Director of
   International Affairs
Lienhard School of Nursing
Pace University
New York, NY
   American Assembly for Men in Nursing

**Jeanette Ives Erickson, RN,
   DNP, FAAN**
Senior Vice President for Patient Care
Massachusetts General Hospital
Boston, MA
   Nurse Satisfaction in the Professional
      Practice Environment
   Professional Practice Model
   Staffing Effectiveness

Linda Q. Everett, PhD, RN, FAAN
Executive Vice President
Chief Nurse Executive
Indiana University Health
Associate Dean Clinical Affairs
Indiana University School of Nursing
Indianapolis, IN
  Accountable Care Organizations

Claire M. Fagin, PhD, RN, FAAN
Leadership Professor Emerita
Dean Emerita
University of Pennsylvania
Philadelphia, PA
  Academic Leadership
  Building Academic Geriatric Nursing
    Capacity

Harriet R. Feldman, PhD, RN, FAAN
Interim Provost and Executive Vice
  President for Academic Affairs
Pace University
New York, NY
  American Association of Colleges of Nursing
  American Association of University
    Professors
  American Association of University Women
  American Nurses Association Hall of Fame
  National Organization of Nurse Practitioner
    Faculties
  Truth About Nursing

Joyce J. Fitzpatrick, PhD, RN, FAAN
Elizabeth Brooks Ford Professor of Nursing
Frances Payne Bolton School of Nursing
Case Western Reserve University
Cleveland, OH
  Associate Degree Nursing Education
  Case Statements
  Foundation Funding of Health Care and
    Nursing
  International Council of Nurses (ICN)
  International Leadership in Nursing
  Management by Objectives

Patricia Franklin
Doctoral Candidate
College of Health and Human Services
George Mason University
Braddock, VA
  Building Academic Geriatric Nursing
    Capacity

David C. Free
Graduate Student
University of Maryland School of
  Nursing
Baltimore, MD
  Advance Care Planning and Advance
    Directives

Terry Fulmer, PhD, RN, FAAN
Erline Perkins McGriff Professor
  and Dean
New York University School of
  Nursing
New York, NY
  Interprofessional Collaboration in Nursing

Diane M. Gengo, MS, RN, ACNS-BC
Cambridge Health Alliance
Cambridge, MA
  Patient Self-Determination Act

Francis Gerbasi, CRNA, PhD
Executive Director
Council on Accreditation
Park Ridge, IL
  Council on Accreditation of Nurse
    Anesthesia Programs

Martha J. Greenberg, PhD, MSN, BSN
Associate Professor and Chairperson
Undergraduate Department
Lienhard School of Nursing
Pace University
Pleasantville, NY
American Holistic Nurses Association
Budget Management
Case Management
Clinical Evaluation
Delegation
Flextime
Human Resource Management
Patient Classification Systems
Planetree Model

Philip A. Greiner, DNSc, RN
Associate Dean for Faculty
  Development in Scholarship &
  Teaching and Professor
College of Health Professions
Pace University
Pleasantville, NY
Peer Review

**Linda Groah, RN, MSN, CNOR, NEA-BC,
  FAAN**
Chief Executive Officer
Association of periOperative Registered
  Nurses
Denver, CO
*Association of periOperative Registered
  Nurses*

Divina Grossman, PhD, RN, FAAN
Dean
Founding Vice President for Engagement
Florida International University
College of Nursing and Health Sciences
Miami, FL
Community Engagement

Patricia S. Groves, PhD(c), RN
University of Missouri
School of Nursing
Columbia, MO
Writing for Publication

Judith Haber, PhD, APRN-BC, FAAN
Interim Dean
Ursula Springer Leadership Professor
  in Nursing
College of Nursing
New York University
New York, NY
Interprofessional Collaboration in Nursing

**Karen Toby Haghenbeck, PhD, FNP-BC,
  RN-BC, CCRN**
Assistant Professor College of Health
  Professions
Lienhard School of Nursing
Pace University
Pleasantville, NY
Technology

Kimberly B. Hall, MSN, RN, NE-BC
Assistant Professor
Department of Nursing
Jefferson College of Health Sciences
Roanoke, VA
Internships
Interprofessional Leadership in Nursing

Edward J. Halloran
Financing Health Care

**Judith A. Halstead, PhD, RN, ANEF,
  FAAN**
Executive Associate Dean for Academic
  Affairs
Indiana University School of Nursing
Indianapolis, IN
Accreditation in Nursing Education

Susan B. Hassmiller, PhD, RN, FAAN
Senior Adviser for Nursing and
  Director of Future of Nursing:
  Campaign for Action
Robert Wood Johnson Foundation
*Robert Wood Johnson Foundation's Initiative
  on the Future of Nursing*

Ada Sue Hinshaw, PhD, RN, FAAN
Dean and Professor
Uniformed Services University
Graduate School of Nursing
Dean and Professor Emerita
University of Michigan, School of
    Nursing
Ann Arbor, MI
    Funding for Nursing Research
    National Institute of Nursing Research
    Research Integrity

Margaret Holder
    Military Nursing

Nancy Hollingsworth, RN, MSN, MBA
President and Chief Executive Officer
Saint Agnes Medical Center
Fresno, CA
    Benchmarking
    SWOT Analysis

William L. Holzemer, PhD, RN, FAAN
Dean and Professor College of Nursing
Rutgers the State University of
    New Jersey
Newark, NJ
    Council for the Advancement of Nursing
        Science

Marilyn Jaffe-Ruiz, EdD, RN
Professor Emeritus
Lienhard School of Nursing
College of Health Professions
Pace University
New York, NY
    Academic Degrees in Nursing
    Assessment of Leadership Styles and Skills
    Distance Education in Nursing
    Image of Nursing
    Leadership Traits

Connie A. Jastremski, RN, MS, MBA
Network CNO
Bassett Healthcare Network
Cooperstown, NY
    Patient Care Delivery Models

M. Christina Johnson, CNM, MS
Director
Professional Practice & Health Policy
    American College of Nurse-Midwives
Silver Spring, MD
    American College of Nurse-Midwives
        (ACNM)

Stacy Hutton Johnson, MS/MBA, RN,
    NE-BC
Nurse Director
Massachusetts General Hospital
Boston, MA
    Leapfrog Group

Joyce Johnston
    Clinical Simulation

Cheryl Bland Jones, PhD, RN, FAAN
Associate Professor
School of Nursing
Research Program Consultant
Nursing Division UNC Hospitals
University of North Carolina
Chapel Hill, NC
    Health Care Systems

Dorothy A. Jones, EdD, RNC,
    ANP, FAAN
Professor of Adult Health
William F. Connell School of Nursing
Boston College
Boston, MA
    Nurse Satisfaction in the Professional
        Practice Environment

Paule V. Joseph MSN, FNP-BC, RN, CRRN, BCLNC-C
Clinical Nurse
Mount Sinai Hospital
New York, NY
Pre-Doctoral Student at the University of
Pennsylvania
Academic Degrees in Nursing
American Association of Colleges of Nursing
American Association of University
Professors
American Association of University Women
American Nurses Association Hall of Fame
Certification
Continuing Professional Education
National Organization of Nurse Practitioner
Faculties
Truth About Nursing

Meredith Wallace Kazer, PhD, APRN, A/GNP-BC
Associate Professor
School of Nursing
Fairfield University
Fairfield, CT
Foundation Funding of Health Care and
Nursing

David M. Keepnews, PhD, JD, RN, FAAN
Associate Professor
Hunter-Bellevue School of Nursing
Hunter College
New York, NY
Lobbying
Political Action Committees

Karlene Kerfoot, PhD, RN
Vice President and Chief Clinical Officer
Aurora Health Care
Milwaukee, WI
Raise the Voice!

Shaké Ketefian, EdD
Director of International Affairs
Professor
University of Michigan
School of Nursing
Ann Arbor, MI
Evidence-Based Practice

Karren Kowalski, PhD, RN, FAAN
Associate Editor
Journal of Continuing Education in
Nursing
Grant Director
Colorado Center for Nursing Excellence
Denver, CO
Clinical Ladder

Phyllis Beck Kritek, PhD, RN, FAAN
Consultant
Conflict Management

Betty R. Kupperschmidt, EdD, RN
Associate Professor
University of Oklahoma Health Sciences
Center College of Nursing
Tulsa, OK
Carefronting

Maryjoan Ladden, PhD, RN, FAAN
Senior Program Officer
Robert Wood Johnson Foundation
Washington, DC
Robert Wood Johnson Foundation Nurse
Faculty Scholars Program

Carol Ledbetter, PhD, APRN, BC, FAAN
Professor and Director
Doctor of Nursing Practice Program
Colonel, USAF, NC Retired Office
University of North Florida
Brooks College of Health
School of Nursing
Jacksonville, FL
Military Nursing

Rebecca C. Lee, PhD, RN, PHCNS-BC, CTN-A
Assistant Professor
University of Cincinnati
College of Nursing
Cincinnati, OH
Human Rights

Kim L. Carnahan Lewis, ARNP
Vancouver, WA
International Leadership in Nursing

Linda Lindeke, PhD, RN, CNP
Associate Professor
Director of Graduate Studies
School of Nursing
University of Minnesota
Minneapolis, MN
   Advanced Practice Registered Nurses

Beverly Louise Malone, PhD, RN, FAAN
Chief Executive Officer
National League for Nursing
New York, NY
   Leadership Development
   National Black Nurses Association, Inc.
   National League for Nursing
   Power and Leadership

Diane J. Mancino, EdD, RN, CAE, FAAN
American Nurses Association and American
   Nurses Foundation
Silver Spring, Maryland
American Organization of Nurse Executives
Washington, DC
Nurses Educational Funds, Inc. and
   National Student Nurses' Association, Inc.
New York, NY
Honor Society of Nursing
Sigma Theta Tau International
Indianapolis, IN
   American Academy of Nursing
   American Nurses Association
   American Nurses Credentialing Center
   American Nurses Foundation
   American Organization of Nurse Executives
   National Student Nurses' Association
   Nurses Educational Funds, Inc.
   Sigma Theta Tau International

Milisa Manojlovich, PhD, RN, CCRN
Associate Professor
University of Michigan School of Nursing
Ann Arbor, MI
   Evidence-Based Practice

Pam Maraldo, PhD
Managing Partner
PGM Consulting
New York, NY
   Gender and Leadership

Angela Barron McBride, PhD, RN, FAAN
Distinguished Professor-University Dean
   Emerita
Indiana University School of Nursing
Indianapolis, IN
   Career Stages
   Constructive Feedback
   Generational Differences in Leadership and
      Mentoring
   Individual Development Plan
   Institute of Medicine
   Letters of Recommendation
   Living Legends
   Mentoring
   Philanthropy/Fund Raising
   Robert Wood Johnson Foundation Nurse
      Faculty Scholars Program

Margaret L. McClure, EdD, RN, FAAN
Professor
College of Nursing
School of Medicine
New York University
New York, NY
   Differentiated Nursing Practice
   Entry Into Practice
   Magnet Hospitals

John McDonough
   Military Nursing

Mary Ann McGinley, PhD, RN
Senior Vice President for Patient Care
Chief Nursing Officer
Thomas Jefferson University Hospital
Philadelphia, PA
   Nurse Residency

Bernadette Mazurek Melnyk, PhD, RN,
   CPNP/PMHNP, FNAP, FAAN
Associate Vice President for Health
   Promotion
University Chief Wellness Officer Dean
College of Nursing
Ohio State University
Columbus, OH
   Faculty Recruitment to Academic Settings

Vickie L. Milazzo RN, MSN, JD
President and CEO of Vickie Milazzo
   Institute
Pioneer of Legal Nurse Consulting
New York Times Bestselling Author
Inc. Top 10 Entrepreneur
Stevie Award—Mentor of the Year
Susan G. Komen's Hope Award for
   Ambassadorship
National Alliance of Certified Legal
   Nurse Consultants
   Legal Nurse Consulting

Paula Milone-Nuzzo, RN, PhD, FHHC,
   FAAN
Dean and Professor
School of Nursing
Pennsylvania State University
University Park, PA
   Resource Development

Ronda Mintz-Binder, DNP, RN, CNE
Assistant Professor
College of Nursing
University of Texas
Arlington, TX
   Agency for Healthcare Research and
     Quality (AHRQ)
   Americans with Disabilities Act
   Associate Degree Nursing Education
   Family Educational Rights and Privacy Act of
     1974 (The Buckley Amendment)
   Health Resources and Services
     Administration
   International Council of Nurses (ICN)
   International Leadership in Nursing
   Malcolm Baldrige National Quality Award
   Management by Objectives
   Nursing Organizations Alliance
   World Health Organization (WHO)

Loretta Molinari
Branch Manager
Visiting Nurse Services
Putnam County, NY
   Emergency Preparedness

Gina M. Myers
Assistant Professor
Le Moyne College
Syracuse, NY
   Consumer Satisfaction
   Employee Satisfaction
   Malpractice
   National League for Nursing Accrediting
     Commission (NLNAC)
   Historical Leadership Figures
   Clarissa Harlowe Barton (1821–1912)
   Karen Buhler-Wilkerson (1944–2010)
   Mary Elizabeth Carnegie (1916–2008)
   Lavinia Lloyd Dock (1858–1956)
   Veronica M. Driscoll (1926–1994)
   Annie Warburton Goodrich (1866–1954)
   Virginia A. Henderson (1897–1996)
   Eleanor C. Lambertsen (1915–1998)
   Rachel Louise McManus (1896–1993)
   Mildred L. Montag (1908–2004)
   Ildaura Murillo-Rohde (1920–2010)
   Florence Nightingale (1820–1910)
   Lucille Elizabeth Notter (1907–1993)
   Mary Adelaide Nutting (1858–1948)
   Estelle Massey Osborne (1901–1981)
   Sophia Palmer (1853–1920)
   Hildegard Peplau (1909–1999)
   Isabel Hampton Robb (1860–1910)
   Jessie M. Scott (1915–2009)
   Laura L. Simms (1919–2009)
   Mabel Keaton Staupers (1890–1989)
   Lillian Wald (1867–1940)
   Harriet Werley (1914–2002)

Deena A. Nardi, PhD
Clinical Nurse
Juliet, IL
   Global Nursing Shortage

Mary D. Naylor, PhD, RN, FAAN
Marian S. Ware Professor in Gerontology
Director, New Courtland Center for
   Transitions and Health
University of Pennsylvania School of
   Nursing
Philadelphia, PA
   Long-Term Quality Alliance
   Transitional Care Model

M. Janice Nelson, EdD, RN
Professor and Dean Emerita,
College of Nursing,
SUNY Upstate Medical University,
Syracuse, NY
  Consumer Satisfaction
  Employee Satisfaction
  Malpractice
  National League for Nursing Accrediting
    Commission (NLNAC)
  Patient Care Delivery Models

Barbara L. Nichols, DHL, MS,
  RN, FAAN
Chief Executive Officer
Commission on Graduates of Foreign
  Nursing Schools
Philadelphia, PA
  Background Screening for Foreign-
    Educated Nurses
  CGFNS International

Stephanie J. Offord, MSN, RN, FNP-BC
Medical College of Wisconsin
Children's Hospital of Wisconsin
Milwaukee, WI
  Centers for Disease Control and
    Prevention

Eileen T. O'Grady, PhD, RN, NP-BC
Certified Nurse Practitioner and Wellness
  Coach
Policy Editor and Columnist, *American*
  Journal for Nurse Practitioners
Visiting Professor Pace University
McLean, VA
  Coaching Nurses
  Health Policy

Ignatius Perkins, OP, PhD, RN, FAAN,
  FNYAM
Professor and Dean
Department of Nursing
Aquinas College
Nashville, TN
  Human Dignity and Ethical Decision Making
    in Nursing

Daniel J. Pesut, PhD RN PMHCNS-BC
  FAAN
Professor of Nursing
Indiana University School of Nursing
Indianapolis, IN
  Change
  Change Agents and Change Agent Strategies
  Complex Adaptive Systems (Chaos Theory)
  Emotional Intelligence
  Self-Renewal
  Strategic Planning

Denise Peterson, RN, BA, MM
Senior Director Risk Management and
  Patient Safety
Cambridge Health Alliance
Cambridge, MA
  Risk Management in the Health Care Setting

Tim Porter-O'Grady, DM, EdD, ScD(h),
  FAAN
Senior Partner
Tim Porter-O'Grady Associates
Atlanta, GA
  Coaching Nurses
  Shared Governance Is Structure Not Process

John C. Preston, CRNA, DNSc
Senior Director, Education & Professional
  Development
American Association of Nurse Anesthetists
Park Ridge, IL
  American Association of Nurse Anesthetists

Mary Ann Radioli, RN, MA
Director of Nurse Recruitment and
  Retention
Maimonides Medical Center
Brooklyn, NY
  Staff Recruitment

Marilyn A. Ray, RN, PhD, CTN-A
Professor Emeritus
Christine E. Lynn College of Nursing
Florida Atlantic University
Boca Raton, FL
  Complexity Science and Nursing

Lesley Reeder, RN, BSN
Senior Manager, Government Programs
Rocky Mountain Health Plans
Denver, CO
   Patient-Centered Medical Home

Cindy A. Reilly
   Accreditation in Nursing Practice

Kelly Reilly
   Participative Leadership

Susan Reinhard, RN, PhD, FAAN
Senior Vice President
AARP Public Policy Institute
Chief Strategist, Center to Champion
   Nursing in America
Washington, DC
   AARP

Hila Richardson, DfPH, RN, FAAN
Clinical Professor
College of Nursing
New York University
New York, NY
   Interprofessional Collaboration in Nursing

Nancy Ridenour, PhD, APRN, BC, FAAN
Robert Wood Johnson Health Policy
   Fellowship
Dean and Professor
University of New Mexico
Albuquerque, NM
   Robert Wood Johnson Health Policy
   Fellowship Program

Carol A. Romano PhD, RN, BC, NEA,
   FAAN, FACMI
Professor and Associate Dean for Academic
   Affairs
Uniformed Services University of the Health
   Sciences
Bethesda, MD
   Electronic Health Record
   Telehealth

Marlene M. Rosenkoetter, PhD, RN, CNS,
   FAAN
Tenured Professor
Medical College of Georgia
School of Nursing
Evans, GA
   Global Nursing Shortage

Marla E. Salmon, ScD, RN, FAAN
The Robert G. and Jean A. Reid Dean in
   Nursing Professor
Psychosocial and Community Health and
   Global Health
University of Washington
Seattle, WA
   Boards and Membership on Boards

Mary Samost, MSN, RN
Associate Chief Nursing Officer
Professional Development & Academic
   Integration
Cambridge Health Alliance
Cambridge, MA
   Certificate of Need
   Gender and Leadership

Julie Schilz, BSN, MBA
Director, Community Collaboratives and
   Practice Transformation
Colorado Beacon & Consortium
Grand Junction, CO
   Patient-Centered Medical Home

Charlotte A. Seckman, PhD, RN, BC
Professor
School of Nursing
University of Maryland Baltimore Research
   Consultant
National Institutes of Health
Clinical Center
Bethesda, MD
   Electronic Health Record
   Telehealth

Deborah Witt Sherman, PhD, CRNP, ANP-BC, ACHPN, FAAN
Professor and Co-Director of the Center for Excellence in Palliative Care Research
University of Maryland School of Nursing
Baltimore, MD
Advance Care Planning and Advance Directives
Palliative Care

Rose O. Sherman, EdD, RN, NEA-BC, FAAN
Director, Nursing Leadership Institute
Associate Professor
Christine E. Lynn College of Nursing, Florida Atlantic University
Boca Raton, FL
Carefronting

Maria R. Shirey, PhD, MBA, RN, NEA-BC, FACHE, FAAN
Associate Professor of Nursing
University of Southern Indiana College of Nursing and Health Professions
University Boulevard
Evansville, IN
Authoritative Leadership

Thomas D. Smith, RN, DNP, NEA-BC
Chief Nursing Officer
Senior Vice President
Maimonides Medical Center
Brooklyn, NY
Institute for Healthcare Improvement

Joan M. Stanley, PhD, CRNP, FAAN, FAANP
Senior Director of Education Policy
American Association of Colleges of Nursing
Washington, DC
APRN Consensus Model & LACE
Clinical Nurse Leader (CNL®)

Kathleen R. Stevens, RN, EdD, ANEF, FAAN
Professor and Director
Improvement Science Research Network and Academic Center for Evidence-Based Practice
School of Nursing
University of Texas Health Science Center
San Antonio, TX
Translational Science

Lillian G. Stokes, PhD, RN, FAAN
Associate Professor Emeritus
Indiana University School of Nursing
Indianapolis, IN
Chi Eta Phi Sorority, Incorporated

Todd D Swinderman, PhD, DNS, RN, NE-BC
North Florida Regional Medical Center
Gainesville, FL
Nursing Informatics

Christine A. Tanner, PhD, RN, FAAN
AB Youmans Spaulding Distinguished Professor Editor
Journal of Nursing Education
Oregon Health & Science University School of Nursing
Portland, OR
Oregon Model: The Oregon Consortium for Nursing Education

Sandra P. Thomas, PhD, RN, FAAN
Professor and Chair of the PhD Program
University of Tennessee at Knoxville
College of Nursing
Knoxville, TN
Managing Anger/Emotions
Staff Retention

Pamela Austin Thompson, MS, RN, CENP, FAAN
CEO, American Organization of Nurse
  Executives (AONE)
Senior Vice President for Nursing, American
  Hospital Association (AHA)
Washington, DC
  Executive Leadership Programs
  Johnson & Johnson Wharton Fellows Program
    in Management for Nurse Executives

Marian C. Turkel, RN, PhD, NEA-BC
Director of Professional Nursing Practice
Albert Einstein Healthcare Network
Philadelphia, PA
  Complexity Science and Nursing

Katherine Vestal, RN, PhD, FACHE, FAAN
President
Work Innovations LLC
Lake Leelanau, MI
  Consultation

Maria L. Vezina, EdD, RN, NEA-BC
Senior Director, Nursing Education and
  Professional Practice
The Mount Sinai Hospital in New York
  Orientation and Staff Development

Joanne Rains Warner, PhD, RN
Dean and Professor
University of Portland
Portland, OR
  Dedicated Education Unit

Barbara Jones Warren, PhD, RN, CNS-BC, PMH
Professor, Clinical and Specialty Director
  Psychiatric Mental Health Nursing
  Program
Ohio State University, College of Nursing
Columbus, OH
  Cultural Competence: An Academic Nursing
    Leadership Imperative

Rachael Watman, MSW
Senior Program Officer
John A. Hartford Foundation
New York, NY
  Hartford Geriatric Nursing Initiative
    (HGNI)

Charlotte Weaver, RN, PhD, FAAN
Sr. VP & Chief Clinical Officer
Gentiva® Health Services
Atlanta, GA
  Health Information Management
    Systems Society

Sharon Stahl Wexler, PhD, RN, BC
Assistant Professor
College of Health Professions
Lienhard School of Nursing
Pace University
New York, NY
  Informed Consent (Research)

Barbara Zittel
Executive Secretary
New York State Boards of Nursing
New York, NY
  National Council of State Boards of
    Nursing, Inc. (NCSBN)
  Regulatory Boards

Eileen H. Zungolo Ed.D., RN, FAAN, CNE, ANEF
Dean and Professor
Duquesne University
Pittsburgh, PA
  Shortage of Nursing Faculty

LIST OF ENTRIES

HISTORICAL LEADERSHIP FIGURES

Thematic List of Entries

INFORMATICS AND TECHNOLOGY

LEADERSHIP IN PRACTICE, EDUCATION, AND RESEARCH

MAJOR LEADERS

MANAGEMENT AND EXECUTIVE SKILLS

ORGANIZATIONAL LEADERSHIP

PROFESSIONAL STANDARDS

QUALITY OUTCOMES

THEORIES AND MODELS

INTRODUCTION

Over the years, I have given a great deal of thought to the topic and concept of leadership. Not a day goes by that issues pertaining to either do not surface. What is your leadership style? What prepared you for your leadership role? Who would you consider a great leader? How do you mentor others to be leaders? What are the key elements of leadership? What is the essence of leadership? What are the characteristics of successful leaders? You have heard these questions as well, and many others. The answers are sometimes complex. I was reminded of this complexity not long ago when I was interviewed for a high-level executive position. The experience gave me a renewed opportunity to think through questions about the nature of leadership and how I lead, a very worthwhile exercise, indeed.

There is not one way to be a successful leader, not one way to develop and hone leadership skills, not one way to mentor others to be leaders. The context of leadership is not only dependent on the person in the leadership role, but on the place where one leads. For example, each organization is different as is each group and individual. Relationships and expectations vary, as do organizational norms and culture.

I believe that success is as much about organizational "fit" as it is about individual leadership skills.

For those of us who are "seasoned" as accomplished leaders, the responsibility to convey our experiences and set the stage for the next generation of leaders is awesome, one that we take very seriously. Sir Isaac Newton said in a letter to Robert Hooke (February 5, 1675), "If I have seen further it is only by standing on the shoulders of giants" (The Quotations Page, 2011). Indeed there are many past giants in nursing. The section on Historical Leadership Figures lists many of the giants who have had great impact on nursing practice, education, and research. We purposely set this group apart in the encyclopedia to signify their importance.

Since the first edition of the encyclopedia was published in 2008, radical changes have taken place in society, most notably those affecting the economy and health care. In 2010, the basis for health care reform was laid when President Barack Obama approved the Patient Protection and Affordable Care Act and the subsequently passed legislation, Health Care and Education Reconciliation Act (Understanding the Affordable Care Act., n.d.). Reforms focus on requiring private health insurers to cover individuals with preexisting conditions, improved prescription drug coverage by Medicare, and other important initiatives.

The Carnegie Foundation for the Advancement of Teaching published their findings on higher education in various professions, calling for "radical transformation" of nursing education and describing its redesign as "an urgent societal agenda" (Schmidt, 2010). The Institute of Medicine issued a number of quality reports. *Keeping Patients Safe* (2003) laid the foundation for the current focus on improving patient safety, emphasizing that nursing leadership is essential to achieving safety goals. This emphasis was clearly made in the 2011 report on the *Future of Nursing*, which grappled with the prevailing concerns of advance practice nursing, noting that "…current conflicts between what APRNs can do based on their education and training and what they may do according to state and federal regulations must be resolved so that they are better able to provide seamless, affordable, and quality care." Scope-of-practice regulations in all states should reflect the full extent not only of nurses but of each profession's education and training. Elimination of barriers for all professions with a focus on collaborative teamwork will maximize and improve care throughout the health care system." This is a call for nursing leadership in its broadest sense.

Also in 2010, New York's then governor-elect, Andrew Cuomo, created a "Medicaid Redesign Team" charged with finding efficiencies in the system and improving quality of care (Gallivan, 2011). The findings led to "opt-out legislation," which means that counties may choose to opt-out of Medicaid programs not mandated by the federal government. The president

of the New York State Nurses Association, a well-respected nursing leader, was part of that team. Nursing has become active in these and similar debates. We are making a difference!

Technology has led to an information explosion, from tweeting to Facebook, to Second Life, creating a new generation of thinkers and different ways to learn and teach. The world has opened, and we can no longer be insular. The new ease of communication also gives new meaning to the following quote:

Think Globally, Act Locally refers to the argument that global environmental problems can turn into action only by considering ecological, economic, and cultural differences of our local surroundings. This phrase was originated by Rene Dubos as an advisor to the United Nations Conference on the Human Environment in 1972. In 1979, Dubos suggested that ecological consciousness should begin at home. He believed that there needed to be a creation of a World Order in which "natural and social units maintain or recapture their identity, yet interplay with each other through a rich system of communications." In the 1980's, Dubos held to his thoughts on acting locally, and felt that issues involving the environment must be dealt with in their "unique physical, climatic, and cultural contexts." (Eblen & Eblen, 1994)

The culture we live in, consisting of many individuals from diverse backgrounds, many languages and customs, and many generations co-existing, has resulted in the need to create new systems of health care delivery—for example, the medical home—with more attention paid to the "greater good" of society. Nursing's emphasis on primary care has been renewed; new roles have emerged—for example, the clinical nurse leader and doctor of nursing practice—and there are new models to focus advanced practice nursing specialties (APRN Consensus Model).

What does this mean for emerging and seasoned leaders? How do we create balance in our lives and continue to accomplish great things? Our leadership roles, which have transcended the boundaries of our profession and our knowledge, require different skill sets. These, and other, changes have called for leaders that are creative, flexible, thoughtful, "other-focused," global thinkers, inter- and multidisciplinary minded, and knowledgeable in areas well beyond the scope of their daily work. All nurses are now expected to be leaders, not solely those in leadership positions. Today's leaders must exert their leadership within 21st-century notions of leadership.

The second edition of *Nursing Leadership: A Concise Encyclopedia*, guided by recent changes and the anticipated future, adds many terms that speak to the new kind and style of leadership that we need. For example, there are entries on transforming nursing education, lobbying, accountable care organizations, academic mobbing, carefronting, transformational leadership, peer review, and editing and reviewing manuscripts. Career development entries include post-baccalaureate nurse residencies, career stages, constructive feedback, self-renewal, and professional presence. The theme of organization leadership has been added, including board membership, chairing committees, and community engagement. In addition to recognizing new nursing roles, we introduce innovative pathways for education, for example, the Oregon Consortium for Nursing Education model. Further, first edition entries have been updated to reflect changes in society as well.

The discussions about leadership will continue for generations to come, each one affected by the external environment in which we live. It is our hope that this enriched edition of the encyclopedia will serve as a resource to inform and guide the current and next generation of aspiring and functioning leaders.

Benner, P., Sutphen, M., Leonard, V., & Day, L. (2010). *Educating nurses: A call for radical transformation.* San Francisco, CA: Jossey-Bass.

Eblen, R. A., & Eblen W. (1994). *The encyclopedia of the environment.* Boston, MA: Houghton Mifflin Company.

Gallivan, P. M. (2011, 14 February). *Major Medicaid Reform Legislation Approved in Social Services Committee.* Retrieved, May 15, 2011, from http://www.nysenate.gov/press-release/major-medicaid-reform-legislation-approved-social-services-committee

Keeping Patients Safe: Transforming the Work Environment of Nurses. (2003, November 3). Retrieved May 23, 2011, from http://www.iom.edu/Reports/2003/Keeping-Patients-Safe-Transforming-the-Work-Environment-of-Nurses.aspx

http://www.quotationspage.com/quotes/Isaac_Newton

Schmidt, P. (2010, January 6). *Carnegie Foundation Calls for "radical transformation" of nursing education.* Retrieved, May 15, 2011, from http://chronicle.com/article/Carnegie-Foundation-Calls-for/63443

The Future of Nursing: Focus on Scope of Practice. (2011, January 26). Retrieved May 23, 2011, from http://www.iom.edu/Reports/2010/The-Future-of-Nursing-Leading-Change-Advancing-Health/Report-Brief-Scope-of-Practice.aspx

The Quotations Page. (2011). Retrieved, May 7, 2011, Understanding the Affordable Care Act. (n.d.). Retrieved May 18, 2011, from http://www.healthcare.gov/law/introduction/index.html

Harriet R. Feldman

Nursing Leadership
A Concise Encyclopedia

Second Edition

AARP

Established in 1958 as the American Association of Retired Persons, AARP is the nation's leading membership organization for people aged 50 and over. AARP is a nonprofit, nonpartisan membership organization with nearly 40 million members. AARP is dedicated to enhancing the quality of life for all, nationally and globally, and leading positive social change by providing information, advocacy, and service to its members and the public. AARP's founder, Dr. Ethel Percy Andrus, was a high school principal in Los Angeles when she retired at the age of sixty to take care of her mother. Her mother recovered, and Dr. Andrus volunteered with the California Retired Teachers Association and led its committee for retired teachers' welfare. Learning that many retired educators had no health insurance and inadequate pensions, Dr. Andrus testified before the California legislature. Her efforts resulted in the formation of the National Retired Teachers Association in 1947, which advocated for educators throughout the United States. Dr. Andrus developed benefits and programs including group health insurance for older persons and a discount mail order pharmacy service. These programs were so popular that thousands of persons asked the association to open its membership to noneducators, and in 1958, the American Association of Retired Persons was founded. In 1999, its name was changed to the four letter acronym AARP since the membership is open to persons age 50 and above, with almost half of the current membership continuing to work. The National Retired Teachers Association continues as a division of AARP.

In 2007, the AARP Foundation established the Center to Champion Nursing in America. Funded by the Robert Wood Johnson Foundation and AARP, the Center's mission is to ensure that all Americans have a highly skilled nurse, when and where they need one. The Center's goals are to (1) strengthen our nation's educational pathways to prepare the nursing workforce of the future, (2) increase the number and diversity of nurses entering and remaining in the profession, (3) remove barriers that limit nurses' ability to provide the health care consumers need, and (4) enhance the influence of nurses in high levels of health care, policy, business, and community decision making. The Center founded the Champion Nursing Coalition, whose member organizations represent the voices of consumers, purchasers, and providers of health care. The coalition is raising awareness of the roles of nurses in increasing access to primary care, transitional care, and chronic care management in a reformed health care delivery system and partnering with the Campaign for Action to implement the recommendations of the Institute of Medicine's report *The Future of Nursing: Leading Change, Advancing Health*. The Center supports state grassroots efforts including building and implementing public education and advocacy initiatives nationwide by providing ongoing technical assistance and convening national and state level stakeholders and providing advocacy training, communications support, and assistance to help them communicate more effectively with policy makers and private-sector leaders.

AARP History. (2009). Retrieved January 30, 2011, from http://www.aarp.org/about-aarp/info-2009/History.html

About AARP. (2011). Retrieved January 30, 2011, from http://www.aarp.org/about-aarp

AARP About Us, Center to Champion Nursing in America. (2009). Retrieved January 30, 2011, from http://championnursing.org/content/about-us

Susan Reinhard

ACADEMIC DEGREES IN NURSING

Anatole France said, "An education isn't how much you have committed to memory, or even how much you know. It's being able to differentiate between what you do know and what you don't" (The Quotations Page, 2007).

An educated nurse has many options with which preparation for a career in nursing can be begun. The American Association of Colleges of Nursing (AACN, 2000, 2010) recognizes three levels of education for the preparation of the professional nurse role. Basic entry into practice can be at the diploma, associate, baccalaureate, or, for those with a previous college degree, generic master's degree level.

The bachelor of science degree in nursing (BSN) is the preferred minimum educational requirement for professional nursing practice. While graduates can begin practice as a registered nurse with an associate degree or hospital diploma, the BSN degree is essential for nurses seeking to perform with the knowledge and skills necessary in today's complex health care environment (AACN, 2004a).

In 2004, the American Organization of Nurse Executives (AONE) Board of Directors released the AONE Guiding Principles for the Role of the Nurse in Future Health Care Delivery. It states, "…This (BSN) educational preparation will prepare the nurse of the future to function as an equal partner, collaborator and manager of the complex patient care journey…" (http://www.aone.org/aone/resource/practiceandeducation.html).

The Tri-Council for Nursing (the AACN, American Nurses Association [ANA], and AONE) and the National League for Nursing issued a consensus statement calling for all registered nurses to advance their education to enhance the quality of nursing practice across health care settings in May 2010. The Tri-Council recognizes the three levels of education for the preparation for the professional nurse role. These are the baccalaureate, master's, and doctoral degrees (www.aacn.nche.edu/Education/pdf/TricouncilEdStatement.pdf).

Nurses enter the profession from different initial educational backgrounds, which include licensed practical nurses (LPN), associate degree (ADN) and diploma-prepared nurses, baccalaureate and generic master's-prepared nurses.

With the demand for more nurses with advanced preparation, creative efforts have to be developed to assist nurses to increase their education and to move along the continuum to advanced practice roles. For example, some nurses who enter nursing profession as an LPN, with AAS degree or diploma-prepared nurse use their employer-sponsored tuition reimbursement programs to obtain the baccalaureate and higher degrees.

Following a study by the committee on the Robert Wood Johnson Foundation Initiative on the Future of Nursing, at the Institute of Medicine, in October 2011, a final report was issued, titled "The Future of Nursing: Leading Change, Advancing Health" (http://www.nap.edu/catalog/12956.html). Among the committee's recommendations are the following:

Increase the proportion of nurses with a baccalaureate degree to 80% by 2020. Academic nurse leaders across all schools of nursing should work together to increase the proportion of nurses with a baccalaureate degree from 50% to 80% by 2020. These leaders should partner with education accrediting bodies, private and public funders, and employers to ensure funding, monitor progress, and increase the diversity of students to create a workforce prepared to meet the demands of diverse populations across the life span.

Double the number of nurses with a doctorate degree by 2020. Schools of nursing, with support from private and public funders, academic administrators and university trustees, and accrediting bodies should double the number of nurses with a doctorate degree by 2020 to add to the cadre of nurse faculty and researchers, with attention to increasing diversity.

AACN has historically supported a career ladder based on different points along the educational continuum. Recognition of nurses prepared at the associate degree level is essential in order to further professionally practice and develop the supply of nurses needed for practice (AACN Media Fact Sheet, April 2002).

The Associate Degree of Science in Nursing Program (ADN), a 2-year degree, focuses on technical skills more than theory. For many seeking to practice nursing, it is a faster and less expensive entry way into the profession; for others, it is a stepping stone to a BSN degree.

The BSN program takes 4 years and provides preparation in science and the humanities as well as in nursing. The BSN curriculum includes a strong focus on the development of intellectual skills, critical thinking, and communication and leadership skills. Community health and research classes are part of the program curriculum. With the growing number of American Nurses Credentialing Center, Magnet-accredited hospitals, the BSN has been made a requirement or strong preference for nurses at Magnet designated hospitals.

The accelerated BSN program was created for those students who hold a degree in another field and choose nursing as a second career. Students who choose this curriculum are enrolled in a rigorous program. Typically, students attend classes full-time and earn a BSN degree in 12 to 18 months.

The RN-to-BSN degree program is designed for nurses who hold an associate degree or diploma, who need to obtain their BSN degree. This program gives advanced standing for the nursing classes already taken. Content is then offered in a curriculum that builds on previous nursing knowledge. The programs are taught in both traditional nursing schools and in online programs. Another variation and option for these are also sometimes called "degree completion" or "articulation programs" in which there is an agreement between two schools, one that has a BSN program and the other, an ADN program. The ADN graduates have the opportunity to continue their education in the program in which their institution has a contract with. The students save both money and credits already earned.

The master's degree in nursing is generally 2 years in length and typically includes a research component. Entry to these programs may be accompanied by the requirement of the Graduate Record Exam and/or the Miller Analogy Test. The master's-prepared nurse functions in advanced practice roles, including health promotion, the management and delivery of primary health care, and case management. This nurse is also prepared for roles in community health care organization, research, health policy, education, and administration. Nurses who hold a master's degree are qualified to become administrators and managers. Master's-prepared nurses are also qualified to teach full-time in community colleges and as clinical faculty or adjuncts in baccalaureate schools of nursing. Among the master's degrees available are those for advanced practice nurses, which is the global term used to include the following specialization: the nurse practitioner, the clinical nurse specialist, the certified registered nurse anesthetist, and the certified nurse midwife.

The doctoral degree in nursing prepares nurses to contribute to nursing knowledge through research, scholarly work, advanced practice, administration, and education. A doctorally prepared nurse is considered a leader in the profession. The doctoral degree has become a preferred degree for some administrative positions and mandatory for tenure track positions in higher education. Research methods are part of the foundation of these program, as well as history, philosophy, and leadership. The doctoral degrees that are usually granted are Doctor of Philosophy, Doctor of Education, and Doctor of Nursing Science. There is also a growing demand for the Doctor in Nursing Practice. Graduates of these programs are highly knowledgeable clinicians who may also do administration and teaching.

American Association of Colleges of Nursing. (2000). *The Baccalaureate Degree in Nursing as Minimal Preparation for Professional Practice.* AACN Position Paper. Retrieved from http://www.aacn.nche.edu/Publications/positions/baccmin.htm

American Association of Colleges of Nursing. (2004a). *Education center.* Retrieved from http://www.aacn.nche.edu/education/career.htm

American Association of Colleges of Nursing. (2004b). *Education center.* Retrieved from www.aacn.nche.edu/Education/pdf/TricouncilEdStatement.pdf

American Association of Colleges of Nursing. (2010). *Fact sheet: The impact on nursing education.* Retrieved from http://www.aacn.nche.edu/media/factsheets/impactednp.htm

American Organization of Nurse Executives. (2004). *Practice and education partnership for the future. Guiding principles for the role of the nurse in future health care delivery.* Retrieved from http://www.aone.org/aone/resource/practiceandeducation.html

Institute of Medicine. (2011). *The future of nursing: Leading change, advancing health.* Washington, DC: National Academies Press.

The Quotations Page. (2007). *Anatole France.* Retrieved from http://www.quotationspage.com/quote/31753.html

Marilyn Jaffe-Ruiz
Paule V. Joseph

ACADEMIC LEADERSHIP

Academic leadership is an anomaly, and should be. Academic leadership is most like leadership of an orchestra rather than a corporation, and should be. Academic leaders, colleagues among colleagues, lead by persuasion rather than mandate. Academic leadership focuses on building excellence, and rewards competition for excellence rather than rewarding competition for personal gratification or pleasing the leader. Academic leadership shows by vision and example that individual differences and personality quirks can be accommodated and even embraced so long as productivity and quest for excellence is maintained.

Leadership means many things to people. Often it gets confused with management or administration. But those are positional while leadership is a qualitative statement of individual capability. Academic leadership does have characteristics that may be different from other forms of organizational leadership. This was truer in the past than at present. In the recognition of excellence for business leaders, the very characteristics that have been defined as the sine qua non of academic leadership are being touted as though the leaders had just reinvented or rather invented the wheel. Many of the descriptions of fine corporate leaders today are straight out of the handbook of academic leadership. These include the encouragement of leaders around you; building and recognizing autonomy in the organization; allowing innovations to rise and be implemented; and the absence of believing that you wear an invisible crown which all must bow to.

But academic leaders are essentially without the hierarchical power of corporate leaders and must achieve goals to the extent to which they are able to influence and support their faculty in individual and school development. The academic leader "must have sufficient ego strengths to recognize that building leaders and sharing leadership does not in any way diminish [her] prestige…" (Fagin, 2000). Nor is reaching for excellence a finite process. But no part of it can be achieved without creating an atmosphere of openness and trust while rewarding excellence in the shared value system of the group. In effect, the academic leader moves the discipline forward and represents the institution in the best way possible. Faculty want their leader to represent them to the administration, help them achieve their full rights and respect, present the discipline in the most reputable way possible, and be able to engage in the broad campus and alumni arenas in a way that brings positive attention to nursing (Fagin, 1983). Thus, the academic leader must be a superb role model of the values espoused, must be able to mentor others, must recognize instances of success, and may manipulate the organizational structure and resources to support goal achievement (Beverly, Maas, et al., 2006). Along the way, a certain degree of ambiguity is inevitable. For some leaders, it is an easy call; for others, it is more uncomfortable.

Ambiguity is a trait that some find difficult to accept; however, for the academic leader, ambiguity is not negative. It has its place in that it gives the leader time to evaluate situations and to change one's own opinions as experience dictates. The faculty member who finds ambiguity intolerable is the one who needs to be encouraged to think creatively and to tolerate differences of opinion. Being unwilling to accept or to demonstrate ambiguity may result in rigidity, which is anathema to leadership in academia or anywhere. By contrast, academic leadership requires strength and fortitude as well as strategy to accomplish institutional goals, which may not be popular with all faculty. The academic leader's ability to balance these traits is best demonstrated in the reverse by those with a rigid belief in "consensus," which in some cases defies the entire notion of leadership.

A

A

"Teaching and research are the main missions of universities and a suitable system of governance should, therefore, make these activities as efficient as possible." Rosovsky's (1990) view of governance is crucial for academic leaders to understand fully. Students are the business of universities and need to be attended to with interest and dedication by faculty who are appointed to tenure holding positions. Although research is vital for advancement of the discipline, it is not an either/or situation. In the quest for new knowledge, the transfer of that knowledge to the next generation is the sine qua non of the fully credentialed faculty member. Attention to research alone is possible if one is employed by a research institute at which the staff may work with postdoctoral trainees and the like, but in an academic institution faculty research must be reconciled with dedication to building future leaders and practitioners. The academic leader must have the vision—defined here as an awareness of current trends and future needs of the profession and health care system— the strategic approach, and the personal skills to make this holistic role possible. In academia, students are the principal business that keeps an institution going and growing.

But in academia, as well as other venues, there seems to be an absence of transformational leaders "who not only respond to their institutional challenges but also speak for their professions and for the public they serve" (Fagin, 2000). The Institute of Medicine (2004) described transformational leadership as benefiting the leader and the led, because it is a process by which both are stimulated to achieve their preferred future. Vision alone does not accomplish the vital tasks of leadership in academia or any other venue. The leader must have the ability to refine and refocus problems and pose a variety of scenarios and solutions. This component of leadership has been described by Foote and Cottrell (1955) as "interpersonal competence." Interpersonal competence is the skill or set of abilities allowing an individual to shape the responses he or she gets from others. Clearly, this is a developmental ability because self-knowledge and experience are necessary to predict the impact of one's own actions on another and having a large and varied repertoire of possible lines of action and appropriate tactics.

Peter Senge's (1990) definition of a learning organization helps to focus the academic mission. "A learning organization…is continually expanding its capacity to create its future. For such an organization, it is not enough merely to survive. 'Survival learning'…is important…. But for a learning organization…[it] must be joined by 'generative learning,' learning that enhances our capacity to create." Leaders in academia are the resource for the future since their primary goals should be building the discipline and developing the next generation of leaders. Leaders can be made, not born.

Beverly, C., Maas, M., Young, H., Richards, K., Scalzi, C., & Kayser-Jones, J. (2006). Leadership development in the John A. Hartford Centers of Geriatric Nursing Excellence. *Nursing Outlook, 54*(4), 204–211.

Fagin, C. (2001). *When care becomes a burden.* New York, NY: Milbank Memorial Fund.

Fagin, C. M. (1983). The dean and faculty development. In M. E. Conway & O. Andruskiw (Eds.), *Administrative theory and practice.* East Norwalk, CT: Appleton, Century, Crofts.

Fagin, C. M. (2000). *Essays on nursing leadership.* New York, NY: Springer Publishing.

Foote, N., & Cottrell, L. (1955). *Identity and interpersonal competence.* Chicago, IL: University of Chicago Press.

Institute of Medicine. (2004). *Keeping patients safe: Transforming the work environment of nurses.* Washington, DC: National Academies Press.

Rosovsky, H. (1990). *The university: An owner's manual.* New York, NY: W.W. Norton & Company.

Senge, P. M. (1990). *The fifth discipline.* New York, NY: Doubleday.

Claire M. Fagin

ACADEMIC MOBBING

Mobbing is an aggressive antagonistic behavior implemented by a group of people toward one or more individuals that aims to humiliate, discredit, and marginalize a targeted individual. The terms mobbing and bullying are often used interchangeably in the literature. Bullying more accurately, however, refers to individual acts of aggression (Davenport, Schwartz, & Elliott, 2005). Mobbing occurs when one or more individuals in the workplace become allies with a bully by provoking or encouraging the bully or by looking the other way and remaining silent. These individuals comprise the "mob" who systematically isolate, marginalize, and emotionally abuse the targeted person until he or she resigns (Twale & De Luca, 2008). Why certain people are targeted for mobbing is incompletely understood. However, victims of mobbing are often creative people who promote change and threaten the status quo (Davenport et al., 2005; Twale & De Luca, 2008).

Leymann (1996) identified five phases of mobbing: (1) a critical incident of conflict with victim, (2) aggressive behavior and psychological assaults of victim, (3) management involvement, (4) labeling of victim as difficult or mentally unstable, and (5) firing of victim or forced resignation (Davenport et al., 2005). When the target is a tenured faculty member who cannot be fired, the mob may use isolation, slander, shunning, and elimination from university governance to prompt the victim to resign (Twale & De Luca, 2008).

Few studies have explored the phenomenon of mobbing in the United States. However, in their review of research conducted in Australia and Europe, Yildirim and Yildirim (2007) found that many nurses experienced a hostile work environment where mobbing behaviors were demonstrated by colleagues but more often by managers.

The impact of mobbing on the individual can be devastating. Mobbing victims often experience high levels of anxiety, stress, and depression that can result in long-term physiological, psychological, and social problems (Yildirim & Yildirim, 2007). Unchecked, mobbing may become part of a toxic organizational culture that results in loss of trust, respect, and/or productivity.

Mobbing is a workplace safety and health issue with serious negative sequelae for nurses, their patients, and health care organizations. Nurse leaders play a key role in establishing the workplace climate and are uniquely positioned to transform organizational structures and processes that inadvertently reinforce a toxic workplace culture and allow it to persist. One of the first steps to changing the culture is to raise consciousness about mobbing. Porter-O'Grady and Malloch (2011) challenge nurse leaders to become more self-aware of dysfunctional behaviors, walk the talk in word and behavior, listen carefully, empower employees, engender organizational health, and transform the culture.

Davenport, N., Schwartz, R. D., & Elliott, G. P. (2005). *Mobbing: Emotional abuse in the American workplace.* Ames, IA: Civil Society Publishing.

Leymann, H. (1996). The content and development of mobbing at work. *European Journal of Work and Organizational Psychology, 5*(2), 165–184.

Porter O'Grady, T., & Malloch, K. (2011). *Quantum leadership: Advancing information, transforming healthcare* (3rd ed.). Sudbury, MA: Jones and Bartlett.

Twale, D. J., & De Luca, B. M. (2008). *Faculty incivility: The rise of the academic bully culture and what to do about it.* San Francisco, CA: Jossey-Bass.

Yildirim, A., & Yildirim, D. (2007). Mobbing in the workplace by peers and managers: Mobbing experienced by nurses working in healthcare facilities in Turkey and its effect on nurses. *Journal of Clinical Nursing, 16,* 1444–1452.

Darlene Del Prato

ACCOUNTABLE CARE ORGANIZATIONS

Redesign of the current health care system is essential. Despite advanced biomedical knowledge, the United States continues to experience wide variation in health care quality and outcomes and unprecedented health care costs (Institute of Medicine [IOM], 2008; McGlynn et al., 2003). With health care spending expected to reach 20% of the nation's GDP by 2015 (IOM, 2008), most understand and support the need for health care reform that includes accountable care organizations (ACOs).

ACOs are designed to shift focus away from expensive, hospital-based acute care to a model centered on preventive care and wellness, coordinated patient care, and disease management. ACOs involve teams of doctors and hospitals working together to achieve higher quality patient outcomes, increased efficiencies, and lower costs. These teams are responsible for providing care to patients while meeting and reporting on various quality and efficiency standards (Shortell & Castalino, 2010).

Providers are compensated according to how well they meet the standards.

Suggested attributes of ACOs include physician-led organizations responsible for coordinated care delivery, health information technology that supports coordination of care delivery, non-physician roles, such as case managers or boundary spanners (Gittell, 2009) to assist with coordination of care, and the use of evidence-based practice as required components of coordinated care delivery (Everett & Sitterding, 2010; Johnson, 2010). An ACO is an interdisciplinary and people-centered model that provides significant provider incentives to coordinate and integrate care with a focus on disease management. Hospitals and their extended medical staff are viewed as a central source of accountability for quality and cost because of their focus on performance measurement, organizational accountability, quality improvement, and cost containment. The model has three key features: local accountability, shared savings, and performance measurement, including quality and cost (Lowell & Bertko, 2010).

ACOs likely will face a variety of challenges prior to adoption. One is health care's limited success (to date) with cooperative governance models. Another is increasing competition between physicians and hospitals resulting in the full-time need for hospital-based physician support. Cultural barriers also exist, including isolated examples of physicians and nurses not accepting responsibility for the care of all patients within their delivery system. Other practical challenges include legal obstacles, variability in degree of alignment, achievement expectations, incentives, and risk management (Dove, Weaver, & Lewin, 2009; Fisher, Staige, Bynum, & Gottlieb, 2006; Fuller, Clinton, Goldfield, & Kelly, 2010; Johnson, 2010; Larson, 2009; Lowell & Bertko, 2010; Rittenhousse, 2009; Taylor, 2010).

While diverse pilot ACO programs (Carilion Clinic Health System in Roanoke, Virginia, the Norton Health System in Louisville, Kentucky, and the Tucson Medical Center in Arizona) will inform future ACO design (Taylor, 2010), there remain numerous unanswered questions for patients, providers, and hospitals. Questions include (Dove et al., 2009; Shomaker, 2010; Tallia, 2010):

1. Who will set benchmark cost targets and how?

2. How will the proper size of an ACO be determined?

3. How will geography and related circumstances influence variations in the model?

4. Will there be real patient choice of ACO?

5. Should patients be concerned about rationing of care and limited innovation?

6. What governance structures will be necessary to bring networks together?

7. Will health information technology deliver on expectations regarding quality?

8. How might academic medical centers become an organizing force in the health of local populations, including medical homes?

Critical design and operational features influencing the organizational and management of ACOs will include leaders willing to challenge the status quo; a local contractual structure conducive to managing budget while allocating payments and bonuses; health care information technology with the capacity for real-time data and feedback; analytic capacity to provide quality feedback with a short turnaround; contracts for provider payment rates and services; and organizational form (Dorn, 2009; Lowell & Bertko, 2010, p. 86).

Although ACOs are not a complete solution to the acute shortage of primary care clinicians in the United States, they may help alleviate the problem by allowing primary care practices to more efficiently care for larger number of patients through team-based practice. Innovative payment incentives offered by ACOs may prompt more medical and nursing school students to pursue careers in primary care (Shortell, Casalino, & Fisher, 2010), further addressing the shortage.

Dorn, S. (2009). United States Health Care Reform in 2009: A primer for gastroenterologists. *Clinical Gastroenterology & Hepatology, 7*(11), 1168–1173.

Dove, J., Weaver, W., & Lewin, J. (2009). Health care delivery system reform: Accountable care organizations. *Journal of American College of Cardiology, 54*(11), 985–988.

Everett, L., & Sitterding, M. (2010). Nursing leadership competencies to implement and sustain evidence-based practice: A multi-hospital system exemplar. *Western Journal of Nursing Research, 33*(3), 398–426.

Fisher, E., Staiger, D., Bynum, J., & Gottlieb, D. (2006). Creating accountable care organizations: The extended hospital medical staff. *Health Affairs, 26*(1), 44–57.

Fuller, R., Clinton, S., Goldfield, N., & Kelly, W. (2010). Building the affordable medical home. *Journal of Ambulatory Care Management, 33*(1), 71–80.

Gittell, J. (2009). *High performance healthcare: Using the power of relationships to achieve quality, efficiency, and resilience.* New York, NY: McGraw-Hill Publishing.

Institute of Medicine. (2008). *Knowing what works in health care: A roadmap for the nation.* Washington, DC: National Academies Press.

Johnson, B. (2010). Accountable care organizations and beyond. Position your practice for a quality-based delivery system. *MGMA Connexion/Medical Group Management Association, 10*(4), 32–35.

Larson, E. (2009). Group Health Cooperative: One coverage-and-delivery model for accountable care. *New England Journal of Medicine, 361*(17), 1620–1622.

Lowell, K., & Bertko, J. (2010). The Accountable Care Organization (ACO) Model: Building blocks for success. *Journal of Ambulatory Care Management, 33*(1), 81–88.

McGlynn, E., Asch, S., Adams, J., Keesey, J., Hicks, J., DeCristofara, A., et al. (2003). The quality of health care delivered to adults in the United States. *New England Journal of Medicine, 348*(26), 2635–2643.

Rittenhousse, D. (2009). Primary care and accountable care—Two essential elements of delivery-system reform. *New England Journal of Medicine, 361*(24), 2301–2303.

Shomaker, T. (2010). Health care payment reform and academic medicine: Threat or opportunity? *Academic Medicine, 85*(5), 756–758.

Shortell, S., & Casalino, L. (2010). Implementing qualifications criteria and technical assistance for accountable care organizations. *Journal of the American Medical Association, 303*(17), 1747–1748.

Shortell, S., Casalino, L., & Fisher, E. (2010). How the Center for Medicare and Medicaid Innovation should test Accountable Care Organizations. *Health Affairs, 29*(7), 1293–1298.

Tallia, A. (2010). Commentary: Academic health centers as accountable care organizations. *Academic Medicine, 85*(5), 766–767.

Taylor, M. (2010). The ABCs of ACOs. Accountable care organizations unit hospitals and other providers in caring for the community. *Trustee, 63*(6), 12–14.

Linda Q. Everett

ACCREDITATION COMMISSION FOR MIDWIFERY EDUCATION

In 1925, Mary Breckinridge brought nurse–midwifery to the United States when she founded the Frontier Nursing Service in Leslie County in eastern Kentucky. The Maternity Center Association in New York City founded the first nurse–midwifery education program in 1932. In 1955, the American College of Nurse–Midwifery was founded in 1957, created a Committee on Curriculum and Approval to develop formal processes of evaluation and approval of nurse–midwifery education programs. In 1969, this college merged with the American Association of Nurse–Midwives to become the American College of Nurse–Midwives (ACNM). The Committee on Curriculum and Approval became a separate division of the ACNM in 1974.

The U.S. Department of Education recognized the ACNM Division of Accreditation (DOA) in 1982 and since then has continuously recognized the DOA, or its successor, the Accreditation Commission for Midwifery Education (ACME). ACME autonomously establishes accreditation standards and conducts accreditation reviews of applicant programs and freestanding institutions whose graduates are then eligible to take the American Midwifery Certification Board's (AMCB) national certification examination. Graduates who are nurses and who pass the examination are certified nurse-midwives (CNMs).

In 1994, the DOA completed the task of identifying those competencies essential to the practice of midwifery that are inherent in nursing education and that would need to be included in any non-nurse–midwifery education program. The resultant document, *The Knowledge, Skills, and Behaviors Prerequisite to Midwifery Clinical Coursework,* was added to those competencies already identified in the ACNM *Core Competencies for Basic Nurse–Midwifery Practice.* In 1996, DOA pre-accredited the first education program for non-nurse–midwives. The first batch of students graduated a year later and the program achieved full accreditation in 1999. Graduates who pass the AMCB examination are certified midwives (CMs).

Since 1980, innovative nurse–midwifery programs have received accreditation from the DOA or its successor, ACME. These programs combine intensive on-campus instruction and simulation experiences, didactic education completed by students in their homes, and clinical education obtained with CNMs/CMs at facilities in the student's community. Currently, many programs combine on-campus and distance education modalities and all meet the same criteria for quality established by ACME.

See also American College of Nurses–Midwives; American Midwifery Certification Board

Adapted from the American College of Nurse–Midwives (http://www.midwife.org/accreditation)

Mary C. Brucker

ACCREDITATION IN NURSING EDUCATION

Accreditation in higher education is both general (as in institutional accreditation) and specialized (as in nursing, law, business, and other disciplines). General accreditation is under the purview of the Council for Higher Education Accreditation (CHEA), a private, nongovernmental organization consisting of institutional membership. "A national advocate and institutional voice for self-regulation of academic quality through accreditation, CHEA is an association of 3,000 degree-granting colleges and universities and recognizes 60 institutional and programmatic accrediting organizations" (Council for Higher Education Accreditation, 2010). There are seven regional (institutional) accrediting bodies for universities and colleges (Council for Higher Education Directories, 2010). The U.S. Department of Education also has a role in the national recognition of accrediting agencies deemed to be reliable authorities in ensuring educational quality (U.S. Department of Education, 2010).

Specialized accreditation in nursing education is a process by which the quality of programs is ensured (Bourke & Ihrke, 2009). Nursing programs voluntarily choose to participate in the accreditation process as one means of publicly demonstrating that program outcomes meet educational standards established by the profession. There are two major evaluative components to the accreditation process: an extensive self-study conducted by the faculty of the program and an accompanying peer review process conducted on site by external reviewers.

Although accreditation is a voluntary process, there are many benefits to nursing programs participating in the process. Besides providing an opportunity to evaluate the quality of program outcomes and develop plans for continuous quality improvement, accreditation can be a recruiting factor in attracting qualified students and faculty, affect a program's eligibility to receive external funding and students' ability to receive federal financial aid, and also influence graduates' ability to enroll in subsequent nursing education programs (Iwasiw, Goldenberg, & Andrusyszyn, 2005). For these reasons, most nursing programs pursue accreditation.

Two national professional nursing accrediting organizations accredit nursing programs. The National League for Nursing Accrediting Commission (NLNAC) accredits all nursing programs including licensed practical (vocational) nursing, diploma, associate's degree, baccalaureate degree, master's degree, and clinical doctorate programs. The Commission on Collegiate Nursing Education (CCNE) accredits baccalaureate, master's degree, and clinical doctorate programs. Research-focused doctoral programs (PhD, EdD, DNS, DNSc) are not subject to accreditation by the professional nursing accrediting organizations. Baccalaureate and higher degree nursing programs can choose to be accredited by either organization; some programs choose to be accredited by both.

The accreditation process provides a thorough evaluative review of all components of the program with an emphasis on program outcomes. Substantive program elements that are reviewed include outcomes related to curriculum, institutional and program mission and governance, fiscal and institutional resources, instructional resources, student support services, qualifications of faculty and students, faculty and student accomplishments, and the systematic program evaluation plan that guides faculty decision making. It is important that faculty have an understanding of the accreditation standards that guide the implementation of their nursing program. The accreditation standards established by NLNAC are found at http://www.nlnac. org/home.htm. The accreditation standards established by CCNE are found at http://www.aacn.nche.edu/Accreditation/ index.htm.

The process by which a nursing program achieves accreditation is similar for both NLNAC and CCNE. Before receiving an on-site visit from external peer reviewers, the program faculty and the chief program officer (e.g., chair, dean) prepare and submit a written self-study report that addresses each accreditation standard. This self-study provides faculty with an opportunity to identify program strengths and areas for improvement and to cite evidence that supports the faculty's findings. After submission of the self-study report, the program receives an on-site visit from a team of peer reviewers, who validate the findings reported in the self-study and review additional data provided by the program during the visit. Following the on-site visit, the team of reviewers prepares a report of their findings, which is submitted to the agency for a decision on the program's accreditation status. It is not the responsibility of the external reviewers to make recommendations regarding the program's accreditation status. The decision regarding program accreditation is made by a review committee that bases its decision primarily upon a review of the team's report.

Programs that meet all standards receive accreditation for the full number of years (8 years for NLNAC applicants, 5 years for first-time CCNE applicants, and 10 years for continuing CCNE applicants), after which time they will need to seek reaccreditation. Programs that do not fully meet all standards may receive accreditation for a limited number of years before they must undergo another visit; it is also possible that a program will be denied accreditation. Programs that receive a limited accreditation term or are denied accreditation are given a report of the standards not met and the improvements that must be made before the program will again be eligible to seek accreditation. The accreditation status of educational programs is publicly reported by the accrediting agency.

Bourke, M. P., & Ihrke, B. A. (2009). The evaluation process: An overview. In D. M. Billings & J. A. Halstead (Eds.), *Teaching in nursing: A guide for faculty* (3rd ed., pp. 391–408). St. Louis, MO: Elsevier Saunders.

Council for Higher Education Accreditation. (2010). *2010–2011 Directory of CHEA recognized organizations.* Retrieved October 5, 2010, from http://www.chea.org/pdf/2010– 2011_Directory_of_CHEA_Recognized_ Organizations.pdf

Council for Higher Education Directories. (2010). *Directories: Regional accrediting organizations 2010–2011.* Retrieved October 5, 2010, from http://www.chea.org/Directories/ regional.asp

Iwasiw, C., Goldenberg, D., & Andrusyszyn, M. (2005). Planning curriculum evaluation. In *Curriculum development in nursing education* (pp. 221–242). Sudbury, MA: Jones and Bartlett.

U.S. Department of Education. (2010). *Overview of accreditation*. Retrieved October 7, 2010, from http://www2.ed.gov/admins/finaid/accred/accreditation.html#Overview

Judith A. Halstead

ACCREDITATION IN NURSING PRACTICE

Accreditation in the practice setting is a formal process of recognition or conformance to standards that are intended to reflect quality and safety in health care settings. Health care organizations in many countries throughout the world voluntarily participate in the accreditation process to demonstrate to the public their accountability to continuously improve the quality and safety of their care. Accreditation is often required for a health care institution or program to be eligible for third-party insurance payment for rendered patient care services. Although there are many organizations that provide accreditation of health care systems, the most well-known and comprehensive is The Joint Commission (TJC) (previously known as the Joint Commission on Accreditation of Healthcare Organizations, or JCAHO). This organization will be described in this entry as an exemplar for accreditation in the practice setting. Other accrediting organizations that also provide valuable information dependant on the health care setting or program are the Commission on Accreditation of Rehabilitation Facilities, Community Health Accreditation Program, Utilization Review Accreditation Committee, Accreditation Commission for Healthcare, American Osteopathic Association and, most recently in 2008, Det Norske Veritas.

Organized health care improvement efforts began with the work of Dr. Ernest Codman, who in 1910 introduced the concept of an "end result system." This system would track each hospitalized patient to determine whether treatment was effective. If treatment was not deemed to be effective, hospital personnel would explore the reasons and implement a new process for improvement. A colleague of Dr. Codman's, Franklin Martin, MD, founded the American College of Surgeons (ACS), which then brought the concept of "end result" to another level. The ACS developed "minimum standards," which were subsequently required for review and assessment when on-site inspections of hospitals for accreditation by the ACS began in 1918.

By 1950, over 3,200 hospitals participated in the inspections, which were intended to promote improvements in care. As a result of these improvements, the American Medical Association, American College of Physicians, Canadian Medical Association, and the American Hospital Association joined forces with the ACS to create the Joint Commission on Accreditation of Hospitals (JCAH) in 1951. JCAH developed standards of performance for a variety of patient care settings, including acute and long-term care, ambulatory care, mental health, laboratory and pathology services, and hospice care. The "minimum standard" threshold developed by ACS was modified and enhanced by JCAH to promote performance that exceeded basic requirements.

In 1987, the JCAH changed their name to JCAHO. This reorganization set the climate for change and further refocused their expectations of institutions seeking accreditation. Health care organizations were required to show comprehensive and continuous improvement efforts through outcome and process metrics that demonstrated performance exemplifying

A

safe and reliable care. In 2002, the JCAHO announced the Shared Visions—New Pathways initiative, which was focused on critical systems to improve and ensure the safety and quality of patient care. A 24/7/365 readiness campaign was established with unannounced surveys. JCAHO continued to refresh their mission, and in 2007 changed their name to The Joint Commission. The Joint Commission currently performs accreditation surveys through the use of a "tracer" methodology for assessment. The on-site surveyors assess the delivery of services throughout episodes of care, observing the patient as she or he touches multiple providers and processes. This format allows for the assessment of the continuity, quality, safety, and patient centeredness of care in a longitudinal fashion.

Opportunities for improvement that are identified during these survey processes have historically carried a burden for organizations to identify ways to improve without assistance from the accrediting body. In 2009, The Joint Commission Center for Transforming Healthcare was established to provide organizations with strategies for solving complex quality and safety problems.

Organizations measure their performance over time through the collection and analysis of data, demonstrating accountability and commitment to continuous high performance. Because of mandated reporting requirements, the public is able to visit multiple Internet sites to view, compare, and subsequently select the organization or provider that achieves the best performance. Accreditation is one mechanism to promote adherence to standards in the practice setting. Survey readiness has become an integral part of the daily operations of health care organizations and has resulted in measurable improvements in patient care delivery.

Additional information is available at these Web sites:

Accreditation Commission for Health Care (ACHC), www.achc.org

American College of Physicians (ACP), www.acponline.org

American College of Surgeons (ACS), www.facs.org

American Hospital Association (AHA), www.aha.org

American Medical Association (AMA), www.assn.org

American Nursing Association (ANA), www.ana.org

American Osteopathic Association (AOA), www.osteopathic.org

Centers for Medicare and Medicaid Services (CMS), www.cms.hhs.gov

Commission on Accreditation of Rehabilitation Facilities (CARF), www.carf.org

Community Health Accreditation Program (CHAP), www.chapinc.org

Det Norske Veritas (DNV), www.dnvaccreditation.com

National League for Nursing (NLN), www.nln.org

The Joint Commission (JC), www.jointcommission.org

Utilization Review Accreditation Committee (URAC), www.urac.org

Cindy A. Reilly

Advance Care Planning and Advance Directives

Advance care planning (ACP) is a dynamic process of preparing for serious, progressive, life-threatening illness and eventual death and is the appropriate context for facilitating the completion of advance directives (ADs). ADs are advantageous to family members, surrogate decision makers, and health care providers because they can help take away some of the burden of difficult end-of-life health care decisions and make it easier to carry out the patient's wishes. ACP occurs over time and does not necessarily occur in a single conversation. It entails introspection about values and what is important to that individual in both living and in dying. ACP enables an individual to make a plan for future care and death that is in keeping with his/her wishes and encourages the communication of those preferences to loved ones, surrogate decision makers, and care providers, in the event that decision-making capacity is lost (Matzo & Sherman, 2010; Samanta & Samanta, 2010). Although ACP should be part of routine health care, it becomes particularly urgent with the destabilization of a chronic disease or the diagnosis of a life-threatening terminal illness.

The nurse's role in facilitating ACP includes:

- Providing information to patients to promote an understanding of potential future health care decisions and the various life-sustaining treatments that are available.

- Encouraging patients to decide what types of treatment they would or would not want if diagnosed with a serious, progressive, life-threatening illness, if they become incapacitated, or at the time of death.

- Asking patients what would be their preferred place for end-of-life care and death.

- Encouraging patients to share their feelings and wishes with loved ones and their health care providers on an ongoing basis.

- Providing information to patients about the types of ADs in their state.

- Encouraging patients to put plans into writing in the form of ADs.

Cultural, ethnic, and religious views can have a significant impact on ACP. One review found that, compared to other races, non-White racial groups are more likely to lack knowledge of advanced directives. The same review found a preference for family centered decision making in Hispanic and Asian cultures, and that African Americans are more likely to prefer the use of life-sustaining therapies (Kwak & Haley, 2005). Variations among racial and ethnic groups do exist—necessitating individualized patient and family cultural assessments (Mitchell & Mitchell, 2009).

As part of the ACP discussion, it is helpful to have patients state their preference of four basic options: (1) "I want to remain in my place of residence with comfort care as the goal and hospice care, if possible;" (2) "If necessary to achieve comfort, I would go to the hospital briefly for symptom relief, then return to my usual place of residence for comfort care;" (3) "If it is unclear whether or not I could respond to a trial of therapy, including life support, I would like to have this trial, but stop the treatment in a few days if it is not working;" (4) "I would like all measures provided to keep me alive as long as possible, regardless of the discomfort this may entail" (Henderson, Hansen, & Reynolds, 2003).

There is clear and convincing evidence that, as part of ACP, health care team members need to take on a leadership role in working with individuals, families, and surrogate decision makers to help them prepare for any subsequent "in-the-moment" treatment decisions that might arise. These in-the-moment decisions should be based on both the patient's preferences and any new information that might inform the decision-making process. This is imperative since people cannot always foresee or predict what their feelings and wishes will be when they are actually faced with a health crisis (Fried, O'Leary, Van Ness, & Fraenkel 2007; Halpern & Arnold, 2008; Sudore & Fried, 2010; Ubel, Loewenstein, Schwarz, & Smith, 2005).

Health care decisions and wishes are best communicated and documented in the

A

form of ADs, before a health crisis occurs. ADs are legal documents signed by individuals with decision-making capacity to direct health professionals and loved ones about their treatment wishes. Depending on the state, ADs may only be applicable when a person is terminally or critically ill or has advanced dementia and is unable to make informed decisions or is in a persistent vegetative state (Guido, 2006).

There are two primary kinds of AD documents. First is the living will, a statement that says, essentially, "If I am terminally and irreversibly ill, or in a persistent vegetative state, I do not want my life prolonged by extraordinary means." In some states, a living will includes specific options, such as, no cardiopulmonary resuscitation attempt in the case of a respiratory or cardiac arrest; no ventilator support; or no tube feeding or artificial hydration. The living will may be a handwritten, personalized directive rather than a formal state-generated form. Second is the health care proxy, or durable power of attorney for health care (DPOAHC), in which an individual appoints someone to speak for him/herself regarding medical treatment when the person cannot make his or her decisions due to incapacitating injury or illness. The DPOAHC may afford more flexibility in health care decision making than the living will. In that health care scenarios that had not been anticipated at the time the living will was written can be addressed by the DPOAHC (Caring Connections, 2005). The DPOAHC must clearly state the patient's end-of-life wishes and advocate for those wishes as the patient intended. The family should be informed of this arrangement and invited to be part of the decision-making process, if possible (Ashley, 2005).

A recent advance in end-of-life care is the Physicians Orders for Life-Sustaining Treatment (POLST) paradigm, or Medical

Orders for Life-Sustaining Treatment (MOLST) in some states (Abrahm, 2010). The POLST is a form of medical order that accompanies and complements the AD and is not intended to replace it. POLST can be completed by a physician, nurse practitioner, physician assistant, or social worker, depending on the state. The POLST translates the treatment wishes of individuals into actionable medical orders and is portable from one health care setting to the next. As of December 2010, there were seven states with endorsed POLST programs and 18 states with developing programs (POLST, 2010).

The Patient Self-Determination Act (PSDA) is a federal law passed by the U.S. Congress in 1990. The PSDA requires all health care providers or facilities receiving Medicare or Medicaid funding to ensure that every newly admitted patient with decision-making capacity or his or her representative is asked if he or she has an AD and, if so, that directive is obtained. They also must provide information to patients and their health care agents in writing about their right to accept or reject any surgical procedure or medical treatment, as per state law. Although the law does not require that patients complete and execute advanced directives, they must be informed of their right to complete an AD and be given the opportunity to do so. ADs must also be documented in each patient record. Finally, the PSDA requires that education on ADs be provided to staff, patients, health care agents, caregivers, and the community (Watson, 2010). It is important to remind patients and families that ADs are not immutable and can be changed as wishes or situations change.

ADs are recognized in all 50 states (Klein, 2005), but must comply with specific state legislation in order to make them legally binding. State-specific laws related to ADs are available from the American Bar

Association Web site (2010) at http://new. abanet.org/aging/Pages/StateLawCharts. aspx. Most states have some form of AD documents available online, with information regarding notarization and witness requirements from the Caring Connections Web site at http://www.caringinfo.org/ stateaddownload.

Further work to promote ADs is needed. The overall completion rate for either a living will or health care proxy document has slowly risen from about 20% in the early 1990s to only 29% in 2007 (AARP, 2008). Some barriers to AD completions include reluctance of patients and health care providers to discuss end-of-life issues, time constraints, denial, procrastination, delaying until crisis occurs, unrealistic expectations of CPR, discomfort with planning palliative care, cultural and health system barriers, not ready for the discussion, overwhelmed with illness, physician worried about burdening patient, access to information, the complexity of end-of-life decision making, inability to choose a proxy, ethnicity, and lack of trust in the AD process (Later & King, 2007).

According to the American Nurses Association (2001), nurses have an ethical responsibility to teach patients about their right to self-determination in care. Nurses can play a vital role in ACP by educating patients about their rights in end-of-life care, informing patients of the benefits of advance planning, helping them navigate the process of ACP, encouraging ongoing communication of wishes with family and health care providers, and by acting as effective patient advocates.

Instead of a possible crisis, the time of dying can be one of gentle closure, with "quality" time and a chance to say good-bye (Byock & Heffner, 2002). Patients with ADs are much more likely to experience end-of-life care that is consistent with their wishes (Silveira, Kim, & Langa, 2010), resulting in increased patient and family satisfaction, and a decreased incidence of stress, anxiety, and depression in surviving loved ones (Detering, Hancock, Reade, & Silvester, 2010).

AARP. (2008). AARP Bulletin Poll: "Getting Ready to Go," Executive Summary. Retrieved November 28, 2010, from http://assets.aarp. org/rgcenter/il/getting_ready.pdf

Abrahm, J. L. (2011). Advances in palliative medicine and end-of-life care. Annual Review of Medicine, 62, 9.1–9.13.

American Nurses Association. (2001). Code of ethics for nurses. Silver Spring, MD: American Nurses Association.

Ashley, R. C. (2005). Why are advanced directives legally important? Critical Care Nurse, 25(4), 56.

Byock, I., & Heffner, J. E. (2002). Palliative and end-of-life pearls. Philadelphia, PA: Hanley & Belfus, Inc.

Caring Connections. (2005). Health care agents: Appointing one and being one. National Hospice and Palliative Care Organization. Retrieved November 21, 2010, from http://www.caring-info.org

Detering, K. M., Hancock, A. D., Reade, M. C., & Silvester, W. (2010). The impact of advance care planning on end of life care in elderly patients: Randomised controlled trial. British Medical Journal, 340, c1345.

Fried, T. R., O'Leary, J., Van Ness, P., & Fraenkel, L. (2007). Inconsistency over time in the preferences of older persons with advanced illness for life-sustaining treatment. Journal of the American Geriatric Society, 55(7), 1007–1014.

Guido, G. (2006). Legal and ethical issues in nursing (4th ed.). Englewood Cliffs, NJ: Prentice-Hall.

Halpern, J., & Arnold, R. M. (2008). Affective forecasting: An unrecognized challenge in making serious health decisions. Journal of General Internal Medicine, 23(10), 1708–1712.

Henderson, M. L., Hanson, L. C., & Reynolds, K. S. (2003). Improving nursing home care of the dying: A training manual for nursing home staff. Philadelphia, PA: Springer Publishing.

Klein, C. A. (2005). The importance of advanced directives. The Nurse Practitioner, 30(4), 11.

Kwak, J., & Haley, W. E. (2005). Current research findings on end-of-life decision making among racially or ethnically diverse groups. *The Gerontologist, 45*(5), 634–641.

Later, E. B., & King, D. (2007). Advance directives: Results of a community education symposium. *Critical Care Nurse, 27*(6), 31–36.

Matzo, M., & Sherman, D. W. (2010). Palliative care nursing: Quality care to the end of life (3rd ed.). New York: Springer Publishing.

Mitchell, B. L., & Mitchell, L. C. (2009). Review of the literature on cultural competence and end-of-life treatment decisions: The role of the hospitalist. *Journal of the National Medical Association, 101*(9), 920–926.

POLST. (2010). *POLST State Programs.* Retrieved November 29, 2010, from http://www.ohsu. edu/polst/programs/state+programs.htm

Samanta, A., & Samanta, J. (2010). Advance care planning: The role of the nurse. *British Journal of Nursing, 19*(16), 1060–1061.

Silveira, M. J., Kim, S. Y. H., & Langa, K. M. (2010). Advance directives and outcomes of surrogate decision making before death. *The New England Journal of Medicine, 362*(13), 1211–1218.

Sudore, R. L., & Fried, T. R. (2010). Redefining the "planning" in advance care planning: Preparing for end-of-life decision making. *Annals of Internal Medicine, 153*(4), 256–261.

Ubel, P. A., Loewenstein, G., Schwarz, N., & Smith, D. (2005). Misimagining the unimaginable: The disability paradox and health care decision making. *Health Psychology, 24*(4 Suppl.), S57–S62.

Watson, E. (2010). Advance directives: Self-determination, legislation, and litigation issues. *Journal of Legal Nurse Consulting, 21*(1), 9–14.

Deborah Witt Sherman
David C. Free

ADVANCED PRACTICE REGISTERED NURSES

Advanced practice registered nurses (APRNs) are registered nurses (RNs) with advanced educational and clinical preparation. APRNs include clinical nurse specialists (CNSs), certified registered nurse anesthetists (CRNAs), certified nurse–midwives (CNMs), and nurse practitioners (NPs). State nurse practice acts delineating APRNs legal parameter vary widely. The APRN Consensus Model (APRN Joint Dialogue Report Group, 2008) defines roles and regulations, and the extensive Institute of Medicine (IOM) report recommends enhancing APRN practice and contributions with health care (IOM, 2011).

CLINICAL NURSE SPECIALISTS

The CNS role originated in psychiatric nursing during a Quaker-led 19th-century reform movement protesting brutal treatment of the insane (Hamric, Spross, & Hanson, 2009). Psychiatric nursing education began at McLean Hospital, Massachusetts, in 1880, and the first psychiatric master's degree was established by Hildegard Peplau at Rutgers University in 1955. The 1964 Nurse Training Act led to a proliferation of clinical nurse specialization (Fulton, Lyon, & Goudreau, 2010; Hamric et al., 2009). In the late 1960s and 1970s, specialty nursing organizations (i.e., American Association of Critical-Care Nurses, Oncology Nursing Society) were established for nurses at entry and advanced levels. Currently, the National Association of Clinical Nurse Specialists unites CNSs from all specialties for practice improvement and advocacy.

CNSs must have graduate degrees with a clinical concentration; their practice focuses on patients and families. CNS certification at an advanced level is available for most specialties and is required in many states. Some specialties do not have national certification exams. Most CNSs practice in hospitals, the community, or independently. Their depth of clinical knowledge and expertise makes them ideal for developing protocols, standards, and care guidelines, and for fostering healthy work environments (Disch, Walton, & Barnsteiner, 2001). CNSs improve care quality through enhancing the care environment and practice of others.

CERTIFIED REGISTERED NURSE ANESTHETISTS

Nurse anesthetist practice can be traced to the late 1800s when a commonly used 1893 textbook (*Nursing: Its Principles and Practices for Hospital and Private Use* by Isabel Adams Hampton Robb) included a chapter on anesthesia administration (Bankert, 1989). CRNAs are RNs with master's degree or doctoral degree preparation to provide anesthesia and anesthesia-related services in a care team with anesthesiologists or independently. CRNA graduates must successfully complete the National Certification Examination (Council on Accreditation of Nurse Anesthesia Educational Programs, 2004). CRNAs are the sole anesthesia providers for approximately 50% of hospital surgeries and more than 65% of rural hospital surgeries (American Association of Nurse Anesthetists [AANA], 2007). The AANA 2005 Practice Profile indicated that CRNAs annually administer approximately 27 million anesthetics in the United States. Because of CRNAs' high-quality and safe anesthesia care, health facilities in medically underserved areas are able to offer obstetrical, surgical, and trauma stabilization services (AANA, 2007). The AANA and CRNA educators have joined forces to ensure the supply of nurse anesthetists keep pace with the demand. Nonetheless, CRNAs face resistance by some physicians and hospitals that restrict their full scope of practice. Research verifies the safety and cost-effectiveness of CNRA practice, thus refuting unsubstantiated claims and practice barriers (Dulisse & Cromwell, 2010; Hogan, Seifert, Moore, & Simonson, 2010).

MIDWIFERY

Nurse–midwifery was founded in the United States by Mary Breckinridge, an RN who received midwifery education in England and brought the British model of nurse–midwifery to the United States in 1925. America's first nurse–midwifery education program began in 1931 in New York City. Today, CNMs are educated in accredited programs in the two disciplines of nursing and midwifery and must be nationally certified by the American Midwifery Certification Board to legally practice. The CNM scope of practice includes prenatal care, labor and birth, well-woman gynecologic care, and basic primary care. The American College of Nurse–Midwives (ACNM) defines Core Competencies for Basic Midwifery Practice, Standards for the Practice of Midwifery, a Code of Ethics, and a Philosophy Statement. ACNM's Accreditation Commission for Midwifery Education began in the 1970s. A direct-entry (non-nursing) midwifery option utilizes the same accreditation and certification mechanisms began in 1997 in New York State, resulting in the certified midwife (CM) credential (legal in New York, New Jersey, and Rhode Island). Other midwives (sometimes called lay, home-birth, or direct-entry midwives) practicing primarily in out of hospital settings are recognized by state licensing agencies in approximately half of U.S. states and by some third-party payers (M. Avery, personal communication, October 27, 2010). Lay midwifery education varies from formal to apprentice-type education and can include accreditation and certification. Current issues for CNMs/CMs are the rising cesarean section rate, technology use for normal births, lack of health insurance for underserved women and their families, and increased recognition of the CM credential.

A

A

NURSE PRACTITIONERS

The NP role was developed in 1965 by Loretta Ford, PhD, RN, and Henry Silver, MD, at the University of Colorado (Ford & Silver, 1967). It focused on health promotion, illness prevention, and increasing access to care for children and their families. Role success led to NPs being adopted for other specialties (adult, family, gerontology, neonatal) and in diverse settings (clinics, critical care units [Kleinpell, 2005], retail spaces [Trossman, 2005]). NPs perform direct patient care, including holistic assessment, health promotion, illness/injury prevention, and disease management. They deliver care that is personalized, cost-effective, and timely (Brown & Grimes, 1995; Burl, Bonner, Rao, & Khan, 1998; Horrocks, Anderson, & Salisbury, 2002; Laurant, Reeves, Hermens, Braspenning, Grol, & Sibbald, 2004; Mundinger et al., 2000; Sarkissian & Wennberg, 1999).

COMMON APRN ISSUES

APRNs have moved from diverse historical beginnings to mainstream acceptance as skilled health care professionals with tremendous career opportunities. APRNs also predictably face barriers to the sustained growth of the APRN workforce (IOM, 2011). Confusion about scope of practice, legal parameters, and models of practice persists (Chevalier, Steinberg, & Lindeke, 2006). The general public, nurse colleagues, regulators, and administrators are challenged to fully understand and accept APRN roles. Relationships between physician and APRN professional organizations continue to be challenging though many physicians are staunch supporters and partners of APRNs. APRNs may be prevented from practicing interdependently and independently within their full scopes of practice thus depriving the public of access to capable, cost-effective APRN providers. APRN educational requirements are moving to doctoral preparation, with a recommended date of 2015 by which the Doctor of Nursing Practice degree would be the entry to ARPN practice (American Association of Colleges of Nursing, 2011). Finding enough qualified faculty to teach in APRN programs is challenging.

See also Accreditation Commission for Midwifery Education; American Association of Nurse Anesthetists; Shortage of Nursing Faculty

American Association of Colleges of Nursing. (2011). *Doctor of nursing practice.* Retrieved from http://www.aacn.nche.edu/DNP/index.htm

American Association of Nurse Anesthetists. (2007). *Certified registered nurse anesthetists at a glance.* Retrieved, from http://www.aana.com/aboutaana.aspx?ucNavMenu_TSMenuTargetID=179&ucNavMenu_TSMenuTargetType=4&ucNavMenu_TSMenuID=6&id=265

APRN Joint Dialogue Report Group. (2008). Retrieved from http://faanp.com/NR/rdonlyres/56292A59–8240-449D-910D-EF331FC7DC86/0/FinalAPRNJointDialogueReport7708.pdf

Bankert, M. (1989). *Watchful care, a history of America's nurse anesthetists.* New York, NY: Continuum.

Brown, S. A., & Grimes, D. E. (1995). A meta-analysis of nurse practitioners and nurse midwives in primary care. *Nursing Research,* 44(6), 332–339.

Burl, J. B., Bonner, A., Rao, M., & Khan, A. M. (1998). Geriatric nurse practitioners in long-term care: Demonstration of effectiveness in managed care. *Journal of the American Geriatrics Society,* 46(4), 506–510.

Chevalier, C., Steinberg, S., & Lindeke, L. (2006). Perceptions of barriers to psychiatric-mental health CSN practice. *Issues in Mental Health Nursing,* 27, 253–263.

Dulisse, B., & Cromwell, J. (2010). No harm found when nurse anesthetists work without supervision by physicians. *Health Affairs, 29,* 1469–1475.

Disch, J., Walton, M., & Barnsteiner, J. H. (2001). The role of the clinical nurse specialist in creating a healthy work environment. *AACN Clinical Issues: Advanced Practice in Acute and Critical Care, 12*(3), 345–355.

Ford, L. D., & Silver, H. K. (1967). Expanded role of the nurse in child care. *Nursing Outlook, 15,* 43–45.

Fulton, J., Lyon, B., & Goudreau, K. (2010). *Foundations of clinical nurse specialist practice.* New York, NY: Springer Publication.

Hamric, A. B., Spross, J. A., & Hanson, C. M. (2009). *Advanced practice nursing* (4th ed.). St. Louis, MO: Elsevier Saunders.

Hogan, P., Seifert, R., Moore, C., & Simonson, B. (2010). Cost effectiveness analysis of anesthesia providers. *Nursing Economics, 28,* 159–169.

Horrocks, S., Anderson, E., & Salisbury, C. (2002). Systematic review of whether nurse practitioners working in primary care can provide equivalent care to doctors. *British Medical Journal, 324*(7341), 819–823.

Institute of Medicine. (2011). *The future of nursing: Leading change, advancing health.* Washington, DC: National Academies Press.

Kleinpell, R. (2005). Acute care nurse practitioner practice: Results of a 5-year longitudinal study. *American Journal of Critical-Care, 14*(3), 211–219.

Laurant, M., Reeves, D., Hermens, R., Braspenning, J., Grol, R., & Sibbald, B. (2004). Substitution of doctors by nurses in primary care. *Cochrane Database of Systematic Reviews,* 4, No: CD001271.

Lindeke, L., Zwygart-Stauffacher, M., Avery, M., & Fagerlund K. (2010). Overview of advanced practice nursing. In M. P. Mirr Jansen & M. Zwygart-Stauffacher (Eds.), *Advanced practice nursing: Core concepts for professional role development* (4th ed.). New York, NY: Springer Publishing.

Mundinger, M. O., Kane, R. L., Lenz, E. R., Totten, A. M., Tsai, W. Y., Cleary, P. D., et al. (2000). Primary care outcomes in patients treated by nurse practitioners or physicians: A randomized trial. *Journal of the American Medical Association, 283*(1), 59–68.

Sarkissian, S., & Wennberg, R. (1999). Effects of acute care nurse practitioner role on epilepsy

monitoring outcomes. *Outcomes Management for Nursing Practice, 3*(4), 161–166.

Trossman, S. (2005, May/June). One-stop shopping—and some help for that strep throat. *The American Nurse, 37*(3), 1, 6.

Linda Lindeke
Joanne Disch

ADVOCACY

Nursing has a long and distinguished history of advocacy from the trenches of Crimea to the halls of the U.S. Congress. Past–American Nurses Association President Dorothy Cornelius once observed, "There is a great recognition of the need for nursing to speak with one voice on social issues in the areas of poverty, malnutrition, hunger and discrimination, all of which profoundly affect the health and well-being of the people of this country...Nursing is the conscience of the health care system" (van Betten & Moriarty, 2004, p. 145). Nurses advocate in their daily nursing practice on behalf of patients and their families—they track down the physician or advanced practice registered nurse for a change in pain medication or treatments, work with the social worker to find a "safe haven" for an abused mother, and request more nursing staff to ensure the delivery of safe care. This is the everyday advocacy that nurses do so well. Increasingly, nurses have taken their advocacy skills into the political arena, supporting social justice issues, promoting grassroots and legislative support, and political activity to advance nursing's agenda for health system reform and for the future of the profession (American Nurses Association, 1995, 2002, 2010).

American Nurses Association. (1995). *Nursing's agenda for health care reform*. Washington, DC: Author.

American Nurses Association. (2002). *Nursing's agenda for the future*. Washington, DC: Author.

American Nurses Association. (2010). *Health system reform*. Retrieved January 23, 2011, from http://www.nursingworld.org/health carereform

van Betten, P. T., & Moriarty, M. (2004). *Nursing illuminations: A book of days*. Chicago, IL: Mosby.

Karen A. Ballard

AFFIRMATIVE ACTION

Affirmative action is about equal opportunity and the use of policies to pave the way for all citizens of the United States to have the chance to be successful. Its purpose is to overcome the history of the subordination and segregation of certain groups of people in our society. President John F. Kennedy first used the term in the early 1960s. On March 6, 1961, he issued Executive Order 10925, which created the Committee on Equal Employment Opportunity and mandated that projects financed with federal funds "take affirmative action" to ensure that hiring and employment practices were free of racial bias. President Lyndon B. Johnson took further action on July 2, 1964, and signed the most sweeping civil rights legislation since Reconstruction, the Civil Rights Act, which prohibited discrimination of all kinds based on race, color, religion, or national origin.

The underlying foundation of the affirmative action concept is that unless positive action is undertaken to overcome the systemic institutional forms of exclusion and discrimination, benign neutral employment practices will perpetuate the status quo indefinitely. The objective is to have equal employment opportunity as a sustaining and permanent feature of the workplace. In an eloquent speech delivered to the graduating class at Howard University on June 4, 1965, President Johnson framed the concept underlying affirmative action, asserting that civil rights laws alone are not enough to remedy discrimination:

You do not wipe away the scars of centuries by saying: "Now, you are free to go where you want, do as you desire, and choose the leaders you please." You do not take a man who for years has been hobbled by chains, liberate him, bring him to the starting line of a race, saying, "you are free to compete with all the others," and still justly believe you have been completely fair…This is the next and more profound stage of the battle for civil rights. We seek not just freedom but opportunity—not just legal equity but human ability—not just equality as a right and a theory, but equality as a fact and a result.

Another move was made by President Johnson in September 24, 1965, when he issued Executive Order 11246, which requires government contractors to "take affirmative action" toward prospective minority employees in all aspects of hiring and employment. Contractors must take specific measures to ensure equality in hiring and must document these efforts. On October 13, 1967, the order was amended to cover discrimination on the basis of gender. President Richard M. Nixon implemented goals and timetables to expand the affirmative action executive order. During the presidency of Gerald R. Ford, the Rehabilitation Act of 1973 and the Vietnam Era Veterans Readjustment Act of 1974 were enacted. These acts guaranteed that federal contractors had affirmative action programs established for recruiting and hiring people with disabilities and Vietnam veterans. The Age Discrimination Act of 1975 was also enacted during Ford's presidency. This act barred discrimination in hiring or firing of older persons.

President Bill Clinton articulated four standards of fairness for all affirmative action programs approximately 40 years after the concept's initial debut:

1. No quotas in theory or practice;

2. No illegal discrimination of any kind;

3. No preference for people who are not qualified for any job or other opportunity;

4. As soon as a program has succeeded, it must be retired. Any program that does not meet these four principles should be eliminated or reformed to meet them.

The scrutiny regarding privileges to some and discrimination eventually permeated two other main sectors of people's lives: education and health care. Accusations were hurled of reversed discrimination by the majority and that unfair preferences toward less qualified minority applicants was displacing and subsequently causing qualified majority college applicants to be rejected for admission. The first significant challenges to affirmative action in educational admissions practices came in the 1970s with the *University of California Regents v. Bakke*. This case officially set the parameters for admissions practices in higher education for almost 25 years. The Supreme Court, in a 5-to-4 decision, upheld the right of universities to use race as one of the many admissions factors to be considered as a part of a holistic review. It specifically prohibited the use of quotas or separate admissions tracks.

Proposition 209 in California, Initiative 200 in the state of Washington, and the Hopwood case (University of Texas) were other significant antiaffirmative action cases that basically prohibited consideration of race, religion, sex, color, ethnicity,

or national origin as criteria for admission. Student body diversity was not considered a feature of "compelling interest" and therefore not a basis for consideration in admissions criteria. Other states followed suit, namely Washington State and Florida. Since the year 2000, the University of Michigan has been center stage on this issue and in the most important affirmative action decision since the 1978 Bakke Case, the Supreme Court (5–4) upheld the University's Law School's policy, ruling that race can be one of the many factors considered by colleges when selecting their students. The Supreme Court went only to rule (6–3) that a formulaic approach utilizing a point system at the undergraduate level had to be modified because it did not provide the "individualized consideration" of applicants deemed necessary in previous Supreme Court decisions on the matter.

Having equal access to good health is critical to having equal opportunity to success.

In terms of health care, evidence abounds that there have been inequities in hiring and firing practices but also in the delivery of health outcomes typically referred to as health disparities. Over 50 years ago, Dr. Martin Luther King, Jr. said, "Of all the forms of inequality, injustice in healthcare is the most shocking and inhumane."

The health care system was not invulnerable to the same forces found outside its walls. Their far-reaching effects are at the roots of many of the factors previously mentioned. With the publication of the Institute of Medicine report *Unequal Treatment* in 2003, health disparities finally was brought from the dark into the light and has become the topic and focus of many research studies, discussions, and target actions. Their landmark report, *Unequal Treatment: Confronting Racial and*

Ethnic Disparities in Health Care, cited a host of contributing factors housed both within the knowledge, skills, and attitudes of individual health care providers, and within the structure and processes of the health-care system.

New challenges to affirmative action have continued to exponentially surface as of late. Some consider the election of President Barack Obama a positive proof that we now live in a race-neutral society making such a legislative action unnecessary. Many hear in the background of any affirmative action discussion, a directive for legalizing entitlement and elevating the unqualified person of color at the expense of those who are hard working and qualified. Those in leadership positions can mitigate such concerns by deploying intentional efforts to teach and expand the operational definition of diversity that includes but moves beyond race and ethnicity. In their respective work environments, it would be worthwhile to make the case for how having diverse perspectives enhance decision making, market share, and cultural relevancy to those who are the recipients of services. In fact when the constellation of decision makers is diverse, considerations and consequences as a result of certain decision occur with more frequency. The assumption that treating everyone the same is treating everyone fairly requires vigilant examination and assault since it erroneously assumes that everyone has the same starting point in their pursuits to live the American dream. Good faith efforts to develop and execute race-, gender-, and sexuality-neutral policies would also be helpful.

Furthermore, it has been posited that increasing minority representation in the health provider workforce is the most effective place to start to rectify the situation. There is substantial evidence showing that minority populations respond and relate quite favorably to having minority providers in charge of their care. Having employment affords one to make a living, to pay for needed services, to obtain education, and to have access to health care. The major obstacles to achieving that goal lie in the domains of employment and education—right where affirmative action policies and concepts had its beginnings and yet the debate for whether such policies and actions are warranted continues. Leaders committed to positive change through diverse leadership have affirmative action laws in their tool kits to assist them. Affirmative action is a stop-gap measure to overcome disparities of power and the distribution of resources. When properly utilized, leaders are demonstrating their responsibility to be prudent stewards of the resources of the organization and the payoff is big—all boats rise.

Affirmative Action: Creating Economic Opportunity and Security For All Americans. Retrieved from U.S. Department of Labor Affirmative Action Fact Sheet (http://www.dol.gov/ofccp/regs/compliance/aa.htm)

Amirkhan, J., Betancourt, H., Graham, S., López, S. R., & Weiner, B. (2003). Reflections of affirmative action goals in psychology admissions. In S. Plous (Ed.), *Understanding Prejudice and Discrimination* (pp. 197–202). New York, NY: McGraw-Hill.

Smedley, B., Stith A., & Nelson A. (Eds.) (2002). *Unequal Treatment: Confronting Racial and Ethnic Disparities in Health Care.* Washington, DC: Committee on Understanding and Eliminating Racial and Ethnic Disparities in Health Care, Board on Health Sciences Policy, Institute of Medicine, National Academy Press.

Ten Myths about Affirmative Action. Retrieved from http://www.understandingprejudice.org/readroom/articles/affirm.htm

Timeline of Affirmative Action Milestones. Retrieved from http://www.DiversityInc BestPactices.com

G. Rumay Alexander

AGENCY FOR HEALTHCARE RESEARCH AND QUALITY (AHRQ)

Agency for Healthcare Research and Quality (AHRQ) is a division of the U.S. Department of Health and Human Services and is located in Rockville, MD. The AHRQ strives to improve all aspects of health care for Americans by supporting research and partnerships within health systems (AHRQ, 2009). AHRQ is classified as a U.S. Public Health Service Agency and was created in 1989. AHRQ has one primary goal: to actualize noted improvements in the nation's health care in relation to improved patient outcomes and overall quality of life (AHRQ, 2009). Therefore, specific competitive grants are made available by the agency to accomplish the priority goals of the organization. AHRQ provides notice regarding the highest priorities for each application year along with consistent updates of the research priorities throughout each year. Grants are made available in the following global categories: *clinical information*, such as evidence-based practice, outcomes and effectiveness, prevention, and technology; *specific populations*, such as women, children, minorities, elderly, disabled, and innercity; *public health preparedness* within the areas of bioterrorism and national and global environmental threats such as hurricanes; *health information technology*, which investigates electronic health records, clinical decision making, and industrial and systems engineering; and *quality and patient safety*, which focuses on areas such as medical errors, quality measurements and improvement, and communication with consumers (AHRQ, 2010). Additionally, the AHRQ Web site maintains a current listing of all recently completed research studies.

Dissemination of research findings is a critical component of this organization. The availability of grants, support for research, and sharing of findings establishes this organization as a leader in establishing communication and collaboration among researchers across disciplines and the nation.

Agency for Healthcare Research and Quality (AHRQ) At a Glance. AHRQ Publication No. 09-P003, May 2009. Agency for Healthcare Research and Quality, Rockville, MD. http://www.ahrq.gov/about/ataglance.htm

Agency for Healthcare Research and Quality. (2010). *FactSheets*. Retrieved September 6, 2010, from http://www.ahrq.gov/news/factix.htm

Ronda Mintz-Binder

AGING IN PLACE

Aging in place is an approach to provide supports and interventions that enable older adults to maintain as much independence and dignity for as long as possible in their preferred setting, typically the home environment. Solutions to support aging in place cross disciplinary boundaries encompassing nursing, medicine, physical therapy, occupational therapy, nutritional science, kinesiology, social work, and fields such as communication science, computer and information science, anthropology, informatics, engineering, architecture, environmental design, and public administration (Benefield, 2010).

Remaining in one's own home allows people to sustain connections to their communities and friends, retain health care providers who know their health history and maintain the security of familiar surroundings (Westchester, 2010). Characteristics of community environments that support aging in place include:

1. Affordable and accessible housing
2. Network of health care services
3. Easy access to affordable transportation
4. Safety assurance
5. Opportunities for recreational activities
6. Social, cultural, and educational enhancement

HOUSING: AFFORDABLE AND ACCESSIBLE

Enabling older persons to age successfully in their homes supports a community's ability to retain a strong tax base and preserve neighborhood stability. Creating affordable housing options and associated property tax relief programs is essential if older homeowners are to remain in their primary residence (Hartsfield, 2007). Older persons often require assistance in making their existing home more accessible, including changes in exits and entrances, stairs, and bathrooms. The National Association of Homebuilders' three-day Certified Aging-in-Place Specialist trains professionals to better work with older adults to remodel their homes (Homebuilders, 2010). Incorporating universal design, the creation of environments meant to be usable by all people without need for adaptation or specialization, is a current trend in housing design.

HEALTH CARE

Services providing health maintenance and chronic disease management, training in self-management of chronic disease, and episodic use of home health care may enhance the ability to remain in one's preferred setting. In-home health and diagnostic technologies can eliminate or reduce health-related travel to diagnostic or primary care clinical settings. Additionally, new technologies available via the Internet and novel wireless communication modes are used by increasing numbers of older adults to encourage behavioral changes that emphasize health rather than the treatment of disease. High- and low-tech in-home sensors and monitors make it easier for family caregivers to monitor distant family members and take action in case of an emergency (Bezatiti, 2009). A local support network of relatives, neighbors, and friends also supports older persons' aging in place.

TRANSPORTATION

The ability to continue driving or a desirable and accessible transportation system is requisite to successful aging in place. Expanding mobility options for older people include enhancements to fixed-route public transportation operations and planned route and stop placement; public transportation vehicles such as low-floor buses, kneeling buses, additional stanchions, and grab bars; and accessibility features including larger letters on head signs and stop announcements. Actions to encourage using existing services and expansion of services including flexible-route and community transportation services, Americans with Disabilities Act (ADA) and non-ADA demand-responsive services, taxi subsidy programs, and volunteer driver programs are required (Koffman, Weiner et al., 2010).

SAFETY ASSURANCE

Safety includes individual, in-residence, and community environment issues. Reducing the risk of falls and fires in the home is necessary if an older adult is to remain at home (Safety, 2010). Although often overlooked, a personal exercise regime is important to improve strength, balance, and mobility (Stafford, 2009) and requisite to engaging in walking activities within community. The surrounding community must provide for personal safety in the physical environment via walkability assessments and pedestrian-friendly neighborhood walkways, and public safety such as adult protective services programs, legal aid, disability rights programs, traffic safety programs, and community watch programs.

SOCIAL, CULTURAL, AND EDUCATIONAL ENHANCEMENT

Communities that support aging in place provide opportunities for lifelong learning and participation in cultural and recreational activities. Socialization in a form that suites the older person, whether intergenerational or among peers, enhances personal health and increases the community's quality of life and economic vitality (Hartsfield, 2007).

Establishing social networks has been successful in both city governmental and private sector initiatives.

Aging in place with a sense of control and dignity can be achieved within settings that incorporate these essential principles. Livable communities incorporate these principles and are characterized by safe environments with easy access to health care, recreation, and socialization. Universal design principles are used in housing and public spaces, networks of friends and others are available for support, incorporating high- and low-tech diagnostic and assistive devices for health and socialization. Model programs include Tiger Place, Beacon Hill, and Fairview Village (http://aginginplace.com/mini-2/other-models-of-aging-in-place/, accessed September 8, 2010).

Benefield, L. E. (2010). Reynolds Center of Geriatric Excellence. Retrieved September 21, 2010, from http://nursing.ouhsc.edu/Geriatric_Nursing

Bezatitis, A. (2009). New technologies for aging in place. *For the Record, 21*(1), 24.

Hartsfield, P. (2007). A blueprint for action: Developing a livable community for all ages. Retrieved August 24, 2010, from http://www.n4a.org/pdf/07-116-n4a-blueprint4action wcovers.pdf

Greenberg, B., & Schwarz, J. (2009). Aging in place…with a little help from our friends. *Grantmakers in Aging Conference.* May 2009. Retrieved September 21, 2010, from http://intergenerational.cas.psu.edu/Docs/AginginPlace.pdf

Homebuilders, N. A. O. (2010). Certified Aging-in-Place Specialist. Retrieved July 28, 2010, from http://www.nahb.org/generic.aspx?genericContentID=9334

Koffman, D., R. Weiner, Pfeiffer, A., & Chapman, S. (2010). *Funding the public transportation needs of an aging population.* San Francisco, CA: Nelson/Nygaard Consulting Associates.

Safety, S. (2010). Senior safety online—Living safely at home. Retrieved August 24, 2010, from http://www.seniorsafetyonline.com/home_safety.html

Westchester. (2010). Informing, enabling and facilitating aging in place in Westchester County. Retrieved July 20, 2010, from http://www.aipsupport.org/index.php?option=com_content&task=view&id=15&Itemid=35

Lazelle E. Benefield

AMERICAN ACADEMY OF NURSING

American Academy of Nursing (Academy), a subsidiary of the American Nurses Association (ANA), serves the public and the nursing profession by advancing health policy and practice through the generation, synthesis, and dissemination of nursing knowledge (http://www.aannet.org). Established in 1973 under the aegis of the ANA, membership is by invitation. Applicants must be sponsored by two Fellows in good standing with the Academy

A

and must be a current member of the ANA or an ANA constituent. Criteria for membership include evidence of outstanding contributions that have made an impact on nursing practice at the national level and evidence of potential to continue contributions to nursing and the Academy.

As of 2010, the Academy comprised approximately 1,500 Fellows of the American Academy of Nursing. Fellows are recognized nursing leaders in education, management, practice, and research. Fellows work with other leaders in health care on expert panels, the Institute of Medicine, American Nurses Foundation, AAN Scholar-in-Residence Program, and the facilitation of appointments to policy positions.

The Academy is constituted to anticipate national and international trends in health care, and address resulting issues of health care knowledge and policy. Not only is the invitation to Fellowship recognition of one's accomplishments within the nursing profession, but also affords an opportunity to work with other leaders in health care in addressing the issues of the day. Fellows come together annually to address crucial health issues and to identify research and policy initiatives to improve health care. The official journal of the Academy is *Nursing Outlook,* published bimonthly by Elsevier. *Nursing Outlook* provides innovative ideas for leaders in the nursing profession through peer-reviewed articles and timely reports.

In 2007, the Academy established the Raise the Voice campaign with the goal of transforming America's health care system through nursing solutions. Showcasing stories of innovative nurses, "Edge Runners," the Academy has raised the voice of nursing with Congress, the general public, and the nursing community.

See also American Nurses Association

American Academy of Nursing (AAN) http://www.aannet.org

Diane Mancino

AMERICAN ASSEMBLY FOR MEN IN NURSING

American Assembly for Men in Nursing (AAMN) provides a national forum for "nurses as a group to meet, discuss, and influence factors which affect men as nurses" (AAMN, 2010). AAMN had its origins in the National Male Nurses Association (NMNA), founded by Dennis Martin in 1971 with the intention of stimulating interest among men in a nursing career. Although initially quite successful as an organization, NMNA later faltered until being revitalized in 1980, largely through the leadership of Dr. Luther Christman. In 1981, it changed its name to AAMN and adopted objectives to encourage (1) men to become nurses and join with all nurses in humanizing health care, (2) nurses who are men to grow professionally and demonstrate the contributions made by men in nursing, and (3) members to participate fully in the nursing profession and its organizations. Later, an additional objective was added supporting men's health issues, and the organization has developed a position statement on a men's health curriculum in schools of nursing (AAMN, 2010). Although not stated, fighting discrimination is an implied goal, and the organization is truly nondiscriminatory, with membership "unrestricted by age, color, creed, handicap, sexual orientation, lifestyle, nationality, race, religion or gender" (Pittman, 2005, p. 156). Thus, there are women and men among the membership, and the current AAMN Board, chaired over the years by

Christman, has female and male members (AAMN, 2010). Overall, the association promotes the idea that every professional nursing position and educational opportunity should be equally available to anyone meeting entry requirements, regardless of gender (Bullough, 2006, p. 567). AAMN sponsors annual conferences consistent with its objectives, produces a quarterly newsletter (*Interaction*), encourages formation of local chapters, provides educational scholarships, and offers annual awards for organizations and individuals who are supportive of men in nursing. The AAMN Web site has a career center, a discussion forum, and links to resources for men in nursing and about men's health.

American Assembly for Men in Nursing (AAMN). (2010). *Welcome to the AAMN*. Retrieved from http://www. aamn.org

Bullough, V. (2006). Nursing at the crossroads: Men in nursing. In P. S. Cowan & S. Moorhead (Eds.), *Current issues in nursing* (7th ed., pp. 559–568). St. Louis, MO: Mosby.

Pittman, E. (2005). *Luther Christman: A maverick nurse—A nursing legend*. Victoria, BC: Tafford.

David N. Ekstrom

AMERICAN ASSOCIATION OF COLLEGES OF NURSING

Founded in 1969, the American Association of Colleges of Nursing (AACN) is the national voice for baccalaureate and higher degree programs in nursing. Over 600 nursing programs are represented by this organization in its efforts to establish quality standards for nursing baccalaureate and graduate education and influence public policy to improve funding and practices for nursing education, health care, and research. "AACN's educational, research, governmental advocacy, data collection, publications, and other programs work to establish quality standards for bachelor's- and graduate-degree nursing education, assist deans and directors to implement those standards, influence the nursing profession to improve health care, and promote public support of baccalaureate and graduate education, research, and practice in nursing—the nation's largest health care profession" (American Association of Colleges of Nursing, 2010a, 2010b). In 1986, a national panel was established by AACN to develop the *Essentials of Baccalaureate Education for Professional Nursing Practice*. Initially, this document was designed to guide nursing schools in developing standards for undergraduate programs; in 2005, the Commission on Collegiate Nursing Education voted to adopt the *Essentials* document as mandatory for its accreditation practices. In 1994, a task force was appointed to develop a companion document for master's education in advanced practice specialties, the *Essentials of Master's Education for Professional Nursing Practice*. In 2006, a task force was appointed to develop the *Essentials of Doctoral Education for Advanced Practice Nursing*. These were adopted in October 2006 by the AACN membership. Master's and doctor of nursing practice guidelines have also been adopted by the Commission on Collegiate Nursing Education as mandatory for accreditation. In March 2010, the AACN established the NursingCAS—the nation's only centralized service for students applying to nursing programs allowing students to apply to multiple nursing programs with a single application; this initiative also serves as an important mean for addressing the national shortage of nurses and faculty by helping to fill vacant seats in nursing school throughout the country. In addition, the AACN has developed position papers and white papers to address issues for nursing education and

A

practice: *Faculty Shortages in Baccalaureate and Graduate Nursing Programs, Differentiated Competencies for Nursing Practice, the Role of the Clinical Nurse Leader, the Clinical Practice Doctorate, Position Statement on Nursing Research, Hallmarks of the Professional Nursing Practice Environment,* and *Indicators of Quality in Research-Focused Doctoral Programs in Nursing* (http://www.aacn.nche.edu).

American Association of Colleges of Nursing. (2010a). Homepage. Retrieved September 19, 2010, from www.aacn.nche.edu

American Association of Colleges of Nursing. (2010b). Nursing's Centralized Application Service Expands to Accommodate Applicants to Both Graduate and Entry-Level Nursing Programs. Retrieved September 19, 2010, from http://www.aacn.nche.edu/Media/NewsReleases/2010/ExpanNursingcas.html

Paule V. Joseph
Harriet R. Feldman

AMERICAN ASSOCIATION OF NURSE ANESTHETISTS

The mission of the American Association of Nurse Anesthetists (AANA) is to advance patient safety and to practice excellence in its members' profession. AANA's vision is to be a preeminent professional association for health care and patient safety. The AANA is the sole professional association for the nation's more than 44,000 Certified Registered Nurse Anesthetists (CRNAs) and nurse anesthesia students who practice in all 50 states, the District of Columbia, Puerto Rico, and the Virgin Islands. Nurse anesthetists provide anesthesia services to all segments of the population including substantial numbers of Medicare, Medicaid, public employee, veteran, and indigent patients. More than 90% of all U.S. nurse anesthetists belong to the professional association. Founded in 1931, the AANA has routinely issued educational and practice standards and guidelines, promoted educational advancement, and played a key role in supporting nurse anesthesia credentialing since its inception. The AANA is actively involved in the development of federal and state healthcare policy and offers consultation and data sources regarding CRNA practice to both public and private entities.

Although nurse anesthetists have been providing anesthesia care to patients in the United States for nearly 150 years, the credential "CRNA" was established by the AANA in 1956. As graduate-level educated advanced practice registered nurses, CRNAs are anesthesia professionals who, working in collaboration with surgeons, physician anesthesiologists, and other qualified healthcare professionals, administer more than 32 million anesthetics to patients each year in the United States, according to the AANA 2009 Practice Profile Survey.

John C. Preston

AMERICAN ASSOCIATION OF UNIVERSITY PROFESSORS

"The mission of the American Association of University Professors (AAUP) is to advance academic freedom and shared governance, to define fundamental professional values and standards for higher education, and to ensure higher education's contribution to the common good. Founded in 1915, the AAUP has helped to shape American higher education by developing the standards and procedures that maintain quality in education and academic freedom in this country's colleges and universities" (AAUP, 2010a, 2010b, 2010c). Membership is represented by individual faculty, librarians, and other academic professionals at public and private universities across the country. The principles and practices of AAUP may be found in its *Statement of Principles on Academic Freedom and Tenure*. The AAUP largely concerns itself with issues of due process and academic freedom. The organization works with legislative leaders to influence higher education legislation. In 2006, the association launched the "Speak Up, Speak Out: Protect the Faculty Voice" on campus because of the unprecedented threats to academic freedom at public colleges and universities. The AAUP publishes statements on such topics as intellectual property, distance education, and the use of part-time and nontenure track faculty and an annual faculty salary report that includes detailed salary and benefit information. AAUP documents that appear to merit continue reference have been collected and compiled in a single set titled *AAUP Policy Documents and Reports* known as the *Redbook*, considered as a reliable source on sound academic practice; this document has been used by both administrators and faculty alike. A range of the policy statements from the *Redbook* is available in the association Web site.

American Association of University Professors. (2010a). *Mission and description.* Retrieved September 19, 2010, from http://www.aaup.org/AAUP/About/mission

American Association of University Professors. (2010b). *Policy documents and reports (the Redbook).* Retrieved September 21, 2010, from http://www.aaup.org/AAUP/pubsres/policydocs

American Association of University Professors. (2010c). *Speak up, speak out: Protect the faculty voice.* Retrieved September 19, 2010, from http://www.aaup.org/AAUP/protectvoice

Paule V. Joseph
Harriet R. Feldman

AMERICAN ASSOCIATION OF UNIVERSITY WOMEN

A

Founded in 1881, the mission of the American Association of University Women (AAUW) is to promote "equity for women and girls, through advocacy, education, philanthropy and research" (AAUW, 2010a, 2010b). Furthermore, the AAUW "contributes to a more promising future and provides a powerful voice for women and girls—a voice that cannot and will not be ignored" (AAUW, 2007b). AAUW sees itself as a "catalyst for change," and in this vein has promoted a number of successful initiatives, for example, *How Schools Shortchange Girls: The AAUW Report* (AAUW, 1992) and the implementation of the Sister-to-Sister summits for teens. AAUW provides educational and professional support, scholarships and awards, grants and fellowships, updates on research, conferences that include opportunities for activism, information on up-to-date issues affecting girls and women, a voice in government, and a community network of colleagues around the world. In 2005, AAUW adopted the theme Education as the Gateway to Women's Economic Security, which "represents a shared commitment [of the AAUW Educational Foundation Board and the Association Board]...to support and engage members and prospective members..." (AAUW, 2007a). AAUW members are also members of the International Federation of University Women, which was founded by the association in 1919, linking women around the world. The association's Web site contains information for members and nonmembers alike.

American Association of University Women. (1992). *How schools shortchange girls: The AAUW report: A study of major findings on*

A

girls and education. Washington, DC: AAUW Educational Foundation and National Education Association.

American Association of University Women. (2007a). *Education as the gateway to women's economic security*. Retrieved August 12, 2007, from http://www.aauw.org/newvision/index.cfm

American Association of University Women. (2007b). *The value of belonging to AAUW*. Retrieved June 14, 2007, from http://www.aauw.org/join/value/index.cfm

American Association of University Women. (2010a). *About us*. Retrieved September 19, 2010, from http://www.aauw.org/about/index.cfm

American Association of University Women. (2010b). *American Association of University Women: A historical summary*. Retrieved September 19, 2010. From http://clubs-orgs.colstate.edu/aauw/AAUWHistory.htm

Paule V. Joseph
Harriet R. Feldman

AMERICAN COLLEGE OF NURSE-MIDWIVES (ACNM)

With roots dating to 1929, the American College of Nurse-Midwives (ACNM) is the oldest women's health care organization in the United States. As the professional association that represents certified nurse-midwives (CNMs) and certified midwives (CMs) in the United States, ACNM provides research, establishes clinical practice standards, determines core competencies for basic midwifery education, promotes continuing education programs, and creates liaisons with state and federal agencies and members of Congress. ACNM accredits midwifery education programs through its autonomous Accreditation Commission for Midwifery Education and publishes the peer-reviewed bimonthly *Journal of Midwifery and Women's Health*.

ACNM's mission is to promote the health and well-being of women and infants within their families and communities through the development and support of the profession of midwifery as practiced by CNMs and CMs. Midwifery practice is the independent management of women's health care, including primary care of women and newborns with a particular focus on pregnancy, childbirth, postpartum period, family planning, and gynecologic needs of women. Midwives are federally recognized as primary health care providers, providing and referring for appropriate health care services, including prescribing, administering, and dispensing pharmacologic agents.

The organizational structure of ACNM includes an active board of directors and numerous member-led divisions, committees, taskforces, state affiliates, and other working groups. ACNM supports its members on regulatory and practice issues, assists consumers in locating midwifery practices, answers queries from the health care stakeholders, the media, and the public, and provides guidance to aspiring midwives.

The standards for graduate level education and national certification in midwifery are identical for CNMs and CMs, with CNMs entering midwifery education as registered nurses. Upon graduation from an Accreditation Commission for Midwifery Education–accredited midwifery education program, individuals are eligible to sit for the certification exam administered by the American Midwifery Certification Board, the national certifying body for CNMs and CMs.

Accreditation Commission for Midwifery Education. Retrieved from http://www.midwife.org/acme.cfm

American College of Nurse-Midwives Code of Ethics. Retrieved from http://www.midwife.

org/siteFiles/descriptive/code_of_ethics_2008.pdf

American College of Nurse-Midwives Core Competencies for Basic Midwifery Practice. Retrieved from http://www.midwife.org/siteFiles/descriptive/Core_Competencies_6_07_000.pdf

American College of Nurse-Midwives Standards for the Practice of Midwifery. Retrieved from http://www.midwife.org/siteFiles/descriptive/Standards_for_Practice_of_Midwifery_12_09_001.pdf

American College of Nurse-Midwives Philosophy Statement. Retrieved from http://www.midwife.org/philosophy.cfm

American College of Nurse-Midwives Mission Statement. Retrieved from http://www.midwife.org/mission.cfm

American Midwifery Certification Board. Retrieved from www.amcbmidwife.org

M. Christina Johnson

AMERICAN HOLISTIC NURSES ASSOCIATION

Founded in 1981 by Charlotte McGuire, the American Holistic Nurses Association (AHNA) is a nonprofit membership association for nurses and other holistic healthcare professionals. Holistic nursing is a mind–body–spirit–emotion approach to practice and is recognized by the American Nurses Association as a nursing specialty with a defined scope and standards of practice. AHNA "promotes the education of nurses, other healthcare professionals, and the public in the philosophy, concepts, practice, and research of holistic caring and healing" (AHNA.org).

AHNA supports policy relating to holistic nursing and integrative health care, educates the professionals and the public about holistic nursing and integrative health care, promotes research and

scholarship in the field of holistic nursing, and provides continuing education in concepts of holistic nursing. The AHNA is affiliated with the American Holistic Nurses Certification Corporation. The American Holistic Nurses Certification Corporation offers certification examinations to become Holistic Nurse-Board Certified (HN-BC), Holistic Baccalaureate Nurse-Board Certified (HNB-BC), or Advanced Holistic Nurse-Board Certified (AHN-BC) (AHNA.org; Dossey, Keegan, & Guzzetta, 2009). AHNA has member chapters called networks in more than 40 of the United States and publishes the quarterly journal *Beginnings*.

Dossey, B., Keegan, L., & Guzzetta, C. (2009). *Holistic nursing: A handbook for practice.* Gaithersburg, MD: Aspen Publishers.

Martha J. Greenberg

AMERICAN MIDWIFERY CERTIFICATION BOARD

The American Midwifery Certification Board (AMCB), formerly the ACNM Certification Council, Inc. (ACC), is the national certifying body for Certified Nurse-Midwives (CNMs) and Certified Midwives (CMs). The certification function is a critical aspect of professional quality assurance in midwifery. Nurse-midwives have been certified by examination since 1971. At that time, certification rested within the American College of Nurse-Midwives (ACNM), first within the Division of Examiners and then within the Division of Competency Assessment. In 1991, in keeping with the professional standard that certification should be separated from the professional organization, the

ACC was incorporated as a distinct organization charged with functions related to the midwifery certificate. These functions include initial certification, recertification (certificate maintenance), and discipline. In 1998, in addition to the CNM certificate, the ACC began to offer certification to professionally educated midwives who were not first educated as nurses. The CM certificate is offered to candidates from ACNM-accredited programs in midwifery. In 2005, the organization's name was changed to AMCB but the mission and goals of the organization have remained the same (http://www.amcbmidwife.org/c/104/about-us).

AMCB's vision statement: AMCB is committed to using progressive, comprehensive educational and professional criteria to certify midwives. The National Commission for Certifying Agencies (NCCA) granted accreditation to the CNM® and the CM® certification programs administered by the AMCB for demonstrating compliance with the *NCCA Standards for the Accreditation of Certification Programs*. NCCA is the accrediting body of the National Organization for Competency Assurance. The NCCA Standards were created in 1977 and revised in 2003 to ensure certification programs adhere to modern standards of practice in the certification industry.

The AMCB consists of officers (president, secretary, and treasurer), board of directors, and committees responsible for the creation of the national certification examination, certificate maintenance, and research and credentialing/reporting.

Additional information is available at the AMCB Web site http://www.amcbmidwife.org

Carrie Bright

AMERICAN NURSES ASSOCIATION

Established in 1896 as the Nurses' Associated Alumni of the United States and Canada, the American Nurses Association (ANA) is today considered to be the voice of registered nurses in the United States. In 1899, the name was changed to Nurses Associated Alumnae of the United States; in 1911, the name was changed to its current name, American Nurses Association (ANA, 2010a). Today, the ANA represents 50 Constituent Member Associations, as well as specialty nursing organizational affiliates, labor affiliates, workforce advocacy affiliates, individual members, and individual affiliates. The ANA serves as the parent corporation for the American Nurses Credentialing Center, the American Nurses Foundation, the American Nurses Association–Political Action Committee, and the American Academy of Nursing. The ANA's purposes include the following: working for the improvement of health standards and the availability of health care services for all people, fostering high standards of nursing, and stimulating and promoting the professional development of nurses and the advancement of their economic and general welfare (ANA, 2010b).

As the only national full-service professional organization representing the nation's 3.1 million registered nurses, ANA engages constituents, affiliates, and members in a variety of programs and activites that address nursing issues from the national perspective. The following examples reflect ANA's commitment to nurse and patient advocacy:

1. Congress on Nursing Practice and Economics: This organized, deliberative body brings together the diverse

experiences and perspectives of ANA members. The Congress focuses on establishing nursing's approach to emerging trends within the socioeconomic, political, and practice spheres of the health care industry by identifying issues and recommending policy alternatives to the ANA Board of Directors (ANA, 2010c).

2. Improving Work Environment: ANA, with its partners and through its organizational relationships, is a leader in promoting improved work environments and the value of nurses as professionals, essential providers, and decision makers in all practice settings. ANA protects, defends, and educates nurses about their rights as employees under the law by addressing the growing number of occupational hazards that threaten nurses, such as needle stick injuries, latex sensitivity, back injuries, and violence (ANA, 2010d).

3. Patient Safety and Nursing Quality: For more than 100 years, ANA has been working to improve patient safety by promoting nursing quality. The National Center for Nursing Quality® has been created by ANA to address patient safety and quality in nursing care and nurses' work lives. The center advocates for nursing quality through quality measurement, novel research, and collaborative learning. Issues such as the nursing workforce and the effect on patient outcomes are tackled through innovative initiatives, which include the National Database for Nursing Quality Indicators® and Safe Staffing Saves Lives, among others (ANA, 2010e).

4. Code of Ethics for Nurses: The Code of Ethics for Nurses was developed as a guide for carrying out nursing responsibilities in a manner consistent with quality in nursing care and the ethical obligations of the profession (ANA, 2010f). In addition, Nursing's Social Policy Statement: The Essence of the Profession, revised in 2010, demonstrates nursing's deep societal commitments of the profession (ANA, 2010g).

5. Federal Government Affairs: ANA monitors legislative and regulatory issues for nurses and others to understand health care reform and related proposals and takes appropriate action to advocate for the nursing profession and health care consumers. ANA advocates for health care reforms that would guarantee access to high-quality health care for all. With the passage of the Health Care and Education Affordability Act, millions of people have greater protection against losing or being denied health insurance coverage and better access to primary and preventive services (ANA, 2010h).

6. Occupational and Environmental Health: ANA's Center for Occupational and Environmental Health provides occupational and environmental health expertise on issues related to the nursing profession and health care industry. The mission of the center is to protect the health and well-being of nurses and their patients and communities through policy advocacy, programs, and training on the prevention and control of occupational and environmental hazards in relation to health care settings (ANA, 2010i).

The ANA offers several publications, including *The American Nurse, American Nurse Today, The Online Journal of Issues in Nursing,* and so forth, addressing standards and principles of various areas of nursing practice. For more than a century, ANA's leadership has advanced the profession of nursing and worked to protect the rights and responsibilities of registered nurses. Through its many programs and services, ANA continues to make progress to strengthen the position of registered nurses and to advocate for patients.

See also American Nurses Foundation; American Academy of Nursing; American

A

Nurses Credentialing Center; Political Action Committees

American Nurses Association. (2010a). *Who we are.* Retrieved December 11, 2010, from http://www.nursingworld.org/FunctionalMenuCategories/AboutANA/WhoWeAre/History/ExpandedHistorical Review.aspx

American Nurses Association. (2010b). *ANA bylaws* (Section 2, p. 3). Retrieved December 11, 2010, from http://www.nursingworld.org/MemberCenterCategories/ANAGovernance/HOD/ANABylaws.aspx

American Nurses Association. (2010c). *Congress on nursing practice.* Retrieved December 11, 2010, from http://nursingworld.org/MainMenuCategories/ThePracticeofProfessionalNursing/NewCNPE.aspx

American Nurses Association. (2010d). *Improving work environment.* Retrieved December 11, 2010, from http://www.nursingworld.org/ndnqi2

American Nurses Association. (2010e). *Patient safety and nursing quality.* Retrieved December 11, 2010, from http://www.nursingworld.org/MainMenuCategories/ThePracticeofProfessionalNursing/PatientSafetyQuality.aspx

American Nurses Association. (2010f). *Code of ethics for nursing.* Retrieved December 11, 2010, from http://www.nursingworld.org/MainMenuCategories/EthicsStandards/CodeofEthicsforNurses.aspx

American Nurses Association. (2010g). *Nursing's social policy statement: The essence of the profession.* Retrieved December 11, 2010, from http://www.nursesbooks.org/MainMenu/Foundation/Nursings-Social-Policy-Statement.aspx

American Nurses Association. (2010h). *Federal government affairs.* Retrieved December 11, 2010, from http://nursingworld.org/MainMenuCategories/HealthcareandPolicyIssues/HealthSystemReform.aspx

American Nurses Association. (2010i). *Occupational and environmental health program.* Retrieved December 11, 2010, from http://nursingworld.org/MainMenuCategories/OccupationalandEnvironmental.aspx

Diane Mancino

AMERICAN NURSES ASSOCIATION HALL OF FAME

In 1976, the American Nurses Association (ANA) established their Hall of Fame, coinciding with the year of the bicentennial of the United States. Fifteen charter members were selected to represent the leadership of nursing, nominated because they "affected the health and/or social history of the United States through sustained, lifelong contributions in or to nursing practice, education, administration, research, economics, or literature" (ANA, 2010). The ANA Hall of Fame serves as an enduring tribute to these dedicated and accomplished nurses. Initially, one criterion for selection was that individuals be deceased; however, following the 1996 induction, it was decided that members could be deceased or living. New members are added at each of the ANA biennial conventions.

American Nurses Association. (2010). *Hall of fame.* Retrieved September 19, 2010, from http://nursingworld.org/FunctionalMenuCategories/AboutANA/WhereWeComeFrom_1/HallofFame.aspx

Paule V. Joseph
Harriet R. Feldman

AMERICAN NURSES CREDENTIALING CENTER

The mission of the American Nurses Credentialing Center (ANCC) is to promote excellence in nursing and health care globally through credentialing programs and related services. The American Nurses Association (ANA) established the ANA Certification Program in 1973 to provide tangible recognition of professional achievement in a defined functional or clinical area of nursing. The ANCC became its own corporation, a subsidiary of the ANA, in 1991. More than 250,000 nurses including 80,000 advanced practices nurses carry ANCC certification. The ANCC certifies health care providers; accredits educational providers, approvers, and programs; recognizes excellence in nursing and health care services; educates the public; collaborates with organizations to advance the understanding of credentialing services; and supports credentialing through research, education, and consultative services.

As offered by the ANCC, the Magnet Recognition Program® is an important and growing effort. It was developed by the ANCC to recognize health care organizations that are successful in recruiting and retaining registered nurses because they provide the very best in nursing care and uphold the tradition, within nursing, of professional nursing practice. The Magnet Recognition Program® also provides a vehicle for disseminating successful practices and strategies among nursing systems. It is based on quality indicators and standards of nursing practice as defined in the ANA's (2009) *Nursing Administration: Scope and Standards of Practice* and qualitative factors in nursing derived from the original Magnet Hospital study (McClure, Poulin, Sovie, & Wandelt, 1983). As a natural outcome of the program, Magnet Recognition elevates the reputation and standards of the nursing profession.

In an effort to recognize health care organizations that create work environments where nurses flourish, the ANCC established the Pathway to Excellence® program. This program, acquired in 2007, is based on the Texas Nurses Association Nurse-Friendly™ program. Organizations earn the designation when they integrate specific Pathway to Excellence standards into operating policies, procedures, and management practices. The Magnet Recognition Program focuses on excellence in nursing and patient care, whereas ANCC's Pathway to Excellence program emphasizes the "fundamental elements of an ideal nursing practice environment."

See also Magnet Hospitals

American Nurses Association. (2009). *Nursing administration: Scope and standards of practice.* Washington, DC: Author.

McClure, M. L., Poulin, M. A., Sovie, M. D., & Wandelt, M. (1983). *Magnet hospitals: Attraction and retention of professional nurses.* Washington, DC: American Nurses Association.

Diane Mancino

AMERICAN NURSES FOUNDATION

Founded in 1955, the American Nurses Foundation (ANF) is the charitable and philanthropic arm of the American Nurses Association (ANA) supporting its mission to promote the welfare and the well-being of nurses and to advance the nursing profession, thereby enhancing the health of the public. ANF raises funds and develops and manages grants to support nursing research, education, and clinical practice.

The nursing research grant program provides funding for beginning and experienced nurse researchers in clinical and academic settings. Since 1955, more than $4 million in grant awards have supported the work of 1,000 nurse researchers. Through its programs and initiatives, ANF advances the work of the profession and improves health care environments and patient care.

A

The research of ANF scholars impacts health outcomes, improves the delivery of nursing services, and enhances the quality of work life for nurses. The ANF also manages grants and contracts funded externally. Funding contributed by private foundations and grants from several government agencies and Nursing Research Grant Partners (including the American Nurses Credentialing Center, the Association of Nurses in AIDS Care, the Association of periOperative Registered Nurses, the Sigma Theta Tau International, etc.) provides funds for ANF's programs and research grants. These funded projects address such concerns as nurse staffing, workplace health and safety, continuing competency, patient safety, and health policy. In 2009, ANF established a Nurses Disaster Fund to assist nurses who are victims of disasters.

One example of an important ANF program is the Nurse Competence in Aging initiative funded by the Atlantic Philanthropies (USA) Inc. Awarded to ANA through ANF, this initiative represents a strategic alliance between the ANA, the American Nurses Credentialing Center, the John A. Hartford Foundation Institute for Geriatric Nursing, and the New York University College of Nursing. Designed to maximize and sustain geriatric competency within national specialty nursing associations, the Nurse Competence in Aging seeks to improve nursing care for older adults. The anticipated outcome of this initiative is to enhance the geriatric competence, knowledge, skills, and attitudes of thousands of national specialty nursing organization members, thereby improving the care of our elderly citizens.

See also American Nurses Association

Diane Mancino

AMERICAN ORGANIZATION OF NURSE EXECUTIVES

Founded in 1967, the American Organization of Nurse Executives[1] (AONE), a subsidiary of the American Hospital Association, is a national organization of more than 7,000 nurses who design, facilitate, and manage care. Its mission is to represent nurse leaders who strive to improve health care. AONE members are leaders in collaboration and catalysts for innovation. The AONE's vision is to shape the future of health care through innovative nursing leadership. The organization provides leadership, professional development, advocacy, and research to advance nursing practice and patient care, to promote nursing leadership excellence, and to shape health care public policy.

The AONE serves its members by (1) providing vision and actions for nursing leadership to meet the health care needs of society; (2) influencing legislation and public policy related to nursing and patient care issues; (3) offering member services that support and enhance the management, leadership, educational, and professional development of nursing leaders; and (4) facilitating and supporting research and development efforts that advance nursing administration practice and quality patient care. A grassroots network of 49 state chapters connected through a listserv keeps AONE informed of the current legislative, regulatory, and practice issues.

For staff nurses who aspire to a career in nursing leadership, nurse managers in a first management position, directors

---

[1] The original name for the group was the American Society of Nursing Service Administrators; the current name was adopted in 1985.

who manage one or many departments, the chief nursing officers of large health care systems, or a nurse consultant or educator, AONE offers the tools, insights, and solutions to help these professionals achieve even more success in their career. AONE offers several publications including a bimonthly journal, *Nurse Leader,* and a member newsletter, *Voice of Nursing Leadership.* Timely information on critical topics is available through the weekly *AONE eNews Update.* An Annual Meeting and Exposition brings AONE members together for continuing education, networking, and leadership development.

Diane Mancino

AMERICANS WITH DISABILITIES ACT

The Americans with Disabilities Act (ADA), which was signed into law in 1990, details the legal rights of disabled U.S. citizens. A significant amendment was signed into law in 2008 with enforcement as of January 2009. The ADA Amendments Act of 2008 has expanded and clarified two parts of the original Act: (a) by giving a broader definition to the term disability and (b) by making it easier for a person to proceed with recognition of a disability (U.S. Equal Employment Opportunity Commission, 2010a).

The ADA is comprised of five titles and is located in volume 42 of the U.S. Code, beginning at section 12101. Although the ADA does not list all impairments that are included in the law, a person with a disability is defined as having a physical or mental impairment that significantly restricts one or more primary life activities,

along with a person who has a history of this impairment or who is seen by others as having an impairment (U.S. Department of Justice, 2005). Title I covers employment, requiring employers with 15 or more workers to offer equal opportunities to disabled qualified potential employees. Therefore, this forbids discrimination in any aspect of the work environment, from initial recruitment and interviewing to promotion, pay, social events, and other benefits of employment (U.S. Department of Justice, 2005). This title also disallows any potential prehire question about a disability before offer of a position occurs. Title I complaints need to be filed with the U.S. Equal Employment Opportunity Commission inside of 180 days of the date of the potential infringement (www.eeoc.gov).

Title II covers two sections: state and local government activities and public transportation. Title II mandates that both state and local governmental agencies provide opportunity for equal access to any or all events, services, and offerings that range from educational to sports to voting options to town meetings (U.S. Department of Justice, 2005). In addition, governments are required to comply with upgraded building codes and standards that take people with disabilities into consideration. Complaints or concerns can be forwarded to the Department of Justice within 180 days of the potential date of concern. The transportation mandates from Title II cover city uses and all public trains and subways. The authorities must assure that public transportation is available and accessible to those with disabilities, especially with new purchases and renovations (U.S. Department of Justice, 2005). Concerns regarding public transportation may be sent to the Office of Civil Rights within the Federal Transit Administration.

Title III addresses the spectrum of public accommodations that covers diverse

A

businesses and nonprofit offerings that cover restaurants, theaters, medical offices, shelters, recreation options, hotels, private education, and so on (U.S. Department of Justice, 2005). Public accommodations must comply with the same nondiscrimination expectations along with adhering to new building codes and regulations. Concerns regarding public accommodations may be sent to the Office of Civil Rights Division within the U.S. Department of Justice (www.ada.gov).

Title IV states regulations regarding telecommunication including telephone and television access for those with hearing and speech disabilities. This Title requires telephone companies to offer telecommunication relay services 24 hours a day, 7 days a week. The relay services offer specialized services for the deaf, which include devices and teletypewriters (U.S. Department of Justice, 2005). For additional information, the Federal Communications Commission would be the contact source (www.fcc.gov/cgb/dro). Title V is a miscellaneous section that contains additional provisions specific to the explanation and enforcement of Title I through the U.S. Equal Employment Opportunity Commission. These additional clarifications address threatening and/or retaliation against people with disabilities as well as technical assistance and other clarifications related to the determinations of disabilities (Equal Employment Opportunity Commission, 2010b).

U.S. Department of Justice. (2005). *A guide to disability rights laws.* Retrieved September 20, 2010, from http://www.ada.gov/cguide.pdf

U.S. Department of Labor, Civil Rights Center. Retrieved from http://www.dol.gov/oasam/programs/crc

U.S. Equal Employment Opportunity Commission. (2010a). *The Americans With Disabilities Act Amendments Act of 2008.* Retrieved September 20, 2010, from http://www.eeoc.gov/laws/statutes/adaaa_info.cfm

U.S. Equal Employment Opportunity Commission. (2010b). *Titles I and V of the Americans With Disabilities Act of 1990 (ADA).* Retrieved September 20, 2010, from http://www.eeoc.gov/laws/statutes/ada.cfm

Ronda Mintz-Binder

APRN Consensus Model and LACE

As nurses, the larger health care community, policy makers, and others work to reform the nation's health care system, there is increased appreciation for the important role that advanced practice registered nurses (APRNs) play in improving access to high-quality, cost-effective care. The lack of common definitions regarding APRN roles, increasing numbers of APRN specializations, differing credentials and scopes of practice across states, and a lack of uniformity in education and state regulations has limited the ability of patients to access APRN care in many areas. The APRN Consensus Model (to be called the Consensus Model) seeks to address these issues.

Initiated by the American Association of Colleges of Nursing and the National Organization of Nurse Practitioner Faculties, the dialogue to reach consensus around these issues spanned 4 years. The Consensus Model is the result of collaborative work of the APRN Consensus Work Group (23 education, accreditation, certification, practice, and licensing organizations) and the National Council of State Boards of Nursing APRN Advisory Committee with extensive input from a larger APRN stakeholder community. To date, 48 nursing organizations have endorsed the Consensus Model and are working to advocate for full implementation of the model within their constituent groups and stakeholders.

The Consensus Model establishes a common understanding about how all APRNs are regulated. Regulation includes essential elements such as licensure, accreditation, certification, and education (LACE). The Consensus Model provides a detailed definition of an APRN and each of the four APRN roles: certified registered nurse anesthetist, certified nurse–midwife, clinical nurse specialist, and certified nurse practitioner. There was consensus that only individuals educated, certified, and licensed in one of these four roles and one of six population foci may use the legal title APRN. In addition, expectations for all APRN education programs, accrediting, certifying, and licensing bodies are delineated in the model.

The target date for full implementation of the Consensus Model is 2015. Implementation will occur sequentially, but education programs, certifying, accrediting, and licensing bodies have been working together since the final adoption of the Consensus Model in 2008 to meet this target date. Since policies will be implemented and changes made throughout this transition period by the various organizations and boards responsible for APRN regulation, nurse leaders are encouraged to remain informed regarding the ongoing implementation of the Consensus Model.

For more detailed description of the APRN roles, population foci, and requirements for education, accreditation, certification, and licensing bodies, as well as a list of the endorsing organizations, see the full document available at http://www.aacn.nche.edu/apn.htm. A set of FAQs and other information can be accessed at http://www.aacn.nche.edu/pdf/APRNReport.pdf.

LACE

LACE is an electronic communication network which includes organizations that represent the LACE components of APRN regulation. The LACE electronic network creates a venue to facilitate transparent communication regarding APRN regulatory issues and implementation strategies and activities. LACE also includes a public site which allows broad dissemination of information regarding the Consensus Model and its implementation.

To access the LACE Web page, go to http://www.APRNLACE.org.

Spector, N., & Echternacht, M. (2010). A regulatory model for transitioning newly licensed nurses to practice. *Journal of Nursing Regulation, 1*(2), 18–25.

Stanley, J. (2009). Reaching consensus on a regulatory model: What does this mean for APRNs? *The Journal for Nurse Practitioners, 5*(2), 99–104.

Stanley, J. M., Werner, K. E., & Apple, K. (2009). Positioning advanced practice registered nurses for health care reform: Consensus on APRN regulation. *Journal of Professional Nursing, 25*(6), 340–348.

Joan M. Stanley

ASSESSMENT OF LEADERSHIP STYLES AND SKILLS

Alvin Toffler said, "The illiterate of the 21st century will not be those who cannot read and write, but those who cannot learn, unlearn, and relearn" (The Quotations Page, 2007). The essential abilities of effective leaders may not be measurable by any particular instrument but more by how the person does in the setting or context of the work environment. That being said, there are a variety of personality assessment tools used by employers and others to assess the strength of leaders.

Some of these tools are as follows: the Multifactor Leadership Questionnaire,

A

which measures a broad range of leadership types, developed by Bass in 1985, and revised in 1990. The Multifactor Leadership Questionnaire is considered the primary quantitative instrument to measure the transformational leadership construct. The concept measures four factors demonstrated by leaders: idealized influence, inspirational motivation, intellectual stimulation, and individualized consideration (Bass & Avolio, 1990). The Myers–Briggs Type Indicator is a commonly used personality test that is a psychometric questionnaire designed to measure psychological preferences in how people perceive the world and make decisions. The Sixteen Personality Factor Questionnaire, which measures key personality characteristics, such as extraversion, anxiety, tough mindedness, independence, and self-control, is another frequently used instrument.

Another form of intelligence considered crucial for effective leadership—emotional intelligence—is measured by the Emotional Intelligence Questionnaire. Emotional intelligence is the ability to manage feelings so that they are expressed appropriately and effectively, enabling people to work together smoothly toward their common goals.

Strengths that are needed by leaders include a capacity to inspire a shared vision, to enable others to act, to challenge the status quo, and to motivate others within an ethical context. Outcomes desired from nurse leaders are improvements in quality of care, compliance with standards, efficient and effective operations, and individual growth and cultural enhancements. Effective leadership is measured by how well the leader manages real-world challenges on a day-to-day basis. The successful leader needs technical skills and emotional competence and the ability to manage one's own emotions

and those of others. The literature consistently emphasizes the "need for technical and cognitive competence while having highly developed emotional and relational skills" (Scott, 2005, p. 24). Some of the day-to-day requirements for successful leadership are to be a visionary, a protector, an evaluator, a negotiator, an evaluator, a selector, a problem solver, and a healer, all of this while managing budgets, conducting strategic and fiscal planning, ensuring high quality of care and compliance with regulatory standards, and contributing to organizational growth. Increasingly, nurse leaders have broader and larger spans of control, which may include non-nursing areas (Arnold et al., 2006). The capable leader provides an environment for people to experience caring, healing, and learning. This leader treats others with dignity, respect, honesty, and fairness. The leader also recognizes the value of individual differences and the collaboration of people with different strengths and expertise (Malloch & Porter-O'Grady, 2009).

Leaders who evidence self-knowledge, strategic vision, risk taking, creativity, interpersonal and communication effectiveness, inspiration, and the ability to lead change ought to be successful transformational leaders (Morjikian & Bellack, 2005).

Arnold, L., Drenkard, K., Ela, S., Goedken, J., Hamilton, C., Harris, C., et al. (2006). Strategic positioning for nursing excellence in health systems: Insights from chief nursing executives. *Nursing Administration Quarterly, 30*(1), 11–20. Retrieved July 11, 2006, from http://infotrac.galegroup.com/itw/informark

Bass, B., & Avolio, B. (1990). *Multifactor Leadership Questionnaire: The benchmark measure of transformational leadership*. Retrieved August 3, 2007, from http://www.mindgarden.com/products/mlq.htm

Goleman, D. (1998). *Working with emotional intelligence*. New York: Bantam Books.

Malloch, K., & Porter-O'Grady, T. (2009). *The quantum leader: Applications for the new world of work*. Sudbury, MA: Bartlett and Jones.

Morjikian, R., & Bellack, J. (2005). The RWJ executive nurse fellows program: Part I. Leading change. *Journal of Nursing Administration, 35*(10), 431–438.

Scott, K. A. (2005, August). The new nurse executive: Thriving in the first 6 months. *Nurse Leader, 3*(4), 24–27.

The Quotations Page. (2007). *Alvin Toffler.* Retrieved August 13, 2007, from http://www. quotationspage.com/quotes/Alvin_Toffler

Marilyn Jaffe-Ruiz

ASSOCIATE DEGREE NURSING EDUCATION

Associate Degree Nursing (ADN) education began in 1952 on the basis of the results of a research project initiated by Dr. Mildred Montag (National Organization for Associate Degree Nursing [N-OADN], 2006; www.noadn.org). The focus of this study was to determine whether placing a program within the community colleges to prepare technical nurses was feasible or not (Haase, 1990). The results substantiated this approach, and ADN nursing programs are now more than 940, with more than 600 within community colleges across the United States (N-OADN, 2006). Associate degree registered nursing programs were designed to average four semesters of theory and clinical content across medical-surgical, maternity, pediatrics, and psychiatric/mental health nursing. Other program content includes pharmacology, communication, nursing process, and leadership. The units, content, theoretical framework, philosophy, and student learning outcomes are state board of nursing approved; programs also are professionally accredited on a voluntary basis by the National League of Nursing Accrediting Commission. As indicated in the position statement of the N-OADN (2006), associate degree education is focused on evidence-based practice while instilling critical thinking, clinical practice competency, and technical expertise. Students completing an ADN program are eligible to take the National Council Licensure Examination for Registered Nurses (NCLEX-RN). In 2008, 45.4% of RNs entering the workforce did so with associate degrees compared with 33.7% with baccalaureate degrees (bachelor of science in nursing [BSN]), 20.4% with diplomas, and 0.4% with graduate degrees (Health Resources and Services Administration, 2010). Registered nurses in practice nationally include an even split with half practicing now at the ADN or diploma level compared with half with BSN degrees or higher (Health Resources and Services Administration, 2010). Within the BSN practicing group, 32% were initially ADN or Diploma graduates. Leadership at the ADN level is primarily spearheaded by organizations such as N-OADN and the National League for Nursing (http:// www.nln.org). N-OADN is the national leader and advocate for ADN. The National League for Nursing represents all accredited academic programs of nursing with many members and board of governor members from associate degree programs. The American Association of Community Colleges also has been a strong proponent for ADN education (www.aacc.nche.edu/ Pages?default.aspx).

Issues regarding ADN education are generally the same across the United States; however, the timing of such issues coming forward often is legislatively driven. The primary issue confronting associate degree education has been the debate over what academic degree should be the basis for entry into nursing practice. ADN proponents believe that this degree is the minimum for entry and should remain as such. Proponents for baccalaureate education as

A

the minimum degree for entry into practice believe that a 4-year education enriched with research, community health, and stronger theoretical knowledge base is essential for entry into practice. Examples of this debate include several attempts in various states and nationally to change entry into practice to the BSN level, starting in 1965 (Smith, 2010). Furthermore, in 2006, legislation was introduced in New York State and later in New Jersey to mandate that associate degree educated nurses graduating after a specific date would be required to obtain the BSN within 10 years after graduation. As of 2011, this legislation has not been passed.

Many issues have faced the leaders of associate degree education, such as unfilled faculty vacancies, titling for administrative heads of ADN programs, faculty retention, and fiscal constraints in college education. For example, in the early to mid-2000s, ADN leaders were faced with limited nursing faculty, overwhelming numbers of applying students, and budgetary constraints (Milone-Nuzzo & Lancaster, 2004), accompanied by an aging faculty and administrative workforce and few anticipated future replacements (Health Resources and Services Administration, 2010). ADN leaders attempted to counter these issues through stronger mentorship programs for new faculty as well as operating programs with smaller budgets and seeking outside funding to provide resources to accommodate increases in the number of students. These pressures and stresses continue today, as community colleges are funded by each individual state and receive yearly budgets on the basis of each state's fiscal priorities. With many states affected by the economic downturn over the last few years, the majority of community colleges in fiscally affected states have received budget cuts and, as such, nursing programs expected to expand have received smaller base budgets. Balancing more students,

fewer faculty and support staff, and competition from other expanding neighboring programs for clinical placements, ADN program directors are facing unprecedented workload demands. A study of program directors reported that 25% of those surveyed in California were in interim status (Mintz-Binder & Fitzpatrick, 2009). In this same study, respondents reported average job satisfaction at the time the study, which was conducted in 2006. Since that time, there have been heightened fiscal constraints across the United States accompanied by a lack of strong leadership for succession planning and training and anticipated leadership turnover in the years to come.

See also Entry into Practice; Licensure

Haase, P. T. (1990). *The origins and rise of associate degree nursing education*. Durham, NC: Duke University Press.

Health Resources and Services Administration. (2010). *The registered nurse population: Initial findings from the 2008 National Sample Survey of Registered Nurse*. Retrieved September 7, 2010, from http://bhpr.hrsa.gov/healthworkforce/rnsurvey/initalfindings2008.pdf

Milone-Nuzzo, P., & Lancaster, J. (2004). Looking through the right end of the telescope: Creating a focused vision for a school of nursing. *Journal of Nursing Education, 43*(11), 506–511.

Mintz-Binder, R.D., & Fitzpatrick, J. J. (2009). Exploring social support and job satisfaction among associate degree program directors in California. *Nursing Education Perspectives, 30*(5), 299–304.

National Organization for Associate Degree Nursing. (2006). *Position statement of associate degree nursing*. Retrieved September 7, 2010, from http://www. noadn.org/component//option,com_docman?Itemid,250/task,doc_view/gid,16

Smith, T.G. (2010). A policy perspective on the entry into practice issue. *Online Journal of Issues in Nursing,15*(1). doi:10.3912/OJIN.Vol15No01PPT01

Ronda Mintz-Binder
Joyce J. Fitzpatrick

ASSOCIATION OF periOPERATIVE REGISTERED NURSES

AORN, Inc., the Association of periOperative Registered Nurses, representing the interests of more than 160,000 perioperative nurses, provides nursing education, standards, and services that enable optimal outcomes for patients undergoing operative and other invasive procedures. AORN's 40,000 registered nurse members facilitate the management, teaching, and practice of perioperative nursing, are enrolled in nursing education, or are engaged in perioperative research. Its members also include perioperative nurses who work in related business and industry sectors.

In its mission to promote safety and optimal outcomes for patients undergoing operative and other invasive procedures, AORN provides practice support and professional development opportunities, including educational resources that enable the safe surgical practices of perioperative nurses working in the inpatient and ambulatory settings. At the core of its educational offerings for patient and workplace safety is the AORN Perioperative Standards and Recommended Practices for Ambulatory and Inpatient Settings. Updated and published annually, it is a compendium of 30 recommended practices that are evidence based and peer reviewed. In 2011, AORN introduced a ranking method for rating the level of collective scientific evidence for AORN recommendations. In addition to the recommended practices, AORN position statements and guidelines enable surgical teams to communicate effectively and achieve optimal patient outcomes.

The association is governed by a board of directors consisting of the officers and seven elected members. It has the power, the authority, and the responsibility to manage the affairs of the association, except to modify actions of the House of Delegates.

AORN monitors nursing and health care laws and regulations and, through its National Legislative Committee and AORN State Legislative Coordinators, coordinates and engages AORN members that are active grassroots advocates to participate in the legislative and regulatory processes. Legislative priorities are established by the AORN board of directors to protect and enhance the profession of perioperative nursing. Its clinical and administrative staff serves on the committees and boards of approximately 30 professional associations to protect and improve safe perioperative practices.

AORN offers several publications including the monthly *Journal*, with peer-reviewed and evidence-based articles. *Connections* is published monthly within the *Journal* pages to also provide members with practical and personal perspectives that affect perioperative practice. *Periop Insider* is a weekly e-newsletter with time-sensitive news briefs, information on critical topics, and educational resources including online and face to face events. In addition to its print and online publications, AORN provides perioperative professionals with the online discussion community, ORNurseLink.

AORN of New York has been credited as being the founder of the national AORN. This group became the charter members of the Association of Operating Room Nurses, Inc., in 1954. The current name was adopted in 1999. Since its founding, the Association has expanded to include more than 300 U.S. chapters and now makes its headquarters in Denver, Colorado. There are 23 specialty assemblies that offer a formal structure within AORN to facilitate national networking of AORN members interested in a subspecialty or interest area.

A

A

The Association's annual national conference, Congress, first presented in New York in 1954, is acknowledged as the largest gathering of perioperative professionals in the world and the largest surgical products trade show in the United States.

Linda Groah

AUTHORITATIVE LEADERSHIP

The term authoritative leadership refers to a leadership style that is also called visionary. Authoritative leaders are known to inspire and mobilize others to buy into a common organizational vision. Individuals who work for an authoritative leader understand how they fit into the overall organizational mission and vision; these employees appreciate that what they do matters. Although often incorrectly referred to as authoritarian (autocratic, commanding, or overbearing), an authoritative leadership style is usually engaging and effective. Although autocratic leaders might often direct followers to *do as I say*, the authoritative leader would more likely use the phrase *come with me*.

Authoritative leadership is one of six leadership styles within Goleman's (2000) seminal framework. Although individuals might want to identify one leadership style as the "right" one, the literature suggests there is not one style that is better than another. Effective leaders are wise and versatile; they can identify when and how to use any or all of the six leadership styles to achieve desired results. An authoritative leadership style is most effective when radical change is needed and current organizational employees lack the expert knowledge and direction a visionary and decisive leader can contribute.

DISTINGUISHING CHARACTERISTICS

Vibrant enthusiasm and clear vision are hallmarks of the authoritative leadership style (Goleman, 2000). Dinham (2007) identifies high responsiveness (supportiveness toward employees) and high demandingness (demands and expectations of employees) as characteristics of the authoritative leader. Authoritative leaders set high expectations for employees simultaneously providing the necessary support to attain those standards (Martin, 2005). Authoritative leaders are productive; they are known to have a bias for innovation and action.

AUTHORITATIVE LEADERSHIP FIT WITHIN A BROADER CONTEXT

Authoritative leadership first described by Goleman (2000) is part of a six distinct leadership style framework (coaching, affiliative, democratic, pacesetting, and coercive are the other five styles). According to Goleman, leaders with the best performance outcomes do not rely on only one leadership style. In fact, effective leaders use the various leadership styles and seamlessly adapt these styles dependent on the business situation.

In terms of mastery, leaders generally prefer one or more styles. Those individuals who can master four or more leadership styles, however, especially the authoritative, coaching, affiliative, and democratic styles, create the very best organizational climate. Goleman (2000) defined organizational climate not as an amorphous term but rather as one that incorporates six key factors: (1) flexibility (how free employees feel to innovate unencumbered by red tape), (2) sense of responsibility for the organization, (3) level of standards people set, (4) sense of accuracy about performance feedback and aptness of rewards, (5) clarity about mission and values, and (6) level of commitment to common purpose.

As noted, all six leadership styles have a measurable effect on each aspect of climate. Although leaders can use all of the leadership styles, four of the six styles (authoritative, coaching, affiliative, and democratic) are consistently associated with positive organizational climate and results. Authoritative leadership in particular "is most effective, driving up every aspect of climate" (Goleman, 2000, p. 6).

Goleman, Boyatzis, and McKee (2002) suggest that a leader's primal task is an emotional one which involves articulating a message that resonates with their follower's emotional reality, builds relationships, moves followers to action, and frees them to do their very best. Goleman et al. established that individuals with the highest emotional intelligence are the most effective leaders because they are capable of switching between the six leadership styles depending on the situation. Each of the six leadership styles embodies an underlying emotional intelligence competence (Goleman et al., 2002) and leadership wisdom (Twentyman, 2007). Authoritative leaders are generally resonant leaders who contribute toward positivity and are self-confident, empathetic, and change catalysts.

STRENGTHS AND WEAKNESSES OF AUTHORITATIVE LEADERSHIP

Authoritative leadership is best used when organizations are adrift, employees are not as experienced as the leader, the organization requires a new strategic vision, and radical change or a clear direction is warranted. One identified weakness of authoritative leadership involves the failure to recognize skills and abilities, denying employees the opportunity to participate in decision making or showcase their talents. Because the authoritative leader derives much power from personal knowledge, this type of leader works best when supervising followers who do not possess more expertise than the leader.

Dinham, S. (2007). *Authoritative leadership, action learning, and student accomplishment.* Retrieved from http://works.bepress.com/stephen_dinham/1

Goleman, D. (2000). Leadership that gets results. *Harvard Business Review, 78*(2), 78–90.

Goleman, D., Boyatzis, R. E., & McKee, A. (2002). *Primal leadership: Realizing the power of emotional intelligence.* Boston: Harvard Business School Press.

Martin, A. J. (2005). The role of positive psychology in enhancing satisfaction, motivation, and productivity in the workplace. *Journal of Organizational Behavior Management, 24*(1/2), 113–133.

Twentyman, J. (2007). Commander one day, coach the next. *Director, 61*(1), 28.

Maria R. Shirey

B

Background Screening for Foreign-Educated Nurses

U.S. law requires that foreign-born health care professionals pass an independent credentials review to qualify for certain occupational visas. Among these professions are registered nurses, licensed practical nurses, occupational therapists, physical therapists, speech language pathologists and audiologists, medical technologists, medical technicians, and physician assistants. A certificate indicating applicants have passed such credentials evaluation is required before the U.S. Citizenship and Immigration Services can issue an occupational visa for them to live and work as a health care professional in the United States. In short, as a foreign-educated nurse, if you are interested in obtaining an occupational visa to work in the United States, you are required by Section 343 of the Illegal Immigration Reform and Immigrant Responsibility Act of 1996 to obtain a VisaScreen™ certificate (Department of Justice, 2003, 2004; Steps to Obtain a VisaScreen Certificate, 2011).

The Visa Credentials Assessment is a program offered by the International Commission on Healthcare Professions, a division of the Commission on Graduates of Foreign Nursing Schools (CGFNS,

1996, 2005, 2010). The VisaScreen™ certificate is issued after a complete evaluation of a professional's credentials to verify that he or she meets the minimum federal requirements. The certificate must be received before the U.S. Citizenship and Immigration Services will issue an occupational visa to the applicants to live and work as professionals in their field in the United States. The VisaScreen™ program is comprised of three parts: a credentials review of the candidate's entire professional education and all registration/licensure that he or she has held and currently holds, a successful completion of either the CGFNS Certification Program or the NCLEX-RN® (for registered nurses), and a successful completion of a group of English-language-proficiency examinations. Minimum passing scores for these examinations are set by the U.S. Department of Health and Human Services and the U.S. Department of Education (CGFNS International., 2007). Criminal background checks and finger printing of foreign health professionals are done at U.S. embassies, where visas are granted. State licensing boards have state-specific requirements regarding criminal background checks and licensing.

See also CGFNS International

CGFNS International. (2007). *Frequently asked questions: VisaScreen™ visa credentials assessment.* Retrieved February 2011 from http://

www.cgfns.org/files//sections/tools/faq/vsfaq.shtml

Commission on Graduates of Foreign Nursing Schools. (1996). *The trilateral initiative for North American Nursing: An assessment of North American Nursing.* Philadelphia, PA: Author.

Commission on Graduates of Foreign Nursing Schools. (2005). *VisaScreen: A crucial step toward working in the U.S.* Philadelphia, PA: Author.

Commission on Graduates of Foreign Nursing Schools. (2010). *2008–2009 Biennial Report: Global Challenges.* Philadelphia, PA: Author.

Department of Justice. Immigration and Naturalization Service. (2003). Section 343, Illegal Immigration Reform Immigrant Responsibility Act of 1996, Final Rules for Certificate for Certain Health Care Workers, vol. 68. no. 103, pp. 43901–43921.

Department of Justice. Immigration and Naturalization Service. (2004). Section 343, Illegal Immigration Reform Immigrant Responsibility Act of 1996, Interim Rule, vol. 69. no. 140, pp. 43729–43732.

Steps to Obtain a VisaScreen Certificate—CGFNS International. (2011). Retrieved February 2011 from http://www.cgfns.org/sections/programs/vs/ussteps.shtml

Barbara L. Nichols

BENCHMARKING

Benchmarking is a method to compare certain aspects of business or clinical performance in order to drive improvement in productivity and quality. The American Productivity and Quality Center describes benchmarking as the process of identifying, understanding, and adapting outstanding practices and processes from organizations anywhere in the world to help organizations improve. The process of benchmarking entails collating an organization's performance data on a wide variety of practices and then comparing that performance with other similar organizations to set goals that will improve quality, efficiency, and profitability. Improvements are accomplished through an increased focus on identifying and replicating best practices from the industry.

Benchmarking can lead organizations to new methods, ideas, and tools to improve effectiveness. Although benchmarks are not necessarily industry standards, regulatory guidelines, or rules, they are a mark against which an organization compares itself in the continuous search for better practices that will lead to superior performance. Investigating the practices of other organizations helps an organization to focus on how to do things better (improve efficiency) and to do things right (improve effectiveness).

For example, a hospital may look at its average length of stay for a particular Diagnostic Related Group, compare it with the length of stay results in a set of similar or comparable facilities, and set a goal of decreasing the average length of stay by a certain percentage. Using benchmarking to help guide improvement targets helps the facility to examine the average length of stay in other hospitals, to gain insights about the factors that are applied in other settings to reduce the length of stay, and then to set an improvement goal on the basis of the data.

Benchmarking methodology includes the following activities:

- Set objectives to define the scope of the effort.

- Select a benchmarking approach.

- Identify benchmarking partners or benchmark sources.

- Determine what constitutes the benchmark calculation.

- Consider both inputs (e.g., labor hours, salary and benefit expense, supply expense) and outputs (e.g., the unit of service statistic, a patient day, a square foot maintained, an emergency visit, an adjusted discharge).

- Compare actual performance data with the benchmark.
- Identify variances. Some variances will be favorable (current performance is better than the benchmark) and some will indicate an opportunity to improve (current performance is not as good as the benchmark).
- Calculate the gap in performance.
- Select ideas for improvement tactics for areas that are not favorable compared with the benchmark.
- Develop an action plan.
- Plan and implement the change.
- Measure the result and compare with the benchmark.

The end goal is not to mimic the practices and goals of other hospitals but rather to understand why their productivity, quality, or processes are performing more effectively or producing better outcomes. In addition, it is not necessarily the case that a higher expenditure compared with the benchmark for a particular service should automatically be labeled as inappropriate. Rather, it would be an area meriting further examination.

Benchmarking should be viewed as a continual process, not limited to once-a-year planning meetings or one-time engagements. Constantly monitoring performance fosters an environment where teams seek to continually improve. Benchmarking, however, is not an easy exercise. The continuous collection of data surrounding competing hospitals can be difficult because most hospitals do not report their statistics publicly. Because of the trend toward greater transparency in the health care industry, benchmark data are more readily available. Several public and private organizations now track various metrics for individual hospitals.

Sources for comparative clinical, financial, and operational benchmarks are available, including Solucient, Premier, and the National Database of Nursing Quality Indicators. These sources allow comparison groups to be composed on the basis of a wide range of possible groupings, such as bed size, teaching status, system affiliation, urban or rural location, profitability, payor mix, or case mix complexity.

Changes and innovations occur constantly within the health care industry. Benchmarking against current and future competitors reduces the risk of becoming a "reactor" to industry changes and allows the organization to take advantage of new applications and leading practices to promote success in their market.

Fuller, J., & Anderson, M. (2009, June). Common ground productivity benchmarking for CFOs and CNOs. *Healthcare Financial Management, 63*(6).

Roberts, A. (2008). A new mindset for hospitals: The value of benchmarking in an era of transparency. *Marketing Health Services, 28*(3).

Shoemaker, W. (2009, April). Benchmarking tools for reducing costs of care. *Healthcare Financial Management, 63*(4).

Solucient. (2007). *The DRG handbook: Comparative clinical and financial benchmarks*. Evanston, IL: Thomson Healthcare.

Stroud, J. (2011). *Understanding the purpose and use of benchmarking*. Retrieved April 12, 2011, from http://www.isixsigma.com/index. php?option=com_k2&view=item&id=225 :understanding-the-purpose-and-use-of-benchmarking&Itemid=166

Nancy Hollingsworth

BOARDS AND MEMBERSHIP ON BOARDS

As a newly educated nurse, one never imagines that the opportunity to improve the health and well-being of millions of Americans would present itself. Imagine being a part of the governing body of a $10 billion corporation. Fortunately, I benefitted from the wisdom and guidance of others who helped me grow into becoming a board member for the nation's largest health foundation, the Robert Wood Johnson Foundation. Through this exceptionally rewarding service, one is able to make unique and valuable contributions to the board, the foundation, and the people of the United States.

Fortunately, board service has become a more common experience for nurses. Nurses are increasingly being seen as having important contributions to make to the governance of not-for-profit and for-profit organizations. There are a number of factors underlying this development, including (1) the increasing presence of nurses in corporate leadership roles, (2) the greater importance of effective boards in nursing's own organizations, (3) the recognition of nursing's potential contributions to governance in other sectors, (4) the nurses' recognition of the value of boards to their own development and that of the profession, and (5) the increasing national emphasis on importance of nurses' presence on boards as a mechanism for improving health and health services. The growing importance of nurses in key governance and advisory roles has resulted in both national dialogue about and support for the development of nurses to serve in these key roles.

As nurses consider engaging in board service, it is important to think carefully about what this really means. Board service is a serious form of leadership that exists to enhance the value of institutions and organizations to the public and/or the institutions involved. There are differences between types of boards and their responsibilities. The consideration of board service begins with understanding types of boards and their functions.

Advisory boards (also referred to as commissions, councils, committees, panels, etc.) are constituted for the purpose of obtaining expert and/or representational advice. Whether ad hoc or ongoing, advisory boards bring together individuals whose expertise, perspective, and/or credibility contribute to advancing the purpose of the organization or entity. Advisory boards can be found in public, private, and voluntary/not-for-profit contexts. Their need for advice can range from particular technical questions or issues to guidance on national or global policy. Although advisory boards usually do not have fiduciary responsibility for organizations, they have important roles to play in shaping the future. For example, both the National Institute for Nursing Research and the Division of Nursing of the Health Resources and Services Administration have congressionally mandated national advisory councils. These councils help to shape the implementation of law, the development of policies, and the planning for the future—all in the public's interest. Although nurses are on both of these groups, members of the public and other disciplines also serve on these bodies. Other important advisory groups are those constituted by the Institute of Medicine of the National Academy of Sciences. For example, the ground breaking report, *The Future of Nursing: Leading Change, Advancing Health* (Committee on the Robert Wood Johnson Foundation Initiative on the Future of Nursing, at the Institute of Medicine: Institute of Medicine, 2010), is the outcome of the work of a commission whose membership included nurses.

Advisory boards can be a good way to begin to engage in board service. The requirement for advisory board members

B

to move from use of technical or specialty expertise to focusing on issues and topics of broader interest and significance helps to develop the skills that are important to being effective on all types of boards. Virtually all board service calls on one to be well prepared, to be well informed, to serve the interests of others, to engage in civil dialogue, and to contribute to the longer term well-being of an institution or program. Although advisory board service is not necessarily a stepping stone to other types of board service, it is can provide a good context for testing out interest in this kind of service and acquiring important skills.

Governing boards are legally constituted bodies that have fiduciary responsibility for a particular entity and legally defined accountabilities for the performance and well-being of the organization. Whether for profit or not-for profit, service on these types of boards carries with it legally defined responsibilities and accountabilities. Board members are not only expected to function in the ways associated with advisory boards, they are legally bound to serve the interests of the organization and its constituencies. When considering board membership, it is crucial to become well versed not only in the types of governing boards that exist but also in their functions, structures, and legal requirements. The roles of directors on governing boards can be thought of as a form of employment. The knowledge and skills required for this type of employment can be acquired through experience, observation, reading, mentoring, and so forth. It is also useful, however, to engage in board training, which is available through such organizations as the National Association of Corporate Directors.

Board service is not for everyone. One must really appreciate the importance of governance, care deeply about the work of the organization, be committed to doing the work required to serve well, and be willing to assume the associated legal and reputational risks. Effective board members are those whose motives transcend personal gain. They are those who are serious about the *service* part of being on a board and care about the impact of their work on the well-being of those for whom they are responsible.

There are many avenues to board service. The key among these are having good networks, good mentors, good experience, and good preparation and viewing the process as part of one's overall career development. Good mentors who are actively engaged in board service can help, as can connections to search firms that are involved in board searches. Participating in board training can provide important insights about approaches and strategies for both preparing for and being selected to serve on boards.

Serving on boards is an important way for nurses to improve health and health care. The incorporation of this type of work into career development for nurse leaders is a significant step in the ongoing improvement of organizational performance and societal good.

BoardSource. (2005). *The source: Twelve principles of governance that power exceptional boards*. Washington, DC: Author. Retrieved from http://www.boardsource.org/Knowledge.asp?ID=4.922

Chinoy, T. L. (2008, June). Don't even think about joining that board unless…*Directors and Boards*. Retrieved from http://directorsandboards.com/DBEBRIEFING/June2008/ColumnJune2008.html

Huskins, P. C. (2007). Questions to consider before joining a board. *Boardroom Briefing: The Consultants Issue*. Philadelphia, PA: Author.

Schmidt, E. (2003, March). Joining a nonprofit board in a post-Enron world. *GuideStar*. Retrieved from http://www2.guidestar.org

rxa/news/articles/2003/joining-a-nonprofit-board-in-a-post-enron-world.aspx?articleId=875

Society of Corporate Secretaries and Governance Professionals. (2007). *Governance for nonprofits: From little leagues to big universities.* New York, NY: Author.

Marla E. Salmon

BUDGET MANAGEMENT

The nursing leadership role in the financial management of an organization or a unit affects the control of nursing practice, nursing service delivery, and program management. Budgeting concepts are focused on money as a resource and for many years were often deemphasized in nursing practice and education. The allocation of resources is an important consideration for the nurse executive and frontline leader-manager because decisions regarding the cost of supplies or personnel have a direct influence on the financial health of an organization as well as the quality of the services that the consumers receive.

A budget is a plan with a timetable that guides an organization's activities (Yoder-Wise, 2007). It is a continuous process of predicting monies needed to provide a service, to implement the service, and to evaluate outcomes of the service. A budget is based on *revenue* (income generated or owed for services) and *expenses* (expenditures and costs of activities needed for the organization's operations). The difference between the projected cost and the actual cost of services is called a *variance*. The major types of budgets include the operating budget (the daily income and costs in 1 year for workload, personnel and labor requirements, supplies, and overhead), the capital budget (buildings, land, long-term

investments, or durable expensive equipment), the cash budget (actual/expected monthly income and cash disbursements), the construction budget (when renovation and/or new structures are planned), and the long-range budget (a strategic plan of goals for more than a 3- to 10-year period). A program budget looks at a certain existing or future program that needs evaluation, a product-line budget analyzes income and costs with a specific patient group, for example, patients with myocardial infarction, and a special-purpose budget is used for an ad hoc service or program that was previously unaccounted for. An organization generally will have a master budget that includes all of the major budgets (Finkler & Kovner, 2000). The master budget will have many sub-budgets, depending on the size of the organization. For example, the operating budget may have a sub-budget for a personnel only that would include the actual worked time (productive time) and the time paid to an employed for not working (nonproductive time) (Kelly, 2008).

Two typical approaches to budgeting that are most often used are the traditional or incremental format, in which the budget is simply increased a certain percentage on the basis of historical operations and projected revenue, and the zero-based format, in which the budget starts anew each cycle with all expenses requiring specific justification (Marquis & Huston, 2009).

The budgeting process is concerned with cost control. Direct costs in nursing service relate to a specific activity (unit) such as provision of nursing care and include the costs of personnel and other resources used in patient care. Indirect costs relate to secondary costs within the organization such as overhead (electricity), administrative and insurance costs, and other support services (housekeeping). The variables of volume and cost measures

B

B

also drive the budget. A *volume* measure is a unit of service adopted by an institution, for example, bed occupancy per day, average daily census, or nursing care hours per patient. A *cost* measure is usually nursing salaries (Huber, 2006).

See also Strategic Planning

Finkler, S. A., & Kovner, C. T. (2000). *Financial management for nurse managers and executives* (2nd ed.). Philadelphia, PA: Saunders.

Huber, D. L. (2006). *Leadership and nursing care management* (3rd ed.). Philadelphia: Saunders.

Kelly, P. (2008). *Nursing leadership & management.* Clifton Park, NY: Thomson/Delmar.

Marquis, B. L., & Huston, C. J. (2009). *Leadership roles and management functions in nursing: Theory and application* (6th ed.). Philadelphia, PA: Lippincott Williams & Wilkins.

Yoder-Wise, P. S. (2007). *Leading and managing in nursing* (4th ed.). St. Louis, MO: Mosby.

Martha J. Greenberg

BUILDING ACADEMIC GERIATRIC NURSING CAPACITY

The Building Academic Geriatric Nursing Capacity (BAGNC) program at the American Academy of Nursing is part of the John A. Hartford Foundation's Geriatric Nursing Initiative. Over the past 14 years, the Hartford Foundation committed $75 million to geriatric nursing, beginning in 1996 with the John A. Hartford Foundation Institute for Geriatric Nursing at New York University (personal communication with R. Watman at the John A. Hartford Foundation, 2010).

The foundation's interest in nursing was stimulated by the paucity of nurses prepared in geriatrics. In 1999, a set of white papers commissioned by Hartford

reported a significant shortage in a geriatric prepared nursing workforce (Belza & Baker, 2000; Fagin, 2000; McBride, 2000; Mezey, Fulmer, & Fairchild, 2000; Strumpf, 2000). At that time, of the 2.56 million registered nurses in the United States, fewer than 15,000 (0.005%) were certified geriatric nurses and less than a quarter of nursing schools required undergraduate courses in geriatrics or had the faculty to teach them. Fewer than 5% of nurse practitioners in training in 1996 were pursuing gerontological specializations, and the lack of faculty to support gerontological training of adult or family nurse practitioners threatened the adequacy of their preparation for the realities of future practice. Of more than 1,000 doctorates awarded by the 43 schools that responded to the foundation-supported survey of doctoral programs, only 16% had a primary interest in geriatrics. Similarly, of the then current National Institute for Nursing Research investigator funded grants, 16% were specifically in geriatrics (Rosenfeld, Bottrell, Fulmer, & Mezey, 1999).

Given these circumstances, geriatric nurses were scarce in the top leadership ranks of both nursing schools and nursing profession. The modest interest in geriatrics of both clinical and academic nurses reflected in these numbers contrasts sharply with the facts that the National Center for Health Statistics reported in 1999 that persons 65 years and older account for 48% of all primary care visits, 19% of ER visits, three times as many hospital days than all younger age groups with those 75 years of age and older reporting four times as many hospital days as younger groups (National Center for Health Statistics, 2011).

There was clear consensus among experts the foundation consulted that the greatest need in advancing the field of gerontological nursing was expansion of academic training capacity, particularly given the progress made by the Hartford Nursing Institute for Geriatric Nursing in advancing undergraduate nursing education and best clinical care practices. Thus, a new program to expand and sustain clusters of geriatric nursing excellence in research intensive universities which had already made major commitments to the field was regarded as the best way to address the field's critical faculty and research shortages. Such centers would create a scientific community, produce a cadre of future researchers, educators and practice leaders, advance knowledge about effective care, and ultimately enhance the well-being of the nation's older adult population.

In 2000, the Foundation significantly increased its commitment to building geriatric nursing capacity and expanded the number of grant funded nursing programs. Over the past 10 years, the John A. Hartford Foundation's Geriatric Nursing Initiative included the BAGNC program, Centers of Geriatric Nursing Excellence located in top-tier Schools of Nursing, and the Hartford Institute for Geriatric Nursing, curriculum and faculty development programs at the American Association of Colleges of Nursing in addition to a number of other smaller grants that focused on leadership development, advanced practice nursing career development, practice competencies, curriculum enhancement, and most recently geropsychiatric health care (John A. Hartford Foundation, 2009).

The BAGNC scholars and fellows program was instituted to work in tandem with the centers and rapidly address the challenge of building academic capacity and is comprised of three major elements. First, it supports both predoctoral students and postdoctoral fellows (later named the Claire M. Fagin Fellows) for the 2-year award terms. Second, an invitational annual leadership program brings together scholars, fellows, faculty, and leaders in the field of nursing, aging, leadership, and policy. Third, a coordinating center established at the American Academy of Nursing manages the operations and facilitates and builds synergies among the participants as well as with the other Foundation's funded geriatric nursing programs.

The BAGNC program completed its 10th year in 2010. At this time, there are nine Centers of Geriatric Nursing Excellence. The original five: the University of Arkansas for Medical Sciences, the University of California, San Francisco, the University of Iowa, the Oregon Health and Science University, and the University of Pennsylvania were joined in 2007 by an additional four Hartford funded Centers: the Arizona State University, the Penn State University, the University of Minnesota, and the University of Utah.

The John A. Hartford Foundation's support of geriatric nursing is a landmark in nursing. Since BAGNC's inception in 2000, the program has awarded more than 200 pre-doctoral scholarships and post-doctoral Claire M. Fagin Fellowships. As of July 2010, 82% hold faculty positions within schools of nursing, teaching close to 33 thousand students in undergraduate and graduate nursing programs. In addition, the scholars, fellows, and alumni received more than $72 million in grant support and published more than 1,000 articles informing the field of geriatric nursing and health care (Sofaer & Firminger, 2010a, 2010b).

Belza, B., & Baker, M.W. (2000). Maintaining health in well older adults: Initiatives for schools of nursing and the John A. Hartford Foundation for the 21st century. *Journal of Gerontological Nursing, 26*(7), 8–17.

Fagin, C. (2000). Guest editorial. Working papers: State of the art in gerontological nursing. The John A. Hartford Foundation meeting, January 11, 2000. New York, NY. *Journal of Gerontological Nursing, 26*(7), 5.

John A. Hartford Foundation Grant Projects. (n.d.). Retrieved from http://www.jhart-found.org/program/index.asp

McBride, A.B. (2000). Nursing and gerontology. *Journal of Gerontological Nursing, 26*(7), 18–27.

Mezey, M., Fulmer, T., & Fairchild, S. (2000). Enhancing geriatric nursing scholarship: specialization versus generalization. *Journal of Gerontological Nursing, 26*(7), 28–35.

National Center for Health Statistics. (2011). *Health, United States, 2010: With special feature on death and dying.* Hyattsville, MD: Author. Retrieved from http://www.cdc.gov/nchs/hus/older.htm#access

Rosenfeld, P., Bottrell, M., Fulmer, T., & Mezey, M. (1999).Gerontological nursing content in baccalaureate nursing programs: Findings from a national survey. *Journal of Professional Nursing, 15*(2), 84–94.

Sofaer, S., & Firminger, K. (2010a). *Evaluation brief: A decade of cultivating leaders in geriatric nursing.* New York: Baruch College. Retrieved from http://www.geriatricnursing.org/110206%20HGNI%20EvaluationBrief_Final%20%282%29.pdf

Sofaer, S., & Firminger, K. (2010b). *John A. Hartford BAGNC Scholar & Fellow Survey Report.* New York, NY: The John A. Hartford Foundation.

Strumpf, N.E. (2000). Improving care for the frail elderly: The challenge for nursing. *Journal of Gerontological Nursing, 26*(7), 36–44.

Claire M. Fagin
Patricia Franklin

C

CAREER STAGES

Patricia Benner's watershed book *From Novice to Expert* (1984) forced the nursing profession to give up any residual expectations that proficiency and excellence can be achieved at the start of a career with a sound education. Her notion that one develops different levels of ability over time—moving from novice to advanced beginner, to competent, then proficient, and eventually an expert—led to more emphasis on stages of a professional career. This career emphasis was, of course, reinforced by the unprecedented number of women entering the workforce in the last third of the twentieth century, which made working fulltime over your peak adult years the norm, rather than an exception. Nurse as careerist became the prevailing image (Kalisch & Kalisch, 1987) as men entered the profession in unprecedented numbers and women ceased to cluster in first-level positions throughout their work lives.

Building on Dalton, Thompson, and Price's classic article (1977) on the stages of a professional career, five career stages can be conceptualized, with mentoring playing a key role in each stage (McBride, 2011). The first career stage is appropriately named *preparation* because the central task is absorbing the values/standards of the nursing profession, learning the basics, and developing the clinical or inquiry skills necessary for your profession or specialty. Different levels of education prepare you for different kinds of practice. Undergraduate education is a typical preparation for licensure as a registered nurse. However, for many nurses, practice as a generalist is not sufficient; so they obtain a graduate degree that prepares for specialization, which is typically confirmed by certification. Because nursing is a learned profession, some nurses will seek a research doctorate, increasingly followed by postdoctoral research training in order to expand the profession's knowledge base. Formal education is the best way to master a body of knowledge, but socialization experiences are also important in learning more and building competencies; they can take many forms: clinical rotations, internships, teaching/research assistantships, apprenticeships, mentoring, workshops, group relations training, serving on committees, and the like. When a professional is becoming prepared, mentoring is crucial in all sorts of ways: modeling values and practices, assessing holes in the mentee's background, providing graded challenges that test abilities without overwhelming; welcoming the individual to the profession/specialty, and helping to set short-term and long-term career goals.

The second career stage is named *independent contributions* because the focus is on demonstrating the ability to work independently and interdependently with nurse colleagues, other health professionals, and a broad array of other kinds of staff and stakeholders. This is the stage where professionals deal with the inevitable gap between ideals learned and the realities of the particular work setting; build a collegial network; demonstrate the ability to think, synthesize and act critically; and focus on meeting institutional and professional benchmarks of success. All nurses must be concerned at this stage with building teams: working with the less-educated and less-experienced staff, learning how to take advantage of peer colleagues who are competent in areas that you are not; and using those who know more than you do as consultants or advisors. At this stage, a mentor can help nurses navigate the inner workings of an institution or profession, open doors of opportunity, and provide direction on resources (human and otherwise).

The third career stage focuses on *development of the home setting*. Though still concerned about how to be more effective, the professional now assumes more responsibility for the development of others and the setting in which he or she operates. In the previous stage, the focus was largely on the "here and now;" in this stage, there is an increasing concern about planning for the future: what needs to be done to expand institutional resources? How does one build a culture of quality and safety? The more the involvement in strategic planning, the more likely it is that the professional is working closely with others in different fields; so, there is expansion to include interdisciplinary work and boundary spanning. As one seeks to build the home setting's image, infrastructure, and resources, it is important to develop greater political savvy because knowing what to do and getting it done involve different competencies. At this stage, a mentor can provide feedback regarding strategy, teach how to delegate, and develop the professionals' mentoring abilities.

In the fourth career stage, *development of the field/health care*, movement is beyond the home setting. It involves taking a more active role in shaping the profession and health care in general. Once the professional becomes known as an expert in a particular area or as someone who has improved the home setting, increased opportunities become available. This leads to even more occasions to shape the future as a consultant or advisor. The nurse may be asked to assume a leadership role in some professional organization, for example, running for office, serving on an editorial board, or developing a practice or research agenda to create a vision. In this stage, there are often more prospects than ever before, partly because she or he is known to others and partly because the boundary-spanning activities reveal even more possibilities. There are many clinical and academic positions that do not belong to any one field—for example, serving as Chief Operating Officer or Provost—and these positions may be opportunities when an individual has demonstrated discipline-specific excellence. Next sentence should then read: At this stage, a mentor can play a role in deciding on strategy and envisioning future scenarios.

Upon reaching the age in which most peers are retired, there can be additional career opportunities. This is the "gadfly stage;" in this stage, it is possible for the professional to take on special assignments that require high-level integrative abilities, continue to serve as a consultant or advisor, coach current leaders, and challenge younger colleagues to new ways of thinking.

Plato saw the gadfly as the truth teller who helps others confront what they might prefer to ignore, and free to be forthright, the seasoned nurse can force important discussions that might not be able to be raised by those still constrained by institutional affiliation. This career stage is not a matter of being salaried or not, but of imagining ways in which to continue to make a contribution, in keeping with one's education, experience, and energy. A mentor can help a professional even at this career stage to envision the postretirement years in less stereotyped ways and recommend new opportunities.

These stages are not meant to be prescriptive, but, like all developmental models, provide a perspective on how the key themes in ascendancy change over the course of a full career. Once some modicum of personal proficiency is developed, the challenge is to branch out and become more engaged in moving your home institution forward, in advancing the profession, and, most of all, in changing health care for the better. As Shirey (2009) has said, it means moving over time from promise to momentum to harvest.

Benner, P. (1984). *From novice to expert: Excellence and power in clinical nursing practice.* (pp. 13–34). Menlo Park, CA: Addison-Wesley.

Dalton, G. W., Thompson, P. H., & Price, R. L. (1977). The four stages of professional careers: A new look at performance by professionals. *Organizational Dynamics*, 6, 19–42.

Kalisch, P. A. & Kalisch, B. J. (1987). *The changing image of the nurse.* Menlo Park, CA: Addison-Wesley.

McBride, A. B. (2011). Orchestrating a career (pp. 51–72). *The growth and development of nurse leaders.* New York, NY: Springer Publishing.

Shirey, M. R. (2009). Building an extraordinary career in nursing: Promise, momentum and harvest. *The Journal of Continuing Education in Nursing*, 40, 394–400.

Angela Barron McBride

CAREFRONTING

One of the most significant challenges that nurse leaders face in today's health care environment is how to effectively manage the conflict that often occurs when individuals have divergent values, beliefs, and attitudes. Guiding individuals and/or teams to get past their day-to-day problems, conflicts, and communication issues toward a goal of high performance takes leadership skill (Sherman & Pross, 2010). "Carefronting" is an important new competency for nurse leaders to help resolve conflict and create healthy work environments. Augsburger (1981), a professor of pastoral care and counseling, coined the term carefronting to refer to the skill of caring enough about oneself, others, and desired goals to confront inappropriate behavior responsibly while offering the opportunity for change. Carefonting is the act of inviting, not demanding, another to change and a creative way through conflict, a way to unite caring and candor in relationships (Kupperschmidt, 2006a).

Carefronting is a skill that can be learned and used in any relationship in which conflict arises. It is appropriate for leaders to apply carefronting in a broad range of settings. The following tenets are encompassed in carefronting (Kupperschmidt, 2006b, 2008):

- *Truthing it: A simplified speech style.* Truthing it encompasses the willingness and ability to listen deeply, empathetically, and accurately to assure understanding of others' points of view. Truthing also encompasses speaking simply, "I want to hear you accurately" and speaking honestly, "I want to share my feelings and attitudes with you; I want to be heard; I care about our relationship."

C

- *Owning anger: Let both your faces show.* Anger is both a positive, self-affirming emotion and a demand. When one feels ignored or rejected, the normal response is anger. "I am a person of worth, I demand that you recognize and respect me." Each person, regardless if the context is a practice or educational setting, is responsible for choosing how they respond and react to others when conflicts occur.

- *Inviting change: Careful confrontation.* Carefronting invites change but does not demand it. Inviting change means focusing feedback on the behavior, not the person; on observations, not conclusions; on descriptions, not judgments; and on ideas and alternatives, not on advice and answers. Inviting change encompasses clear, simple descriptions and observations couched in concern and caring. Invite change by carefronting caringly, gently, constructively, and clearly.

- *Giving trust: A two-way venture.* Trust undergirds, connects, and integrates all human emotions. Trust, which is essential in work relationships, is grounded in authentic self-disclosure. Trust confronts openly, frankly, respectfully, and responsibly, trusting that the other person will assume his or her responsibility to be equally honest and frank. Such trust releases demands and accepts apologies.

- *Ending blame: Forget whose fault the conflict is.* Confrontation that endeavors to place blame inevitably evokes resistance and resentment. Carefronting ends the blame game, leading to the real questions: What is the respectful thing to do now? Where do we go from here? When do we start to discuss the conflict? If not now, when? If not us who cares enough about our goals, such as patient safety, who will end blame and work toward the professional practice we deserve?

- *Getting unstuck: The freedom to change.* Getting unstuck means owning responsibility for one's part in the conflict and refusing to waste time in assigning blame. Getting unstuck means accepting accountability for behavioral changes that accept responsibility for the present conflict and focusing on what can be is shared.

- *Peacemaking: Getting together again.* Nurse leaders who are peacemakers are caring people who dare to be truly present in conflict situations, listening and caring for all stakeholders. Peacemakers care enough to confront and drop the demands of the past. Peacemakers are nurse leaders who value others and who have rediscovered that the values that shape their decisions must be lasting values consistent with the values of the profession.

Carefronting is an alternative to traditional conflict resolution. The use of carefronting is especially important in healthcare environments where team synergy and interdependence are required for high quality and safe patient care. The development of trust among team members on teams begins with communication in relationships, especially, when there is disagreement. Relationships live within the context of conversations that individuals have or do not have with one another (Sherman & Pross, 2010). To be successful today, nurse leaders should develop the skill of carefronting and apply it in interactions with their staff. Carefronting is a skill that should be taught also to interdisciplinary team members and expected in team interactions.

Augsburger, D. (1981). *Caring enough to confront.* Ventura, CA: Regal Publications.

Kupperschmidt, B. (2006a). Carefronting: Caring enough to confront. A reprint. *The Oklahoma Nurse,* 51(2), 22–23.

Kupperschmidt, B. (2006b). Addressing multigenerational conflict: Mutual respect and carefronting as a strategy. Retrieved from http://www.nursingworld.org/Main MenuCategories/ANAMarketplace/ANA

Periodicals/OJIN/TableofContents/Volume 112006/No2May06/tpc30_316075.aspx

Kupperschmidt, B. (2008). Conflicts at work? Try carefronting. *Journal of Christian Nursing,* 25(1), 10–17.

Sherman, R. & Pross, E. (2010). Growing our future nurse leaders to build and sustain healthy work environments at the unit level. *Online Journal of Issues in Nursing,* 15(1), Manuscript 1. http://www.nursingworld.org/MainMenuCategories/ANAMarketplace/ANAPeriodicals/OJIN/TableofContents/Vol152010/No1Jan2010/Growing-Nurse-Leaders.aspx

Betty R. Kupperschmidt
Rose O. Sherman

CASE MANAGEMENT

Case management is a type of nursing care delivery or work design to organize patient care and meet patient needs. The Case Management Society of America (CMSA) defines case management as "a collaborative process of assessment, planning, facilitation, and advocacy for options and services to meet an individual's health needs through communication and available resources to promote quality cost-effective outcomes" (CMSA, 2006).

In the United States, case management originated from managed care and prospective payment reimbursement and is used by many health care providers and systems. Although the nursing profession has a long history of using case management in community and other settings, contemporaneous nursing case management focuses on individual patients rather than populations of patients, and manages patient care by major medical diagnoses or diagnosis-related groups (DRGs). DRGs are predetermined payment schedules reflecting anticipated costs for treatment of specific patient conditions.

In nursing case management, patient care is planned using predetermined patient outcomes with specific time frames and the use of specific resources through the use of critical pathways (also called clinical pathways or care pathways) and multidisciplinary action plans (MAPs). Critical pathways are tools or guidelines, developed by interdisciplinary teams, that provide direction for managing the care of a specific patient concern with specific and expected care outcomes and strategies at certain points in time. A MAP is a combination of a nursing care plan and critical pathway (Kelly, 2008). Regardless of the nomenclature, critical pathways identify crucial and predictable occurrences that (1) must take place at established times, (2) organize time-dependent multidisciplinary provider interventions, (3) utilize best practices, (4) aid the standardization of care, and (5) reduce health care costs. A variance on a critical pathway is any deviation from the standard or expected time frame that alters the patient's progress through the pathway. Case managers track variances, documenting when and why a patient care varies from the pathway, and may recommend changes to the plan.

There are many case management frameworks, perspectives, and meanings because case management exists in many settings. Case management is a *service* for insured patients aimed at identifying the most financially effective health care service providers, treatments, and settings for individuals. The *role* of a case manager is coordination of a patient care. Case management is a *system* that focuses on the continuum of care across settings with a patient's specific episode of illness. The system uses and evaluates time-dependent patient outcomes, strategies, and resources. Case management occurs in acute care settings and outpatient settings such as hospice, home health, psychiatry,

C

and insurance companies. CMSA reiterates, "Case management serves as a means for achieving client wellness and autonomy through advocacy, communication, education, identification of service resources and service facilitation."

Further, CMSA states, "the case manager helps identify appropriate providers and facilities throughout the continuum of services while ensuring that available resources are being used in a timely and cost-effective manner in order to obtain optimum value for both the client and the reimbursement source. Case management services are best offered in a climate that allows direct communication between the case manager, the client, and appropriate service personnel, in order to optimize the outcome for all concerned." To be effective, the nurse case manager must coordinate and evaluate multidisciplinary care, integrate clinical nursing practice, communicate care concepts, direct others, and influence policy and organizational systems. The study by Kelly (2008) also includes the expansion of case managers' involvement in coordinating disease management or population-based health with the focus on populations of patients rather on the individual.

Case Management Society of America. Retrived from http://www.cmsa.org

Huber, D. L. (2006). *Leadership and nursing care management*. (3rd ed.). Philadelphia, PA: Saunders.

Kelly, P. (2008). *Nursing leadership & management*. Clifton Park, NY: Thomson/Delmar.

Marquis, B. L. & Huston, C. J. (2009). *Leadership roles and management functions in nursing: Theory and application*. (5th ed.). Philadelphia, PA: Lippincott, Williams & Wilkins.

Sullivan, E. J. & Decker, P. J. (2005). *Effective leadership and management in nursing*. (6th ed.). Upper Saddle River, NJ: Pearson Prentice Hall.

Martha J. Greenberg

CASE STATEMENTS

Case statements are formal printed documents that are used in fund-raising campaigns to communicate the institution's vision to the public, primarily those who are prospective donors. The Council for Advancement and Support of Education (CASE; 2006), which is an organization serving many institutions of higher education as well as non-profit organizations throughout the United States, recommends that the case statement include attention to the following questions: What about your institution would make a prospect want to donate? How does a donor go about giving to your institution? What makes your institution a good financial investment?

The campaign case statement typically begins with the mission statement of your institution and includes your vision for the future. Many case statements include a brief history of accomplishments so that the prospective donor understands the institution's past success and can be comfortable that there will be future successes. Basic facts about the institution are included. For example, for schools of nursing, it would be important to include types of academic programs offered, overall enrollment within each academic program, percentage of students who receive financial aid, and graduation and pass rates on the required licensing and certification examinations. The case statement often includes information about past successes with fund-raising, even if it is minimal. Donors like to know that there is a beginning infrastructure for accomplishing the institution's goals. The specific fund-raising goals are often detailed in the case statement, although at times, these are included as inserts so that the case statement can be used for a number of requests. Most important, the case statement must include a compelling message of why the institution needs additional support. Donors invest where there is both vision and need, so it is important to tie these components together in the case statement and let the donor know what difference their investment will make. In the case statement, it is most important for the institution or organization to distinguish itself from other like institutions or organizations as fund-raising is extremely competitive and there are many places for possible investment by donors. Prospective donors often choose to invest based on the distinguishing factors that they perceive.

The case statement is used externally with prospective donors. It may be accompanied by an internal case statement that includes more details and is made available to the volunteers who will help with the fund-raising initiative. The internal case statement should be consistent with the external case statement; it serves as a resource document for the Board, volunteers, and staff.

CASE is a membership organization that provides many useful tools for fund-raising campaigns. This organization also makes available sample case statements for campaigns and sponsors an awards program for excellent case statements (CASE, 2006).

Council for Advancement and Support of Education. (2006). *Write-minded: Is anyone reading your case statement?* Retrieved December 10, 2010, from http://www.case.org

Joyce J. Fitzpatrick

Center to Champion Nursing in America

The Center to Champion Nursing in America (CCNA) is a joint initiative of AARP, the AARP Foundation, and the Robert Wood Johnson Foundation (RWJF). The Center, a consumer-driven national force for change, works to increase the nation's capacity to educate and retain nurses who are prepared and empowered to positively impact health care access, quality, and costs. Its mission is to ensure that all Americans have a highly skilled nurse, when and where they need one. In order to ensure a 21st-century nursing workforce with the skills and knowledge Americans need, the Center works to

- strengthen our nation's educational pathways to prepare the nursing workforce of the future;
- increase the number and diversity of nurses entering and remaining in the profession;
- remove barriers that limit nurses' ability to provide the health care consumers need;
- enhance the influence of nurses in high levels of health care, policy, business and community decision making.

The Center uses multiple strategies to create positive change including

- Building coalitions: The Center convenes multidisciplinary health care, business, and consumer organizations at the national level. The Champion Nursing Coalition represents the voices of consumers, purchasers, and providers of health care to support nursing solutions that improve healthcare access, quality, and cost effectiveness. Its purpose is to raise awareness about nurses' roles in health care reform and achieve permanent solutions to the looming crisis of inadequate numbers of nurses with the right skill sets. The Center also convenes the Champion Nursing Council, an advisory group made up of national nursing organizations, which provides high-level input from the nursing community.

C

- Cohosting national summits and forums: CCNA has collaborated with Health Affairs and the Robert Wood Johnson Foundation on two national forums on the role of nurses in health care reform and related workforce development issues. The Center also collaborated with RWJF, the U.S. Department of Labor and the Division of Nursing in the Health Resources and Services Administration to design and implement two national summits on strategies for expanding increasing nursing education capacity.

- Providing ongoing technical assistance to support state/grassroots efforts: Following the national forums on nursing education, CCNA provided continuing technical assistance to multi-stakeholder teams in 30 states, all working to increase education capacity and in redesigning nursing education in order to prepare the nurse of the future. The majority of states that had both baseline (2008) and 2009 data increased statewide enrollment in entry level RN education programs, despite a severe budget crisis.

- Strengthening nursing workforce data: CCNA supported the Forum of State Nursing Workforce Centers in developing a minimum data set for on-going measurement on nurse supply, demand, and pipeline indicators through a consensus process. Implementation across a majority of states holds the promise of not only producing nursing workforce data that can be used to advocate for support of nursing in state legislatures, but that can be used for state-to-state comparisons and holds the potential for national aggregation.

- Acting as a repository of information on nursing in America: The Center is currently collaborating with AARP to raise awareness of the roles of nurses in health care reform, including increasing access to primary care, transitional care, and chronic care management. CCNA's Web site (http://championnursing.org) was launched in October 2009 and is organized around five issue areas (skills for the future, education capacity, recruitment and retention, practice and access to care, and leadership). It includes regularly updated news items, internal and guest blogs, and Champion Nursing TV as well as an "About Nursing" section and pages dedicated to state efforts.

- Other/future initiatives: Due to a lack of photographic images that accurately reflect the important work that nurses do every day, CCNA launched a national photo contest in 2010 in order to build a public Web-based repository of images that better represent the profession of nursing. The repository is available on the champion nursing Web site.

Moving forward, the Center to Champion Nursing in America is expanding its focus on advanced practice registered nurses, especially in primary care. We are engaging stakeholders in understanding the nursing implications of health care reform and promoting nursing leadership in improving health care access, quality, and cost-effectiveness, as well as retention strategies among new graduates and older nurses. With a second funding stream from RWJF for AARP's involvement in the implementation phase of the Initiative on the Future of Nursing, CCNA and the Future of Nursing Teams are working collaboratively under the umbrella of Nursing Initiatives in the Public Policy Institute of AARP, to support RWJF's roll out of the Institute of Medicine's recommendations on the future of nursing.

Brenda L. Cleary

CENTERS FOR DISEASE CONTROL AND PREVENTION

The Centers for Disease Control and Prevention (CDC) is an agency of the U.S.

Department of Health and Human Services located in Atlanta, Georgia. Recognized as the leading U.S. government agency for protecting the health and safety of its people, the CDC "identifies and defines preventable health problems and maintains active surveillance of diseases through epidemiologic and laboratory investigations and data collection, analysis, and distribution" (CDC, 2009). The CDC continues to have strong partnerships with state health departments and other reputable organizations that help enforce health promotion, health protection, and health diplomacy. In addition, the CDC also directs quarantine activities, conducts epidemiological research, and provides consultation on an international basis for the control of preventable diseases.

The CDC was established in 1946 as the Communicable Disease Center in Atlanta. It quickly acquired an epidemiology division when it took over the Public Health Service Plaque Laboratory in San Francisco. Within a year, the CDC gained worldwide recognition for quality and quantity of its contributions to the taxonomy of the Enterobacteriaceae. In the mid-1950s, two major health crises helped establish the CDC's credibility: identifying poliomyelitis and correcting it, and developing national guidelines for an influenza vaccine. Over the next two decades, the CDC was successful in eradicating smallpox and measles. In addition, it traveled overseas in response to health care needs, made advances in research, and continued to grow. In 1970, the agency was renamed the Centers for Disease Control to reflect its expanding role in public health. This agency continued to advance working globally, eradicating diseases, and diagnosing new diseases, such as AIDS. In the past six decades since its founding, the CDC has grown dramatically in size and stature, scope and science, and reputation and reach. In addition,

the CDC addresses the issues related to chronic diseases, disabilities, workplace hazards, injury control, threats to environmental health, and terrorism preparedness. Today, the CDC is considered the nation's premier health promotion, prevention, and preparedness agency and a global leader in public health.

There are 12 centers, institutes, and offices that make up the CDC. Individually, they each respond to their area of expertise, but they pool all of their resources and expertise on crosscutting issues and specific health threats (CDC, 2010). In the last decade, the CDC has reorganized its centers, institutes, and offices to meet 21st-century health and safety threats, such as the 2009 H1N1 pandemic. From the time of the first case on April 15, 2009, it took the CDC less than two weeks until treatment was made available and only four months to develop a vaccine. Through this pandemic the CDC has proven to be a more integrated, adaptable and faster agency.

The goal for the CDC is for people around the world to live safer, healthier, and longer through health promotion, health protection, and health diplomacy. Health promotion consists of improving global health by sharing knowledge, tools, and other resources with people and partners around the world. Implementing protection strategies involves a transnational prevention, detection, and response network that protects Americans from health threats at home or abroad (CDC, 2010). Also, the CDC and U.S. government want to be seen as a trusted and effective resource for health promotion and health protection globally.

One way the CDC plans to spread health promotion is through its partner *Healthy People 2020. Healthy People 2020* provides evidence-based, 10-year objectives for promoting health and preventing disease. It builds on initiatives pursued over the past three decades. *Healthy People 2020* provides health objectives in a way that enables different groups to combine their effects and work as a team. The objectives are integrated into current programs, special events, publications, and meetings involving health care or health promotion. Schools can carry out activities to further the health of the community. Health care providers, specifically nurses, can encourage patients to pursue healthier lifestyles and to participate in community programs.

As the largest group of health care professionals, nurses may be viewed as important leaders for implementing the stated objectives of the CDC. Nurses are uniquely positioned to assist in prevention and promotion efforts in a multitude of health care settings and in various levels of the community. The CDC works with nurses in "state and local health departments to implement disease prevention and health promotion on a variety of issues on an ongoing basis" (CDC, 2009). Because of their high level of public trust, nurses have been effective communicators, counselors, educators, advocates, and mentors to individuals and groups striving to maintain healthier lifestyles. Nurses demonstrate an important leadership role by their involvement in the prevention of diseases and promotion of health as well as being equipped to respond to disaster situations.

The CDC remains committed to its vision of healthy people in a healthy world. It consistently applies research findings to improve people's daily lives. Although the CDC has grown in tremendous ways since 1946, the heart of the CDC is still its people. They are still determined to make a difference in the lives of people around the world.

Centers for Disease Control and Prevention. (2010). *The 2009 H1N1 pandemic: Summary highlights, April 2009*

Centers for Disease Control and Prevention. (April 2010). Retrieved August 15, 2010, from http://www.cdc.gov/h1n1flu/cdcresponse.htm

Centers for Disease Control and Prevention. (2009). *Center for disease control and prevention mission statement.* Retrieved August 3, 2010, from http://www.cdc.gov/maso/pdf/cdc-miss.pdf

Centers for Disease Control and Prevention. (2010). *Our history—Our story.* Retrieved August 3, 2010, from http://www.cdc.gov/about/history/ourstory.htm

The New Georgia Encyclopedia. (2010). *Centers for disease control and prevention.* Retrieved August 8, 2010, from http://www.georgiaencyclopedia.org/nge/Article.jsp?id=h-1209

U.S. Department of health and human services. (2009). *Healthy people 2020: The road ahead.* Retrieved August 3, 2010, from http://www.healthypeople.gov/hp2020/default.asp

Stephanie J. Offord

CERTIFICATE OF NEED

A Certificate of Need (CON) standard is established by state law. It prohibits identified health facilities/services/equipment from being initiated, upgraded, modernized, expanded, relocated, or acquired without a certificate from that state determining that the need exists in the specified area. According to the National Conference of State Legislatures (Cauchi, 2010), the CON programs are aimed at restraining health care facility costs and allowing coordinated planning of new services and construction. Criteria for the approval or denial of a CON are established by law or regulation as review standards, and they include cost, quality, and access considerations. The types of facilities, services, and equipment that are covered, as well as the review standards, vary from state to state. More than half of the U.S. states use this concept with regard to the health care services that they provide (Citizens Research Council of Michigan, 2005). The CON applications are reviewed against the following criteria: public need, financial feasibility, character, and competence (New York State Department of Health, 2005).

Public need: Determination of public need is based on a variety of factors, including population, demographics, and service utilization patterns, epidemiology of selected diseases and conditions, and access to services.

Financial feasibility: Financial feasibility is based on expenses, projected revenues, current financial status, and capacity to retire debt.

Character and competence: Assessment of the character and competence of an applicant is based on experience and past performance in operating a health care service, including records of violations, if any, and whether a substantially consistent high level of care was maintained. Applicants without experience in health care services are evaluated based on compliance with laws and practices pertinent to their professional experience.

By using a CON evaluation system, the government can evaluate the need for specific health care services in a specific region, determining whether there is a lack or surplus of services provided. Although attention is given to the construction and related costs of capital expansion and improvements, the focus of participating states is on the increase in health care costs that can arise from the availability of unneeded service capacity and total operating expenses that are more costly than necessary. Applicants are required to demonstrate that the service is needed, that it is not duplicative, and that the service will be provided at the lowest cost possible (Citizens Research Council of Michigan, 2005).

Health care service providers are also required to demonstrate the need for the initiation, upgrading, expansion, relocation, and acquisition of services and beds, which are all subject to CON review. The basic assumption underlining CON regulation is "that excess capacity (in the form of facility overbuilding) directly results in health care price inflation" (Cauchi, 2010). Each state's certificate of need program has individual features that differentiate it from other states with similar programs. Categories regulated by certificate of need programs include: acute care, air ambulance, burn care, cardiac catheterization, CT scanners, gamma knives, long-term care, mobile hi-tech, MRI scans, neonatal care, obstetric services, open heart services, organ transplant services, PET scans, psychiatric services, rehabilitation, renal dialysis, rescue care facilities, subacute care, substance abuse, swing beds, and ultrasound diagnostic tests (CON Application, State of Alaska, 2006; Citizens Research Council of Michigan, 2005). Some states evaluate projects according to general criteria, whereas others make distinctions as to what entity provides the service, usually including hospitals while excluding other providers.

Cauchi (2010) has developed a map that reflects the state CON laws. In Pennsylvania, Indiana, Kansas, Texas, North Dakota, South Dakota, Minnesota, Colorado, Wyoming, New Mexico, Arizona, Utah, Idaho, and California, state law may be required with respect to CON. In all other states, the CON law was either appealed or is not in effect.

Cauchi, Robert. (2010, January 28). CON-Certificate of Need State Laws. *NCSL Home.* Retrieved September 26, 2011, from http://www.ncsl.org/default.aspx?tabid=14373

C

Certificate of Need Application, State of Alaska. (2006). *Health and social services, office of the commissioner, health planning and systems development.* Retrieved March 11, 2007, from http://www.hss.state.ak.us/commissioner/ Healthplanning/cert_of_need/forms/ default.htm

Citizens Research Council of Michigan. (2005). *The Michigan Certificate of Need Program.* Retrieved September 28, 2006, from http:// www.crcmich.org/PUBLICAT/2000s/2005/ rpt338.pdf#search=%22who%20needs%20 a%20certificate%20of%20need%22

New York State Department of Health. (2005). *Introduction to the CON process.* Retrieved September 28, 2006, from http://www.health. state.ny.us/nysdoh/cons/cons_application/ page_00_intro_to_con_process.htm

Mary Samost

CERTIFICATION

What does certification mean for nurses today? Today's health care demands require nurses to proactively embrace the constant changes of the industry in order to provide the utmost quality of care. The American Nurses Association (ANA) recognizes the importance of nursing certification and defines it as "a means of measuring competency, and the identification of competent nurses that will promote the public welfare for quality in health care" (Thomas, 2002). Quality of practice is enhanced through education. The ANA's Nursing Scope and Standards of Practice (2004) highlights in its eighth standard of nursing practice (*Education*) that "the registered nurse attains knowledge and competency that reflects current nursing practice" (ANA, 2004, p. 35). The measurement criteria of this standard are that the nurse participates in ongoing educational activities and demonstrates a commitment to lifelong learning. Another measurement

criterion is that nurses acquire knowledge and skills appropriate to the specialty area, practice setting, role, or situation. Nurses are ethically and professionally responsible for obtaining specialized knowledge or skills as their careers progress (American Association of Colleges of Nursing, 2006).

Certification, as defined by the American Association of Critical Care Nurses, is "the process by which a nongovernmental agency validates based upon predetermined standards, an individual registered nurse's qualifications and knowledge of practice in a defined functional or clinical area of nursing" (American Association of Critical Nurses Certification Corporation, 2010). Credentialing organizations verify that the nurse applying for certification has completed all eligibility criteria and earned a specific credential. Private voluntary certification reflects the achievement of standards beyond licensure (minimum knowledge required) for specialist nursing practice. Certification often lasts from two to five years, requiring certified nurses to renew their certification or soon after providing evidence that they have maintained the required level of knowledge of their specialty, as well as proof of ongoing participation in activities that support the maintenance of competence in that specialty (American Board of Nursing Specialties, 2005). There are several certification programs, some of which are part of the different professional nursing associations representing specialty areas such as National Certification Board for Diabetes Educators, the Board of Certification for Emergency Nursing, the American Board of Certification for Gastroenterology Nurses, and the HIV/AIDS Nursing Certification Board among others. The American Nurse Credentialing Center (ANCC) is the largest nurse credentialing organization in the United States, offering 42 specialty

certifications for nurses, nurse practitioners, and advance practice nurses.

In early 2000, research from the Nursing
Credentialing Research Coalition (NCRC)
found that certification had a great impact
on personal attitudes and confidence as
well as on the professional and practice
outcomes of certified nurses (American
Nurse Credentialing Center, 2010). It was
reported in this study that nurses who
held certification felt more confident in
their practice and that it allowed them to
initiate early and prompt interventions
when detecting early signs and symptoms of complications in their patient. The
NCRC study also revealed an increase in
patient satisfaction ratings and more effective communication and collaboration
with other health care providers for those
nurses who were certified. On December
11, 2002, the American Association of
Colleges of Nursing (AACN) released a
report about the benefits that specialty certification had for nurses titled *Safeguarding
the Patient and the Profession: The Value of
Critical Care Nurse Certification*. This paper
corroborates the evidence released by the
NCRC, stating that nurses whose clinical judgment has been validated through
certification make decisions with greater
confidence, and increased their knowledge resulting in fewer medical errors
(Redd & Alexander, 2003). Years after the
publication of mentioned research, new
evidence continues to be published about
the importance of certification in quality
patient care, encouraging nurses of distinct specialties to become certified.

American Association of Colleges of Nursing.
(2006). *Advancing higher education in nursing:
2006 Annual report: Annual state of the schools.*
Retrieved June 8, 2006, from http://www.
aacn.nche.edu/2006AnnualReport.pdf

American Nurses Association. (2004). *Scope and
standards of nursing practice.* Washington, DC:
Author.

American Nurse Credentialing Center (2010).
ANCC Certification. Retrieved on September
27th, 2010 from http://www.nursecredential-
ing.org/certification.aspx

American Association of Critical Care Nurses
Certification Corporation (2010) Certification.
Retrieved on September 27th, 2010 from http://
www.aacn.org/WD/Certifications/Content/
consumer-whatiscert.pcms?menu=Certificati
on&lastmenu=

American Board of Nursing Specialties (ABNS).
(2005). *A position statement on the value of
specialty nursing certification.* Retrieved on
September 28th, 2010 from www.nursingcerti-
fication.org/pdf/value_certification.pdf

Redd, M. L., & Alexander, J.W. (2003).
Safeguarding the patient and the profession:
The value of critical care nurse certification.
American Journal of Critical Care, 12, 154–164.

Thomas, L (2002). Letter to the Editor: Response
to Necessity for Subspecialty Certification in
Hepatology for Nurses. *Journal Gastroenterology
Nursing.* Volume 25 Number 4 pp. 174 – 175.
Retrieved on September 28th, 2010 from
http://www.nursingcenter.com/library/
JournalArticle.asp?Article_ID=285667

Paule V. Joseph

CGFNS INTERNATIONAL

CGFNS International, formerly the
Commission on Graduates of Foreign
Nursing Schools (CGFNS), is a not-for-
profit, immigration-neutral, internationally recognized, leading authority on the
education, registration, and licensure of
nurses and other health care professionals
worldwide. The organization was founded
in 1977.

CGFNS protects the public by assuring
the integrity of professional credentials in
the context of global migration. CGFNS
offers certification, verification, evaluation,
and examination that meet U.S. immigration and state licensure requirements. These
services and programs validate credentials

C

and enhance international regulatory and educational standards for health care professionals around the globe.

These programs are as follows:

- Certification Program
- Credentials Evaluation Service
- VisaScreen®: Visa Credentials Assessment
- Credentials Verification for New York State

CERTIFICATION PROGRAM

The CGFNS certificate is recognized by most U.S. State Boards of Nursing as a prerequisite for licensure in the United States and may be required to obtain certain occupational visas to practice nursing in the United States. The CGFNS Certification Program is a three-part program designed for first-level, general nurses educated outside the United States. The program includes a credentials review, CGFNS Qualifying Exam of nursing knowledge, and test of English language proficiency. Upon successful completion of all three parts of the program, the applicant is awarded the CGFNS certificate.

CREDENTIALS EVALUATION SERVICES

As with the CGFNS Certification Program, the CGFNS Credentials Evaluation Service (CES) is a prerequisite for state licensure in certain states and territories in the United States. CES is also used by schools in the United States to determine academic placement of international students; however, there is no examination component in the CES. The program is based on an evaluation of a health care professional's educational and professional licensure or registration credentials. The resulting report compares the health care professional's education

and licensure credentials in terms of U.S. comparability.

VISASCREEN: VISA CREDENTIALS ASSESSMENT

The federal government oversees immigration. Noncitizens must comply with immigration requirements to enter the country. A valid visa is required. Immigrants who are entering the United States to work must have an occupational visa. To receive a valid visa, an immigrant must meet several criteria—criminal background checks, medical examination, fingerprinting, etc. Immigrants who are health care workers are subject to additional criteria.

Section 343 of the Illegal Immigration Reform and Immigrant Responsibility Act of 1996 requires that foreign-born health care professionals who wish to practice in the United States successfully complete a screening program before receiving an occupational visa. This includes registered and licensed vocational nurses, physical therapists, speech language pathologists, audiologists, medical technologists, medical technicians, occupational therapists, and physician assistants.

VisaScreen: Visa Credentials Assessment is a program administered by the International Commission on Healthcare Professions—a division of CGFNS—enabling health care professionals to meet this requirement by verifying and evaluating their credentials to ensure that they meet the U.S. government's minimum requirements. The VisaScreen program is comprised of an education analysis, licensure validation, English-language proficiency assessment, and in the case of registered nurses, an exam of nursing knowledge. Those seeking an occupational visa must have an employer sponsor their petition. The employer is required to show (labor certification) to the Department

C

of Labor that he or she has met all criteria to demonstrate that everything has been done to find a U.S. resident to fill the vacant position. Once the Department of Labor has approved the petition, it must be forwarded to and reviewed by the Department of Homeland Security (DHS), Citizenship and Immigration Service, which will process the visa application. The Department of State grants the visa when all required documents have been submitted. Production of the VisaScreen certificate is required before the Department of State issues an occupational visa.

An occupational visa can be permanent and is known as the "green card." There are also temporary visas, which have a limited duration. The H-1B visa, which has a validity of 3 years, is for those who are filling vacant positions which require a person to have at least a baccalaureate degree. It can be renewed one time, for 3 years. Few nurses are eligible for the H-1B visa because there are three entry level nurses—diploma, associate degree, and baccalaureate. Advanced practice nurses and managers would qualify for H-1B visas. H-1C is another temporary visa, but only applies to 500 registered nurses per year who will work in hospitals in underserved areas, with a designated percentage of Medicare and Medicaid beds. In its 20-year history, no more than 150 nurses have been admitted because few hospitals (11) meet the criteria. It is limited to 3 years of duration and cannot be renewed.

A third temporary category is that for workers from countries under the North American Free Trade Agreement—Canada and Mexico. Initially, Trade North American Free Trade Agreement (TN) workers had to renew their TN status every year. However, in 2008, the DHS extended the TN status duration up to 3 years. TN status can be renewed indefinitely.

TN status is limited to specific workers. Health care workers are registered nurses, medical technologists, physical therapists, and occupational therapists. The majority of TN nurses are from Canada, many of whom are daily commuter workers to U.S. border states. The Canadian nurse or health care worker need only show their offer of employment, required licenses, and a valid VisaScreen certificate at a Canadian border crossing or airport. The process takes less than a day. The TN status process is more complex for Mexican workers. It requires both a visa and processing at a U.S. Consulate, which means the worker must meet all visa criteria; however, the process can be completed in a week.

A VisaScreen certificate is valid for 5 years. If the health care worker has not acquired a permanent visa or has not entered the United States, he or she will have to renew his or her VisaScreen certificate. Without a current VisaScreen certificate, a health care worker cannot renew his or her visa or TN status. He or she would be denied entry to work or be required to return to his or her country.

To receive a VisaScreen certificate, the health care worker must meet the criteria set in Section 343. The education must be comparable to that of the entry level U.S. graduate, all licenses ever held must be validated as unrestricted or unencumbered, meet English proficiency requirements by passing approved English proficiency exams or having been educated in countries deemed exempt by the DHS, and in the case of nurses, passed designated tests of nursing knowledge (CGFNS Qualifying Exam or the National Council Licensure Examination [NCLEX]). All documents, transcripts, and licenses must come directly from the issuing source.

In November 2009, CGFNS was reauthorized through 2014 by the U.S. DHS to continue conducting visa credentials assessment certifications for health care workers who are not U.S. citizens and are seeking a visa to work in the United States.

CREDENTIALS VERIFICATION FOR NEW YORK STATE

For health care professionals, specifically registered and licensed practical nurses, physical and occupational therapists, and therapy assistants, wishing to practice in the state of New York, the CGFNS Credentials Verification Services collects and verifies the authenticity of an applicant's educational and licensure or registration credentials so they can be evaluated by the New York State Education Department.

In addition, CGFNS also offers the International Standards for Professional Nurses Program in designated countries, with the core component being the CGFNS Qualifying Exam for first level, registered nurses.

Another division of CGFNS International, the International Consultants of Delaware, a charter member of the National Association of Credential Evaluation Services, reviews foreign educational credentials for individuals wishing to pursue academic or employment opportunities.

See also Background Screening for Foreign-Educated Nurses

CGFNS International 2008–2009 *Biennial Report.*

Barbara L. Nichols

CHAIRING KEY ORGANIZATIONAL COMMITTEES

Chairing key organizational committees is a responsibility that nurses are well suited for, yet often lack the opportunity to do. A study by the Health Research and Educational Trust (HRET) found that nurses comprised 2.3% of the membership, much less the leadership, of health system boards, compared with 22.6% for physicians (Prybi et al., 2009, p. 8). Other studies have reported similar findings (Prybil et al, 2005; Disch, Dreher, Davidson, Sinioris, & Wainio, 2011). Don Berwick, director of the Centers for Medicare and Medicaid Services has stated: "It is key that nurses be as involved as physicians…the performance of the organization depends as much on the well-being, engagement, and capabilities of nursing and nursing leaders, as it does on physicians" (Prybil et al., 2009, p. 8). The HRET study recommended that "*All* boards…should consider the appointment of highly-respected and experienced nursing leaders as voting members of the board to complement physician members and strengthen clinical input in board deliberations" (Prybil et al., 2009, p. 41). Yet nurses continue to be under-represented on boards, or as chair of key organizational committees. A recent study by Gallup on behalf of the Robert Wood Johnson Foundation (http://www.rwjf.org/pr/product.jsp?id=54488, 2009) queried national opinion leaders who strongly stated that nurses should have greater influence on increasing the quality of care, improving efficiency and promoting health. Disch (2008) has recommended that nurses *lead* the quality journey, not just be influential.

Many nurses have served, and do now, as members of health system boards, as chairs of important organizational committees, or lead national organizations and universities. What distinguishes these leaders is *the nursing lens*, the perspective that nurses bring to any situation whether it relate to nursing, health care or business. The nursing lens is holistic, person-centered, system-oriented, and pragmatic. The leader using a nursing lens skillfully establishes effective interpersonal relationships, quickly sizes up challenging situations, views a problem in the larger context, and engages the input of others in crafting workable solutions.

The National Center for Healthcare Leadership identified 26 competencies for health leaders in administrative and clinical positions (http://www.nchl.org/static.asp?path=2852,3238). These are clustered into three domains (transformation, execution, and people) and portrayed in Figure 1. It is readily apparent that nurses, through education and experience, have well-developed competencies in these areas

and can perform well in chairing committees and serving on boards of directors. What will help nurses gain access to these positions, and perform well, is (1) identifying a mentor in the organization who can coach the leader, make important connections and recommend them for key assignments; (2) cultivating strong interpersonal relationships with colleagues across the organization; (3) developing skills in meeting and management, such as establishing the agenda, conducting the meeting, handling conflict, and building consensus; (4) assuring that timelines are met and goals accomplished; (5) conveying outcomes from the committee's work to key stakeholders and audiences; and (6) sharing

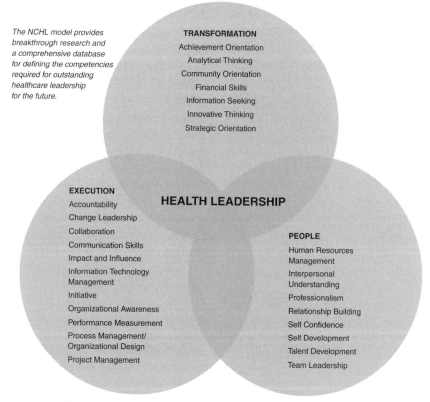

Reprinted with permission from the National Center for Healthcare Leadership (www.nchl.org) Chicago, Illinois.

FIGURE 1: NCHL health leadership competency model.

praise generously and giving constructive feedback privately.

Disch J. (2008). Who should lead the patient safety/quality journey? In R Hughes (ed.), *Advances in patient safety & quality: An evidence-based handbook for nurses*. Washington, DC: Agency for Healthcare Research & Quality.

Disch, J., Dreher M., Davidson P., Sinioris M., & Wainio J. (2011). The role of the chief nursing officer in quality and safety. *Journal of Nursing Administration, 41*(4), 179–185.

National Center for Healthcare Leadership. (2010). *NCHL Health Leadership Competency Model*, Retrived January 23, 2011, from http://www.nchl.org/static.asp?path=2852,3238

Prybil L., Levey S., Peterson R., Heinrich D., Brezinski P., Zamba G., Amendola A., Price J., & Roach W. (2009). *Governance in high-performing community health systems: A report on trustee and CEO views*. Chicago, IL: Grant Thornton LLP.

Prybil L., Peterson R., Price J., Levey S., Kruempe D., & Brezinski P. (2005). *Governance in high-performing organizations: A comparative study of governing boards in not-for-profit hospitals*. Chicago, IL: Health Research and Educational Trust.

Robert Wood Johnson Foundation. (2010). *Nursing leadership from bedside to boardroom: Opinion leaders' perceptions*. Retrieved January 23, 2011, from http://www.rwjf.org/pr/product.jsp?id=54488

Joanne Disch

CHANGE

A simple definition of change comes from Dictionary.com: "to make the form, nature, content, future course, etc., of (something) different from what it is or from what it would be if left alone" (dictionary.reference.com/browse/change). In fact, there are many types of changes. For example, there is a classic distinction to be made between a first-order change and second-order change (Watzlawick & Weakland, 1974). First-order changes are differences that occur in a system that remain unchanged itself. An example of first-order change is water boiling in a pot on a stove. As the water boils, first-order change is taking place. The water is becoming different as the molecules jostle together because of the heat of the stove. In this instance, even though there is change taking place, the water remains water. So second-order change is a state change from water to steam. If there is no change in the state, rules or structure, one is dealing with first-order and not second-order change.

First-order change generally involves the application of a problem-solving model. First-order change is rule- or principle-based, and is circular in nature. First-order change is often incremental and more frequently than not maintains the status quo—hence the adage—"the more things change, the more they stay the same." First-order change often involves a search for a singular antecedent cause or problem to solve. Characteristics of first-order change identified by the National Academy for Academic Leadership (n.d.) include adjustments within existing structures, doing more or less of something. First-order change is reversible, nontransformational, and does not involve new learning or understanding of the systems thinking required in a second-order change effort.

Large system changes involve attention to multiple players, roles, rules, levels, values, beliefs, issues, and questions of politics and resources. Therefore, second-order change requires a shift in thinking to other logical levels. Second-order change exists when there is a change in the state, structure, rules, or principles by which a system operates. Second-order change may seem illogical, however, because it focuses on a system of causes with multiple effects and consequences. Second-order change

C

answers questions of what, how, and why with attention to systems thinking and patterns of relationships between and among elements in a system dynamic (Bellinger, 2004) Second-order change requires an understanding of the Web of reciprocal causality among the variables involved. Causes and effects are linked together in loops and become dynamic rather than static. Consider what happens when the water in the pot reaches a certain temperature. The water changes state, and operates with a different set of rules as the water is transformed into steam. Water turning to steam is an example of second-order change.

As the National Academy for Academic Leadership notes, other characteristics of second-order change involve new ways of seeing things, and shifting gears. Second-order change involves new learning and transformational change. In organizational development change circles, there is a growing awareness that focusing on problems and first-order change efforts may not be that useful.

A problem-oriented approach to change mostly poses these questions: What is wrong? Why is it wrong? How does the problem limit us? This is in contrast to an appreciative approach to change that focuses on what is working and specifying desirable outcomes instead of focusing on the problems. An outcome approach to change poses these questions: What is the change that is wanted? How will the change be defined and made explicit? Where, when, and with whom is the change desired? If the change is achieved, what else will be affected or changed? What stops a group from realizing the changes desired? What are the resources that exist to make the change possible?

Appreciative inquiry (appreciativeinquiry.case.edu) is one approach to change that focuses more on what is working

rather than on what is broken or not working. Appreciative inquiry is about desired results or second-order changes rather than attention to problems, which is a first-order change. Outcome-oriented thinking requires attention to a second-order change rather than first-order change problem-identification frame of mind. For more information about change access, see the Free Management Library Web site (managementhelp.org), especially the Change Management 101 Resource by Fred Nicklos (2010).

Appreciative Inquiry, http://appreciativeinquiry.case.edu/

Bellinger, G. (2004). *Mental model musings: Understanding the way of systems.* Retrieved September 10, 2010, from http://www.systems-thinking.org/index.htm

Dictionary.com Retrieved September 10, 2010, from http://dictionary.reference.com/browse/change

Free Management Library: http://managementhelp.org/

National Academy for Academic Leadership. (n.d.). *Leadership and institutional change resource page.* Retrieved September 10, 2010, from http://www.thenationalacademy.org/ready/change.html#defining

Nicklos, F. (2010). *Change management 101.* Retrieved September 10, 2010, from http://www.nickols.us/change.pdf

Watzlawick, P., & Weakland, J. (1974). *Change: Principles of problem formation and problem resolution.* New York, NY: Norton.

Daniel J. Pesut

CHANGE AGENTS AND CHANGE AGENT STRATEGIES

Change agents are people who lead change projects or business-wide initiatives by defining, researching, planning, and

C

building coalitions and networks as part of a business or organizational change effort. Change agents value and create climates that support change and know how to use appreciation, power, and influence (Smith, 2009). They deal with the analytic, psychologic, strategic, and emotional aspects of change. They start the change process with themselves rather than with others. They facilitate rather than force change. They are able to let go of old ideas and experiment with alternatives that support their own enthusiasm. They seek out and accept criticism of their ideas. They are able to get others to "buy into" their ideas for change. Given this set of characteristics, change agents need the following skill set. Change agents need to be appreciative, trustworthy, reliable, honest, competent, and credible within respective organizations. They must possess persuasion, influence, negotiation, and effective listening skills. Successful change agents embody leadership through the demonstration of a strong work ethic supported by enthusiasm and respect for individual differences. They have the ability to think conceptually and organize thoughts logically as well as the skill to plan and execute activities and plans. They have good judgment and strong communication skills and are able to coach and facilitate others. Change agents are purpose driven and know how best to use appreciation, influence, and control or personal action agendas, as a means to accomplish transformation in the organizations in which they work (Smith, 2009).

Change agents are the masters of change management, and posess the knowledge, skills, and abilities to align people, processes, and purposes to achieve the desired outcomes. Change management consists of a four-phase process of visioning, planning, implementing, and reviewing and learning. In each phase,

both strategies and competencies are needed to influence and achieve effective change. In the visioning phase, the strategies of information-gathering, conceptualizing, and pattern recognition are integrated into coalition building, diagnosis, and outcome specification. In the planning phase's recruitment, team development and delegating parallel and dovetail with the change agent competencies of team building, coalition building, influencing, communicating, and project implementation. In the implementation phase, the change strategies of influencing, negotiating, communicating, listening, monitoring, controlling, and delegating support project management and performance standard setting. Maurer (2010) observes that nearly 70% of change efforts fail because of three levels of resistance and a change agent's lack of appreciation and understanding of the cycle of change. The best way to navigate the change process is to (1) make a compelling case, (2) get started on the right foot, (3) keep the change alive, (4) get back on track if derailed, and (5) know when to move on. Change agents are likely to appreciate Maurer's online resources. Change agents use influence to manage resistance and anxiety. Change agents learn to appreciate, influence, control, reflect, and develop self and others throughout a change management project.

Change agents are "bridgers" and boundary spanners or purposeful network weavers in organizations. That is, change agents connect and weave together people and information or "nodes" in a network of relationships in a way that links the social and intellectual capital of the network in service of well-defined outcomes and the desired change. Change agents build smart communities through actively managing their networks. Network weavers (Krebs & Holley, 2006) know their networks and weave the network together in an iterative connecting and bridging process of communication and interaction in service of an identified vision, goal, or change.

Krebs, V., & Holley, J. (2006). *Building smart communities through network weaving.* Retrieved September 29, 2010, from http://www.orgnet.com/BuildingNetworks.pdf

Maurer, R. (2010). *Beyond the wall of resistance.* Austin, TX: Bard Press. Retrieved September 29, 2010, from http://www.Askboutchange.com

Smith, W. (2009). *The creative power: Transforming ourselves, our organizations andour world.* New York, NY: Routledge.

Daniel J. Pesut

CHI ETA PHI SORORITY, INCORPORATED

Chi Eta Phi Sorority, Incorporated is a professional nursing organization guided by the motto, *Service for Humanity.* This motto is embedded in the mission of promoting higher education, collaborating with other professional groups, developing leaders, and stimulating friendly relationships. The organization was established in 1932 by Aliene Carrington Ewell and 11 other courageous nurses of color at Freedman's Hospital in Washington, DC. Chi Eta Phi is shaped by the attributes of character, education, and friendship. The headquarters is in Washington, DC.

From the inception of the organization, members have implemented national programs in their communities to support the mission of service. The national programs are the vehicle by which members engage in service activities, one of which is to encourage wellness through disease prevention and health promotion programs. Through these programs, members engage in activities such as health screenings in targeted communities to identify potential and actual health problems and health education programs to address these problems, with the goal of facilitating wellness and appropriate disease management. Similarly, programs for youth and young adults may include health education sessions, as well as mentoring and peer forums that encourage the sharing of health care experiences. In addition to health education, support is provided to seniors in the form of travel and assistance with navigating health care systems.

In light of increasing health disparities in underrepresented populations, especially the increasing aging population, partnerships with national organizations such as the American Heart Association, American Stroke Association, National Kidney Education Project, Association of SIDS and Infant Mortality Programs, the National Eye Health Education Program and the Newsreel of California (films and videos for social change, *Unnatural Cancer: Is Inequality Making Us Sick?*) to improve health problems.

In addition to these health-related programs, the sorority engages in recruitment activities to promote interest in nursing careers and to support students who are enrolled in undergraduate and graduate programs. A research development program was added in recent years, designed to assist both novice and seasoned members with projects that address health promotion and health maintenance in underserved populations.

An additional national program awards educational scholarships that support the retention of undergraduate and graduate nursing students in professional nursing programs. Moreover, financial, tutoring, and mentoring activities relating to recruitment and retention of student nurses are also addressed.

Three leadership development programs are designed to assist members and officers by fostering effective leadership skills. In addition, the Leadership Fellows Program is available on a competitive basis for members who are interested in enhancing their leadership skills with the assistance of a mentor.

The organization sponsors biannual leadership and educational conferences and produces journals and newsletter that focus on scholarship and the reporting of programs and the work of the local chapters. The sorority has also published biographies of Mary Eliza Mahoney, America's first Black professional nurse, and Lillian Harvey, nurse leader and former dean of Tuskegee University School of Nursing.

Chi Eta Phi's members include both men and women. Membership is extended by invitation to African American registered nurses, and student nurses who are enrolled in professional schools and have a commitment to service. As of 2011, the organization has approximately 8,000 members located throughout the United States, St. Thomas, U.S. Virgin Islands, and Liberia, West Africa.

Since its founding, Chi Eta Phi Sorority, Inc. has been led by 19 visionary leaders who have focused and dedicated themselves to provide for the viability of the organization. Each administration has made concerted efforts to build on past work in order to better define a viable future and to sustain the organization with an intent for the pursuit of excellence. These leaders are Aliene C. Ewell, Sadie Spradley, Anita K. Bass, Fay O. Wilson, Mazelle D. Dickerson, Minnie J. Whitfield, Fostine Riddick Roach, Leota P. Brown, Helen S. Miller, Verdelle B. Bellamy, Peola H. McCaskill, Essie L. Rowser, Josephine Alexander, Mary Helen Morris, Catherine Binns, Dana Lopez, Carolyn W. Mosely, Lillian G. Stokes, and Mildred Fennal.

Additional information is available from these sources:

The History of Chi Eta Phi Sorority, Inc., Vol II, 1968–1997, Chi Eta Phi Sorority, Inc.

The Legacy of Supreme Leadership (2009). Ed. Fostine Riddick Roach, Chi Eta Phi Sorority, Inc. Retrieved from www.chietaphi.com

Lillian G. Stokes

CLINICAL EVALUATION

Nursing educators, like those in other fields, are concerned with outcomes. Clinical evaluation is one way to measure the outcomes of a nursing program. The work of the educator is not complete until there is an appraisal of how well the students have met course objectives and eventually the overall outcomes of the program. Evaluation is the capstone activity of nursing faculty. Faculty need to learn early in their careers about the art of talking to students about their performance. Clinical days, mid-semester, and end-of-semester activities include the responsibility of student evaluations. Teachers must determine if students have or have not met the course objectives. In addition, faculty has to determine a grade, distinguishing among below average, average, above average, and excellent. The use of a rubric that distinguishes excellent to failing performances is a superb tool that enables faculty to be objective and fair when grading students. Use of a rubric by faculty for grading leads to less confusion about grades, as it is easier to explain and/or defend grade variations that may otherwise be perceived by others as too subjective. The rubric can be norm-referenced or criterion referenced. Norm-referenced evaluation compares an individual's performance with others in the course or cohort, while criterion-referenced compares the individual's performance with a set of defined criteria (Lowenstein & Bradshaw, 2001). In order to increase the likelihood of validity in the evaluation, educators use multiple and varied data gained from the student's written work, observations, staff and/or patient input, and student comments.

A major portion of faculty time is spent evaluating student performance and providing feedback to students. In nursing education, this assessment is very detailed and is ongoing throughout the semester. Most clinical nursing faculty begin evaluation process on the first day of the clinical practicum. The regular use of anecdotal notes that carefully describe the assignment and how well the student met the objectives is necessary, as it is difficult to remember all of the specifics for each student in a clinical group. It is important to write positive comments as well as negative comments. These notes need to be written as soon after clinical evaluation as possible and shared on a weekly basis with students. It is important to include students in this process, asking them to self-evaluate their performance throughout the semester. Mid-semester for most students is a major turning point. This is when students talk in depth with faculty about how well they are meeting the objectives and what they have left to accomplish. Clinical evaluation at this point of time is referred to as a *formative* evaluation. At the time, any student who is failing didactic or clinical coursework should be notified both in writing and in person. Department chairs, deans, and lead teachers also may be notified of an impending failure, depending on the organizational structure and individual school policies and procedures. There also may be systems of remediation in place to assist the students, and these may be included in the notice.

At the end of the semester, a final student evaluation is filed in the student's record. This *summative* evaluation should identify whether or not the student met the objectives, if there are any strengths and/or weaknesses in the student's performance, and any recommendations for improvement going forward. These evaluations must be signed by the student. This does not mean that the student agrees with the findings; rather, it signifies that the student has talked to the faculty member about his or her performance. Course evaluations must be filed in a timely fashion, as it is imperative that all students have complete records; incomplete records may affect financial aid opportunities, future enrollment, and employer requirements. These records become part of the permanent file and are used throughout the student's career, including during the preparation of after-graduation references. Faculty also examines records as the student progresses throughout the curriculum. The record may demonstrate consistent growth or indicate a behavioral trend that is problematic. Deans also may return to the records years after students graduate if they are asked to write recommendations or answer questions about past clinical and classroom experiences.

Additional information is available from these sources:

DeYoung, S. (2003). *Teaching strategies for nurse educators.* Upper Saddle River, N.J.: Prentice Hall.

ILTE Workshop: *Creating grading rubrics.* Retrieved March 24, 2006, from http://ilte.ius.edu/pdf/creating_a_grading_rubric.pdf

Kearns, L. E., Shoaf, J. R., & Summey, M. B. (2004). Performance and satisfaction of second-degree BSN students in Web-based and traditional course delivery environments. *Journal of Nursing Education, 43*(6), 280–284.

Liberto, T., Roncher, M., & Shellenbarger, T. (1999). Anecdotal notes: Effective clinical evaluation and record keeping. *Nurse Education, 24*(6), 15–18.

Lowenstein, a. J. & Bradshaw, M. J. (2001). *Fuszard's innovative teaching strategies in nursing.* 3rd *edition.* Gaithersburg, MD: Aspen.

C

Neary, M. (2000). Supporting students' learning and professional development through the process of continuous assessment and mentorship. *Nursing Education Today*, 20(6), 463–474.

O'Connor, A. (2006). *Clinical instruction and evaluation: A teaching resource*. Salisbury, MA: Jones and Bartlett.

Reising, D.L., & Devich, L.E. (2004). Comprehensive practicum evaluation across nursing program. *Nursing Education Perspective*, 25(3), 114–119.

Ruthman, J., Jackson, J., Cluskey, M., Flannigan, P., Folse, V. N., & Bunten, J. (2004). Using clinical journaling to capture critical thinking across the curriculum. *Nursing Education Perspective*, 25(3), 120–123.

Schaffer, M. A., Nelson, P., & Litt, E. (2005). Using portfolios to evaluate achievement of population-based public health nursing competencies in baccalaureate nursing students. *Nursing Education Perspective*, 26(2), 104–112.

Winters, J., Hauck, B., Riggs, C. J., Clawson, J., & Collins, J. (2003). Use of videotaping to assess competencies and course outcomes. *Journal of Nursing Education*, 42(10), 472–476.

Martha J. Greenberg

CLINICAL LADDER

Because one of the greatest threats to nursing staff satisfaction is lack of recognition for excellent work, it became clear in the 1980s that some new creative ways to acknowledge staff nurses should be developed. Until this time, most nurses were recognized for quality work by gaining administrative positions. Even in the 1980s, job satisfaction translated into nurse retention. With the advent of Patricia Benner's (1984) work, *From Novice to Expert*, however, it seemed possible to develop additional pathways to recognize outstanding clinical nurses. One of these methods became known as the clinical ladder. In the clinical ladder concept, nurses advanced in the organization by demonstrating their growth in knowledge and experience. They were recognized and rewarded for excellent bedside nursing practice (Burket et al., 2010). Each additional level of recognized skills advanced the financial remuneration of the nurse. Often, skills were divided into descriptions of practice, such as beginner, advanced beginner, competent, proficient, and expert. Skill sets describe the various levels of accomplishment. For example, in the area of recognizing and responding to clinical emergencies:

- Beginner: learns by observing and asking questions and understands that critical thinking is involved.

- Advanced beginner: has practice skills required in emergent situations but may lack experiential knowledge to fully appreciate the situation.

- Competent level: has developed necessary skills to function in the emergent situation but may become overwhelmed by multiple tasks or the pressures of leading in the situation.

- Proficient nurse: organization for patient care is automatic and dynamic; picking up on changes in condition and taking appropriate action.

- Expert nurse: is able to take immediate action in the situation, access both nursing and interdisciplinary team resources quickly, function seamlessly and automatically in the situation, and calm others in the midst of a crisis (Schoessler et al., 2005).

Each level builds on knowledge and skills from the previous level as well as adding continuously increasing critical thinking and reasoning, holistic intuition, and experience-guided behaviors. These levels of functioning are on a continuum.

Numerous clinical ladder models exist today. Some have outcome-based criteria, and staff selects a specific number of behaviors from among various categories. For example, categories could include competency, customer service, teamwork, quality, and continuous learning. Within the quality category, the nurse might choose one of the following behaviors:

- assume an active role in the quality or practice outcome project;
- complete special projects with leadership approval and communicate outcomes to the staff;
- participate in an approved research study;
- attend research or quality educational workshop and share learning with other staff members;
- review a nursing research article and present to staff;
- initiate a cost-saving initiative on the unit with documentation of outcomes (Burket et al., 2010).

Hospitals and other health care facilities have traditionally had no salary differential for baccalaureate and higher degree education for nurses. This lack of differentiation may have evolved from the cycles of severe nursing shortages. When such practices are in place for extended periods of time, it is often difficult to change them. Consequently, many health care facilities have used the clinical ladder as a means of rewarding additional education. For example, if an associate degree nurse or a diploma nurse goes back to school to obtain their bachelor of science in nursing (BSN), many clinical ladder programs provide additional points for continuing academic education. Some of these programs allow BSN-prepared nurses without experience to enter the clinical ladder at an additional level, which increases the salary. This is an interesting example of thinking "outside of the box" to be able to reward nurses for education when the general system in which the facility operates does not differentiate one registered nurse from another. This exemplifies creative uses of the clinical ladder concept (Pierson, Ligget, & Moore, 2010).

In many institutions, formal education is a significant part of the program. Thus, masters of science in nursing (MSN)—prepared nurses, who still provide direct patient care, may find themselves at the top of the clinical ladder. Likewise, national certification is a major criterion in many clinical ladder programs (Watts, 2010) and rewards nurses for this continuing effort. In addition, clinical ladder programs for ambulatory care providers have been developed (Nelson & Cook, 2008). Regardless of how the program is structured, the clinical ladder concept encourages and rewards nurses who develop in-depth expertise and professionalism while choosing direct patient care involvement.

Benner, P. (1984). *From novice to expert*. Menlo Park, CA: Addison Wesley.

Burket, T., Felmlee, M., Greider, P., Hippensteel, D.,Rohrer, E., & Shay, M. (2010). Clinical ladder program evolution: Journey from novice to expert to enhancing outcomes. *Journal of Continuing Education in Nursing, 4*(8), 369–374.

Nelson, J., & Cook, P. (2008). Evaluation of a career ladder program in an ambulatory care environment. *Nursing Economics, 26*(6), 353–360.

Pierson, M., Ligget, C., & Moore, K. (2010). Twenty years of experience with a clinical ladder: A tool for professional growth, evidence based practice, recruitment, and retention. *Journal of Continuing Education in Nursing, 41*(1), 33–40.

Schoessler, M., Akin, R., Body, R., Falconer, K., Kaiel, C., Moore-Stout, D., et al. (2005). Remodeling a clinical ladder: An action research design. *Journal for Nurses in Staff Development, 21*(5), 196–201.

Watts, M. (2010). Certification and clinical ladder as the impetus for professional development. *Critical Care Nursing Quarterly, 33*(1), 52–29.

Karren Kowalski

C

CLINICAL NURSE LEADER (CNL®)

Calls to transform the health care system and evolve the preparation of health care professionals have grown louder over the past decade. In 1999, the Institute of Medicine released its landmark report, *To Err Is Human: Building a Safer Health System*, which called on health care systems to reduce medical errors and improve patient safety. The American Hospital Association and the Joint Commission released similar reports in 2002. In 1998, the Pew Health Professions Commission called for new ways of educating future health professions. In 2002, the Robert Wood Johnson Foundation called for developing new practice models and enhancing collaboration between education and practice, and in 2003, the Institute of Medicine released its set of five core competencies that all clinicians should possess, regardless of their discipline, to meet the needs of patients in the 21st-century health care system.

Furthermore, several studies have demonstrated that more nurses educated at baccalaureate or higher levels produced better patient outcomes, specifically, reduced mortality and failure-to-rescue rates. Although there is ample evidence for the need to produce many more nurses to meet the pressing health care needs of society, this is not just a matter of increasing the number of nurses in the workforce. The nursing profession must also produce more skilled and competent graduates who can more effectively lead the care of patients who have much more complex and critical needs.

EVOLUTION OF THE CLINICAL NURSE LEADER'S (CNL) ROLE

To evolve the way nursing care is provided and the way nurses are educated for contemporary practice, the clinical nurse leader (CNL), the first master's-prepared new role for nursing in 35 years, was developed by the American Association of Colleges of Nursing in collaboration with leaders from the education and practice arenas. American Association of Colleges of Nursing is advancing the role to improve the quality of patient care and to better prepare nurses to thrive in the health care system. The CNL role emerged following research and discussion with stakeholder groups inside and outside nursing as a way to engage highly skilled clinicians in outcomes-based practice and quality improvement.

In practice, the CNL oversees the care coordination of a distinct group of patients and may actively provide direct patient care in complex situations. This master's degree–prepared clinician puts evidence-based practice into action to ensure that patients benefit from the latest innovations in care delivery. The CNL evaluates patient outcomes, assesses cohort risk, oversees transitions of care, and has the decision-making authority to change care plans if necessary. The CNL is a leader and lateral integrator of care in any health care setting; however, the implementation of this role varies depending on the type of setting and patient population.

Currently, there are more than 110 schools of nursing partnering with more than 200 health care practice settings to implement the CNL initiative. These partnerships span 38 states and Puerto Rico. The Department of Veterans Affairs has set 2016 as the target date for implementation of the CNL in all of its health care facilities. The success of CNL partnerships hinges on having academia and practice working together to design and implement the CNL education program and to integrate this new role within the health care delivery model.

Evidence from the early adopters of the CNL has shown tremendous cost and quality benefits in a variety of settings. These early outcomes include decreased readmission rates, patient falls, postsurgical infection rates, pressure ulcers, ventilator-acquired pneumonia, and nursing turnover, in addition to increased nurse and physician satisfaction.

CNL CERTIFICATION

The Commission on Nurse Certification (CNC) offers the only professional certification for graduates of the CNL master's or post-master's degree programs. As of September 2011, more than 1,600 CNLs have been certified nationwide. Only individuals who successfully pass the national certification examination may use the CNL title or credential. Additional information on CNL certification can be found at www. aacn.nche.edu/CNC.

CNLA MEMBERSHIP ORGANIZATION

CNL graduates have created a membership organization, the Clinical Nurse Leader Association (CNLA), which currently has 260 members. The purpose of the CNLA is to provide a national forum for CNLs to support, collaborate, and celebrate this unique and evolving role in all practice settings. Additional information regarding this new and growing membership organization can be found at www.cnlassociation.org.

See also American Association of Colleges of Nursing

A regularly updated bibliography on the CNL can be found at http://www.aacn.nche.edu/cnl/pdf/cnlbib.pdf

Additional Resources on the CNL for Educators, Nursing and Healthcare Administrators, Clinicians, and Consumers.

Detailed information regarding the CNL role, FAQs, presentations, publications, and education programs can be found at http://www.aacn.nche.edu/cnl/index.htm

The *CNL White Paper* (http://www.aacn.nche.edu/Publications/WhitePapers/ClinicalNurseLeader.htm) outlines the background, role, expected competencies, and CNL curriculum

Joan M. Stanley

CLINICAL SIMULATION

Nurses have been using different types of simulators for half a century. Two of the most common are models, which have been used to practice intravenous line placement, and mannequins, which have used in cardiopulmonary resuscitation. Simulation is now being widely incorporated as a teaching method in nursing school curricula as well as the education and training of employed nurses and other clinicians in practice. This new approach includes the use of prepared scenarios with simulators that allow learners to respond to a variety of patient care situations and presentations, for example, cardiac arrest, shock, ventricular tachycardia, and diabetic coma. The use of simulation is also a means to develop and enhance teamwork and team communication, increase confidence, and gain acumen in addressing complex situations.

Gaba (2004) states that simulation is a technique to substitute real experiences with guided ones. Improving the way nurses are educated has the potential to enhance the provision of safe clinical care for patients. For example, it has often been a challenge to effectively teach nurses to think critically. The use of simulation training exposes nurses to situations that they

C

may not have previously experienced and assists them to think critically (Durham & Alden, n.d.). Using simulation as part of a student nurse's clinical education creates a safe environment in which the student can make mistakes, learn from them, and build self-confidence (Ryan et al., 2010). One of the most important aspects of simulation, debriefing, follows this scenario (Laster, 2007). The facilitator of the simulation becomes a crucial part of the debriefing and, through debriefing, guides the learners to think critically (Laster, 2007).

The shortage of nurse faculty has added to the challenge of being able to prepare students for the realities of beginning their nursing practice (Jeffries, 2005). Each organization that employs nurses may wish to weigh the costs and benefits of implementing the use of simulation to help support a nurse's entry into practice. In preparation for using this approach, facilitators will have to be specifically taught to incorporate simulation in the education of student nurses as well as employees in various clinical settings.

There is a current and future need for research in many areas of simulation use, including determining whether the use of simulation is beneficial from a learning perspective. It will also be necessary to establish if simulation is a method that can extend and enhance the role of nurse faculty during a period of faculty shortage. Cost–benefit analysis of using simulation is another area that requires examination. There are many unknown challenges as well. One thing is clear, there is a significant and growing role for simulation in preparing clinicians for practice.

Durham, C. F., & Alden, K. R. (n.d.). Enhancing patient safety in nursing education through patient simulation. *Patient safety and quality: An evidence-based handbook for nurses* (pp. 3-221–3–260). Retrieved from www.ncbi. nlm.nih.gov

Gaba, D. M. (2004). The future vision of simulation in health care. *Quality and Safety in Health Care, J3*(Suppl. I), i2–i10. doi: 10.1136/qshc.2004.009878

Jeffries, P. R. (2005). A framework for designing, implementing, and evaluating simulations used as teaching strategies in nursing. *Nursing Education Perspectives, 26*(2), 96–103. Retrieved from www.ncbi.nlm.nih.gov

Laster, K. (2007). High-fidelity simulation and the judgment: Student's experiences. *Journal of Nursing Education, 46*(6), 269–276. Retrieved from www.joumalofnursingeducation.com

Ryan, C. A., Walshe, N., Gaffney, R., Shanks, A., Burgoyne, L., & Wiskin, C. M. (2010). *Using standardized patients to assess communication skills in medical and nursing students.* Retrieved from http://www.biomedcentral.coml1472–6920/10/24

Joyce Johnston

COACHING NURSES

Coaching creates an environment, through conversation, inquiry, and a way of being, that facilitates the coachee to move toward the desired goals in a fulfilling way (Moore & Tschannen-Moran, 2010). When those goals are concerned with improving the nursing practice or building ones' nursing career, coaching becomes a key skill set for the nurse leader. Nursing, for the most part, has been so consumed with the single topic of how humans respond to illness that we have neglected the science of happiness and what makes people find meaning and fulfillment in their lives. Most nurses spend the majority of their lives working and interacting with others, with little apprenticeship in the art and science of conversation. Nurse leaders who are well acquainted in diseases of the mind, body, and subsequent human response to such assaults, can apply the coaching model as they lead nurses. As growth and positive development are essential goals for all nurses, leaders must cultivate nurses to become more thoughtful, reflective, mature, creative, and resourceful clinicians who are able to self-manage. Positivity, grounded in coaching not only has a grand purpose in our evolution, but also it makes a more productive workforce because a fulfilled workforce experiences diseases and disability to a lesser extent than those who dislike their work (Csikszentmihalyi, 1990; Fredrickson, 2009).

The coaching model involves two components, creating awareness and moving to action. We create awareness by asking powerful questions or identifying their inner critic (Whitworth, Kimsey-House, Kimsey-House, & Sandahl, 2007). This involves an evocative, more than didactic approach, an emphasis on listening rather than talking, more asking then telling, and more reflecting than commenting. Familiarity with the Prochaska cycle of change will help the nurse leader identify where the nurse is in the cycle of change. It is within this cycle of change context that the highest degree of self-efficacy can be reached. If a nurse is resistant about some needed change, it is important for leaders to move away from correction to connection. That is, the more we seek to correct people, the more they resist. The more we claim to know, the more resistance is provoked. Making the relationship field between coach and coachee as safe and interesting as possible is the key to the opening up new possibilities and promoting change in nurses. A number of coaching tools bring out nurses' core strengths and authenticity and are essential in creating a team of fulfilled nurses who describe their work as meaningful.

Leadership presence. A nurse leader is responsible for developing nurses by ensuring that they are in a growth mindset. Nursing presence will foster an open

dialogue for coaching to occur, which includes suspending judgment and having unconditional positive regard for the person being coached. This creates an environment in which the nurse leader can uncover the heart of the matter, to identify what is really going on, behind the story, issue, conflict, or poor performance.

Acknowledging. As a leader, it is important to acknowledge the coachees by really seeing who they are and by noticing their core strengths. This includes making sure the role and the work the nurse is doing is large enough for them to grow. Acknowledging nurses for who they are *being* and not what they are *doing* strengthens the nurse's foundation. It recognizes the inner character of the person who is being acknowledged, and is very different from praise or complements, which highlights only their outcomes and relies on the opinions of others. Acknowledging highlights deep values held by the coachee and it is usually an honor to hear. It is important in the coaching context because the nurse leader is acknowledging who the nurse must be in order to make the changes they want. For example, they may have had to be courageous or stand up to fear or show a great degree of tenacity, or determination, or an enormous degree of compassion or creativity (Whitworth et al., 2009). The nurse's way of being and noticing their core strengths, and not necessarily the outcome, is a key coaching strategy.

Level III listening. Everything in a coaching relationship hinges on the leaders' mastery of listening skills. Level III listening involves listening with all of our senses as well as to what is not being said. It involves relying on intuition, and using information that is not directly observable. You may notice the changes in their voice, which reflects changes in their emotions. Once you share your intuition, you observe how the intuition "lands" with the coachee.

Knowing what the nurses' core strengths are as well as what he or she wants in his or her future, along with Level III listening, gives the nurse leader an enormous amount of information (Whitworth et al., 2009). To be really listened to is an astonishing experience and is remarkably rare. Level III listening is a skill that must be developed by nurse leaders, so that the nurses can expand their awareness.

Asking powerful questions. Coach leaders must approach nurses with curiosity, expressed as a question rather than a demand. At the foundation of good coaching is the nurse leader's ability to ask powerful questions, which invites the nurse to be more introspective and to look at a huge range of possibilities with creativity and insight. For example, "When a family situation in the ICU begins to escalate, what can we do to consistently diffuse it or provide comfort to them?" is a powerful question, whereas "Why is it that every week, I am called in to an out-of-control family when you are on duty?" The powerful question invites the nurse to reflect and look into the future, whereas the latter question is blaming and likely to shut down possibilities and force the nurse to defend herself.

Celebrating failure. A prominent part of executing large ideas and a huge obstacle for nurses in taking more leadership is the nurse's pervasive fear of failure. Failure is a tool that accelerates learning, as any toddler learning to walk falls, they may fail at walking but they are not failures. For nurses to make significant changes, they will need to step to the edge of their capability or ability, irrespective of the nurse that failed or did not go far enough, the learning that occurs from failures is enormous. A nurse leader can mine these highly valuable lessons gleaned from disappointment, bringing the core strengths of the individual to the fore, and ensure that the nurse's authenticity is maintained and strengths are intensified.

Csikszentmihalyi, M. (1990). *Flow.* New York, NY. Harper-Perennial.

Fredrickson, B.L. (2009). *Positivity.* New York, NY: Crown Publishing Group.

Moore, M., & Tschannen-Moran, B. (2010). *Coaching psychology manual.* Baltimore, MD: Lippincott, Williams and Wilkins.

Whitworth, L., Kimsey-House, K., Kimsey-House, H., & Sandahl, P. (2009). *Co-active coaching: New skills for coaching people toward success in work and life* (2nd ed.). Boston, MA: Davies-Black.

Eileen T. O'Grady

COLLECTIVE BARGAINING AND UNIONS

Staff nurses in many hospitals have been organizing themselves into unions since World War II. In the 1940s, nurses in New York, California, Pennsylvania, and Ohio formed nursing unions. In 1946, with urging from state nurses' associations representing nurses for collective bargaining, the American Nurses Association started its national economic security program (Foley, 2002). In 1999, the American Nurses Association formed an independent affiliate known as the United American Nurses, which was also a member of the AFL-CIO; this relationship ended in 2008 when five of the major state nurses' associations, representing approximately 75,000 registered nurses, left the United American Nurses to form the National Federation of Nurses (2009). In 2010, approximately 15% of all registered nurses (3.1 million) in the United States were represented by unions. They may be represented by nurses' unions (New York State Nurses Association,

California Nurses Association, Oregon Nurses Association, and Washington State Nurses Association) traditional labor organizations (United Steel Workers [USW], CSEA, and Service Employees International Union [SEIU]), or independent unions.

The National Labor Relations Act governs proprietary and not-for-profit health care facilities. Some states have additional laws that govern employee relations in public health care facilities. The Fair Labor Standards Act sets minimum wages, overtime rules, and workweek hours. The Equal Pay Act of 1963 addresses wage disparities based on sex, whereas the Equal Employment Opportunity Act (1972) prohibits discrimination on the basis of age, race, color, religion, sex, or national origin. The Americans with Disabilities Act (1990) prohibits discrimination against an otherwise qualified individual by reason of a physical or mental disability and requires that the employer bring the physical environment into compliance with the requirements of the Americans with Disabilities Act.

Employee rights include the right to organize and bargain collectively, solicit and distribute union information during nonworking hours, picket and strike, grieve and arbitrate issues, be free from termination unless there is "just cause," and negotiate benefits and conditions of employment. Management rights include the right to a 10-day advanced notice of a bargaining unit's intention to strike, picket, or engage in other concerted work activity; hire replacement workers in the event of a strike; prohibit employees from engaging in union activity during working hours; reasonably restrict union organizers to certain locations and time periods to avoid interference with facility operations; and prohibit supervisors from participating in union activity.

See also Americans with Disabilities Act

Foley, M. F. (2006). Collective action in the workplace. In D. Mason, J. Leavitt, & W. Chaffee (Eds.), *Policy and politics in nursing and health care* (4th ed., pp. 387–397). Philadelphia, PA: W.B. Saunders.

National Federation of Nurses. (2009, April 15). *Coalition of state nursing associations announce an innovative new national nurses union: The National Federation of Nurses.* Retrieved January 22, 2011, from http://www.nfn.org/media/A-NEW-DAY-FOR-NURSING.pdf

Karen A. Ballard

COMMISSION ON COLLEGIATE NURSING EDUCATION

The Commission on Collegiate Nursing Education (CCNE) is a nationally recognized accrediting organization for baccalaureate, graduate, and residency programs in nursing. Established in 1996, CCNE is the autonomous accrediting arm of the American Association of Colleges of Nursing—the national voice for baccalaureate and graduate degree nursing education programs since 1969 (www.aacn.nche.edu/Accreditation/index.htm). CCNE is formally recognized by the U.S. Secretary of Education and serves the public interest by assessing and identifying programs that engage in effective educational practices. With a national scope, CCNE accredits nursing programs in 49 states, the District of Columbia, and the Commonwealth of Puerto Rico. For a complete listing of CCNE-accredited baccalaureate and graduate nursing programs, go to the CCNE Web site: www.aacn.nche.edu/CCNE/reports/accprog.asp. For a complete listing of CCNE-accredited post-baccalaureate nurse residency programs programs, go to the CCNE Web site: www.aacn.nche.edu/CCNE/reports_residency/resaccprog.asp.

C

Within the higher education arena, CCNE's scope of review includes baccalaureate degree nursing programs, master's degree nursing programs, and professional doctorates with the title, "Doctor of Nursing Practice." These programs must be offered by an institution of higher education that is accredited by an organization recognized by the U.S. Secretary of Education. In the practice setting, CCNE evaluates post-baccalaureate nurse residency programs offered by an acute care hospital that is accredited by a nationally recognized accrediting agency.

CCNE is governed by a 13-member Board of Commissioners that includes chief nurse administrators (e.g., deans and directors), nursing faculty, practicing nurses, professional consumers, and public consumers. The work of CCNE is supported by a professional and administrative staff, nearly 800 volunteer evaluators who are trained by the organization to serve as peer reviewers in the accreditation process, and several committees. For educational programs, CCNE accreditation is conferred for up to 5 years for new programs and for up to 10 years for programs pursuing continuing accreditation. Nurse residency programs are eligible for an accreditation term of up to 5 years. Programs are evaluated against a set of established standards during a comprehensive on-site evaluation. A systematic monitoring process ensures that a program's compliance with the standards continues between evaluations. This process includes submission of annual reports, continuous improvement progress reports, substantive change notifications when warranted, and special reports on areas of noncompliance. CCNE accreditation activities are designed to reflect good accreditation practices and are premised on a statement of principles or values that are published by the organization. CCNE is a member of the Association of Specialized and Professional Accreditors—an organization that supports the community of U.S. agencies that assess the quality of specialized and professional higher education programs and schools.

American Association of Colleges of Nursing, http://www.aacn.nche.edu/Accreditation/index.htm

Jennifer Butlin

COMMUNITY ENGAGEMENT

Community engagement is defined as the process of working collaboratively with and through groups of people affiliated by geographic proximity, special interest, or similar situations to address issues affecting the well-being of those people (Centers for Disease Control/Agency for Toxic Substances as a Disease Registry, 2011). It is the "collaboration between institutions and their larger communities (local, regional/state, national, and global) for the mutually beneficial exchange of knowledge and resources in the context of partnership and reciprocity" (Carnegie Foundation for the Advancement of Teaching, 2011).

Community engagement requires power sharing, maintenance of equity, and flexibility in pursuing goals, methods, and time frames to fit the priorities, needs, and capacities within the cultural context of communities (Jones & Wells, 2007). It is operationalized through partnerships, collaboratives, and coalitions that help mobilize resources and influence systems, change relationships among partners, and serve as catalysts for changing policies, programs, and practices (Fawcett et al., 1995). Strategies for community engagement include community partnerships, service learning, community-based participatory research, community-engaged scholarship, training and technical assistance, and capacity building.

Historically in nursing, the spirit of community engagement is embodied in the works of Florence Nightingale, Clara Barton, Lillian Wald, and other nurse pioneers who responded to societal needs during periods of social change; their work exemplified the nursing profession's contract with society in the attainment of health (Kelley, Connor, Kun, & Salmon, 2008). In the last decade, nursing and health professions have increasingly enacted community engagement as a key strategy to improve health status and health education in communities, to increase the diversity of the health care workforce, and to reduce health disparities.

Consistent with Boyer's (1996) challenge to establish a broader framework that integrates engagement and academic scholarship, nursing schools have developed mutually beneficial partnerships with communities that enhance the translation of knowledge into practice and create opportunities for learning and scholarship for faculty, students, and community partners. Echoing Boyer (1996), Duke and Moss (2009, p. 39) assert that "nursing scholarship and schools of nursing cannot afford to remain islands of disengaged teaching and research in seas of ever increasing health inequalities and disparities."

With growing recognition addressing the health care needs of underserved communities experiencing health disparities requires community engagement, the conduct of nursing research has to be "with" rather than "to" the community (Bringle, Games, & Malloy, 1999) and involve the community in collaborative formulation of research questions and identification of appropriate research procedures as well as collaborative data collection, analysis, and dissemination (Duke & Moss, 2009). For nursing and health professions schools, the Commission on Community-Engaged Scholarship in the Health Professions (2005) set forth nine recommendations, including recruitment and retention of community-engaged faculty, the increased extramural support for community-engaged scholarship, and the adoption of promotion and tenure policies and procedures that value community-engaged scholarship, among others.

The implementation of community engagement through service-learning has been found to significantly increase nursing students' understanding of their role as community resources and enhance their knowledge of needs and barriers encountered by communities (Narsavage et al., 2002). Community engagement has been successfully used in health education and outreach to immigrant (Meade, Menard, Thervil, & Rivera, 2009) and marginalized communities (Ramal, 2009) and the identification and management of individuals and groups at risk for cardiovascular disease (Capper, 2009). Future research is promising about the effect of engagement on the health of communities and nursing.

Boyer, E. (1996). The scholarship of engagement. *Journal of Public Service and Outreach, 1*(1), 1–20.

Bringle, R., Games, R., & Malloy, E. (Eds.). (1999). *Colleges and universities as citizens.* Boston, MA: Allyn & Bacon.

Capper, G. (2009). Community engagement for health improvement. *British Journal of Cardiac Nursing, 4*(3), 103–106.

Carnegie Foundation for the Advancement of Teaching. (2011). *Community engagement elective classification.* Retrieved May 2, 2011, from http://classifications.carnegiefoundation.org/descriptions/community_engagement.php

Centers for Disease Control/Agency for Toxic Substances as a Disease Registry. (2011). Community engagement: Definitions and organizing concepts from the literature.

C

C

Retrieved May 2, 2011, from http://www.cdc.gov/phppo/pce/part1.htm

Commission on Community-Engaged Scholarship in the Health Professions. (2005). *Linking scholarship and communities: Executive summary*. Seattle, WA: Community-Campus Partnership for Health.

Duke, J., & Moss, C. (2009). Re-visiting scholarly community engagement in the contemporary research assessment environments of Australasian universities. *Contemporary Nurse, 32*(1–2), 30–41.

Fawcett, S. B., Paine-Andrews, A., Francisco, V. T., Schultz, J. A., Richter, K. P., Lewis, R. K., et al. (1995). Using empowerment theory in collaborative partnerships for community health and development. *American Journal of Community Psychology, 23*, 677–697.

Jones, L., & Wells, K. (2007). Strategies for academic and clinician engagement in community-participatory partnered research. *Journal of the American Medical Association, 297*, 407–410.

Kelley, M. A., Connor, A., Kun, K. E., & Salmon, M. E. (2008). Social responsibility: Conceptualization and embodiment in a school of nursing. *International Journal of Nursing Scholarship, 5*(1), 1–16.

Meade, C. D., Menard, J., Thervil, C., & Rivera, M. (2009). Addressing cancer disparities through community engagement: Improving breast health among Haitian women. *Oncology Nursing Forum, 36*(6), 716–722.

Narsavage, G. L., Lindell, D., Chen, Y. J., Savrin, C., & Duffy, E. (2002). A community engagement initiative: Service-learning in graduate nursing education. *Journal of Nursing Education, 41*(10), 457–461.

Ramal, E. (2009). Integrating caring, scholarship, and community engagement in Mexico. *Nurse Educator, 34*(1), 34–37.

Divina Grossman

COMPLEX ADAPTIVE SYSTEMS (CHAOS THEORY)

In 2001, the Institute of Medicine (IOM) published the second in a series of reports on the quality of health care in America. The committee's first report, *To Err Is Human: Building a Safer Health System*, focused on patient safety as a systems issue that needs attention. However, patient safety is embedded in a context of complexity. *Crossing the Quality Chasm*, the second IOM report, focused on the need to redesign health care systems to foster innovation and to improve care. Quality was defined as a system property, and the IOM established an agenda for change that intends to recast and recraft the American health care system for the 21st century. Zimmerman, Lindberg, and Plsek (2001), in an appendix to the *Crossing the Quality Chasm* report, suggest that the redesign of the health care system for the 21st century may well be strategically accomplished through the use of complex adaptive systems thinking. The redesign of health care through complexity science-inspired innovations is an interesting and useful theoretical framework.

Complex adaptive systems consist of context-sensitive adaptable elements, which respond to simple rules. The emergent evolutions of complex systems reveal that they are nonlinear and support emergence through novel behavior, which is nonpredictable yet inherently orderly. Complexity science provides a new paradigm to guide systems design and suggests a series of questions to consider when confronted with wicked and sticky problems. In 2008, the first book devoted to complexity science applictions to nursing was published (Lindberg, Nash, & Lindberg, 2008). To learn more about complexity science, visit the Plexus Institute (http://www.plexusinstitute.com) and the nursing learning network information on the Plexus Web site (http://www.plexusinstitute.org/complexity/index.cfm?id=2). The mission of this not-for-profit organization is to foster the health of individuals, families, communities, organizations, and our natural environment by helping people through the new science of complexity. Plexus offers a complexity science primer for those new to the concepts and science (http://www.plexusinstitute.com/services/E-Library/show.cfm?id=150).

Institute of Medicine. (2001). *Crossing the quality chasm: A new health system for the 21st century.* Washington, DC: National Academies Press.

Lindberg, C., Nash, S., & Lindberg, C. (2008). *On the edge: Nursing in the age of complexity.* Borden Town, NJ: Plexus Institute.

Zimmerman, B., Lindberg, C., & Plsek, P. (2001). *Edgeware insights from complexity science for health care leaders.* Irving, TX: Voluntary Hospital Association.

Daniel J. Pesut

COMPLEXITY SCIENCE AND NURSING

Complexity science is the culmination of the advance of science over the past three centuries; an advance focused on five major developments in the effort to discover the "truth" about nature. First, nature was interpreted as law-governed processes that could be understood in terms of objective *mechanical causality.* Second, Einstein's discovery of the *theory of relativity* dealt "…with the issue of how phenomena appear different to observers moving at different speeds" (Peat, 2002, p. 4) with no absolutes and no preferred viewpoint. The laws of nature that underlie relative appearances were to be unified into a four-dimensional background called space–time (Peat, 2002). The third advance in science came with the development of *quantum mechanics,* which revealed a physical reality that is holistic: the universe as indivisible, interconnected and relational—where the observer is not separated from the observed. In the quantum realm, particles are governed by the principles of coordination between elements that result in correlated order extending over time and space. The fourth advance came in the 1960s and 1970s, with the realization that the laws governing the motion of the planets and the dynamics of the weather and other phenomena include what is called *deterministic chaos* (communicative reciprocity between disorder and order or how order unfolds as self-organizing through turbulence in systems). The fifth development was the emergence of *complexity theory* in the 1980s and 1990s, portraying dynamical relational system patterning, which extends from physics to biology, economics, organizational science, social sciences, and health sciences, including nursing (Briggs & Peat, 1989; Davidson, Ray, & Turkel, 2011; Goodwin, 2003; Peat, 2002; Smith, 2011; Wheatley, 2006).

Complexity science examines complex systems that are defined as those made up of many diverse elements that interact within networks of relationship; it seeks to discover and understand the dynamics, principles, and rules that affect how such systems evolve and maintain order (Lindberg, Nash, & Lindberg, 2008). Thus, complexity science "…studies how relationships [and choice] between parts cause the collective behaviors of a system and how the system interacts and forms relationships with its environment" (Bar-Yam, 2004, p. 24).

Nursing is a holistic, relationship-centered discipline focused on human caring and leadership in the human health experience (Smith, 2011). From a complex systems perspective, nursing was ahead of its time. Although there are many nursing philosophers and theorists who began to understand nursing as complex and as an integrated science and art, it was Florence Nightingale's (1859/1992) theory in 1859 that first identified the importance of the human–environment relationship and the role that nature played in health, healing, and well-being.

In 1970, Rogers advanced the Science of Unitary Human Beings, a conceptual system that illuminated the concept of the irreducible whole and the unitary and integral nature of the human–environment process as an open system and energy field patterning (Smith, 2011). Rogers postulated and defined the principles of resonancy, helicy, and integrality as central to unitary nursing science. Resonance is a continuous change in wave patterns in human and environmental fields, helicy is the increasing diversity and unpredictability of human and environmental field patterns, and integrality is the continuous mutual human and environmental field processes (Rogers, 1990).

At the same time that many nursing theorists began to appreciate the unitary or holistic features of Rogers's thought, they also began to appreciate the meaning of nursing as caring in the human health experience, a complex process of seeking to understand the role of nursing as a moral ideal for the "…protection, enhancement, and preservation of the person's humanity which helps to restore inner harmony and potential healing" (Watson, 1985, p. 58). Caring is also a transcultural, ethical, and spiritual way of being, knowing, and doing, a caritas or loving process (Leininger, 1981; Ray, 2010; Watson, 2005, 2008) that illuminates the dynamic caring patterns of relationship (commitment, compassion, conscience, competence, confidence, and comportment—the six Cs of Roach, 1987/2002).

These phenomena are continuously evolving and emerging as nurses seek deeper understanding of the meaning of health, healing, well-being within their role as leaders within complex health care organizations (see theorists' views in Alligood & Marriner Tomey, 2010; Davidson et al., 2011; Ray, 2010; Parker & Smith, 2010). The study and practice of caring gives nurses insights into the holistic nature and natural creativity of the human–environment relationship and encourages them to be mindful of the quality (the choice-making capacity) of their interactions. As leaders in patient care and organizational change, nurses must understand health care organizations as *living systems* because moral and spiritual communities where the choices that are made affect the lives of so many. The continued study of nursing as a complex, holistic, and creative caring science and art will facilitate the clarification of the complex issues facing individuals, families, communities, ecosystems, organizations, and global relationships.

Alligood, M., & Marriner Tomey, A. (2010). *Nursing theorists and their work.* St. Louis, MO: Mosby/Elsevier.

Bar-Yam, Y. (2004). *Making things work: Solving complex problems in a complex world.* Boston, MA: NECSI, Knowledge Press.

Briggs, J., & Peat, F. (1989). *Turbulent mirror: An illustrated guide to chaos theory and the science of wholeness.* New York, NY: Harper & Row, Publishers.

Davidson, A., Ray, M., & Turkel, M. (Eds.). (2011). *Nursing, caring, and complexity science: For human–environment well-being.* New York, NY: Springer Publishing Company.

Goodwin, B. (2003). Patterns of wholeness: Holistic science. *Resurgence, 1*(216), 12–14.

Leininger, M. (Ed.). (1981). *Caring: An essential human need.* Thorofare, NJ: Charles B. Slack, Inc.

Lindberg, C., Nash, S., & Lindberg, C. (2008). *On the edge: Nursing in the age of complexity.* Bordentown, NJ: Plexus Press.

Nightingale, F. (1992). *Notes on nursing: What it is and what it is not.* Philadelphia, PA: J. B. Lippincott Company. (Original work published in 1859).

Parker, M., & Smith, M. (Eds.). (2010). *Nursing theories & nursing practice* (3rd ed.). Philadelphia, PA: F. A. Davis Company.

Peat, F. (2002). *From certainty to uncertainty: The story of science and ideas in the twentieth century.* Washington, DC: Joseph Henry Press.

Ray, M. (2010). *Transcultural caring dynamics in nursing and health care.* Philadelphia, PA: F. A. Davis Company.

Roach, M. (2002). *Caring, the human mode of being* (2nd rev. ed.). Ottawa: Canadian Hospital Association. (First edition published in 1987)

Rogers, M. (1970). *An introduction to the theoretical basis of nursing.* Philadelphia, PA: F. A. Davis Company.

Rogers, M. (1990). Nursing: Science of unitary, irreducible human beings: Update 1990. In E. Barrett (Ed.). *Visions of Rogers' science-based nursing* (pp. 5–11). New York, NY: National League for Nursing Press.

Smith, M. (2011). Philosophical and theoretical perspectives related to complexity science in nursing. In A. Davidson, M. Ray, & M. Turkel (Eds.), *Nursing, caring, and complexity science: For human–environment well-being.* New York, NY: Springer Publishing Company.

Watson, J. (1985). *Nursing: Human science and human care: A theory of nursing.* Norwalk, CT: Appleton-Century-Crofts.

Watson, J. (2005). *Caring science as sacred science.* Philadelphia, PA: F. A. Davis Company.

Watson, J. (2008). *Nursing: The philosophy and science of caring* (rev. ed.). Boulder, CO: University Press of Colorado. (Original work published 1979).

Wheatley, M. (2006). *Leadership and the new science* (3rd ed.). San Francisco, CA: Berrett-Koehler Publishers, Inc.

Marilyn A. Ray
Marian C. Turkel

CONFLICT MANAGEMENT

Conflict management is a comprehensive term indicating the range of attitudes and behaviors individuals, groups, and organizations manifest in dealing with conflict.

Like conflict, conflict management is always present and can range from denial, suppression, and retaliation to creative proactive programs. The field of endeavor focused on constructive approaches to conflict management, alternative dispute resolution (ADR), provides an array of processes designed to achieve that goal, negotiation, mediation, and arbitration being the most familiar to health care providers. It also has steadily built a body of literature documenting best practices and empirical findings to guide both students and practitioners of ADR (Gerardi, 2010; Kritek, 2005).

The field of ADR came of age in the 1990s and permeates all sectors of the United States, primarily through mediation programs and policies. ADR practitioners considered health care the "last frontier," persistently resistant to self-examination and action that might enhance existing conflict management practices. Robson and Morrison (2003) posit several reasons for this resistance: health care environments are complex adaptive systems, have widespread inequalities and imbalances in power, include numerous subcultures with significant variance, and have difficulty determining who should be assured a "seat at the table." Historically, health care relied on litigation and has a pattern of conflict aversiveness, avoidance, suppression, and blame.

This historical resistance to ADR is undergoing a rapid shift throughout health care because of the convergence of an array of forces. The restructuring of health care organizations during the 1990s, with both significant reductions in the numbers of nurses in acute care settings coupled with shortened length of stay that increased patient acuity occurred concurrent with increased emphasis on patient safety. These countervailing forces culminated in the report of the Institute of Medicine

C

(IOM), *To Err Is Human: Building a Safer Health Care System* (IOM,1999), documenting the magnitude and severity of preventable medical errors (adverse events). This further catalyzed the patient safety movement, including the creation of patient safety organizations that generated substantial data sets, documenting that problematic relationships among providers was a primary causal factor in adverse events (Kritek, 2012).

Rather abruptly, health care professionals were confronted with overwhelming evidence that moved constructive conflict management from a desired and worthy aspiration to a necessity for patient care safety and quality. The Joint Commission reinforced this shift through the introduction of several standards and sentinel event alerts focused on conflict and communication. These created accreditation expectations, many taking effect in 2009, well before the health care community had prepared for them. The desire for a quick and easy "fix" to address the conflicts that shape health care environments continues; its likelihood of success is questionable.

Professional nursing plays a unique role in this unfolding drama. As noted in the IOM report *Keeping Patients Safe: Transforming the Work Environment of Nurses*, nurses integrate patient care requiring communication and coordination with an array of diverse health care workers (IOM, 2004). This increases both the possibility of conflict and the opportunity to craft enhanced collaborative relationships. The educational preparation of nurses emphasizing relationship-based care and effective communication ensures basic conflict skills, although nursing has not yet focused systematically on the more sophisticated and nuanced training nurses need to become conflict competent.

The Thomas–Kilmann Conflict Mode Instrument, used extensively in ADR research, identifies five potential responses to conflict: avoidance, compromise, accommodation, competition, and collaboration, each appropriate given specific situational factors (Thomas & Kilmann, 2004). All have identifiable costs and benefits, although collaboration is the only mode that demonstrates both high cooperativeness and assertiveness and provides a long-term solution to a conflict. Valentine (2001) analyzed studies conducted on nurses using the Thomas–Kilmann Conflict Mode Instrument, reporting that the nurses' preferred response was avoidance, followed by compromise and accommodation. It is perhaps noteworthy that each of these styles offers short-term solutions and to some degree disadvantages persons using them. These findings contrast with the ethical stance taken in the American Nurses Association (2001) Code of Ethics, which requires that nurses pursue conflict resolution, and links this commitment to patient advocacy and the fundamental values of the profession. The code also supports several ethical stances that nurses must take that will obviously evoke conflict. Conflict competence is prescribed, although without provision for the prerequisite training, which has often been superficial, cursory, aspirational, and prescriptive.

Nurses and their health care colleagues are, however, advantaged in exploring ADR at a time when a robust body of ADR literature exists to guide this exploration (Gerardi, 2005). Conflicts in health care once focused on select individuals can be traced, through careful conflict analysis, to unveil system problems that create the conditions for the conflict and can more appropriately be addressed at the system level. Policy statements as attempted conflict interventions can be revealed as inadequate to the challenge. Interest-based conflict models, incongruent with health care professionals' values and practices, can be replaced by the ADR field's emergent relationship-based value congruent models (Scott & Gerardi, 2011a). The ADR field is also exploring the concept of "conflict engagement" (Mayer, 2004), which de-emphasizes conflict resolution and shifts the focus to competent engagement: a blueprint for collaboration. Professional nursing has always endorsed and supported collaboration; conflict engagement competencies provide the tools to do so successfully.

Some responses to the shift are already apparent, framed by farsighted nurse leaders, frontrunners with imagination. The American Association of Critical Care Nurses (2005) sponsored the landmark study "Silence Kills," identifying conversations especially difficult for health care professionals and concurrently developed related standards for healthy work environments. The Center for American Nurses conducted a national online survey of nurses and found that 53% of respondents reported that conflict while on the job was "common"; they initiated an introductory program on bullying with useful resources about conflict engagement. The American Organization of Nurse Executives Nurse Manager Fellowship Program has integrated conflict engagement training into its program, and the American Nurses Credentialing Center's program "Pathways to Excellence" requires its participants have ADR mechanisms in place.

Although these "first steps" are both proactive and encouraging, nursing will require a much more substantive investment in conflict competence for all nurses and nursing students. An emergent "community of practice" of ADR in health care has already identified the parameters and best practices for that investment (Gerardi, 2010). Most recently, the Joint Commission leadership standards focused on conflict have encouraged the use of Dispute System Design programs that integrate conflict management's proactive efforts into organizational strategic planning (Scott & Gerardi, 2011a, 2011b). Nurse leaders are uniquely positioned to play a key role in such efforts. The more sophisticated their levels of conflict competence mastery, the more impact they will have on this next step in creative conflict management.

Gerardi, D. (2005). The culture of health care: How professional and organizational cultures impact conflict management. *Georgia Law Review, 21*(4), 857–890.

Gerardi, D. (2010). *Conflict engagement training for health professionals: Recommendations for creating conflict competent organizations—A white paper for healthcare and dispute resolution professionals.* Retrieved January 11, 2011, from http://www.ehcco.com

Institute of Medicine. (1999). *To err is human: Building a safer health care system.* Washington, DC: National Academies Press.

Institute of Medicine. (2004). *Keeping patients safe: Transforming the work environment of nurses.* Washington, DC: National Academies Press.

Kritek, P. B. (2005). Alternative dispute resolution: A tool for managing conflict. In D. Mason, J.K. Leavitt, & M. W. Chaffee (Eds.). *Policy and politics in nursing and health care* (5th ed.). St Louis, MO: Saunders Elsevier.

Kritek, P. B. (2012). Conflict management in health care: The tipping point arrives. In D. Mason, J.K. Leavitt, & M. W. Chaffee (Eds.). *Policy and politics in nursing and health care* (6th ed). St Louis, MO: Saunders Elsevier.

Mayer, B. (2004). Beyond neutrality: Confronting the crisis in conflict resolution. San Francisco, CA: Jossey-Bass.

Mediate.com—the world's leading mediation Web site that bridges professionals offering mediation services and people seeking mediation services. Retrieved from http://www.mediate.com

Robson, R., & Morrison, G. (2003, Spring). ADR in healthcare: The last big frontier. *ACResolution*, 1–6. Retrieved April 1, 2010 from http://mediate.com/articles/robmorr1.cfm

Scott, C., & Gerardi, D. (2011a). A strategic approach for managing conflict in hospitals: Part 1. Responding to the joint commission leadership standard. *The Joint Commission Journal on Quality and Patient Safety, 37*(2), 59–69.

Scott, C., & Gerardi, D. (2011b). A strategic approach for managing conflict in hospitals: Part 2. Responding to the Joint Commission Leadership Standard. *The Joint Commission Journal on Quality and Patient Safety, 37*(2), 70–80.

Thomas, K. W., & Kilmann, R. H. (2002). *Thomas–Kilmann Conflict Mode Index*. Palo Alto, CA: CPP.

Valentine, P. E. B. (2001). Gender perspective on conflict management strategies of nurses. *Journal of Nursing Scholarship, 30*(2), 69–74.

Additional information is available from the following Web sites:

American Association of Critical-Care Nurses. (2005). *Silence kills: The seven crucial conversations for healthcare*. Final report cosponsored by Vitalsmarts. Retrieved January 7, 2011, from http://www.aacn.org/WD/Practice/Docs/PublicPolicy/SilenceKillsExecSum.pdf

American Nurses Association. (2001). *Code of ethics for nurses with interpretive statements*. Washington, DC. Retrieved February 21, 2011, from www.nursingworld.org/mods/mod580/cecdevers.htm

Association for Conflict Resolution—U.S. major professional organization for ADR scholars and practitioners. Retrieved from http://www.acrnet.org/about/CR-FAQ.htm

Conflict Resolution Information Source—information resource managed by the Conflict Resolution Consortium at the University of Colorado. Retrieved from http://www.crinfo.org

EHCCO LC—Emerging Health Care Communities—a learning community dedicated to the transformation of healthcare organizations, exploring emerging approaches for addressing conflict and building capacity for effective interprofessional engagement; it is the only company of its kind specializing in health care specific programming. Retrieved from http://www.ehcco.org

Phyllis Beck Kritek

CONFLICT OF INTEREST IN RESEARCH

CONFLICT OF INTEREST FOR INDIVIDUAL SCIENTISTS

One of the critical underlying assumptions of science is that researchers conceptualize, implement, and disseminate their research free from bias. Scientists building on and extending others' research must trust that the findings from previous studies are as reflective of actual reality as possible and that neither the data reported nor the interpretations of the data were influenced by outside forces (Pryor, Broome, & Habermann, 2007). A conflict of interest (COI) in research exists "when the individual has interests in the outcome of the research that may lead to personal advantage and that might, therefore, in actuality or appearance, compromise the integrity of the research" (Rubenstein, 2002, p. 38).The National Institutes of Health (NIH) defines COI as "a significant financial interest that could directly and significantly affect the design, conduct, or reporting of NIH funded research" (www.grants.nih.gov/grants/policy/coi). COI has the potential to bias a researchers' conduct of research in a variety of ways (Lo, 2009).

There are several types of situations that can create a COI for an individual scientist. These COIs can include those based on financial interests, competitive goals to be first to discover and report findings, or concurrently held roles such as grant reviewer and grant writer. The most common are financially related conflicts in which an investigator has a financial interest in a source that funds the research itself. This conflict might be present for someone who is a member of a governing board of a company funding the research, an investigator who holds stock in the company that

C

supports the research, or an investigator who is a paid speaker for a company that funds his or her research (Lo, 2009). If successful recruitment of an adequate number of participants is crucial and an investigator has a financial investment that relies on the outcomes of a particular study, many different aspects of a study can be affected. Throughout the research process, from the conceptualization of the problem through the dissemination of findings, a COI on the part of any investigator has the potential to influence:

- how potential participants are recruited (e.g., application of inclusion/exclusion criteria);
- how the informed consent process is implemented (e.g., subtle coercive techniques applied);
- how requests by participants to withdraw from a study are handled;
- how decisions are made about what data represents true outliers;
- which findings are chosen for inclusion (or exclusion) in a report; and
- the timeliness of a published report.

Strategies for managing COIs at the individual level include (1) institutional reviews for potential COIs for investigators and research staff (Federman, Hanna, & Rodriguez, 2003), (2) disallowing individuals who hold significant financial interest in research involving human subjects from conducting the research (Lo, 2009), and (3) promoting disclosure and transparency of financial interests (Lo, 2009; National Institutes of Health, 2011).

CONFLICTS OF INTEREST AT THE INSTITUTIONAL LEVEL

There is a clear expectation that institutions in which research is conducted will provide oversight of scientific activities and researchers by creating an ethical environment that promotes research integrity and discourages scientific misconduct (Lo, 2009; Rubenstein, 2002). Institutional COIs include relationships with agencies or industries that promote a real or perceived impression that could compromise the trust the public places in them as credible sources of information and protection of human subjects.

Every institution should have a written policy and procedures that address COI on both the part of the individual investigator and the institution. This policy should include the following:

- offering educational opportunities to all employees engaged in research about research integrity;
- providing for external review of arrangements or relationships that could represent a potential compromise or COI;
- having procedures to oversee the commitments of those involved in the conduct, design, and review of research, including all levels of personnel such as research assistants, principal investigators, students, and administrators;
- listing acceptable activities and financial relationships and those that require review;
- having a plan to evaluate the ethical climate of the institutional environment and monitor compliance of individuals equitably; and
- implementing procedures that guide investigations of allegations of scientific misconduct or potential COI (Rubenstein, 2002; National Institutes of Health, 2011).

The ethical climate of an institution is thought to be one predictor of the strength of research integrity held by the investigators who conduct science and the administrators and trustees of the organization

C

itself (Gaddis, Healon-Fauth, & Scott, 2003). The development of educational venues and policies and procedures about COI are primary responsibilities of an institution. However, monitoring COI is the responsibility of all individuals involved in research. An ethical climate that promotes research integrity will help assure that the public's trust is maintained in the credibility of research findings and those who conduct research.

Federman, D. D., Hanna, K., & Rodriguez, L. (2003). *Responsible research: A systems approach to protecting research participants*. Washington, DC: National Academies Press.

Gaddis, B., Helton-Fauth, W., & Scott, G. (2003). Development of two measures of climate for scientific organizations. *Accountability in Research, 10*, 253–288.

Lo, B. (2009). *Conflict of interest in medical research, education, and practice*. Washington, DC: Institute of Medicine of the National Academies Press.

National Institutes of Health, Office of Integrity. Retrieved September 12, 2011, from www.nih.gov

Pryor, E.R., Habermann, B., & Broome, M. (2007). Scientific misconduct from the perspective of research coordinators: A national survey. *Journal of Medical Ethics, 33*, 365–369.

Rubenstein, A. (2002). *Integrity in scientific research*. Washington, DC: National Academies Press.

Marion E. Broome

CONSTRUCTIVE FEEDBACK

Feedback is the key to all learning in a practice profession. You learn how to become an expert clinician, teacher, researcher, writer, and/or manager by getting feedback about your strengths and your areas in need of improvement. However, that feedback needs to be constructive to be effective. If feedback is specific, considerate, and does not attribute poor performance to some immutable internal cause, the individual will profit from the criticism (Baron, 1988). Emphasizing improvable performance and incremental development fosters remediation; implying that the person does not have the ability to meet the challenge encourages defensiveness (Nussbaum & Dweck, 2008).

Dweck (2007) has been critical of the prevailing mindset in American society whereby the emphasis is on indiscriminate praise. Wholesale compliments do not necessarily change behavior positively, particularly if the commendation is for something fixed like intelligence, because the person might become fearful of challenges that hold the possibility of disconfirming the current good opinion. What is effective in reinforcing positive behaviors is commenting on what people do well that is under their control, for example, the approach taken, the thoroughness of the preparation, and the amount of effort exerted. The more the primary emphasis is on learning, rather than smartness, then intrinsic motivation is activated, and the person is more likely to persevere in the face of prolonged challenges or setbacks (Grant & Dweck, 2003).

Constructive feedback is important to mentoring (Kalet, Krackov, & Rey, 2002) and a skill to be learned by nurse leaders (Gershenson, Moravick, Sellman, & Sommerville, 2004). The focus of feedback should be on learning, as opposed to correcting discreet performance. In providing feedback, there are a number of points to keep in mind: feedback should be clear, purposeful, and meaningful; it should be specific about what was effective and what was not effective rather than using code like "you were brilliant" or "you were sloppy"; speak for yourself using "I" statements—for example, "I liked the way you drew out the silent members of the committee at yesterday's meeting"... "I don't think you intended it, but I thought your response to that patient was abrupt, implying that you didn't care; what was going on in that situation from your point of view?" In giving feedback, use "and"— "I thought you responded sensitively to his concerns *and* in the future you need to remember to follow up later on to see how he is doing"—more than "but"—"I thought you responded sensitively to his concerns *but* in the future need to remember to follow up later on to see how he is doing"—because the latter implies "to the contrary" and may leave the person doubting anything positive already said because of the negative connotation of "but" (Zsohar & Smith, 2009).

Peer feedback that is an integral part of training can be useful to both the recipient of the comments and the person providing the pointers because the tips can be helpful and learning to give constructive criticism in an ego-enhancing way is an essential leadership skill (Cushing, Abbott, Lothian, Hall, & Westwood, 2011). The process of learning from experience can be enhanced by asking: What did you learn from the experience? What would you do differently next time? Such self-reflections build the person's ability to self-correct in the future. It also helps to remember that a mistake can be constructive—"That was a great mistake; it helped you see _____."

Constructive feedback serves many purposes. Seeking advice on a first draft of a paper or grant proposal can save time in the long run; ideas always get more comprehensive with commentary. Evaluation is a feature of all aspects of nursing, and feedback provides information about the needed course corrections. Building regular feedback into ordinary processes provides face-saving opportunities for rethinking matters without having to declare that what is in place is inadequate.

Baron, R. A. (1988). Negative effects of destructive criticism: Impact on conflict, self-efficacy, and task performance. *Journal of Applied Psychology, 73*, 199–207.

Cushing, A., Abbott, S., Lothian, D., Hall, A., & Westwood, O. M. (2011). Peer feedback as an aid to learning—What do we want? Feedback. When do we want it? Now! *Medical Teacher, 33*, e105–e112.

Dweck, C. S. (2007). *Mindset: The new psychology of success.* New York, NY: Random House.

Gershenson, T. A., Moravick, D. A., Sellman, E., & Somerville, S. (2004). Expert to novice: A nurse leader's evolution. *Nursing Management, 35*(6), 48–52.

Grant, H., & Dweck, C. S.(2003). Clarifying achievement goals and their impact. *Journal of Personality and Social Psychology, 85*, 541–553.

Kalet, A., Krackov, S., & Rey, M. (2002). Mentoring for a new era. *Academic Medicine, 77*, 1171–1172.

Nussbaum, A. D., & Dweck, C. S. (2008). Defensiveness versus remediation: Self-theories and modes of self-esteem. *Personality and Social Psychology Bulletin, 34*, 599–612.

Zsohar, H., & Smith, J. A. (2009). The power of *and* and *but* in constructive feedback on clinical performance. *Nurse Educator, 34*, 241–243.

Angela Barron McBride

CONSULTATION

Nurses are all consultants. There are many different types of consultants, both internal and external to the organization. Nurses are consulting every time they recommend a change to make something better, often without real control over the implementation of the changes. If you are advising or teaching, but have little control over the process of implementation, you are consulting. If you *do* have control over the implementation, you are managing. Hence, in the

C

broadest sense of consultation, nurses are routinely involved in advising and consulting. Consultants usually are in a position of having little direct control or authority to implement recommendations, and this can be a very frustrating position in which to be. The challenges of consulting are to have practical and knowledgeable advice that can be used and implemented to make a positive impact. In general, nurses make good consultants and the profession is improved by their expertise.

The *Merriam-Webster Desk Dictionary* (McKechnie, 1995, p. 118) defines consultation as "the process of using an expert for professional or technical advice or opinions." An expert is further defined as someone who is very "skilled; having much training and knowledge in a special field." Although it can be debated what makes an expert and what knowledge is needed, in general, nurses who function as consultants have an area of expertise that is valued and needed by others. The role of the consultant is to transfer knowledge, be a trainer or problem solver, or enable others to better accomplish their role to ensure the needed results.

Broadly, consulting can cover many functions. Nurses who teach patients, advise other employees, or have staff roles in the organization are internal consultants. They offer expertise and advice to others but usually do not have the positional power to make sure something is done. That is the role of the manager. Organizations today have many staff roles that support specific areas, and the nurses in these roles are in effect consulting to bring a level of expertise and advice that is needed to improve results. Outside consultants are experts who are not employed by the organization and are invited in to provide expertise and advice in areas where the organization does not have internal expertise or capacity. It is increasingly common that health

care organizations cannot afford to employ someone with niche knowledge on a full-time basis, or support a major project such as a technology installation which takes many experts for a short intense time. Hence, it is appropriate to be able to contract with those experts on an "as needed" basis.

INTERNAL CONSULTATION

Internal consultation takes place every day in organizations. As an internal consultant, you have a job in the organization and need to juggle respect for and challenge of the status quo. You must work through the line manager to get things done so all of the organization's managerial, clinical, and political issues may come into play. You are, in effect, expected to "sell your solutions" so that they are implemented and make a difference. In addition, in some ways, it is more difficult to be "a prophet in your own land," so getting changes adopted may be frustrating and challenging. As health care organizations rapidly add more complex technology and major clinical information systems, the number of internal consultants will undoubtedly increase.

EXTERNAL CONSULTATION

Consultation is considered "external" if the advisors are not employed by the organization and bring expertise into the organization on a contractual basis. External consultants can be solo consultants or employees of a consulting firm. Nurse consultants are employed in a variety of companies that focus on managerial consultation, clinical consultation, financial consultation, or technology consultation. In addition, there are many niche companies that focus on a narrower spectrum of health care, such as case management or recruitment. The variety of consulting opportunities for nurses is enormous, given the complexity of health care and nursing. For example, consultation associated with such areas as information systems often requires a nurse that has expertise in clinical delivery, technology, and change management to support major initiatives involved in implementing a new system.

External consultants are often viewed as a threat because they are unknown to the staff and are often involved in disruption to the status quo by the nature of the consultation. External consultants spend time learning about the organization, understanding the issues surrounding the consultation, and soliciting information and knowledge from staff and managers. With what they learn about the organization and their own expertise and experience, they work to craft a plan to implement changes that will address the issues they were hired to solve. One of the advantages of external consultants is that because they are not a part of the formal organization, they have the freedom to think and act independently of the internal hierarchy. This independence in thinking enables them to honestly design the best approaches to the situations that are under consultation. Because staff initially may be very wary of the questions that consultants ask, full information may not be conveyed or the nurses may be afraid to engage in the process itself. It is important to understand clearly the nature of the consultative process, the input needed from staff, and the expected outcomes. This clarity will go a long way toward facilitating the process and ensuring good results.

CONSULTATION PROCESSES IN NURSING

Because of the complexity of nursing, there will always be a need for consulting expertise in organizations. Consultation in nursing generally focuses on areas of clinical, education, research, and administration/management. Although rarely is a consulting assignment purely in one area, it is usually based on mainly one of the four. For instance, consultation may be used to determine the optimal model of care needed for defined patient populations. Alternatively, consultation may be used to facilitate research processes that will guide clinical innovation. Increasingly, consultants provide support to the installation of clinical technology and information systems. Whatever the need, it is possible to find experts in the field who are engaged in consulting. Internally, expert nurses such as educators, clinical nurse specialists, and advanced practice nurses are employed by the organization to support learning and practice on an ongoing basis. These experts typically have a reporting relationship to a manager of education and practice but deliver consultation to nurses who are practicing in the delivery sites in the organization. In this case, the expert nurses advise, teach, and support nurses but have no direct control or authority to implement. In seeing the value of their advice, the manager hopefully will follow through to be sure that changes are made and evaluated.

THE CONSULTATION PROCESS

The consultation process is similar to the nursing process, beginning with discussions to clarify the issues to be resolved. Who will be involved in defining the problems and framing the consultation? What methods of consultation will be used? And what kind of information and data will be necessary to support the decision making? Next, the data collection and problem diagnosis phase will typically involve a lot of people who will be interviewed, questioned, and observed to gather as much information as possible. The ability to efficiently gather data is a

C

big determinant of how rapidly the project can be done. Collected data will need to be organized and reported in some fashion. The consultant will synthesize data into a manageable number of issues. The client will then be able to give feedback, think through potential resistance, and determine the most acceptable way to proceed with the project. Goals can be clearly set and action plans developed. Only after this important groundwork is laid can the project proceed. The last phase involves implementation and measurement of results. The consultant may or may not be involved in the implementation phase, which will be accomplished by the line organization under the direction of a director or manager. Because the actual changes are taking place, the plan and the process are continuously reviewed to ensure that desired outcomes are being met. This is also the time when there is a degree of anxiety in the organization and there may be resistance to change. Therefore, it is an imperative that measurement systems are in place to monitor progress and document results.

The process of consultation is clearly a commitment to find the best ways to build and start new plans, or may be conducted to improve existing processes or define and implement innovation. Whatever the impetus, it is the role of the consultant to support and facilitate the process in a way that brings expertise to the organization and streamlines the work to be accomplished. It is more than just another pair of hands. Rather, consultation involves melding expert knowledge with the strengths of the organization.

PREPARATION TO BECOME A CONSULTANT

A nurse who is interested in becoming a consultant will need to develop an inventory of skills necessary to be successful. Although the skills may vary widely depending on the area of expertise, there are some basic skills that should be a part of every consultant's tool kit. First, there are skills and knowledge specific to one's discipline and in some cases clinical area of expertise, which should be well grounded in evidence and current for the practice area. Second, skills specific to the processes and phases of the consultation must be developed, including negotiation skills, dealing with conflict, extensive analytical ability, presentation skills, and the ability to see things from many vantage points. In all situations, consultants must be able to act assertively, express support, listen and learn, confront issues, and manage group process. Most of these characteristics can be learned and mastered with experience. For the person who is introverted, developing a public persona and confidence may require experience and practice. By contrast, for the extrovert, learning to step back and listen may be the biggest challenge. Above all, a consultant must be authentic, genuine, and honest. Learning when to walk away from opportunities that may not fit one's skill set is an important lesson. No one can be an expert in everything so an honest assessment of skills and attributes is essential to build a portfolio of successful consultation.

Successful consultation is a complex blend of gaining an understanding of the client's need, outlining a process for the consultation, developing a budget, and designing a contract to guide the project. It is important to get the agreement of all parties to the consultation in writing so that it is clear what the deliverables will be so that all expectations are met. It is common during consultations to have the scope of the project expand. This will require an addendum to the original contract. Consultation is a serious endeavor and should be guided by clear and achievable goals and contractual agreements. The business skills of developing work plans and contracts can be learned from a variety of sources including written guidance, other experienced consultants, or lawyers.

In summary, consultation is a fascinating career path for nurses, which expands with expertise in one's field. As an early career pathway, it is possible to receive extensive training in tools and methodologies as a member of a consulting firm. Or one can take on a consulting role within an organization to fill a need for focused expertise and guidance. Regardless of the route, the process is always interesting and challenging. Whether consulting internally or externally arriving at recommendations is much the same and includes a carefully crafted set of activities that define needs, determine approaches, provide data support, and develop implementation plans. The discipline of project management will help any initiative to come in on time, on budget, and with good results. With the ever declining reimbursement in health care, the need for focused consultation that can produce *rapid* results will increase and nurse consultants will be a part of many solutions.

Block, P. (1981). *Flawless consulting.* San Diego, CA: Pfeiffer & Company.

McKechnie, J. (Ed.). (1995). *Merrian-Webster desk dictionary.* New York, NY: Simon and Schuster.

Norwood, S. (1998). Making consultation work. *Journal of Nursing Administration, 28*(3), 44–47.

Smeltzer, C., & Hope, C. (2002). Can I be a healthcare consultant? *Journal of Nursing Administration, 32*(1), 12–14.

Wong, L. (2000). *The Harvard Business School guide to careers in management consulting.* Boston, MA: HBS Press.

Katherine Vestal

CONSUMER SATISFACTION

C

Consumer satisfaction is key to the financial success of any marketing enterprise, regardless of the profit or nonprofit status, the religious or secular affiliation, and the product, whether it is automobiles, computers, cosmetics or hair products, or health care. Given the competitive nature of health care facilities over the last 30 years or so, it is imperative that these organizations concentrate on quality improvement strategies that will "capture" a certain population needing health care services and will concomitantly lead to a high level of consumer satisfaction, often called *patient satisfaction.* Further, health care organizations, especially hospitals, are mandated to collect and report customer satisfaction data using standardized tools and also given financial incentives to achieve acceptable consumer satisfaction levels (Kutney-Lee et al., 2009). Although organizations strive to provide the best quality of care to meet the needs of their patients, it is necessary to determine if the consumer perceives the service or care to be at the same level that the organization believes it to be. The organization may provide a service that is at the highest quality; however, if patients are not satisfied and perceive the service as inferior, they will pass that information to their family and friends (Kelly, 2007).

Some of the most widely used standardized consumer satisfaction tools are Press-Ganey and the Consumer Assessment of Health Care Providers and Systems. Press Ganey is able to assess patient satisfaction in hospitals, medical offices, outpatient settings, and homecare. The company promises to assist organizations in improving quality and efficiency and increasing market share by collecting consumer satisfaction data and analyzing the results (Press Ganey Associates, Inc., 2011). The Consumer

C

Assessment of Healthcare Providers and Systems program provides a national standard for collecting patient's perspectives of care to assist hospital facilities and ambulatory care centers to assess the patient-centered aspects of the organization, to learn about performance from a patient perspective, and also to improve the quality of care (Agency for Healthcare Research and Quality, 2011). Mandated reporting of patient satisfaction scores gives consumers the ability to access Web sites such as U.S. News (http://health.usnews.com/best-hospitals) to review the scores of over 5,000 hospitals in the United States. Thus, it is imperative that health care organizations measure and address satisfaction; however, measurement should be done in multiple formats to determine an accurate picture of what is truly satisfying or dissatisfying to the consumer (Kelly, 2007).

In addition to standardized questionnaires, consumer satisfaction can also be determined in a number of ways:

- Face-to-face interviews: this is particularly effective when the consumer has registered a complaint; process improvements that address satisfaction for all consumers can be made.
- Telephone interviews: to ascertain more qualitative data about service satisfaction.
- Consumer surveys: surveying the community at large, whether or not they have sought or received services at a given institution.
- Focus groups: bringing together a group of consumers to take part in a facilitated discussion of the aspects of a service or quality of care (Yoder-Wise, 2007).

It is important for leaders to appreciate the role that nursing plays in consumer satisfaction. Administrators or administrative teams (including the chief nursing officer) have a dual responsibility: employee satisfaction and consumer satisfaction. Research supports that a higher quality working environment for nurses in terms of leadership, nurse–physician relationships, and high nursing standards along with lower nurse–patient ratios are related to increased consumer satisfaction (Kutney-Lee et al., 2009). Stopper (2004) asserts that trusting the people you work for, having pride in what you do, and enjoying the people you work with has a positive effect on employee morale and results in a high level of patient satisfaction. Consumers are more likely to respond favorably to employees who enjoy what they are doing, and they are more likely to return for additional services. Dissatisfied employees will more than likely cause dissatisfaction among consumers (Neff, 2002).

The majority of studies that have been conducted to assess patient satisfaction view it as one of the many outcomes of care, not necessarily as impacting clinical outcomes. Although there is little research that directly links consumer or patient satisfaction to patient outcomes, it is suggested that the more satisfied patients are, the more likely they are to adhere to their medical regimens and return to the facility for care needs in the future (Wagner & Bear, 2008). One study found that for patients who were experiencing lower back pain, the higher their satisfaction, the more likely they were to go into remission, regardless of receiving chiropractic or medical care. However, this link was only found during the first 6 weeks of treatment (Hurwitz, Morgenstern, & Yu, 2005). The limited number of studies conducted in this area provides direction for nurses to carry out research that will support the belief that consumer satisfaction is not only good for an organization's bottom line but also necessary for excellent clinical outcomes.

See also Employee Satisfaction

Agency for Healthcare Research and Quality. (2011). *CAHPS: Survey tools to advance patient care.* Retrieved January 7, 2011, from https://www.cahps.ahrq.gov/default.asp

Hurwitz, E. L., Morgenstern, H., & Yu, F. (2005). Satisfaction as a predictor of clinical outcomes among chiropractic and medical patients enrolled in the UCLA Low Back Pain Study. *Spine, 30*(19), 2121–2128.

Kelly, P. (2007). *Nursing leadership and management* (2nd ed.). New York, NY: Delmar Cengage Learning.

Kutney-Lee, A., McHugh, M. D., Sloane, D. M., Cimiotti, J.P, Flynn, L., Felber-Neff, D., et al. (2009). Nursing: A key to patient satisfaction. *Health Affairs, 28*(4), w669–w667.

Neff, T. M. (2002). What successful companies know that law firms need to know: The importance of employee motivation and job satisfaction to increased productivity and stronger client relationships. *Journal of Law and Health, 17*(2), 385ff.

Press Ganey Associates, Inc. (2011). *Creating high performance health care organizations.* Retrieved January 7, 2011, from http://www.pressganey.com/aboutUs.aspx

Stopper, W. G. (2004). Creating a great place to work [R]—Lessons from the "100 Best." *Human Resources Planning, 27*(2), 20ff.

U.S. News. (2011). *Best hospitals.* Retrieved January 7, 2011, from http://health.usnews.com/best-hospitals

Wagner, D., & Bear, M. (2008). Patient satisfaction with nursing care: A concept analysis within a nursing framework. *Journal of Advanced Nursing, 65*(3), 692–701.

Yoder-Wise, P. S. (2007). *Leading and managing in nursing* (4th ed.). St. Louis, MO: Mosby.

Gina M. Myers
M. Janice Nelson

Continuing Professional Education

Continuing professional education (CPE) "refers to the inculcation, assimilation and acquisition of knowledge, skills, proficiency and ethical and moral values, after initial registration of a professional, that raises and enhances the profession-al's technical skills and professional competence. PRC. Res. #381 s. 1995" (Loretto, 1996, p. 79).

In today's ever changing world, CPE has become an increasingly important topic in many professions, especially for those that exist in environments of increased complexity and accelerating change. In general, CPE is intended for adult learners, especially for those beyond the traditional undergraduate college level. In professions like nursing, it is expected that nurses are competent to care for patients, provide the highest standard and quality of care, and stay current. The rapid changes in health care, the diminished life span of useful information, and the increasing complexity of practice make it essential that nurses maintain competence by continuing to learn throughout their careers (Williams, 2004, p. 277).

Nurses are constantly challenged to update old knowledge; indeed, nurses more than ever are expected to embrace new and upcoming research and changes relevant to the profession. CPE has become the way that professionals gain new information and is a requirement for many organizations. For professionals who hold licenses to practice as well as certifications, CPE also has been found necessary for the renewal process. In the United States, CPE can be obtained in programs often found in college/university credit-granting courses or online classes and conferences where individuals obtain continuing education units (http://www.iseek.org/static/awards.htm; http://www.iseek.org/education/fieldOfStudy). Many nursing professionals recognize the need to make a strong commitment to education. Expanding and deepening the knowledge base enriches the profession. CPE, which provides a route to that enrichment, has become an imperative in nursing along with other disciplines.

ISEEK Solutions. (2011). Field of study: Adult and continuing education teaching. Retrieved from http://www.iseek.org/education/fieldOfStudy?id=470100

Loretto, M. (1996). Midwifery law and ethics. Quezon City, Philippines: Rex Printing Company. Retrieved from http://books.google.com/books?id=YHUCZS

Williams, B. (2004). Self direction in a problem based learning program. *Nurse Education Today*, 24(4), 277–285.

Paule V. Joseph

CONTINUOUS QUALITY IMPROVEMENT

Quality and safety are major foci in health care today and are important not only professionally for nursing but also strategically across the continuum of care in this era of health care reform (The Patient Protection and Affordable Care Act, 2010). Continuous quality improvement (CQI) combines quality improvement initiatives involving multiple disciplines with evidence-based practice to provide the best possible care for patients. Although CQI has a long history, quality and safety became forefront issues following the reports of the Institute of Medicine (IOM; http://www.iom) *To Err Is Human* and *Crossing the Quality Chasm* (IOM, 2001; Kohn, Corrigan, & Donaldson, 1999). Many health care facilities use the six aims for improvement cited in *Crossing the Quality Chasm* as a framework for quality improvement. The report cited that a health care system that achieves gains in six areas will be focused on meeting patients' needs. These six core needs are for care to be safe, effective, patient centered, timely, efficient, and equitable. Numerous additional reports such as *Preventing Medication Errors, Future Directions for National Healthcare Quality and Disparities Reports, Leadership Commitments to Improve Value in Healthcare: Finding Common Ground*, and *The Future of Nursing: Leading Change, Advancing Health* all have continued to stimulate interest and concern about quality and safety in health care (IOM, 2006, 2009, 2010a, 2010b).

Today, terms such as CQI, performance improvement (PI), and quality improvement are used to describe a process and common thread, regardless of the name, which is to improve the care and outcomes of patients or clients regardless of the setting. Parenthetically, it should be noted that higher education in nursing has taken a similar path with CQI (see Yearwood, Singleton, Feldman, & Colombraro, 2001). CQI mandates a top-down promulgation of quality and a cultural change for the organization. CQI focuses on processes and systems of care, not individuals, requiring a multidisciplinary approach and focusing on all aspects of care related to structure, process, and outcome. CQI requires the health care organization to constantly evaluate and revise processes to better meet the needs of patients and stakeholders.

CONTINUOUS QUALITY IMPROVEMENT IN NURSING

Nursing has long been involved in CQI initiatives, reporting not only to evaluate specific nursing practice but also to evaluate patient care in the broader context. Nursing-sensitive measures must be quantifiably influenced by nursing personnel, but the relationship is not necessarily causal. Nursing has specific indicators that are monitored; examples include the National Database for Nursing Quality Indicators (NDNQI™) and the Veterans Administration Nursing

Outcomes Database (http://vaww.collage. research.med.va.gov/collage/VANOD). The NDNQI™ is a proprietary data base for acute care inpatient hospitals started by the American Nurses' Association in the early 1990's. The nursing-sensitive indicators in this database reflect the structure, process, and outcomes of nursing care. For more information about NDNQI™, visit the Web site (https://www.nursingquality.org).

FUTURE TRENDS

CQI will continue to be a focus for health care organizations, and in the future, several concepts will continue to grow and new ones will emerge. Transparency in health care quality will become more common as institutions strive to distinguish themselves in this era of health care reform, bundling of payments, and accountable care organizations. In addition, an institution's quality performance is readily available to the public. One example of transparency is quality data on the Centers for Medicare and Medicaid Services' Hospital Quality Measures (previously known as Core Measures and now referred to as National Hospital Inpatient Quality Measures). Data are available on the Hospital Compare Web site (http://www.healthcare.gov/compare) and include not only process and outcome measures for specific conditions but also patient satisfaction data (U.S. Department of Health and Human Services, 2010).

Value is an emerging concept in health care that nursing, physicians, and all can support. Health care providers, providers, patients, payers, and policy makers all support the goal of improving outcomes as efficiently as possible (Lee, 2010). However, the measurement of value is difficult from the patients' perspective. How do we measure or capture data on outcomes that matter to patients as well as the costs for a patient over an episode of care? One way value can be enhanced is by improving one or more outcomes without compromising others or by reducing the costs required to achieve the same levels of outcome (Lee, 2010).

The number of quality indicators that institutions are required to monitor either voluntarily or via mandates is increasing at a frenetic pace, and these external pressures continue to grow. Examples of organizations with quality indicators include the Centers for Medicare and Medicaid Services, the Agency for Healthcare Research and Quality, the accrediting agencies (The Joint Commission, National Committee on Quality Assurance), the purchasers of care, and the coalitions (Leapfrog Group, http://www.leapfroggroup.org).

Pay for performance (value-based purchasing) is receiving increasing attention in the era of health care reform. Hospitals have been required to report quality measures to Medicare to receive their full annual payment update since the Medicare Modernization Act of 2003 (pay for reporting). However, beginning in October 2012, the health care reform law will actually begin to tie hospitals' Medicare reimbursements on their performance on quality measures. Initially, hospitals will be assessed on a set of 12 clinical process of care measures (70% of score) and eight patient experience of care measures taken from the Hospital Consumer Assessment of Healthcare Providers and Systems (HCAHPS) survey. Starting in FY 2013, hospitals will be paid for their performance as compared with their peers and for their improvement in quality over time. Going forward, additional new measures (including outcome measures) will be added to the value-based purchasing program.

Last is an increasing focus on patient-centered systems of care versus patient-centered individual care. Institutions will

C

focus on the entire episode of care across all settings, especially with chronic diseases. The accountability for quality processes and outcomes will no longer be focused in one setting (e.g., hospital) but will focus on the coordination of care across the continuum of care.

Nursing leadership plays a key role in the successful development and implementation of programs related to quality and safety. Nursing has an in-depth understanding of systems and the ability to lead teams and bring together multiple stakeholders toward a common goal. The essentials of nursing leadership in quality include the knowledge of CQI techniques, the use of quality tools such as those of Six Sigma or lean techniques, the current knowledge of external organizations driving the quality reporting agenda nationally, the benchmarking techniques, and the knowledge of health information technology. Nursing education must also be involved in this process. It is crucial that undergraduate and especially graduate programs in nursing incorporate information on CQI and a working knowledge of the national agenda related to health care quality and safety.

See also Agency for Healthcare Research and Quality (AHRQ); Leapfrog Group

Healthcare Reform. Retrieved from http://www.healthcare.gov

Institute for Healthcare Improvement. Retrieved from http://www.ihi.org

Institute of Medicine. (2001). *Crossing the quality chasm: A new health system for the 21st century.* Washington, DC: National Academies Press.

Institute of Medicine. (2006). *Preventing medication errors.* Washington, DC: National Academies Press.

Institute of Medicine. (2009). *Leadership commitments to improve value in healthcare: Finding common ground.* Washington, DC: National Academies Press.

Institute of Medicine. (2010a). *Future directions for the national healthcare quality and disparities reports.* Washington, DC: National Academies Press.

Institute of Medicine. (2010b). *The future of nursing: Leading change, advancing health.* Washington, DC: National Academies Press.

Kohn, L. T., Corrigan, J. M., & Donaldson, M. S. (Eds.). (1999). *To err is human: Building a safer health system.* Washington, DC: National Academies Press.

Lee, T. H. (2010, December 8). Putting the value framework to work. *New England Journal of Medicine, 363,* 2481–2483. doi:10.1056/NEJMp1013111.

National Database of Nursing Quality Indicators. Retrieved from http://www.nursingworld.org/quality/database.htm

National Quality Forum. Retrieved from http://www.qualityforum.org

The Patient Protection and Accountable Care Act (the Affordable Care Act), Pub. L. No. 111–148 (2010, March).

U.S. Department of Health and Human Services. (2010). *Hospital compare.* Retrieved December 1, 2010, from www.hospitalcompare.hhs.gov

Yearwood, E., Singleton, J., Feldman, H. R., & Colombraro, G. (2001). A case study in implementing CQI in a nursing education program. *Journal of Professional Nursing, 17,* 297–304.

Jo Ann Brooks

COUNCIL FOR THE ADVANCEMENT OF NURSING SCIENCE

After the American Nurses Association restructured and disbanded the Council of Nurse Research, the American Academy of Nursing (AAN) Board members in the late 1990s recognized the need to create a national nursing research organization. Thus, the Council for the Advancement of Nursing Science (CANS), an open-membership entity of the AAN, was established in 2000 to foster Better Health through Nursing Science. In addition,

CANS became the research policy and facilitation arm for the AAN. The goals of the Council are to be a strong voice for nursing science at national and international levels by developing, conducting, and using nursing science to disseminate research findings across individuals and groups in scientific and lay communities and to facilitate lifelong learning opportunities for nurse scientists.

Prior to and coincidental with the formation of the council, the national biennial State of the Science Congresses in Nursing Research were held, originally through university sponsorships but ultimately with the support of the National Nursing Research Roundtable and through a consortium of nursing organizations with rotating leadership. In 2002, the meeting was chaired by the American Association of Colleges of Nursing and Sigma Theta Tau International. To ensure and build consistency and planning by active nursing scientists and to further its mission, the council received support to spearhead and sustain ongoing State of the Science Nursing Research Congresses, starting with the 2004 meeting. The State of the Science meeting along with Special Research Topics Conferences on the alternate (odd number) years forms the main Council agenda platform, along with funding a seed money grant through the American Nurses Foundation, participating in the National Nursing Research Roundtable, and analyzing and speaking out on research development and policy issues on behalf of and in concert with the AAN. In 2010, the Council hosted its largest State of the Science Congress on Nursing Conference, which hosted 400+ abstracts from nursing researchers nationally to present at the podium through poster presentations and was attended by more than 1,000 nursing researchers. In addition, the council also continued to support

and fund research grants to its partners, the Sigma Theta Tau International, the American Nursing Foundation, the National Institute of Nursing Research, the Eastern Nursing Research Society, the Midwest Nursing Research Society, the Southern Nursing Research Society, and the Western Institute of Nursing.

For information about attending Council conferences or learning about its contributions to nursing research, visit the Council for the Advancement of Nursing Science Web site at www.nursing science.org.

William L. Holzemer

COUNCIL ON ACCREDITATION OF NURSE ANESTHESIA PROGRAMS

The Council on Accreditation of Nurse Anesthesia Educational Programs (COA) was established in 1975 as an autonomous, multidisciplinary body under the corporate structure of the American Association of Nurse Anesthetists (AANA), representing the various publics within the nurse anesthesia community of interest in which the profession resides. The mission of the COA is to (1) grant public recognition to nurse anesthesia programs and institutions that award post master's certificates, master's and doctoral degrees that meet national established standards of academic quality (quality assessment) and (2) assist programs and institutions in improving educational quality (quality enhancement). The COA has been continuously recognized to accredit nurse anesthesia programs and institutions by the U.S. Department of Education (USDE) since 1975, as well as the Council for Higher Education Accreditation (CHEA) since 1985. The USDE recognition identifies

C

the COA as a reliable authority for the quality of training that is offered by educational institutions and programs as the basis for ascertaining eligibility for federal funding under selected legislation. The CHEA recognition demonstrates the COA's effectiveness in assessing and encouraging improvement and quality in programmatic accreditation. In February 2009, the COA separately incorporated as a 501(c3) nonprofit organization. As of November 1, 2010, there were 110 accredited nurse anesthesia programs located throughout the United States and its territories. The over 5,000 students enrolled in these programs obtain a wide variety of clinical experiences in over 2,000 COA-approved clinical sites. Since January 1, 1998, all nurse anesthesia programs are required to award a master's or higher degree upon graduation. In 2009, the COA established the requirement that students accepted into a nurse anesthesia program on January 1, 2022, and thereafter, must graduate with doctoral degrees. This requirement is consistent with the AANA's 2007 position statement that supports doctoral education for entry into practice by 2025.

Additional information is available at the following Web sites:

http://www.coastandards.org/about.php
http://www.aana.com/councilaccreditation. aspx

Francis Gerbasi

CREDENTIALING

Credentialing is a process through which registered nurses who have developed expertise in a particular specialty have this specialized knowledge base acknowledged. One such mechanism is certification, "the formal recognition of specialized knowledge, skills, and experience demonstrated by the achievement of standards identified by a nursing specialty to promote optimal health outcomes" (American Board of Nursing Specialties, 2010). To become certified by the American Nurses Credentialing Center (ANCC, 2010; nursescredentialing.org) or one of the specialty nursing organizations offering such a process, the nurse usually has to submit a professional portfolio demonstrating applicable education, years of work experience, a nursing license, references, and evidence of successful completion of the organization's certification examination. Certifications are usually renewed every 5 years by completion of continuing education requirements or submission of professional accomplishments and/or additional examination.

According to ANCC, certification does not confer a protected, legal scope of practice but does aid the public by identifying competent nurses within a nursing specialty (ANCC, 2010). In addition, certification recognizes professional achievement within the profession, in the workplace, and among one's peers and enhances professionalism; in some federal and state statutes such as the federal Balanced Budget Act of 1996, credentialing serves as a criterion for third-party reimbursement of the nurse specialist's practice.

See also Certification

American Board of Nursing Specialties. (2010). *ABNS fact sheet*. Retrieved January 24, 2011, from www.nursingcertification.org

American Nurses Credentialing Center. (2010). *Overview of ANCC nursing certification: Achieve your professional best with ANCC certification*. Retrieved January 24, 2011, from http://www.nursecredentialing.org/Certification/Certification-Overview-Brochure.aspx

Karen A. Ballard

CULTURAL COMPETENCE: AN ACADEMIC NURSING LEADERSHIP IMPERATIVE

Cultural competence is an ongoing educational process that includes a proficiency in acknowledging the value of culture within the lives of persons and then understanding the importance of addressing cultural norms and beliefs of persons in conjunction with outcomes development within educational, work, and health care settings (Warren, 2009). As a multifaceted construct, culture may be defined by individuals, groups, and communities for themselves or by persons outside a specific cultural group. Of course, everyone is part of a culture or cultures, including cultures rooted in diversity of thought, sexual orientation, socioeconomic class, religion, age, gender, race, and ethnicity as well as many other self-determined cultures (Lutz & Warren, 2007; Warren & Lutz, 2007). Population statistics also indicate that, in the United States, demographics are now more racially and ethnically diverse than in the past (U.S. Department of the Census, 2010). Hence, the immersion of cultural competence is a salient component within academic settings.

Nonetheless, the inclusion of culturally competent strategies within education, practice, and research remains controversial for many academicians across all specialty disciplines. Nursing is no exception to this controversy. Nursing academicians, however, have even more responsibility to help students and themselves understand the importance of culturally competent strategies within nursing education, practice, and research to address the health care needs of culturally and ethnically diverse individuals, groups, and populations. Failure to address these needs will diminish the quality of life for culturally and ethnically diverse persons and place more burden upon society and the health care systems and organizations (U.S. Department of Health and Human Services, 1999, 2001).

This entry delineates barriers that create cultural incompetence within nursing academic settings and proposes solutions that enhance the immersion of cultural competence within nursing academic settings.

The nursing discipline faces challenges in the education of students at undergraduate (UG) and graduate (G) levels, and these barriers often stifle the implementation of cultural competence in curricula. There is an acknowledgment regarding health care disparities but understanding the role of cultural perspectives outside of race and ethnicity may not be part of nursing curricula. Kossman (2009) describes the presence and misunderstanding regarding cultural issues as the lack of "cultural fit" between nursing students and faculty (p. 29). Other scholars of cultural competence describe the presence of health care inequities as a lack of understanding between health care professionals regarding their worldviews. Worldviews encompass communication patterns and the value that persons consign to relationships, interactions, and educational approaches (Campinha-Bacote, 2007; Munoz & Luckmann, 2005; Munoz, Primm, & Ananth, 2007; Purnell, 2007; Warren & Lutz, 2007).

Another challenge for the nursing discipline involves increasing the numbers of diverse nursing students within academic institutions of nursing at the UG level. Research indicates that increasing cultural and ethnic diversity in academic settings facilitates the intellectual growth of all students (Smedley, Butler, & Bristow, 2004). The lack of diverse students at the UG level

C

decreases the available diverse pool for the doctoral pipeline and subsequent faculty availability. This lack of diverse doctoral faculty often affects the perception of "cultural fit" between students and faculty. Students assess the faculty mix and equate this mix as being reflective of whether they will be understood, accepted, and welcomed. For many diverse students, the lack of cultural and ethnic diversity among the faculty ranks indicates that culture may not be valued within an academic setting (Pharris, 2009).

Finally, there is the issue of financial impact for schools and colleges of nursing as balancing budgets become a paramount goal for many. Revising curricula is a common faculty solution when budgets are decreased. Part of the revision process generally includes the identification and elimination of "nonessential" courses. Unfortunately, courses that focus on culture, ethnic diversity, and cultural competence may be viewed within this "nonessential" category. Content from these courses is either folded into other courses or completely eliminated. Thus, valuable and important discussions regarding culture and diversity are lost and this compounds the problem of "cultural fit." As such, what solutions are available to meet the challenges that nursing academicians face when they want to enculturate cultural competence within their curricula?

First, is to increase the number of faculty with expertise in understanding and teaching the process of cultural competence. It is imperative that nursing academicians become scholars of cultural competence and take the lead in developing and teaching courses that nurture nursing students' development of cultural competence. Reflective and mindfulness techniques aimed at understanding and discussing cultural similarities and differences need to be components of content across all courses. These techniques help students and faculty understand each other, facilitating the "cultural fit" between them (Warren, 2009). Nursing academicians need to become involved in the development of recruitment and retention strategies that are aimed at creating a more diverse cadre of students. Faculty members do not need to do recruitment, but they can collaborate with the staff members primarily responsible for it. The development of a diversity committee composed of students, staff, and faculty at UG and G levels can facilitate culturally competent discussions and develop programming. There are also educational and sensitizing culturally competent programs that faculty members can attend to learn educational exercises and techniques that they can use in their interactions and discussion with other faculty and students. The National Coalition Building Institute, for example, is composed of a group of students, faculty, and staff that are trained in specific techniques aimed to eliminate cultural bias and intergroup conflict.

Finally, there are some basic reports that are recommended for nursing faculty to use in helping themselves and their students grow in learning the process of cultural competence. Among these are:

- *Cultural Diversity in the Nursing Curriculum: A Guide for Implementation* (American Nurses Association, Council on Cultural Diversity in Nursing Practice, 1986)
- *Mental Health: A Report of the Office of the Surgeon General* (U.S. Department of Health and Human Services, 1999)
- *Mental Health: Culture, Race, and Ethnicity: A Supplement to Mental Health: A Report of the Office of the Surgeon General* (2001)
- *In the Nation's Compelling Interest: Ensuring Diversity in the Health-Care Workforce* (2004)

In conclusion, the issues of culture and cultural competence are essential to the successful development of quality outcomes within health care systems and organizations for all persons. The tackling of health care disparities is a multifaceted issue that needs to begin in nursing academic settings. The word imperative means urgent and important. These words aptly describe the rationale why nursing faculty scholars need to be at the forefront of becoming culturally competent and then facilitating the growth of the process for their faculty peers and nursing students.

American Nurses Association, Council on Cultural Diversity in Nursing Practice. (1986). *Cultural diversity in the nursing curriculum: A guide for implementation.* Kansas City, MO: Author.

Campinha-Bacote, J. (2007). *The process of cultural competence in health care in the delivery of healthcare services: The journey continues.* Cincinnati, OH: Transcultural C.A.R.E. Associates.

Kossman, S. P. (2009). The power of nurse educators: Welcoming and unwelcoming behaviors. In S. D. Bosher & M. D. Pharris (Eds.), *Transforming nursing education: The culturally inclusive environment* (Chapter 2, pp. 27–60). New York, NY: Springer Publishing Company.

Muñoz, C. C., & Luckmann, J. (2005). *Transcultural communication in nursing* (2nd ed.). Clifton Park, NY: Thomson Delmar Learning.

Munoz, R., Primm, A., & Ananth, J. (2007). *Life in color: Culture in American psychiatry.* Chicago, IL: Hilton Publishing Co.

Pharris, S. D. (2009). Understanding inclusivity in the current nursing culture. In S. D. Bosher & M. D. Pharris (Eds.), *Transforming nursing education: The culturally inclusive environment* (Chapter 1, pp. 3–26). New York, NY: Springer Publishing Company.

Purnell, L. D. (2009). *A guide to culturally competent health care* (2nd ed.). Philadelphia, PA: F.A. Davis.

Smedley, B. D., Butler, A. S., & Bristow, L. R. (2004). *In the compelling interest: Ensuring diversity in the health-care workforce.* Washington, DC: National Academies Press.

U.S. Department of the Census. (2010). *Current demographic census data.* Retrieved October 4, 2010, from http://www.census.gov/popest/datasets.html

U.S. Department of Health and Human Services. (1999). *Mental health: A report of the Surgeon General.* Rockville, MD: DHHS, Substance Abuse and Mental Health Services Administration, Center for Mental Health Services, National Institutes of Health, National Institutes of Mental Health.

U.S. Department of Health and Human Services. (2001). *Mental health: Culture, race, and ethnicity. A supplement to mental health: A report of the Surgeon General.* Rockville, MD: U.S. Department of Health and Human Services, Public Health Services, Office of the Surgeon General.

Warren, B. J. (2009). Teaching the fluid process of cultural competence. In S.D. Bosher & M. D. Pharris (Eds.), *Transforming nursing education: The culturally inclusive environment.* New York, NY: Springer Publishing Company.

Warren, B. J., & Lutz, W. J. (2007). The state of nursing science—Cultural and lifespan issues in depression: Part I. Focus on adults. *Issues in Mental Health Nursing, 28*(7), 707–748.

Barbara Jones Warren

C

CULTURAL DIVERSITY

Cultural diversity is about embracing and valuing differences due to cultural forces. It includes beliefs, lived experiences, practices, behaviors, and perspectives that include race, ethnicity, age, gender, gender orientation, sexuality, physical, mental and intellectual abilities, religion, language, body size, generational group, family configuration, socioeconomic status, and other characteristics, which can potentially shape one's approach to life circumstances. The knowledgeable leader works with others to facilitate safe, culturally competent practice for patients. Cultural competence suggests awareness, sensitivity, and

C

knowledge about different cultural groups and the conscious attention to managing these differences in a respectful, responsive, and skillful manner in various settings. It also connotes an awareness that differences exist in access and delivery of care to various people, thus making some more vulnerable and likely to experience health care disparities.

Major health care accreditation organizations now recognize the importance of treating diverse patients in a culturally competent way. The Joint Commission (TJC) is scheduled to publish standards in 2011 intended to focus on communication, cultural competence, and patient centered care. Areas addressed in the draft standards include "(1) the collection and use of demographic data for both service provision and strategic planning, (2) assessing patient communication needs and providing resources to meet those needs and (3) developing systems of care that promote equity, respect and inclusion" (Wilson-Stronks, 2009).

Culture shapes the way in which individuals approach and make sense of their world and provides a lens through which they create meaning. Culture helps to distinguish virtues, gives substance to the terms of discourse, and defines courage, generosity, strength, moderation, and equality. We are all influenced by and belong to multiple cultures that extend beyond the usual cultural variables. They typically place us into a deep emotional space of understanding human variations and sometimes competing values, practices, languages, and dimensional factors whether physical, philosophical, perceived, socially imposed, power referenced, or permutations of any of the aforementioned. Cultural assertion in the context of cultural struggles is often a struggle over forms, although struggle over forms is often a struggle for power. For example, organizationally speaking, culture will eat strategy for lunch. When speaking of individuals, many of the rules that govern the determination of race are still rooted in social and cultural traditions rather than sound biological reasoning, hence the proliferation of "races" in the literature and the ambiguity often observed between such groupings in the contemporary scientific literature. In fact, one's national culture is a powerful differentiator often, greater than ethnicity, gender, or language. Burgeoning is the wide range of cultural diversity based on place of birth alone. Put this with the realities of "the world is flat," and exponentially there are so many instances of unchecked assumptions, stereotypes, bias, and lack of personal awareness about bias.

Cultural diversity calls for making cultural adjustments and continues to present many challenges for health providers and the system at large. Such occurrences are inevitable because all encounters are cultural encounters. Every culture will exhibit its biases, and this is particularly poignant in the health care encounter, which involves the intersection of the following:

- the culture of the provider, which includes their profession and its codes of conduct, their generational classification, gender, and primary language;
- the culture of the institution, that is, rural, urban, academic, metropolitan, and religious affiliated;
- the culture of the patient including the generational classification of the patient's occupation, degree of migration, religion, level of education, and so forth; and
- the culture of the country in which the institution exists.

Cultural assessments tend to be the exception rather than the norm, and cultural rules are often not discussed until a difference often labeled a problem between the provider and the patient occurs. Proactive behaviors on the part of the provider to gain an understanding of the patient's explanatory model of his or her illness are fundamental and also efficacious. There are many models available, such as Kleinman's model, the addressing framework, respect, and the live and learn model. It seems prudent to put in place cultural brokers, that is, individuals who construct bridges between different cultures and also develop positive approaches to manage the differences of diverse cultures. Emphasizing corporate values and biases can pay off in the long run. Zero tolerance for assaults on anyone's self-esteem when executed without exception provides a solid platform for many courageous acts of walking the talk regarding valuing cultural diversity. Encouraging curiosity and minimizing certainty are practices that will also bode well in this global milieu of today. Providing to the workforce growth opportunities such as continuing education regarding different cultures and establishing book clubs or travel clubs can also increase an individual's cultural competency. The development of mentorship programs, diversity training for search committee members, and inviting community or faculty members to participate in employment searches can assist in recruitment and retention efforts to attract diverse applicants. Bringing speakers who are either practitioners or researchers from different cultures can be quite enlightening and allows the opportunity to explore in depth questions one may have about cultural behaviors, beliefs, and practices.

Alexander, G. R. (2008). Cultural competence models in nursing. *Critical Care Nursing Clinics of North America, 20*(4), 415–421

Betancourt, J., Green, A. R., Carrillo, J. E., & Park, E. R. (2005). Cultural competence and health care disparities: Key perspectives and trends. *Journal of Health Affairs, 24*(2), 499–505.

Brett, J., Behfar, K., and Kern, M.C. (2006). Managing multicultural teams. *Harvard Business Review,* 84–91.

Institute of Medicine. (2002). Unequal Treatment Committee on understanding and eliminating racial and ethnic disparities in healthcare, board on health sciences policy. *Unequal Treatment: Confronting racial and ethnic disparities in healthcare.* Washington, DC: The National Academies Press.

National Center for Cultural Competence. Retrieved from http://nccc.georgetown.edu

Nunez, A. E. (2000). Transforming cultural competence into cross-cultural efficacy in women's health education. *Academic Medicine,* 75(11), 1071–1080.

Pew Research Center. (2008). *Immigration to play lead role in further U.S. growth.* Retrieved from http://pew research.org/pibs/729/United_States_population-projections

Wilson-Stronks, A. (2009). *Advancing effective communication, cultural competence & patient-centered care. Principal Investigator of the Hospitals, Language and Culture study.* Oak Brook Terrace, IL: The Joint Commission. Retrieved from http://www.patientprovider-communication.org/index.cfm/article_5.htm

G. Rumay Alexander

D

DEDICATED EDUCATION UNIT

A dedicated education unit (DEU) is a "client unit developed into an optimal teaching/learning environment through the collaborative efforts of nurses, management, students and faculty" (Warner & Moscato, 2009, p. 60). This model of clinical teaching was initiated to maximize resources needed to expand enrollment and prepare a robust workforce. The model is sustained through the mutual benefits across the academic and service partnership.

When a school of nursing has exclusives use of a DEU, it maximizes the understanding of curriculum, clinical paperwork, and calendars. Because of increased efficiency, fewer clinical units are needed by the school. Clinically expert staff selected by the nurse manager, and oriented by the school, serve as the primary clinical instructors (CIs) for the students. One or two students are paired with each CI for the entire rotation granting continuity and increased accountability for clinical performance. Patient assignments for the CI vary depending on the student level, generally lighter at the beginning and heavier at the end of the rotation. Nursing faculty coach and mentor the CIs in best practices in clinical teaching, facilitate connections between didactic and clinical learning, and assess attainment of student outcomes. All partners commit to the shared goals of excellent patient care, optimal student learning, and ongoing career fulfillment for all (Moscato, Miller, Logsdon, Weinberg, & Chorpenning, 2007).

Costs incurred in a DEU model are shared. The CIs' salary is paid by the service organization, including a per hour supplement equivalent to the preceptor rate. They also pay the CI salary for time off the unit for orientation and ongoing development. Nurse managers report that being a DEU is budget neutral because students at the end of the rotation contribute to the productivity of patient care. The school pays the salary of academic nurse faculty and a DEU coordinator. They also assume the costs of partnership infrastructure, for example, quarterly dinner meetings with key stakeholders and expenses for ongoing communication and that sustain the relationships.

Each partner experiences benefits. DEUs report increased CI professionalism and career advancement and have been cited in the Magnet process as evidence of innovation and exemplary practice. The agencies see reduced orientation costs and time when new hires were DEU students. The financial efficiency of the faculty to student ratio is a significant benefit to the school. State regulation governing this ratio can be as high as 1:24, easing the challenge of the faculty shortage. Students benefit from a learning environment where a team of professionals

D

from service and academe are invested in their optimal learning. Most importantly, patients and families receive stellar care.

Extensive information and tools are found on the University of Portland School of Nursing Web site (nursing.up.edu) in a DEU section. Together with their clinical partners, they have successfully used the DEU model since 2003. All who implement the DEU model have unique characteristics or arrangements that match the institutional cultures of their organizations.

An effective DEU requires a cooperative and collaborative partnership between academe and service. Inherent in this partnership are political dynamics, policy issues, and negotiated practices that must be managed through mutual respect and transparent communication (Warner & Burton, 2009).

Moscato, S., Miller, J., Logsdon, K., Weinberg, S., & Chorpenning, L. (2007). Dedicated education unit: An innovative clinical partner education model. *Nursing Outlook, 55*(1), 31–37.

Warner, J. R., & Burton, D. J. (2009). The policy and politics of emerging academic-service partnerships. *Journal of Professional Nursing, 25*(6), 329–334.

Warner, J. R., & Moscato, S. R. (2009). Innovative approach to clinical education: Dedicated education units. In N. Ard & T. Valiga (Eds.) *Clinical nursing education: Current reflections. National League for Nursing* (pp. 59–69). New York: National League for Nursing.

Joanne Rains Warner

DELEGATION

Delegation is an essential skill, process, and art learned by nurses, managers, and leaders. In today's world of nursing practice, management, and leadership, delegation is a necessity. Although definitions of delegation may differ, the purpose of delegation remains constant, that is, to get the work done efficiently. The nurse, manager, and leader do this through others by directing the work or performance of others to accomplish patient or organizational goals. The American Nurses Association (www.nursingworld.org) defines delegation as transferring responsibility of performing a task from one person to another. The National Council of State Boards of Nursing (www.ncsbn.org) specifies that delegation is transferring authority to a competent person to perform a select nursing task in a select situation. The National Council of State Boards of Nursing further describes steps in the process of delegation, which include (1) identifying the task to be done, (2) selecting the most capable/competent person, (3) using clear communication of the goals and purpose of the task, (4) establishing a time frame for task completion, (5) monitoring the progress of the job, (6) providing guidance, and (7) assessing the performance and accomplishment of the goal or task.

The key components of delegation are legal liability or accountability, responsibility, and authority (Kelly, 2008). In direct patient care, a registered nurse (RN) is liable for his or her actions and must be cognizant of the state nurse practice act, standards of practice, organizational policies, and legal-ethical behaviors. Generally, acceptable delegated tasks fall within the implementation phase of the nursing process. Direct patient care activities include assisting the patient with activities of daily living and collecting and documenting relating to these activities. The RN may not delegate the other phases of the nursing process involved in direct patient care, for example, assessing, analyzing, diagnosing, teaching, and evaluating. Nurses may delegate tasks that do not involve direct patient care which may carry fewer legal risks.

D

Delegation involves responsibility and the duty for the person accepting the task to follow through and accomplish the task at an appropriate level. The person who the nurse has delegated the task to must have an appropriate level of education and skill or training to assume the task.

Several factors and contexts influence the delegation of authority. In patient care, the state nurse practice act gives the RN the authority to delegate. In organizations, managers and leaders have legitimate authority to direct personnel and anticipate compliance. Nurses in direct patient care, management, and leadership positions may transfer responsibility and authority for the delegated task; however, each retains accountability for the process. Because many organizations use unlicensed assistive personnel such as nurses' aides, orderlies, and technicians, it behooves the nurse leader to be cognizant of the state nurse practice act, job description, knowledge and training, and skill level of each unlicensed assistive personnel before delegating.

Errors and pitfalls in delegation can occur particularly when the manager or leader is in a new position. The most common errors include over-delegation, under-delegation, and improper delegation (Kelly, 2008). Over-delegation often occurs when time management skills are poorly developed in an individual or when one is insecure in his or her own ability to perform a task. Under-delegation can occur when a leader manager lacks trust in subordinates' ability, may assume their subordinates will resent or feel overburdened with delegated work, or thinks that delegation connotes weakness and inability to get the work done. Improper delegation is delegating to the wrong person, or at the wrong time, or for the wrong reason or delegating beyond the capability of a person.

Lastly, delegation is highly impacted by cultural diversity (Marquis & Huston,

2009; Poole, Davidhizar, & Giger, 1995). Poole, Davidhizar, and Giger (1995) identify six cultural phenomena to consider when delegating: communication, space, social organization, time, environmental control, and biological variations. These can potentially affect the process and outcome of delegation because a select culture may have differing expectations concerning these behaviors or values. Communication refers to dialect, volume, eye contact, and touch. Interpersonal space differs between cultures. Social organization, particularly the family unit, is of greatest importance in some cultures. Cultures tend to be past, present, or future oriented to time. Cultural groups have internal or external locus of control or environmental control. Biological variations such as susceptibility to disease and physical stamina or physical differences, for example, size, should be considered when delegating.

See also American Nurses Association; Cultural Diversity; National Council of State Boards of Nursing, Inc. (NCSBN)

Kelly, P. (2008). *Nursing leadership & management.* Clifton Park, NY: Thomson/Delmar.

Marquis, B. L., & Huston, C. J. (2009). *Leadership roles and management functions in nursing: Theory and application* (6th ed.). Philadelphia, PA: Lippincott Williams & Wilkins.

Poole, V. L., Davidhizar, R. E., & Giger, J. N. (1995). Delegating to a transcultural team. *Nursing Management, 26*(8), 33–34.

Martha J. Greenberg

DIFFERENTIATED NURSING PRACTICE

The term "differentiated practice" entered the nursing lexicon in the mid-1950s, at the time when associate degree preparation for the registered nurse (RN) license came into being. The original plan was that professional practice would be within the realm of the nurse prepared at the baccalaureate-degree level and the new associate degree graduates, along with their colleagues prepared in hospital diploma programs, would practice as "technical" nurses.

Since the middle of the 20th century, there has been interest in developing models of care delivery that differentiate practice scope and responsibilities, based on the educational differences of the practitioners involved. It should be noted that the terms "professional" and "technical" are no longer the labels used in such differentiation discussions.

While this conceptual idea has long been discussed, there has never been a successful and lasting model of differentiated nursing practice implemented. There are several likely causes for this failure. First and probably foremost, there has always been an uneven distribution of graduates from the several programs. Over the years, hospital diploma schools have all but disappeared and in their place associate degree programs have been established in most geographical areas, thus providing a consistent supply of nurses to their respective communities. On the other hand, baccalaureate programs are less available, particularly in certain areas of the country and, therefore, cannot produce the number of graduates necessary for health care organizations to adequately fill the differentiated roles that they might wish to create.

Second, and equally important, is the fact that patients and clients do not tend to emit their needs in neat bundles that might be labeled as requiring the presence of either the bachelor of science in nursing (BSN) or the associate degree in nursing (ADN) prepared nurse at any given time. Rather, they generally emit their needs in "...muddled, unsorted and quite unpredictable bundles..." (McClure, 1976), making suitable staffing plans for differentiated models all but impossible.

Third, and perhaps least important, early on, the profession made the decision to license the graduates of the differentiated educational programs with an identical credential, that is, the RN. Although, to some, this may seem like a technicality, this has contributed to the view that there is, in fact, a single RN practice that is similar enough in most respects to make any differentiation an academic exercise.

As a result of this view, there has been very little movement toward the creation of differentiated practice models. One effort worth noting was attempted in South Dakota during the 1980s. It was a large demonstration project that was mounted over several years and involved intense work between a major health care provider and several nursing education programs (Koerner & Karpiuk, 1994). Other smaller efforts have also proven unsuccessful, and this track record, coupled with the predicted nursing shortage, will undoubtedly make the pursuit of differentiated models less attractive in the years to come.

American Association of Colleges of Nursing, American Organization of Nurse Executives & National Organization for Associate Degree Nursing. (1995). *A model for differentiated nursing practice.* Washington, DC: American Association of Colleges of Nursing.

Koerner, J. & K. Karpiuk. (1994). *Implementing differentiated practice: Transformation by design.* Gaithersburg, MD: Aspen.

McClure, M. L. (1976). Entry into professional practice: The New York proposal. *Journal of Nursing Administration. 6*(5), 12–17.

Margaret L. McClure

D

DISTANCE EDUCATION IN NURSING

Distance education is a broad term that describes teaching and learning when the student and the teacher are separated by time and space. Various types of information technology are used to connect the student and teacher and to create a virtual classroom. Distance education is used to facilitate access to education for learners who cannot easily travel to the source of instruction, to provide convenience for learners who are working during times when instruction is offered, and to recruit learners. Distance education is widely used in nursing education, particularly to offer graduate degrees, to provide continuing education, to orient new staff and update nurses' competencies in clinical agencies, and for client instruction.

FORMS OF DISTANCE EDUCATION

Early forms of distance education included print media (correspondence courses; independent study modules), broadcast television, videoconferencing, and audio-conferencing using a dial-up telephone with multiple connecting ports (Billings, 2007). With the advent of the Internet, online teaching (full Web courses or online courses blended with on-site learning experiences) and Internet videoconferencing have replaced these formats. Emerging technologies such as Second Life (secondlife.com/whatis) and other virtual excursions follow the basic concepts of distance education by promoting learning just-in-time regardless of proximity of learner and educator.

Distance education can be offered in synchronous or asynchronous modes. With *synchronous learning*, the teacher and the student meet together at the same time using "chat" software or videoconferencing programs, thus facilitating real-time interaction, dialogue, and document sharing. In *asynchronous* formats, learners and faculty interact independent of time constraints and communicate through discussion forms. *Blended* learning has both asynchronous work and at other times synchronous work online or on campus. Most recently, educators are adding mobile learning or m-learning. Mobile devices are helpful for people on the go and as an adjunct to other devices for learning. These handheld devices can be used for homework, looking up best practices while on a clinical service, communicating with classmates and instructors, course announcements, and other functions that are currently managed by computer (Huffstutler, Wyatt, & Wright, 2002).

ADVANTAGES AND DISADVANTAGES OF DISTANCE EDUCATION

The primary advantage of teaching and learning at a distance is the ability to make education accessible. Because learning at a distance can increase the use of best practices in teaching and learning such as active learning, interaction, and feedback, there can be pedagogical advantages as well (Billings, Connors, & Skiba, 2001). Disadvantages include high cost, time required to orient users to technology and new modes of teaching and learning, and teacher and learner preferences for face-to-face instruction for particular types of learning.

STRATEGIC PLANNING

To offer distance-accessible courses and programs requires a substantial investment in hardware or software, ongoing technology and user support, course design or redesign, and user orientation; leaders are well advised to develop thoughtful strategic plans before implementation. Strategic plans should include a proposed budget; although difficult to calculate, cost and benefit should be considered before initiating a distance education course or program.

QUALITY STANDARDS FOR OFFERING DISTANCE EDUCATION PROGRAMS

Several organizations have developed standards, guidelines, and peer review processes for offering quality distance delivered courses and programs (Little, 2009). These include the Council for Higher Education Accreditation (2002) and the American Association of Colleges of Nursing (1999, 2005), Distance Technology in Nursing Education and Alliance for Nursing Accreditation Statement on Distance Education Policies, which advise that schools of nursing seeking accreditation for distance education programs should meet the same standards as their on-campus programs.

EFFECTIVENESS OF DISTANCE EDUCATION IN NURSING

Numerous studies and recent analytic reviews of the literature indicate that distance education is effective (Mancuso-Murphy, 2007). The learning outcomes of distance-delivered education are the same as those when the instruction is offered on campus (Bata-Jones & Avery, 2004; Coose, 2010; Mills, 2007). Learners who participate in distance education are satisfied with the learning experience, particularly because of the access and convenience of remaining employed in their community while studying at a well-regarded school of nursing miles away (Leners, Wilson, & Sitzman, 2007). Data also indicate that the intended outcomes of professional

development and socialization can be obtained when learners work with mentors and preceptors during clinical components of distance education offerings (Billings et al., 2001; Lerners, Wilson, & Sitzman, 2007). Increased leadership effectiveness and efficiency using tablet technology is now being touted for the different types of business, including health care delivery (Helft, 2011).

American Association of Colleges of Nursing. (1999). *Distance technology in Nursing Education.* Retrieved from http://www.aacn.nche.edu/Publications/WhitePapers/whitepaper.htm

American Association of Colleges of Nursing. (2005). *Alliance for nursing accreditation statement on distance education policies.* Retrieved from http://www.aacn.nche.edu/Education/disstate.htm.

Billings, D. (2007). Distance education in nursing: 25 years and going strong. *Computers, Informatics, Nursing, 25*(3), 121–123.

Billings, D., Connors, H., & Skiba, D. (2001). Benchmarking best practices in Web-based nursing courses. *Advances in Nursing Science, 23*(3), 41–52.

Coose, C. S. (2010). Distance nursing education in Alaska: A longitudinal study. *Nursing Education Perspectives, 31*(2), 93–96.

Helft, M. (2011, February 21) IPad and other tablets make push into corporate world. *New York Times.* Retrieved from http://www.nytimes.com/2011/02/21/technology/21tablet.html?_r=1&ref=todayspaper

Huffstutler, S., Wyatt, T. H., & Wright, C. P. (2002). The use of handheld technology in nursing education. *Nurse Educator, 27,* 271–275.

Leners, D. W., Wilson, V.W., & Sitzman, K. L. (2007). Twenty-first century doctoral education: Online with a focus on nursing education. *Nursing Education Perspectives, 28*(6), 332–336.

Little, B. B. (2009).Quality assurance for online nursing courses. *Journal of Nursing Education, 48*(7), 381–387.

Mills, A. C. (2007). Evaluation of online and on-site options for master's degree and post-master's certificate programs. *Nurse Educator, 32*(2), 73–77.

Mancuso-Murphy, J. (2007). Distance education in nursing: An integrated review of online

D

nursing students' experiences with technology-delivered instruction. *Journal of Nursing Education, 46*(6), 252–260.

http://www.aacn.nche.edu/Education/pdf/MacyReport.pdf

http://www.brighthub.com/education/online

Diane M. Billings
Marilyn Jaffe-Ruiz

DOCTOR OF NURSING PRACTICE

In October 2004, the members of the American Association of Colleges of Nursing (AACN) passed a position statement endorsing the view that all nurses prepared for advanced nursing practice should acquire their education in a doctor of nursing practice (DNP) program, which prepares clinicians for the highest level of nursing practice. This monumental decision was accompanied by a second vote to approve the goal that the transition of all advanced nursing practice programs from the master's degree to the DNP level should be complete by 2015, thus providing a decade of advance notice for planning and transition.

In the intervening years, a groundswell of activity has occurred with the majority of academic institutions that prepare nurses for advanced practice having already made the transition or planning to do so. Why did this recommendation to move to the DNP come forward? How was the proposed position created? What is the potential impact on patient care? These are fundamentally important questions that the discipline must answer to assure the relevance of this evolution in nursing education.

The study of the potential transition to the practice doctorate in nursing began more than 2 years before the approval of the recommendations outlined in AACN's (2004) *Position Statement on the Practice Doctorate in Nursing.* During those discovery years, the task force charged with studying the issue met with multiple stakeholders from nursing education and practice, the higher education community, and health professionals from multiple disciplines. The recommendation to grant the DNP was also stimulated by an assessment of the changes that had occurred in nursing programs at the master's level. Master's programs had grown in the number of credits and clinical training required to earn a graduate degree in nursing. These changes were in direct response to the increasingly complex nature of health care delivered by nurses. Thus, graduates of master's programs were not awarded degrees that reflected the intense time and resource commitment required for program completion.

Upon endorsement of the DNP position statement by its membership, the AACN Board established a task force charged with setting the standards for these programs, and in October 2006, the *Essentials of Doctoral Education for Advanced Nursing Practice* (AACN, 2006a) was endorsed by the AACN members. These standards clearly articulate the expectations for the design and implementation of high-quality DNP programs and have since been endorsed by the Commission on Collegiate Nursing Education as a required set of standards to achieve DNP program accreditation. In addition, the AACN Board created a separate task force to develop an online tool kit and resources for educators seeking to implement DNP programs. This task force's final report continues to serve as an important resource for academic programs that are making the transition to the DNP (AACN, 2006b).

In an effort to enhance clarity around the practice doctorate in nursing, several important issues were addressed in the DNP position statement. First, the DNP is the only title that should be used in granting degrees. Similar to the expectations for medical doctors who receive only the MD degree, the recommendation was made that using multiple degree designations is confusing to the public and will hinder efforts to assure high-quality and safe patient care by similar professionals. Second, the position statement made clear that the DNP is a degree for individuals receiving preparation for practice in nursing. As defined in this document, only those areas of nursing that have a direct impact on patient care can be the focus of a DNP program. Thus, the DNP is not a degree for individuals who may want to specialize in education as their primary emphasis. The *DNP Essentials* document provides further articulation of this expectation, noting that individuals who desire a faculty role should have additional education beyond that required for the DNP to assure their effectiveness as educators (AACN, 2006a, p. 20).

The *DNP Essentials* were created with a strong focus on assuring that advanced clinicians would have continued expert preparation in the practice of nursing with an added capacity to engage in systems evaluation, evidence-based practice, quality improvement, and capacity to collaborate with nurse scientists to identify evidence gaps for future study. These skills assure that a more nuanced and sophisticated level of care interventions will be provided by DNP-prepared nurses.

The evolution of the DNP has been shaped by the discipline's widespread acceptance of the need to transition to the practice doctorate. Multiple organizations representing advanced nurses have endorsed the move to the DNP and established frameworks for the education of nurse practitioners, nurse anesthetists, clinical nurse specialists, and other advanced roles. In addition, the American Association of Nurse Anesthetists has endorsed the expectation that by 2015, no new master's-level nurse anesthetist programs will be accredited. In addition, by 2022, students may only enter nurse anesthetist programs that award the DNP to be eligible to sit for the nurse anesthetist certification examination, which is a requirement for practice in every state in the United States.

Currently, 72% of U.S. nursing programs that prepare advanced practice registered nurses have either begun the transition or have already made the move to the DNP (AACN, 2010). Clearly, the goal articulated by AACN's members, that the transition to the DNP occur by 2015, may not be met fully, although great progress has been made. However, the evidence is strong that the transition to this important new phase of education for advanced nursing practice is well underway and will continue to gain momentum into the foreseeable future.

American Association of Colleges of Nursing. (2004). *Position statement on the practice doctorate in nursing.* Washington, DC: Author. Retrieved from http://www.aacn.nche.edu/ DNP/DNPPositionStatement.htm

American Association of Colleges of Nursing. (2006a). *Essentials of doctoral education for advanced nursing practice.* Washington, DC: Author. Retrieved from http://www.aacn. nche.edu/DNP/pdf/Essentials.pdf

American Association of Colleges of Nursing. (2006b). *DNP Roadmap Task Force Report.* Washington, DC: Author. Retrieved from http://www.aacn.nche.edu/DNP/pdf/ DNProadmapreport.pdf

American Association of Colleges of Nursing. (2010). *The doctor of nursing practice: A progress report.* Retrieved from http://www.aacn.nche. edu/DNP/pdf/DNPForum3–10.pdf

Geraldine Bednash

E

Editing and Reviewing

The dissemination of knowledge is foundational to the relevance, currency, and growth of any profession. That is, activities engaged in by practitioners should be based upon the latest evidence and current thinking in the field. Dissemination can take many forms, including sharing of ideas among individuals and presentation at conferences via the Internet and in print journals. Dissemination via the written word has the potential to reach a greater number of professionals over varying periods of time, and if the work is peer reviewed, then the credibility of the knowledge is established. To ensure that the knowledge disseminated is accurate, unbiased, and up to date, a system of peer review developed in which experts in the field are asked to review, usually blinded to the authors of the manuscript and who are asked to make judgments about the disposition of the material, that is, reject, accept, revise, to the editor (Godlee & Jefferson, 2003; The British Academy, 2007). Editors, often referred to as "voice of the profession" (Kearney & Freda, 2006) then decide what, when, and how the information will be disseminated in the journal.

PEER REVIEW

The shaping of knowledge for use in a practice discipline is the responsibility of all experts in the field. Peer review provides authors with unbiased, objective opinions of the accuracy, significance, rigor, and usefulness of the content and presentation. Peer reviewers are asked to make recommendations about the significance of an idea, the rigor of the methods used, the appropriateness of the analysis, and the interpretation of the data. For non-data-based papers, reviewers are also asked to consider action or clinical. More recently, reviewers are often asked to report any ethical concerns they may have with a manuscript related to the plagiarism, the falsification, or the fabrication of data or reviewers also focus on the presentation, flow, and clarity of the presentation of material.

One often is asked why professionals will take the time to review manuscripts. A typical manuscript review will take an average of 5 hours of a reviewer's time, with no financial remuneration (Freda, Kearney, Baggs, Broome, & Dougherty, 2009). Most editors acknowledge their reviewers annually in an annual issue of the journal or on the journal Web site. Many individuals who review learn that reviewing helps them to be better writers themselves, keeps them abreast of new and exciting ideas, and enable a "payback" for those anonymous reviewers who provided them with substantive critique.

EDITING

The role of editor (of a book, journal, or any other dissemination venue) is to set the vision for the publication and to work with reviewers and authors to shape the scholarly products to support that vision. Editors of journals in particular play a unique and important role in most disciplines. Editors usually have extensive experience in their field and are well known within either the specialty or the profession for broader based journals.

The responsibilities of an editor include inviting papers from scholars in the field as well as accepting submissions from authors who believe their work is a good fit with the journal. An editor of a peer-reviewed journal will make often initial decisions about whether a manuscript is appropriately fit with the editorial purpose of the journal. If not, they typically notify the author soon after inquiry or submission, and many provide suggestions for journals that may be a better fit. If a manuscript is a "good fit," then the editor assigns the manuscript to peer reviewers, experts in a topic who can evaluate the manuscript for significance, rigor of method and thought, and the relevancy of recommendations for future research and/or practice. When all the referees' recommendations are received, a decision is made by the editor about the disposition of the manuscript—accept, revise, or reject. Editors, along with the authors, have responsibility for ensuring, as far as possible, that the content in an article is accurate, the sole intellectual property of the authors of the paper (Broome, 2009).

In cases where these conditions have not been met, editors have guidelines set by international organizations, such as the International Committee of Medical Journal Editors (icmje.org), that provide guidance about the next steps, including not publishing the paper and notifying the author(s) and the institutions they work for. Finally, one of the most challenging responsibilities of an editor is to write scholarly, thought-provoking, and substantive editorials for the journal. Most editors are employed full time in other roles in nursing. Although the time commitment varies depending on the size and number of issues published each year, the average editor spends up to 6 to 8 hours per week in the role. The compensation of editors for their time varies considerably—from no compensation to reimbursement for office expenses and an honorarium. There are numerous other satisfiers in the role that have been identified by editors, including helping to develop authors and helping to shape the profession's knowledge base for practice (Kearney & Freda, 2006).

Broome, M. (2008). The truth, the whole truth and nothing but the truth. *Nursing Outlook, 56*(4).

Freda, M., Kearney, M., Baggs, J., Broome, M., & Dougherty, M. (2009). Peer reviewer training and editor support: Results from an international survey of nursing peer reviewers. *Journal of Professional Nursing, 25*(2), 101–108.

Godlee, F., & Jefferson, T. (2003). *Peer review in the health sciences* (2nd ed.). London: BMJ Publishing Group.

Kearney, M., & Freda, M. (2006). Voice of the profession: Nurse editors as leaders. *Nursing Outlook, 54*, 263–267.

The British Academy. (2007, September). *Challenges for the humanities and social sciences: A British Academy Report* (Peer review). London: Author.

Marion E. Broome

E

ELECTRONIC HEALTH RECORD

The U.S. Department of Health and Human Services defines the electronic health record (EHR) as "An electronic record of health-related information on an individual that conforms to nationally recognized interoperability standards and that can be created, managed, and consulted by authorized clinicians and staff across more than one health care organization" (National Library of Medicine, 2010). It is noted that there are no universal definitions for related terms such as electronic medical record, computerized patient record, or computer health record. A personal health record is not the same thing as an EHR. The main difference is that a patient/consumer controls who can see or use the information in the personal health record, whereas the provider (or hospital) controls the information in the EHR (Centers for Medicare & Medicaid, 2010). These terms can refer to systems with distinctive purpose, content, and functional differences. In many cases, present-day EHRs contain patient demographics, financial data, orders, results, and clinical documentation.

In 2003, an Institute of Medicine (IOM) report identified eight care delivery functions that are essential for such records to promote greater safety, quality, and efficiency. The eight core functions are health information and data, result management, order management, decision support, electronic communication and connectivity, patient support, reporting and population health, and administrative processes and reporting. The secure exchange of information between various providers, including radiologists, laboratories, and other clinicians, would allow for comprehensive information to be available at the point of care. The federal Department of Health and Human Services has worked to establish criteria for the function, interoperability, security, and privacy features essential to a certifiable EHR (www.hhs.gov/healthit). Additional information about EHR certification can be found at www.CCHIT.org.

BENEFITS

Many organizations are introducing key components and functionality toward meeting the goal of a fully implemented EHR system. EHRs can provide many benefits for providers and patients including complete and accurate information, better access, and patient empowerment. With an EHR, providers have the information they need and know more about their patients before they walk into the examination room. They have needed information to diagnose problems earlier and improve patient health outcomes. An EHR also allows information to be shared more easily across health systems, leading to better coordination of care. With an EHR, patients are empowered to take a more active role in their health and can receive electronic copies of their medical records. Currently, most health care providers still use paper-based medical record systems; however, new government incentives are helping providers make the switch to EHRs (www.hhs.gov/healthit).

KEY ISSUES

Human factors research has begun to uncover unintended consequences of computerization. The complexities of the technology that make up an EHR add to the concern that new types of errors are emerging. A landmark study conducted by Ash, Berg, and Coiera (2004) reported two categories of errors that occur with the use of EHR systems; errors in data entry and retrieval and errors in communication and coordination. Data entry and retrieval errors occurred with outdated or complex human–computer interfaces, overly structured data entry requirements, imposing clerical tasks, and fragmented data retrieval formats that intensified the workload of an already busy clinician. This had a significant impact on communication and coordination of patient care. A poorly designed computer system may not reflect the reality of the care tasks or workflow causing the clinician to seek alternative approaches. Decision support tools designed to prevent errors can have the opposite effect when misused or poorly designed. Too many alert messages or overreliance on the system can lead to error and impact patient safety.

The privacy and confidentiality of patient information continues to be a concern. The Health Insurance Portability and Accountability Act is the federal law that has established a foundation to address some aspects of the protection of privacy in EHRs (Tang, 2000); however, there is still variability in the privacy laws across states. Another key issue with EHRs is related to the training required to use such systems; user instruction may not always be adequate to optimize patient privacy protections. In addition, many clinicians have not been exposed to the use of EHRs in their educational programs, which increases the learning curve for mastering use of such systems in the clinical practice environment.

STATE OF THE EVIDENCE

The management of medical orders is considered the connective tissue in any EHR. Orders are necessarily complex and integrate patient-specific interventions across departments. Orders management in an EHR crosses customary boundaries and is just as likely to integrate applications and functions as it is to disintegrate traditions when new work processes are crafted. A synthesis of the research on electronic medical orders, referred to as computerized provider order entry (CPOE), notes that the term CPOE is used imprecisely in the literature, which limits our ability to translate the findings of research. CPOE can refer to electronic systems that do or do not include the electronic transmission of orders to ancillary departments, the use of order sets, capabilities for complex intravenous, total parental nutrition (TPN) or oncology protocol orders, integrated alerts and reminders, pharmacy interfaces, or connections with clinical documentation (Hughes, 2006).

The implementation of an EHR as a means of reducing medical errors has received a lot of attention (Ash et al., 2004; Bates et al., 1999; Kohn, Corrigan, & Donaldson, 2000). Koppel et al. (2005) researched CPOE-related factors that may increase the risk of medication errors and found that clinicians reported new errors with CPOE because of fragmented data and processes, lack of integration among systems, and human–computer interaction issues. Recommendations to address these issues focus on providing communication and education to providers and consumers, system designs that support communication and clinical work processes, user participation in the implementation and ongoing monitoring of safety, and the use of qualitative multidisciplinary research methods to provide deeper insight into the benefits and issues surrounding EHR (Ash & Bates, 2005; Ash et al., 2004). The evidence from 23 studies that focused on efficiency, medication errors, or quality suggests that transcription errors can be eliminated with electronic communication and interfaces and structured order entry.

E

E

CPOE can substantially reduce overall and many serious medication errors if (a) electronic communication and automatic order interfaces are in place, (b) basic order checks for completeness are present, and (c) decision support at its most basic level is available—interaction checking for drug/drug, drug/allergy, and dosing ranges (Hughes, 2006).

The investigation of the challenges and barriers to implementing clinical decision support revealed problems with insufficient clinical evidence to develop complete medical knowledge bases, low clinician demand related to lack of integration into workflow, concerns about autonomy, legal and ethical ramification of overriding recommendations of clinical decision support in an EHR, and its usability (Eichner & Das, 2010).

NATIONAL INITIATIVES

The major challenges in health care including high costs, medical errors, variable quality, administrative inefficiencies, and lack of coordination are all often connected to inadequate use of health information technology (HIT) as an integral part of health care (Thompson & Brailer, 2004). In April 2004, a Presidential Executive Order called for widespread adoption of interoperable EHRs within 10 years. The adoption of interoperable EHRs and a nationwide network for appropriate sharing of health information is the means for realizing the vision of medical information that follows the consumer across settings, of clinicians that have complete, computerized patient information, of quality initiatives that measure and drive performance, and of public health and bioterrorism surveillance that are seamlessly integrated into care. Within the context of a strategic framework, four goals were asserted for the HIT Decade, each with specified strategies intended

to contribute to the vision for improved health care.

These goals include informing clinical practice to improve patient care, connecting clinicians, personalizing care, and improving population health.

In 2009 the Health Information Technology for Economic and Clinical Health Act authorized programs to improve health care through the promotion of HIT, including EHR and secure electronic health information exchange. This law allows eligible health care professionals and hospitals to qualify for Medicare and Medicaid incentive payments when they adopt certified EHR technology for "meaningful use" (Blumenthal, 2010). It also identifies the technical capabilities required for certified EHR technology (healthit.hhs.gov/portal/server.pt?open=512&objID=2996&mode=2). The 2010 Patient Protection and Affordable Care Act also addressed the need to increase adoption of EHRs.

NURSING IMPLICATIONS

The use of EHRs has the potential to improve quality, safety, and efficiency of care delivery. Further research is needed in the areas of nursing impacts in CPOE and EHR, human–computer interaction, and the science of implementation of such systems (Hughes, 2006). Nurses need to be aware of the specific functionality of EHRs that they use and provide diligent clinical and administrative monitoring if decision support and interfaces are not available in such systems. Because EHRs create professional interdependence, work design, roles, and communication changes need to be carefully analyzed. In addition, the design of such systems must be tailored for patient safety, and nurses need to play an important role in the development and implementation of the EHR to ensure success in health care settings. Finally, it is critical for nurses to be informed and involved in national initiatives directed to improve the health and safety of the nation through the safe and appropriate application of the tools of our time.

See also Meaningful Use Rule; Technology; Transforming Care at the Bedside

Ash, J. S., & Bates, D. W. (2005). Factors and forces affecting EHR system adoption: Report of a 2004 ACMI discussion. *Journal of the American Medical Informatics Association, 12*(1), 8–12.

Ash, J. S., Berg, M., & Coiera, E. (2004). Patient care information system-related errors. *Journal of the American Medical Informatics Association, 11*(2), 104–112.

Bates, W. D., Teich, J. M., Lee, J., Seger, D., Kuperman, G. J., Ma'Luf, N., et al. (1999). The impact of computerized physician order entry on medication error prevention. *Journal of the American Medical Informatics Association, 6*(4), 313–321.

Blumenthal, D. (2010). The "meaningful use" regulation for electronic health records. *New England Journal of Medicine.* Retrieved July 13, 2010, from http://www.nejm.org

Centers for Medicare and Medicaid Services. (2010). *Learn more about person health records.* Retrieved August 12, 2010, from http://www.medicare.gov/navigation/manage-your-health/personal-health-records/learn-more-phr.aspx

Eichner, J., & Das, M. (2010, March). *Challenges and barriers to clinical decision support (CDS) design and implementation experienced in the Agency for Healthcare Research and Quality CDS Demonstrations* (AHRQ Publication No. 10–0064-EF). Rockville, MD: Agency for Healthcare Research and Quality, U.S. Department of Health and Human Services.

Hughes, R. G. (2006). *Patient safety and quality: An evidence-based handbook for nurses.* Rockville, MD: Agency for Healthcare Research and Quality.

Institute of Medicine. (2003). *Key capabilities of an electronic health record system: Letter report* (Committee on Data Standards for Patient Safety: Board of Health Care Services). Washington, DC: The National Academes Press. Retrieved August 30, 2010, from http://www.nap.edu/catalog.php?record_id=10781

Kohn, L. T., Corrigan, J. M., & Donaldson, M. S. (Eds.). (2000). *To err is human: Building a safer health system.* Washington, DC: Institute of Medicine.

Koppel, R., Metlay, J. P., Cohen, A., Abaluck, B., Localio, A., Kimmel, S. E., et al. (2005). Role of computerized physician order entry systems in facilitating medication errors. *Journal of the American Medical Association, 293*(10), 1197–1203.

National Library of Medicine. Retrieved August 10, 2010, from http://www.nlm.nih.gov/services/ehr.html#nlm

Tang, P. C. (2000). The HIPAAcratic oath: Do no harm to patient data. *Physician Executive, 26*(3), 50–56. Retrieved July 31, 2006, from http://www.findarticles.com/p/articles/mi_m0843/is_3_26/ai_102450894

Thompson, T. G., & Brailer, D. J. (2004). *The decade of health information technology: Delivering consumer-centric and information-rich health care.* Washington, DC: U.S. Department of Health and Human Services.

Carol A. Romano
Charlotte A. Seckman

EMERGENCY PREPAREDNESS

Nurses, regardless of the health care sector or their assigned role in an organization, are in excellent position to participate in and, in many cases, assume leadership status in emergency preparedness response. Most would agree that after September 11, 2001, much more attention has been focused on emergency preparedness, and the nursing profession was challenged, as were many other professions, to rise to the occasion.

Although there is much more that needs to be accomplished in terms of both clinical practice and educational preparation relative to emergency and disaster preparedness in nursing, as well as in many other facets related to community preparedness planning overall, one must also acknowledge the achievements of nurses in the field who have applied creative approaches to emergency response under difficult, time-sensitive circumstances, often without previous formalized education or training. This has been particularly evident in the community health nursing sector, both in public health and to a lesser degree in home health.

PUBLIC HEALTH

Building upon their population-oriented skill sets, public health nurses, who represent the largest group of professionals in this field, have been among the innovators and foot soldiers in response to biological emergencies. As a direct result of 9/11, followed closely by the threat of anthrax releases thought to be a precursor to biological warfare, mass emergency planning was already in full swing at the local level. After 9/11, the Centers for Disease Control and Prevention had years before assigned biological preparedness and response to the states and their corresponding local health departments. Guided by the Centers for Disease Control and Prevention, states all across the nation in coordination with their local health departments and community partners achieved numerous preparedness-related deliverables, many involving nursing leadership. This was particularly apparent during the H1N1 influenza outbreak that began in 2008 and was formally declared a global pandemic in June 2009. In collaboration with their community partners, hundreds of public health nurses in New York State can be credited with the following during the recent H1N1 influenza pandemic:

- Developing and implementing complex plans to quickly stand up points of dispensing clinics for the mass dispensing of vaccine. In one New York county,

individuals were vaccinated within 8 to 10 minutes, including time for registration, medical interviewing, and clearance by public health nurses to assure safe vaccination. In many instances, public health nurses assumed leadership status as points of dispensing managers in directing mass clinic activities whereby hundreds and even thousands of residents were treated.

- Taking local responsibility for heightened surveillance activities to detect patterns of infectious illness in its earliest stages on a daily and real-time basis in coordination with state officials.

- Investigating infectious disease reports to determine confirmation of illness, contacting exposed individuals for follow up, and taking other measures to prevent or limit the scope of the outbreak.

- Extensive teaching to health providers and community members on a one-to-one and broader basis regarding the infectious agent and prevention and control measures.

- Coordinating with physicians to assess their need for vaccine, and providing it to ensure as widespread a distribution as possible.

HOME CARE

In the home health care industry, progress in emergency preparedness and response can also be recognized. Although not nearly to the same level as in the public health nursing sector, there is clearly a raised consciousness of the role of the home care nurse vis-à-vis emergency preparedness.

In New York State, certified home health agencies implement a patient classification system that assesses and prioritizes a patient's risk level in the home setting under emergency circumstances. In this system, there are three levels of risk from highest to lowest need. Once entered into an agency's information system, a list of patients in greatest need of assistance during an emergency can be immediately identified. In addition, home health agencies in New York State monitor the Health Provider Network (HNP) on a daily basis; the HPN is a statewide secured, electronic communications system that notifies health care providers of critical information including emergency situations.

Of primary significance, home care organizations are in position to outreach to special needs populations, a critically important and challenging segment in terms of emergency preparedness. Special needs populations, of major concern to emergency partners, include the homebound frail elderly and physically disabled populations among others. These individuals account for the majority of those on service with home care agencies and are at their most vulnerable because of the current acute episode of illness that preceded the need for home care services in the first place. One-to-one education regarding personal and family preparedness by home care nurses is opportune in this setting. Has the client or family considered a plan in the event of power and telephone outages? Are there adequate provisions in the home should sheltering in place becomes necessary? What other factors are critical to consider that may impact on their health and well-being? In a pandemic influenza scenario and during other emergency events as well, there is a growing sense of urgency among nursing leaders regarding emergency preparedness and awareness of the need to engage this population of special needs clients.

CONCLUSION

- Nurses play a critical role in emergency planning and response that is exponentially enhanced through collaboration with key partners such as departments of emergency services, local hospitals, law enforcement, state and federal officials, academic institutions, medical reserve corps, and other entities.

- Public health nurses are advancing population health and safety through mass distribution of vaccine, heightened surveillance, and educational outreach among other activities.

- Home care nurses play a critical role in reaching special needs populations on a one-to-one and family-oriented basis and underscoring the need for personal preparedness planning. They are in position to effectively coordinate with their emergency partners in providing names of individuals and families who are at most risk. During surge circumstances, home care nurses can be an invaluable part of the community's emergency response team by managing the care of clients already on service and those being prematurely discharged from local hospitals.

- These strategies must be systematically extended to all home care organizations to reach as many individuals as possible during emergency events.

- Academic and clinical sectors must intersect and collaborate so that lessons learned in the field can be incorporated into nursing curricula and in turn future nurses can enter their chosen clinical workplaces with basic knowledge regarding emergency preparedness and the understanding that this is a critical nursing role in today's uncertain world.

- The public health and home care sectors serve as ideal clinical training sites for nursing students at all levels of education. There are numerous preparedness activities in these settings; however, there must be some flexibility built into nursing curricula to allow students to take advantage of the many opportunities for learning that exists.

- In spite of progress, many barriers still exist in community health nursing emergency

E

preparedness that nursing leaders must continue to address.

Additional information is available from the following sources:

Aldrich, N., & Benson, W. (2008, January). Disaster preparedness and the chronic disease: Needs of vulnerable older adults. *Preventing Chronic Disease, 5*(1), 1–7.

Barney, C. E., et al. (2009). Emergency preparedness and considerations for the geriatric population. *Texas Public Health Association Journal, 61*(4), 39–41.

Baron, S., McPhaul, K., Phillips, S., Gershon, R., & Lipscomb, J. (2009). Protecting home health care workers: A challenge to pandemic influenza preparedness planning. *American Journal of Public Health, 99*(Suppl. 2), S301–S307.

Davies, K. (2005). Disaster preparedness and response: More than major incident initiation. *British Journal of Nursing, 14*(16), 868–871.

Doherty, M. (2004). An emergency management model for home health care organizations. *Home Health Care Management Practice, 16*, 374.

Fox, M. H., White, G. W., Rooney, C., & Rowland, J. L. (2007). Disaster preparedness and response for persons with mobility impairments: Results from the University of Kansas "Nobody Left Behind" Study. *Journal of Disability Policy Studies, 17*, 196.

Gershon R. R. M., et al. (2007). Home health care challenges and avian influenza. *Home Health Care Management Practice, 20*, 58.

Hendriks, L., & Bassi, S. (2009, August). Emergency preparedness from the ground up: A local agency perspective. *Home Health Care Management & Practice, 21*(5), 346–352.

Hughes, F., Grigg, M., Fritsch, K., & Calder, S. (2007) Psychosocial response in emergency situations—The nurse's role. *International Nursing Review, 54*, 19–27.

Jakeway, C. C., LaRosa, G., Carry, A., & Schoenfisch, S. (2008). The role of public health nurses in emergency preparedness and response: A position paper of the association of state and territorial directors of nursing. *Public Health Nursing, 25*(4), 353–361.

Knebel, A., & Phillips, S. J. (2008). *Home health care during an influenza pandemic: Issue and resources* (ARHQ Publication No. 08-0018). Rockville, MD: Agency for Healthcare Research and Quality.

Laditka, S. B., Laditka, J. N., Cornman, C. B., Davis, C. B., & Chandlee, M. J. (2008). Disaster preparedness for vulnerable persons receiving in-home, long-term care in South Carolina. *Prehospital and Disaster Medicine, 23*(2), 133–142.

McHugh, M. D. (2010). Hospital nursing staff and public health emergency preparedness: Implications for policy. *Public Health Nursing, 27*(5), 442–449.

National Association of Home Care & Hospice. (2008). *Emergency preparedness packet for home health agencies.* Washington, DC: Author.

National Center for Disaster Preparedness (2007, March). *Emergency preparedness: Addressing the needs of people with disabilities.* New York, NY: Mailman School of Public Health: Columbia University.

Nick, G. A., et al. (2009, March–April). Emergency preparedness for vulnerable populations: People with special health-care needs. *Public Health Reports, 124*, 338–343.

O'Brien, N. (2003, January–February). *Emergency preparedness for older people.* New York, NY: International Longevity Center.

Office of Homeland Security. (2008). *Disaster planning guide for home health care providers.* Washington, DC: Author.

Rebmann, T., Carrico, R., & English, J. F. (2008). Lessons public health professionals learned from past disasters. *Public Health Nursing, 25*(4), 344–352.

Turale, S. (2008). How prepared are nurses and other health professionals to cope in and manage disaster situations? *Nursing and Health Sciences, 10*, 165–166.

Weeber, S. C. (2007). Home health care after Hurricanes Katrina and Rita: A report from the field. *Home Health Care Management Practice, 19*, 104.

Loretta Molinari

EMOTIONAL INTELLIGENCE

Emotional intelligence (EI) developed as a topic of scientific interest when Salovey and Mayer (1990) used the term to refer to people's ability to monitor emotions in themselves and others and then to use this information to guide actions. Rooted in the work of Edward Thorndike on social intelligence, the recent popularity of EI stems from writings of supporters who believe EI is important for personal and professional success, represents a component of effective leadership, and can be enhanced through training. Cooper and Sawaf (1997) define EI as "…the ability to sense, understand and effectively apply the power and acumen of emotions as a source of human energy, information, connection and influence" (page xiii). These authors go on to define four cornerstones of EI. They are (1) emotional literacy, (2) emotional fitness, (3) emotional depth, and (4) emotional alchemy. Emotional literacy involves attention and self-management of one's emotional honesty, emotional energy, emotional feedback, and practical intuition. Emotional fitness requires attention and focus of one's authentic presence, skill at radiating trust, management of constructive discontent, and attention to resilence and renewal. Emotional depth relates to mastery of one's unique purpose and potential coupled with commitment, accountability, and use of influence without authority, resulting in applied integrity. Finally, emotional alchemy is supported by a leader's development of intuition, reflective time shifting, and sensing opportunities to create the future. EI is a critical success factor that supports decision making, communication, strategic thinking, team work, customer loyalty, creative thinking and innovation, and leadership success.

There is considerable interest in three models and measures (Cherniss, 2004) of EI, which are Salovey and Mayer (1990), Goleman (1995), and Bar-On (2000). John D. Mayer, one of the authors of the Mayer–Salovey Caruso Emotional Intelligence Test has created and collaborated with others on the development of a Web site

(http://www.unh.edu/emotional_intelligence/index.html) dedicated to communicating scientific information about EI including information about cognition, motivation, emotions, and personality.

Bar-On, R. (2000). Emotional and social intelligence: Insights from the Emotional Quotient Inventory. In R. Bar-On & J. D. A. Parker (Eds.), *The handbook of emotional intelligence* (pp. 363–388). San Francisco, CA: Jossey-Bass.

Cherniss, C. (2004). Intelligence, emotional. In C. Spielberger (Ed.), *Encyclopedia of applied psychology* (Vol. 2, pp. 315–319). Oxford, UK: Elsevier Academic Press.

Cooper, R., & Sawaf, A. (1997). *Executive EQ: Emotional intelligence in leadership and organizations*. New York, NY: Putnam.

Emotional Intelligence. Retrieved September 11, 2010, from http://www.unh.edu/emotional_intelligence.

Goleman, D. (1995). *Emotional intelligence*. New York, NY: Bantam Books.

Salovey, P., & Mayer, J. D. (1990). Emotional intelligence. *Imagination, Cognition, & Personality, 9*(3), 185–211.

Daniel J. Pesut

EMPLOYEE PERFORMANCE APPRAISAL

One of the most important responsibilities of leaders, who are also managers, is evaluating the work performance of individuals that they supervise. The employee appraisal provides the opportunity to review goals and the attainment of these expectations. This formal time is devoted to a review of past work and culminates with a discussion of future direction and opportunities for growth and professional development; it is also a valuable opportunity to look toward the future and to assess alignment with organizational priorities.

Ideally, the process is a two-way communication designed to motivate and encourage the employee and stimulate professional growth. The time should also be used to clarify the mission and goals of the institution and whether and to what extent the employee is contributing to achieving these goals.

The public has long demanded patient safety and fiscal accountability from health professionals. The Centers for Medicare and Medicaid Services (2010) initiated mandates for patient care outcomes that are tied to financial incentives. The Hospital-Consumer Assessment of Health Plans Survey (2010), designed by the Centers for Medicare and Medicaid Services and the Agency for Healthcare Research and Quality, makes patient satisfaction scores transparent. The Joint Commission (2010) standards call for a culture of safety. Further, the Institute of Medicine of the National Academies (2010) calls on nurses to be full partners with physicians and other health care professionals in providing patient care. Currently, the public demand that health care professionals who are accountable also need to play a role in ongoing employee evaluations. Employees need to be appraised of how they are meeting the challenges of their roles. If the employees are ultimately accountable, this needs to be acknowledged in employee evaluations.

APPRAISER ANXIETY

The appraiser has the responsibility of evaluating feelings and preconceived ideas about the employee and focusing on clear measurable outcomes with concrete examples. This may be complicated by anxiety experienced by both the manager and the employee. What gets in the appraiser's way emotionally? The appraiser's own anxiety about anticipated results based on past history with a particular employee or other employees, or personal feelings or biases may affect the assessment process and, ultimately, the outcomes. Most health care managers have risen to their positions because they are clinically competent. Many have not had formal management training and have had little experience in giving employee evaluations. In the role of appraiser, the manager may also worry about anticipated and unanticipated results. For example, what should the manager do if there is an emotional reaction such as crying, denial, or defensiveness?

The evaluation process requires specific interpersonal and counseling skills (Chandra, 2006). If the manager has been attentive all year, addressed concerns when they occurred, and offered praise when appropriate, there should be no surprises for the employee. The meeting can be used for a productive look at performance and future goals. Performance reviews are not the time to give negative criticism for things that have gone wrong all year long. The review is not an opportunity to place blame. Failure of an employee to reach targets should be addressed when the failure is discovered, not at the time of the annual review (Armstrong, 2006). If the formal review is viewed in a negative light by the employee, it is likely to cause more apprehension, especially if the review is tied to compensation. Therefore, it is wise to give prior thought to handling employee tension and possible emotional reactions should they occur.

EMPLOYEE ANXIETY

Anxiety for the employee is caused by a fear of the unknown. Even if they have open communication with their manager, the anticipation of an evaluation causes tension. To eliminate some of this fear and tension, a standard approach is used for evaluating employees. The position description specifies preemployment competencies and what competencies the employee needs to attain. This becomes the basis for the annual evaluation. In addition, there may be annual institutional and/or employee goals that the employee is required to accomplish. Agency human resource policies guide the manager and provide standardized forms for each position description. A standardized measurement-based performance evaluation process creates objectivity and makes the process predictable. When the manager has solid measures, employees are more focused (de Koning, 2005). Outcome measures instill clarity of role expectations.

Evaluating employees is an ongoing process. It takes the form of the required annual appraisal mandated by the organization and regulatory agencies and the ongoing evaluation of work and performance to be addressed whenever the employee is not fulfilling role expectations. In addition, incorporated into a manager's routine is the praise and recognition of a job well done. The Gallup Organization researchers and others have reported that people remember criticism but respond to praise. Feedback that focuses on the negative makes people defensive, whereas praise produces confidence and a desire to be more productive (Morgan, 2005).

EMPLOYEE SELF-ASSESSMENT

A proactive approach for the employee has been recommended by Jackman and Strober (2003). Their four manageable-step approach consists of self-assessment, external feedback, absorbing the feedback, and absorbing the change. In the Jackman and Strober method, the feedback is from trusted colleagues. The organization benefits when employees are open and deal with feedback constructively; their work better aligns with the mission and goals of the institution. Employees can improve communication throughout their department by openly seeking feedback from management and coworkers. This approach is not to be confused with the 360-degree method described by Peiperl (2001).

The popular 360-degree feedback approach focuses on feedback from peers, supervisors, and subordinates and self-evaluation. Although time consuming, it has value in that it is comprehensive. This kind of feedback is a work in progress because all employees need coaching to understand the method and potential hidden conflicts (Peiperl, 2001). Ideas from this method should be incorporated into employee evaluations in health care settings, including consumer satisfaction, a valuable outcome measure. Every employee is responsible for patient satisfaction. Also, peer review is useful to evaluate teamwork. When the health care team works well together, everyone benefits. The classic work regarding employee self-assessment by Drucker still has validity today. McGregor (1957) described this process as part of objective review that ensures employee participation in the process. The employee starts the process with a self-analysis, identifying strengths and weaknesses and defining short-term goals or targets. The manager enters the process by helping the employee relate the self-appraisal to targets that are in alignment with organization goals. The employee, with coaching from the manager, identifies specific steps to take to achieve these targets. This is to be accomplished within a specific time frame. The approach described by McGregor shifts the emphasis from appraisal to analysis, which is a more positive approach. Performance is tied to goals or targets rather than employee personality. This allows the manager to focus on coaching the employee.

Although evaluation of employees is time consuming and labor intensive, it is an

E

E

opportunity for the manager and employee to connect and revitalize their work relationship. Successful appraisals yield positive results with motivated workers. Take the time to provide a quiet, confidential environment and focus on the opportunities for the coming year.

Armstrong, M. (2006). Performance management key strategies and practical approaches (3rd ed.). Philadelphia, PA: Kogan Page.

Centers for Medicare and Medicaid Services. (2010). *Reporting hospital quality data for annual payment update.* Retrieved on November 22, 2010, from http://www.cms.gov/Hospital QualityInits/08_HospitalRHQDAPU.asp

Chandra, A. (2006, Spring). Employee evaluation strategies for healthcare organizations— A general guide. *Hospital Topics: Research and Perspectives on Healthcare, 84*(2).

de Koning, G. (2004, December). Evaluating employee performance: Part 2. *Gallup Management Journal*, 1–5. Retrieved November 24, 2010, from http://gmj.gallup.com

Hospital-Consumer Assessment of Health Plans Survey. (2010). Retrieved November 24, 2010, from http://www.hcahpsonline.org/home.aspx

Institute of Medicine of the National Academies. (2010). The future of nursing leading change, advancing health report brief. Retrieved November 20, 2010, from http://www.nap.edu/catalog/12894.html

Jackman, J. M., & Strober, M. H. (2003, April). Fear of feedback. *Harvard Business Review*, 101–107.

McGregor, D. (1957, May–June). An uneasy look at performance appraisal. *Harvard Business Review*, 89–94.

Roberts, L. M., Spreitzer, G., Dutton, J., Quinn, R., Heaphy, E., & Barker, B. (2005, January). How to play to your strengths. *Harvard Business Review, 83*(1), 74–80.

Peiperl, M. (2001, January). Getting 360-degree feedback right. *Harvard Business Review*, 142–147.

The Joint Commission. (2010). National Patient Safety Goals (NPSGs). Retrieved November 24, 2010, from http://www.jointcommission.org/PatientSafety/NationalPatientSafetyGoals

Christine Coughlin

EMPLOYEE RESOURCE GROUPS

Employee resource groups (ERGs) are the miner's canaries in today's organizations and one of the most formidable workplace engagement strategies in today's successful companies. Ninety percent of Fortune 500 companies have them in place (Frankel, 2010). ERGs are called different things in different companies—business resource groups, associate resource groups, and sometimes employee networks or affinity groups. Regardless of the nomenclature, they are defined as a group of employees who come together for a common business mission and reflect a common characteristic, for example, ethnicity, race, age sexual orientation, life situation, organizational level, and religion. Participation is open to all employees who are in good standing with the company. The relationship is mutually beneficial for employees and for the agenda of the company.

Because they are not social enclaves, many believe they create a sense of community and connectivity, both internally and externally, and many consider ERG members to be partners to an organization. They can break down barriers on understanding or mistrust or misinformation that exist not only between colleagues but also between members of particular communities and to a larger community external to the organization. The needs and interests of the participants come together so that their knowledge and lived experience can be tapped

- to raise awareness of cultural and demographic shifts that impact the business;
- to identify opportunities to capitalize on changing market conditions;
- to drive problem solving for issues impacting the organization;

- to support recruitment and retention of a diverse workforce;

- to provide peer coaching;

- to model behaviors that demonstrate the organization's ideals; and

- to enhance the cultural competency of the organization.

ERGs are often used to nurture talent and to validate human resource processes for talent development and retention and typically product development, customer service enhancements, and marketing campaigns geared toward traditionally underrepresented groups. Three key benefits of ERGs are leadership development, customer outreach, and improving corporate culture. To avoid them from becoming griping sessions, the purpose of ERGs should be tied to support of an organization's mission. They should not be used to set strategy, to make or embrace policy, to make or transmit grievances, and to investigate discrimination or harassment charges, nor should they be used to engage in activities that address terms and conditions of employment, employee evaluations, or employee discipline.

History and circumstances are asking new things from us, and diversity is yet another fundamental human experience that is always intruding itself into our lives. The fact of the matter is who we are today is different from who we were yesterday, challenging organizations to be culturally responsive. Most of us are communicating with persons from other cultures, either in person or electronically. One of the greatest requests is to embrace a deeper insight of the new norm of constant change in this flatter world. Constant change places us in a continual state of transformation and is unsettling, unnerving, and intimidating (Rosen, 2008). Gripped in fear about having to confront the differences that diversity

brings, society focuses on numbers and statistics to frame the ground sweeping changes rather than to hold the courageous and robust dialogues that would truly bring transformative understandings of our different lived experiences and the subsequent impact of tapping available resources of existing colleagues. A just society, however, brings issues out into the open and so does a smart organization.

Stephan Strasser (1969), in *The Idea of Dialogical Phenomenology*, points out in his third law of dialogue that "in knowing, evaluating, and striving I must approach the matter under discussion in a way that is formally the same as that of the 'you' with whom I am in dialogue." Framing realities, which by the way are invented not discovered, means facing the complexities, challenges, and opportunities of a global world, ready or not. When it comes to the lived experience of difference, they help us to know and to be familiar with the world of others on the basis of their being in the world (Gendlin, 1973).

There's a reason ERGs are called "resource" groups. They are key to finding and developing organizational leaders and reaching increasingly diverse markets; they help to maximize curiosity and minimize certainty with everyone encountered. Patterned responses have no place in today's global society and offer very little to the work that presents itself to the nurse leader of today. Philosophers like Karl Jaspers and Martin Buber devoted their works to the value of dialogue in human relationships. For example, Jaspers (1957) stated that "conversation, dialogue, is necessary for the truth itself which by its very nature opens to an individual only in dialogue with another individual" (Halling, Leifer, & Rowe, 2006). The German hermeneutic philosopher, Hans-George Gadamer (1975), portends that "a conversation has a spirit of its own, and

E

that the language used in it bears its own truth within it" (p. 345). ERGs are all about the currency of dialogue and taking the information, wisdom, and insights to make great organizational decisions and strategies for success. Their benefits far exceed their risks.

Frankel, B. (2010, September/October). *Reach your business goals through increased participation* (pp. 21–35). Newark, NJ: DiverstyInc.

Gadamer, G. H. (1975). *Truth and method*. New York, NY: Crossroad.

Gendlin, E. T. (1973). Experiential phenomenology. In M. Natanson (Ed), *Phenomenology and the social science* (pp. 281–322). Evanston, IL: Northwestern University Press.

Halling, S., Leifer, M., & Rowe, J. (2006). *Emergence of the dialogical approach: Forgiving another. Qualitative research methods for psychologist*. New York, NY: Elsevier.

Jaspers, K. (1957). *The great philosopher*. New York, NY: Harcourt, Brace, and World.

Rosen, R. H. (2008). *Embracing uncertainty and anxiety. Leader to leader* (Vol. 50, pp. 34–38). San Francisco, CA: Jossey-Bass.

Strasser, S. (1969). *The idea of dialogical phenomenology*. Pittsburgh, PA: DuQuesne University Press.

G. Rumay Alexander

EMPLOYEE SAFETY

Under the workers' rights section of the Occupational Safety and Health Act (OSHA) of 1970, all workers in the United States have the right to a safe workplace, and OSHA requires employers to provide a workplace that is free of serious recognized hazards and is in compliance with the mandatory OSHA standards. Occupational health surveillance for health care workers is targeted to specific exposures (e.g., chemicals, hazardous drugs, blood-borne pathogens, airborne infections). A medical surveillance program should be in place to minimize worker exposure and to include appropriate elements of a hierarchy of controls (including engineering, administrative, and personal protective equipment). Rogers (1997), a nursing expert in occupational health, delineated five categories of safety risk hazards encountered in health care—biological/infectious risks, chemical risks, environmental/hazards risks, physical risks, and psychological risks. The American Nurses Association (ANA, 2010a, 2010b) through various surveys of its members, for example, the Registered Nurse Population Survey (2000) and the Nurses' Health and Safety Concerns (2001), has concluded that nurses are increasingly in "harm's way" in health care settings. Nurses report job stress as a top health concern, followed by back injuries, contracting HIV or hepatitis from a needle stick injury, becoming infected with TB or another disease, sustaining an on-the-job assault, developing a latex allergy, and having a fatigue-related car accident after leaving work (IOM, 2004). In response to the significant number and severity of work-related back injuries and other musculoskeletal disorders among nurses, ANA sponsors a highly successful *Handle with Care Campaign* (de Castro, 2004), an award-winning health care industry-wide effort to prevent back and other musculoskeletal injuries. In addition, ANA supports Safe Needles—Save Lives, Tobacco-Free Nurse, Nurse Immunization, RN No Harm, and Healthy Nurse programs. ANA has made nurses' health, environmental, and workplace safety issues an organizational core issue addressed by its Center for Environmental and Occupational Health. Nurse leaders have the responsibility of ensuring that vulnerabilities in the workplace are minimized. According to ANA's *Code of Ethics for Nurses*, Provision 6, nurses should address concerns about the health care environment through appropriate channels and, if not successfully resolved, then it is essential to have whistleblower protections in place to ensure proper reporting of unsafe work conditions and patient safety issues.

See also American Nurses Association

American Nurses Association. (2010a). *Safe needles, save lives*. Retrieved January 23, 2011, from www.nursingworld.org/MainMenu Categories/OccupationalandEnvironmental/ occupationalhealth/SafeNeedles.aspx

American Nurses Association. (2010b). *Safe patient handling*. Retrieved January 23, 2011, from http://www.anasafepatienthandling. org/

de Castro, A. B. (2004). Handle With Care®: The American Nurses Association's campaign to address work-related musculoskeletal disorders. *Online Journal of Issues in Nursing, 9*(3), 45–54.

Institute of Medicine, Committee on the Work Environment for Nurses and Patient Safety. (2004). *Keeping patients safe: Transforming the work environment of nurses*. Washington, DC: National Academies Press.

Rogers, B. (1997). As I see it: Is health care a risky business? *The American Nurse, 29*, 5–6.

The Registered Nurse Population. (2000, March). In E. Spratley, A. Johnson, J. Sochalski, M. Fritz, & W. Spencer, *Nurses' Health and Safety Concerns* (2001). Retrieved March 30, 2011, from http://www.nurs-ingworld.org/MainMenuCategories/ OccupationalandEnvironmental/occupa-tionalhealth/HealthSafetySurvey.aspx

Karen A. Ballard

EMPLOYEE SATISFACTION

One of the critical conditions of organizational success is employee satisfaction. Although this particular phenomenon is true of any business enterprise, it is particularly true of health care organizations. Employee satisfaction is a cornerstone, as it were, of organizational stability and continuity of patient care. Employee satisfaction can lead to loyalty to and pride in the organization, creativity in the workplace, and mutual interchange between employer and employee; also, it can certainly influence patient satisfaction with his or her quality of care.

Employee satisfaction is important to health care organizations because it can reflect the climate of a healthy facility and a high level of organizational productivity, employee motivation, and employee performance. Satisfied employees convey a certain level of confidence to clients, which, in turn, generates a level of trust in the competence and quality of care provided by the caregiver(s) in particular, and by the organization, in general.

Circumstances that lead to a reduction in nurse satisfaction revolve around staffing, specifically coworker absenteeism or high turnover, which leaves the workplace chronically short staffed, increasing stress. Adequate staffing is an integral part of job satisfaction for nurses. Other dissatisfiers include a lack of supplies to care for patients, work overload, poor communication with physicians, and negative relationships with coworkers. Conversely, strong coworker bonds can be a satisfier. Employee satisfaction is enhanced when organizations have open and clear lines of communication to administrators and provide those working directly with patients the ability to participate in decision making. Further, nurses who are able to practice autonomously, providing a high level of care to patients on the basis of clinical judgment, experience greater satisfaction. Work areas that do not provide both autonomy and accountability lead to discontent (Patronis Jones, 2007; Yoder-Wise, 2007). In reexamining the characteristics of "Magnet" hospitals as published in 1983 (McClure, Poulin, Sovie, & Wandelt, 1983), McClure and Hinshaw (2007) reiterate the critical components of what it is

E

that identifies those health care organizations commonly referred to as "Magnet" hospitals. These characteristics have tended to attract and retain professional nurses and certainly increase job satisfaction, even in the midst of a cyclical nursing shortage. The characteristics of "magnetism" include nurse staffing, nursing autonomy, and control over nursing practice—all of which "require strong administrative and organizational support of the nursing staff" (McClure & Hinshaw, 2007). Clearly, the key to employee satisfaction depends largely on an administration that is open to suggestion, demonstrates support of its employees, and fosters an environment conducive to collaboration and creativity on the part of its employees. Research supports that nurses who are satisfied with their work environment and administrators are more likely to be content and remain in their current position (Smith, Hood, Waldman, & Smith, 2005; Sourdif, 2004).

See also Magnet Hospitals

McClure, M. L., & Hinshaw, A. S. (2007). Spotlight on nurse staffing, autonomy, and control over practice. *American Nurse Today*, 2(4), 15–17.

McClure, M., Poulin, M., Sovie, M., & Wandelt, M. (1983). *Magnet hospitals: Attraction and retention of professional nurses*. Washington, DC: American Nurses Association.

Patronis Jones, R. A. (2007). *Nursing leadership and management: Theories, processes and practice*. Philadelphia, PA: F.A. Davis Company.

Smith, H. L., Hood, J. N., Waldman, J.D., & Smith, V. L. (2005). Creating a favorable practice environment for nurses. *Journal of Nursing Administration*, 35(12), 525–532.

Sourdif, J. (2004). Predictors of nurses' intent to stay at work in a university health center. *Nursing and Health Sciences*, 6, 59–69.

Yoder-Wise, P.S. (2007). *Leading and managing in nursing* (4th ed.). St. Louis, MO: Mosby.

Gina M. Myers
M. Janice Nelson

ENTRY INTO PRACTICE

The term "entry into practice" generally refers to the educational preparation that is required for basic practice within a profession. In nursing, however, it has become a shorthand manner for referring to the long, ongoing debate that the profession has engaged in regarding the appropriate level of education that should be required for entry into registered nurse (RN) practice.

Historically, nurses in the United States were educated in hospital schools of nursing patterned after the Nightingale schools that were introduced in Europe during the late 19th century (*see also* Florence Nightingale). By the early 20th century, a few colleges and universities were beginning programs designed to prepare nurses at the baccalaureate level, but these never became very popular or numerous. Then in the mid-20th century, the community college movement started and quickly spread across the nation and nursing became one of the earliest and most successful majors to be offered by this new form of education. For many years, the hospital schools continued to flourish as well.

Today, the large majority of the nation's nurses are prepared in community college programs, graduating with associate degrees, while diploma programs have all but disappeared. Baccalaureate programs have become numerous and are generally graduating more than 30% of the new nurses in most states. Moreover, a small number of universities and colleges offer entry preparation at the master's level.

Over the years, many efforts have been made to standardize basic nursing preparation, most of which have attempted to require at least a baccalaureate degree in order for new nurses to qualify for licensure. For example, in 1965, the American

Nurses Association went on record endorsing such a change in standards (American Nurses Association, 1965). Then, in 1975, the New York State Nurses Association attempted to have legislation introduced that would require the baccalaureate for all new RN candidates and the associate degree for all new licensed practical nurse (LPN) candidates. In spite of rigorous efforts, the bill died in committee and was, therefore, never introduced into the legislative body. South Dakota is the only state that was actually successful in changing their standards and required the baccalaureate degree for a period of years. However, early in this century, that change was rescinded and the baccalaureate degree is not currently mandated for licensure in any of the 50 states.

The most recent attempt to change the education for entry into nursing began in New York State just after the turn of this century. However, this legislation is focused on continuation of licensure and not specifically the entry point. The proposal would require that all nurses prepared at the diploma or associate degree level attain a baccalaureate degree in nursing within 10 years of their initial licensure (Murray, 2006). This idea has been explored by other states as well, but there has been substantial opposition to the plan—chiefly arising from hospital administrators—and it remains to be seen whether the effort will prove successful.

Of interest is the fact that a large number of developed and developing countries already require the baccalaureate degree for entry into nursing practice and a number have done so for many years. At present, this trend is spreading across Western Europe as the need for better-educated nurses becomes evident to health care influentials (Spitzer & Perrenoud, 2006). Most comparable professions report that they have gone through similar struggles whenever they have proposed an elevation of their educational standards. What is striking is the fact that nursing is the only occupation that has been unsuccessful in making such changes to date.

New movement on this issue began in 2010, with the publication of a study conducted by the Institute of Medicine and published under the title, *The Future of Nursing* (IOM, 2011). A number of important, evidence-based recommendations were contained in the report. Among the goals is that the percentage of nurses in the United States holding the baccalaureate degree in nursing should be increased from 50% to 80% by 2020. There are several reasons why this goal has such promise for change at this point in our history:

- The study was conducted by an interdisciplinary panel composed of highly influential leaders.

- There is increasing recognition that any reform of the health care system will require many more well-prepared nurses to make such reform possible, both from a workforce and a quality point of view.

- The Robert Wood Johnson Foundation is actively providing support for the implementation of the study findings.

In addition to these formal efforts, there are anecdotal reports that increasing numbers of employers are pressing hard to raise the percentage of their staff that hold a baccalaureate or higher degree in nursing.

With these multiple pressures to improve the basic educational requirements for nursing, it is possible that the term "entry into practice" will actually disappear as a topic for professional debate later in the 21st century.

American Nurses Association. (1965). *Educational preparation for nurse practitioners* and assistants to nurses: A position paper. New York, NY: ANA.

Institute of Medicine. (2011). *The future of nursing: Leading change, advancing health*. Washington, DC: National Academies Press.

Murray, C. (2006). Advancing the profession of nursing: A new approach. *Journal of the New York State Nurses Association, 37*, 22–25.

Spitzer, A. & Perrenoud, B. (2006). Reforms in nursing education across Western Europe: From agenda to practice. *Journal of Professional Nursing, 22*, 150–159.

Margaret L. McClure

EPIGENETICS

Epigenetics, the study of changes in gene activity that do not include alterations to the genetic code, leads to an alternative to the race model, ethnogenetic layering (EL). EL relies on geographic information system computational technology to digitize and horizontally layer various data (e.g., genetic, toxicological, historical, demographic, etc.) on a particular geographical region for subsequent multilayer vertical analysis. Historical patterns of gene flow and defined opportunities for genetic drift have produced interesting human variations. Epigenetics addresses gene expression changes due to factors on top of or in addition to genetics. In some ways, epigenetics is the lived experience of genes being manifested in changes of their expression. In some circles, it is used to describe anything other than DNA sequence that influences the development of an organism.

The molecular basis of epigenetics is complex because the modifications in a gene are acknowledged, yet the basic structure of the DNA remains unchanged. In other words, there is no change in the underlying DNA sequence of the organism; instead, nongenetic factors cause the organism's genes to express themselves differently and even behave differently. Most epigenetic changes only occur within the course of one individual organism's lifetime.

Over the last 17 years, the Genomic Models Research Group in the Department of Anthropology at the University of Maryland has crafted a reproducible method for reconstructing and examining the human biocultural mosaic with the goal of predicting disease susceptibility and risk in specified microethnic groups (MEGs). In EL, the level of analysis is the MEG. In the research literature, socially constructed geographical designations referred to as local MEGs have been theoretically identified.

An MEG is a local constellation of genetically related biological lineages with shared cultural practices, environmental exposures, geographical residence, demographic status, and historical backgrounds (Jackson, 2008). Augmenting these shared ways of approaching the world are also shared health-related exposures to environmental toxins and communicable disease agents. As products of the environment, human beings are impacted by the environments in which they live and move as well as by the behaviors of those with whom they regularly interact. There is perhaps nothing in the universe that escapes the consequences of the environment including gene expression. The end result can be modifications to genetic expression due to the sociocultural, abiotic, and biotic filters encountered as human beings go about living their lives, resulting in what, when, and how genes may be expressed.

For human beings, the number of direct ancestors increases with each generation (approximately every 20 years), whereas the number of humans alive on the planet decreases as we travel back in time (Cloud,

2010). Each human being starts off with two parents, then four grandparents, then eight great grandparents, and so forth. Therefore, it is evident that the further back in time we go, the higher the probability that human beings share common ancestors and are in fact one family.

Cloud, J. (2010, January 6). Why your DNA isn't your destiny. Retrieved November 9, 2010, from http://www.time.com/time/health/article/0,8599,1951968–2,00.html

Jackson, F. L. (2008, March–April). Ethnogenetic layering (EL): An alternative to the traditional race model in human variation and health disparity studies. *Annals of Human Biology, 35*(2), 121–144.

G. Rumay Alexander

EVIDENCE-BASED PRACTICE

The strong emphasis on research within the nursing profession is based on an implicit expectation that the results of such research will be used to improve patient care and outcomes. Yet, for many years, no particular attention has been paid to the idea of knowledge use and how it was to be done.

The mid-1970s saw a spurt of discussion that appeared in the nursing literature about the need to systematically use knowledge generated through research in patient care. This may have been stimulated in part by the work being done by social scientists at the time about approaches to "research utilization." In examining the work of these early social scientists, the fact that their discourse had a distinctly organizational dimension to knowledge application did not seem to have an impact on nursing for quite some time. It would take several decades before the issue of research utilization made a comeback, this time in the form of evidence-based practice (EBP). The profile of the current literature on EBP, however, is different than the emphasis on research utilization of the 1970s, as is the climate within which the discussions are occurring. Several other health professions are engaged in major efforts to implement EBP and to teach EBP in their educational programs. As well, there is an emphasis within federal agencies on EBP, with a number of institutes within the National Institutes of Health dedicating significant amounts of funding to address issues in EBP.

Research utilization is defined as the use of research to guide clinical practice (Estabrooks, Winther, & Derksen, 2004), whereas EBP is "the conscientious and judicious use of current best evidence in conjunction with clinical expertise and patient values to guide health care decisions" (Titler, 2008, p. I–113). Although EBP extends beyond research utilization by including patients' perspectives and a focus on decision-making, EBP and research utilization may exist on a continuum. The distinction, however, does not seem to be especially relevant, given that the literature conflates both research utilization and EBP in describing theoretical models used to advance knowledge in the field (Estabrooks et al., 2004; Titler, 2008).

Nursing has enthusiastically embraced the movement of EBP. The literature reveals that health care organizations are now dedicating highly qualified personnel teams and developing systematic strategies to facilitate the implementation of EBP on the part of their staffs. This is one of the most significant and productive movements within nursing, with the potential to transform the profession and the quality of care it provides the public. The formation of several centers on EBP such as

E

E

the Joanna Briggs Institute (Adelaide, Australia), now partnered by Sigma Theta Tau International, and the Cochrane Collaboration at York University (UK) focusing on meta-analytic studies, have further stimulated the EBP movement in nursing both within the United States and internationally.

Most research findings are not immediately ready to be implemented into practice, nor should the findings of any single study be implemented. A variety of steps are necessary to determine the applicability of research findings (evidence) into practice within specific settings with particular populations. The nature and quality of the research need to be carefully evaluated and corroboration sought from multiple studies. Best evidence can come from randomized controlled trials, but also from expert opinion, depending on whether or not a sufficient research base is available in a particular topic (Titler, 2008). With this in mind, *translation research* is expected to play a key role in moving research from bench to bedside. Translation research is defined as testing the effect of interventions on the extent of adoption of EBP by health care providers, including nurses and physicians (Titler & Everett, 2001). Attention is now given to approaches to translate research into forms that render findings applicable to practice. Importantly, translation research includes testing the effect of interventions on *promoting* and *sustaining* the adoption of EBP (Titler, 2004).

When reviewing the literature for relevant research, all types of research must be considered. Quantitative, qualitative, outcomes focused, and intervention studies are all potentially useful and should be evaluated for their applicability to the practice change being considered. All research studies are not equal in the strength of the evidence they provide. The strength of research evidence is on a continuum, with descriptive surveys providing the weakest evidence and meta-analyses of experimental studies providing the strongest evidence. In addition to the strength of the research evidence, the expertise of the practitioners who will be implementing the change, the values and needs of the patients who will be the recipients of change, and finally the unique characteristics of the organization must be considered as well.

Most critically, supportive leadership is crucial to successful use of EBP (Titler, 2008). Leadership support includes providing necessary resources, materials, and time to incorporate EBP into daily activities (Titler, 2008). Embedding EBP into a practice setting requires other leadership activities as well. An organization's mission, vision, and strategic plan should reflect the use of EBP. Aligning staff performance criteria with the use of EBP can be an incentive to staff to continue with the use of EBP, helping to promote the sustainability of EBP (Titler, 2008).

There are also specific areas within the EBP movement that would benefit from leadership guidance. Nursing leaders who are interested in developing EBP may want to use an interdisciplinary approach to practice change, depending on the change being considered. For example, reducing the incidence of ventilator-associated pneumonia in mechanically ventilated, critically ill patients is an important organizational initiative. Ventilator-associated pneumonia (VAP) is a leading cause of morbidity and mortality in critically ill patients (Hilinski & Stark, 2006). Although nursing has developed evidence-based intervention bundles to reduce the incidence of VAP (Hilinski & Stark, 2006), nursing is not the sole health care profession that manages mechanically ventilated patients. Both physicians and respiratory therapists also manipulate ventilators and therefore should be included in the development and implementation of practice changes aimed at reducing VAP.

The evidence base for many areas of nursing practice is relatively strong, whereas research evidence to assist with nursing leadership decision making is relatively weak. More specifically, there is a paucity of consistent research findings available to help nurse leaders make informed decisions regarding staffing levels that optimize patient outcomes. For example, several studies have examined the relationship of hours per patient day (HPPD) to various patient outcomes (Blegen, Goode, & Reed, 1998; Cho, Ketefian, Barkauskas, & Smith, 2003; Needleman, Buerhaus, Mattke, Stewart, & Zelevinsky, 2002). Both Blegen et al. (1998) and Cho et al. (2003) found an unexpected positive relationship between total HPPD and the prevalence of pressure ulcers, but when Cho et al. isolated RN-HPPD, they found an inverse relationship with pneumonia. Needleman et al. (2002) also found an inverse relationship between RN-HPPD and pneumonia. Contradictory findings across studies suggest that more research on this topic is needed before nursing leaders can use the research evidence to make informed staffing decisions. Furthermore, this reality of contradictory findings highlights the importance of meta-analytic studies of research related to specific phenomena. Meta-analysis enables the synthesis of many studies on a topic, in which studies with positive and negative results are included and analyzed; the effect size from meta-analytic studies of multiple research reports points the way to the particular research evidence and practice innovation to be implemented.

Although evidence is emerging of the influence of nursing leadership on EBP, the evidence base for a broader understanding of nursing leadership's role in patient care is lacking. For example, it is unclear which leadership style can best promote positive patient outcomes. A recent systematic review of this topic was inconclusive because few studies have reported a relationship between leadership and patient outcomes (Wong & Cummings, 2007). There was some evidence to suggest that positive leadership behaviors such as being relationship-oriented could be instrumental in increasing patient satisfaction and reducing adverse events (Wong & Cummings, 2007).

In summary, nursing leaders now have many templates to choose from in helping them institute EBP. Nurse leaders should institute broad organizational initiatives as well as specific approaches to embed EBP in practice settings and promote sustainability of EBP. Depending on the practice issue being considered, other disciplines may need to be part of the process. By promoting EBP, nursing leaders can make a powerful impact on the nursing profession and patient care.

Blegen, M. A., Goode, C., & Reed, L. (1998). Nurse staffing and patient outcomes. *Nursing Research, 47*(1), 43–50.

Cho, S. H., Ketefian, S., Barkauskas, V. H., & Smith, D. G. (2003). The effects of nurse staffing on adverse events, morbidity, mortality, and medical costs. *Nursing Research, 52*(2), 71–79.

Estabrooks, C. A., Winther, C., & Derksen, L. (2004). Mapping the field: A bibliometric analysis of the research utilization literature in nursing. *Nursing Research, 53*(5), 293–303.

Hilinski, A. M., & Stark, M. L. (2006). Memory aide to reduce the incidence of ventilator-associated pneumonia. *Critical Care Nurse, 26*(5), 80–81.

Needleman, J., Buerhaus, P., Mattke, S., Stewart, M., & Zelevinsky, K. (2002). Nurse-staffing levels and the quality of care in hospitals. *New England Journal of Medicine, 346*(22), 1715–1722.

Titler, M. G. (2004). Overview of the U.S. invitational conference "Advancing Quality Care Through Translation Research." *Worldviews on Evidence-Based Nursing* (Suppl. 1), S1–S5.

E

E

Titler, M. G. (2008). The evidence for evidence-based practice implementation. In R. G. Hughes (Ed.). *Patient safety and quality: An evidence-based handbook for nurses* (Vol. 1, pp. 1–113–1–161). AHRQ Publication No. 08–0043. Rockville, MD: Agency for Healthcare Research and Quality.

Titler, M. G., & Everett, L. Q. (2001). Translating research into practice: Considerations for critical care investigators. *Critical Care Nursing Clinics of North America, 13*(4), 587–604.

Wong, C. A., & Cummings, G. G. (2007). The relationship between nursing leadership and patient outcomes: A systematic review. *Journal of Nursing Management, 15*, 508–521.

Milisa Manojlovich
Shaké Ketefian

EXECUTIVE LEADERSHIP PROGRAMS

Nurses in executive practice require expertise in a broad spectrum of knowledge and skills. The American Organization of Nurse Executives' Nurse Executive Competencies identifies five domains that include leadership, business skills and principles, knowledge of the health care environment, communication and relationship management, and professionalism (www.aone.org/aone/resource/home.html). There are formal leadership development programs that are available to nurses who seek to augment their skills as executive leaders.

Nationally, there are two well-established programs. The highly competitive Johnson & Johnson Wharton Fellows Program at the University of Pennsylvania focuses on cutting edge business and management science during an intensive 3-week session (www.executivefellows.net). The equally competitive Robert Wood Johnson Foundation Executive Nurse Fellows Program is a 3-year fellowship that focuses on the experience and skills necessary to be a leader in the health care system, both locally and nationally. Fellows remain in their permanent jobs while completing this fellowship (www.executivenursefellows.org). Both of these programs offer participants the opportunity to learn with a diverse cohort of colleagues.

There are several programs that are state based. Two examples include the Midwestern Institute for Nursing Leadership, sponsored by the Illinois Organization of Nurse Leaders and the Boston-based, Harvard-affiliated Institute for Nursing Healthcare Leadership. The former offers a 5-day session, which includes executive decision making, strategic management, high performance teams, and change theory (www.ionl.org). The latter offers a yearly conference that focuses on current issues impacting nurse executive leaders (www.inhl.org/inhl.html).

Several universities offer multidisciplinary leadership programs. Two examples are the Harvard Management Development Program (www.gse.harvard.edu/ppe/programs/higher-education/portfolio/management-development.html) and the Leadership Development Program at the University of Maryland (www.umuc.edu/prog/nli/ldp.html).

Most leadership development programs target the individual learner and use small class sizes, experiential learning, and expert faculty. Given the variety of programs available, it is critical that nurse executives be clear about their individual goals, preferred learning style, financial resources, and time commitment to select the best program to meet their needs.

Pamela Austin Thompson

Executive Search

In the vernacular, the term "headhunter" is used to describe the work done by an individual who searches for a qualified candidate for a specific position. According to the thesaurus, the headhunter is a recruiter or a talent scout (Kipfer, 2006). A headhunter also may be a search consultant, one who has experience in the profession and subsequently uses this experience to become a consultant. Another way of describing what the consultant does is "matchmaking." For this entry, search consultant is the term used to describe this work.

The search consultant can work with a search firm or can be employed by an institution. When working with applicants for a position, the consultant can take the role of mentor, career counselor, or career coach. The role will depend on the needs of the applicant. Nursing leaders or aspiring nursing leaders may have the occasion to work with a search consultant either as an applicant or as an employer. Among the considerations involved in an executive search are the following: (1) whether or not a search firm is essential for finding the best qualified applicant, and if so, what qualities does the employer look for when selecting a search firm; (2) what is the process used by the search consultant to find the best candidate for the position; and (3) what are the benefits of working with a search consultant. Both the applicant and the employer should expect working with a search consultant to be a positive experience.

SELECTING A SEARCH FIRM

An institution may select from dozens of search firms. They may use word of mouth in selecting a firm or choose to contact an organization by searching online to learn what firms are available. Examples of Internet addresses used to identify some of these are included at the end of this entry. Posting the position in various organizational publications is also a means of advertising the position. Search firms do require a fee for their service, and for this reason the institution may use them only for a specialized search. After taking into account the advantages, the administrator will determine if the institution can best be served by use of a search firm. If that is determined, the decision needs to be made about the type of firm that will best suit the needs of the institution. Some search firms work on a retainer basis, and others work on a contingency basis. Search firms that require a retainer will have an exclusive arrangement with the employing institution. They bring in applicants until the position is successfully filled. These firms receive the first part of their fee when the contract is signed, the second part when the interview process takes place with the search committee, and the third part when an agreement is signed and the selected candidate assumes the new position. Firms working on a contingency basis receive a fee only if the employing agency hires an applicant they bring in. There are search firms that specialize in health care searches and those who have a broader venue. Currently, private and corporate businesses are frequently engaging search firms for assistance in exploring the job market for the best-qualified person to fill a position.

Are search firms the most expedient way to find the best-qualified applicants? The time it takes to complete a search depends on many things, including the time of year it is started, the institution, where it is located, and how well known are its stakeholders. Freedom of interaction between the consultant and the

E

institutional representative also influences the length of time for a search. In the last few years, many books have been written and Web sites have been established that give information about job searches. In spite of the vast amount of information available, many positions are filled through personal contacts. Networking is one tool among many that may be used in searching for the "best" applicant. Meshel and Douglas (2005), along with many others, consider networking to be an essential means of searching for a position.

Although a fee for service is required, the use of a search firm may actually save money for the institution by expediting the search, relieving the staff of the many search activities, and providing a greater pool of qualified applicants. To acquire names of applicants, an experienced search consultant will have developed a database of well-qualified potential applicants as well as resources. The work of the search consultant includes the review of all applications and referring only those who match the position profile to the search committee or institutional representative for a decision to interview or reject. Those applicants who do not match the qualifications for the position are kept in the database of the consultant. Experienced search consultants know the institutions that they work with and the people who work there; they also maintain a cadre of potential persons for positions and resource persons to suggest potential qualified applicants. The fee for a search consultation comes from the institution and direction also come from the institution.

SEARCH CONSULTANT PROCESS

One long-standing process in nursing searches is as follows: The search consultants will use their experience and connections as teachers or administrators, in addition to involvement in national nursing organizations, to seek the "best"-qualified applicants for a position. In addition to working with a committee of stakeholders or an institutional representative, another role of the consultant is to prepare the applicant for the position. This can best be done when the consultant knows the institution, the people who work there, and the kind of person needed to fill the position. To learn this, the consultant visits the institution and talks with many stakeholders. After that visit, a profile of a qualified candidate is determined by the consultant and approved by the search committee or the designated representative. The search consultant will bring to the committee's attention several individuals who are qualified and appear to "fit" the position. Although the consultant provides information about the applicants to the institutional committee, it is also important that the consultant provide support so that the applicant is well prepared for the interview. The consultant suggests to the applicants issues to consider when looking at a position; for example, (1) Are the core values of the institution consistent with yours? (2) What are the personal attitudes and work style at the institution? (3) Are they congruent with yours? (4) What are the critical issues facing the institution? (5) What are opportunities and challenges facing the person accepting the position? Applicants are reminded that there are more important things they need to know about the position than salary because this can be negotiable.

The process for applying for the position is discussed with those candidates whose curriculum vitae are well done, whose experience, characteristics, and qualifications make them a good fit for the position and who meet the position requirements. In other words, their data reflect a potential good fit (a match) with the profile of the person being sought by the institution. The consultant suggests a format for applying for the position. For example, applicants should review the position announcement and other materials that they receive. The letter of application should indicate those areas described in the position announcement where the candidates have had experience. The letter of application should be no more than two pages and should give strong evidence of the applicant's qualifications as they relate to the position. Additional information about background is provided in the resume or curriculum vita. Applications should not be encouraged from those who do not meet the basic requirements for a position.

Information obtained from the qualified applicant and provided to the committee and/or institutional representative by the search consultant includes letters of reference, results of a telephone interview conducted with the applicant, and telephone references from a list the candidate provides. Questions asked of the applicant and references are based on information learned by the consultant in discussion with the stakeholders. This information is compiled and provided to the committee as background information. If an applicant is invited to the institution for a personal interview, the consultant assists in preparing for that visit. Applicants are encouraged to learn as much as possible about the institution and the city in which it is located. They will receive the names of the members of the search committee and the Internet URL for the institution to learn more about the members of the committee. The consultant will also offer suggestions to the members of the search committee about ways in which they can enhance the visit of the applicant.

BENEFITS OF WORKING WITH A SEARCH CONSULTANT

Working with a search consultant should be a learning experience for the applicant. Whether or not the position is attained, the experience should be a positive one. The applicant will be given information about making application for a position from the time of the first contact until a decision has been made. It should help the applicant know better what to expect in future recruitment. The applicant should also learn from interactions with stakeholders in what is important in presenting oneself, which helps narrow down to greater certainty the kind of position to which he or she aspires. The institution benefits are related to time, cost, and quality of applicants.

The search consultant works with the committee or institutional representative in the capacity of a staff person. The consultant keeps the institutional representative informed and encourages the committee or representative to keep stakeholders informed about the process and the progress of the search. The consultant systematically collects information, confirms its accuracy, and provides relevant details about serious and qualified applicants to the designated institutional representative or committee. The consultant provides the information and the committee makes the decisions about applicants. The search consultant assists in the search throughout the search process, until a qualified individual signs a letter of agreement or a contract.

The applicant may choose to post a résumé on a Web site, for example, http://www/monster.com. To find a recruiter, *Consultants News* publishes the Directory of Executive Recruiters. The URL for this group is http://www.jobjunction.com/recruiters.htm. This site lists all types of recruiters, retained, contingent, or corporate. If you are a person who feels that you do not wish to be

E

E

involved with a search firm and you want to find a job on your own, go to http://highly-effectivejobsearch.com. You will learn about the Pierson Method and the book about a systematic approach to job search (Pierson, 2006). It describes how one prepares to find a job (http://www.academickeys.com).

AACN Career Link. Retrieved from www.aacn.nche.edu/careerlink

Employment opportunities for Hispanic. Retrieved from http://www.hispanicoutlook.com

How to Get the Best Job You Ever Had. Retrieved from http://www.jobmiracle.com

Kipfer, B. A. (2006). *Roget's new millennium™ thesaurus* (1st ed., vol. 1.3.1). Los Angeles, CA: Lexico Publishing Group.

Meshel, J. W., & Douglas, G. (2005). *One phone call away*. New York, NY: Portfolio, Penguin Group.

Pierson, O. (2006). *The unwritten rules of the highly effective job search*. New York, NY: McGraw-Hill.

Recruiters Online Network. Retrieved from http://www.recruitersonline.com/Workquest.com, http://www.workquest.com

Resource for Minority Nursing Professionals. Retrieved from www.minoritynurse.com

Serve those seeking positions and employers. www.jobtarget.com

Sigma Theta Tau. Reflections. *Journal of Nursing Scholarship*. Retrieved from www.nursingsociety.org

SUGGESTED READING

Comeford, P. A., & Sauer, G. (2006). *Lessons from a headhunter*. Edina, MN: Beaver's Pond Press.

Kennedy, J. L. (2008). *Job interviews for dummies* (3rd ed.). New York, NY: Hungry Minds. Inc.

Billye J. Brown

EXTERNSHIPS

Originally developed in the 1970s and 1980s to address recruitment and retention issues, nurse externships continue to fill a crucial role in the changing health care landscape of the 21st century. Before computerized examination for nurse licensure became common in the mid-1990s, a new nurse would function in the role of "graduate nurse" under the licensure of another nurse. The current licensure process does not allow for the gradual transition to the role; a nurse today can graduate and become licensed in mere weeks. These nurses are thrust immediately and directly into roles of full responsibility under their own licenses (Dyess & Sherman, 2009).

Although there are many variations in both the definition and content of extern programs, externships are generally defined as employment experiences targeting nursing students in the final year of academic preparation (Cantrell & Browne, 2006; Salt, Cummings, & Profetto-McGrath, 2008). Many extern programs are designed to begin as summer employment and may continue as part-time employment during the school year. Student nurse externships differ from internships in that the latter are typically designed to provide academic credit and meet defined learning objectives.

Benner, Sutphen, Leonard, and Day (2010) indicate that a "practice-education" gap exists within nursing today. This gap represents the increasing difficulty of nursing curricula to keep pace with changes in technologies and practice. By providing learning experiences on a wide range of topics, externships help to fill that gap through training and the development of clinical competence (Salt et al., 2008). A key concept of clinical role maturity is developing an understanding of the culture within a clinical unit. Externships provide opportunities for nursing students to participate in and appreciate the complexities of caring for patients in the acute care environment. Developing an understanding of the teamwork and communication necessary for patient care is the key element in this transitional role between student and practitioner; gaining this understanding early may positively influence participants' professional socialization (Durrant, Crooks, & Pietrolungo, 2009).

In creating an effective program, consideration needs to be given in creating an environment that is safe and supportive for the extern (Dempsey & McKissick, 2006). In terms of skills, externs often function in a role similar to that of a nursing assistant. However, because of their nursing knowledge, externs should be provided opportunities to advance the knowledge and technical skill acquisition. A well-designed program will provide for the observation of procedures, participation in rounds, conferences, and educational sessions, which all serve to enrich the extern experience. Along with providing supervision, the nurse preceptor can further the extern's critical thinking skills, organizational abilities, priority setting, and effective communication skills (Dempsey & McKissick, 2006). Supervision, outcome evaluation, and continuous, constructive feedback to the extern facilitate the transfer of theoretical knowledge to professional nursing practice.

Externships can be a valuable recruitment and retention tool. Throughout the extern experience, managers have the opportunity to assess the potential of the extern to be successful as a staff nurse and thereby reduce the likelihood of hiring someone who will not match unit or hospital needs. A reported 50% to 79% of graduate nurses accepted positions in the facility where they had been externs (Cantrell & Browne, 2006; Dempsey & McKissick, 2006; Stinson & Wilkinson, 2004). Evidence suggests that extern experience reduces the time and cost of orientation (Courtney, 2005; Dempsey & McKissick, 2006) and

facilitates transition to the role of a staff nurse (Durrant et al., 2009). In a systematic review of externships, two studies report an increased retention rate at 1 and 2 years in nurses that participated in an externship program versus those who did not (Salt et al., 2008). Self-reports from program graduates indicate that as a result of the extern experience, students have a better understanding of the role of the staff nurse, increased skill, knowledge, and experience, and more self-confidence (Dempsey & McKissick, 2006; Salt et al., 2008). Externships are an important tool in recruitment, retention, and leadership development. By providing a solid foundation of experiential learning future, nurses are able to gain confidence in their abilities and greater understanding of the many professional roles within nursing.

Benner, P., Sutphen, M., Leonard, V., & Day, L. (2010). *Educating nurses: A call for radical transformation*. San Francisco, CA: Jossey-Bass.

Cantrell, M. A., & Browne, A. M. (2006). The impact of a nurse externship program on the transition process from graduate to registered nurse: Part III. Recruitment and retention effects. *Journal for Nurses in Staff Development, 22*(1), 11–14.

Courtney, R. J. (2005). A look at a successful perioperative nurse extern–intern program. *AORN, 81*(3), 577–578.

Dempsey, S. J., & McKissick, E. (2006). Implementation of a medical-surgical nurse extern and student nurse aide programs in critical care. *Critical Care Nursing Quarterly, 29*(3), 182–187.

Durrant, M., Crooks, D., & Pietrolungo, L. (2009). A clinical extern program evaluation. *Journal for Nurses in Staff Development, 25*(6), E1–E8.

Dyess, S., & Sherman, R. (2009). The first year of practice: New graduate nurses' transition and learning needs. *The Journal of Continue Education in Nursing, 40*(9), 403–410.

Salt, J., Cummings, G., & Profetto-McGrath, J. (2008). Increasing retention of new graduate nurses: A systematic review of interventions by healthcare organization. *Journal of Nursing Administration, 38*(6), 287–296.

E

Stinson, S., & Wilkinson, C. (2004). Creating a successful clinical extern program using a program planning logic model. *Journal of Nursing Staff Development, 20*(3), 140–144.

Tritak, A. B., Ross, B., Feldman, H., Paregoris, B., & Setti, K. (1997). An evaluation of a nurse extern program. *Journal of Nursing Staff Development, 13*(3), 132–135.

Additional information is available at these Web sites:

http://www.vpul.upenn.edu/careerservices/
nursing/extern.html

http://www.choosenursingvermont.org/
extern/externship_manual.pdf

Rachel Behrendt

F

Faculty Recruitment to Academic Settings

The nursing profession is experiencing an acute shortage of qualified faculty to teach and conduct research in academic settings. As a result, recruitment of faculty to academic institutions is a high priority for nursing schools. Major keys to successful recruitment of faculty to academic settings are (a) an exciting, visionary strategic plan; (b) personal contact with potential candidates; (c) an ability to generate enthusiasm in potential candidates regarding how they can be an instrumental part of the team in accomplishing the strategic plan; (d) a well-organized and interesting interview schedule; (e) timely follow-up; and (f) an excellent recruitment package.

An exciting long-range strategic plan is essential for any organization (Melnyk, 2011; Melnyk & Davidson, 2009), because it creates the road map for future success and also recruitment of new faculty should match key areas of the strategic plan. Advertisements that capture the excitement of the strategic plan should be created and disseminated widely through professional journals, the *Chronicle of Higher Education,* and electronic and Web media as they are an important strategy to alert potential faculty to open positions.

Advertisements are no substitute for and are typically not as effective in recruiting faculty as personal contacts with targeted individuals to explain why they were on your radar screen. Personal contacts/conversations should create an excitement in potential candidates about your school's strategic plan and end with an invitation to visit your school. For targeted senior faculty, an excellent strategy to spark their interest is to invite them to your school as a visiting scholar or consultant. Immediately following the initial personal contact, mail an attractive packet of exciting information about your school with a follow-up letter.

Once potential candidates commit to an interview, they should be asked whether there are specific individuals with whom they would like to meet during the course of their interview or places that they would like to visit (e.g., local medical centers, community agencies, interdisciplinary departments). The interview schedule should be composed of faculty, associate deans/chairs/academic program directors, and collaborating research or clinical partners. It makes an outstanding impression on candidates for the dean to have personal, individual time with them during the interview process. It also is important for the first and last individuals who meet with the candidate to be passionate about the direction of the school and be able to create excitement about their potential future on the team. Remember, you never get a second chance to make a great first impression on the candidate. Personal touches, such as placing a welcome card or small basket of fruit in the hotel room and having a faculty member meet the candidate at the airport, will create lasting good impressions, even if the candidate chooses not to accept a position at your school.

All faculty recruits, whether being interviewed for clinical/teaching intensive or tenure track positions in which research is an expectation of the position, will want to know whether there are adequate supports and resources in place for them to have a successful career in teaching, research, and/or clinical practice. Potential research active faculty desire a solid research infrastructure (e.g., a research office/center that assists with pre- and post-award grant activities), outstanding intra- and transdisciplinary collaborators, access to clinical sites where they can obtain their samples and conduct their studies, research start-up funds with designated research space, and substantial time to conduct their research (e.g., limited teaching loads). Formal mechanisms of mentorship for teaching and research/scholarship within a school are important for all new faculty, whether in the clinical or tenure track, to assist them in being successful in the new system as well as to prevent burnout (Shirey, 2006).

Offer potential recruits good salary, or at least one that is commensurate with similar positions in the geographic region. Every year, the American Association of Colleges of Nursing collects and publishes salary data for all tenure track and clinical track faculty as well as for administrators in colleges of nursing (see http://www.aacn.nche.edu). If the candidates are not familiar with the geographic location of the school, it also is a good idea to have a realtor tour them through a few living areas and provide them with information regarding the average cost of housing during the course of their visit. For stellar candidates who you are prepared to make an offer, it is important to inform them of your intent to provide them with the offer letter in the near future and have an exchange with them regarding their desired package (e.g., salary, research start-up funds, percentage of time devoted to teaching). Negotiate and save time in the hiring process by sending draft letters of offer to candidates as terms of the offer are negotiated.

Shortly following the visit, it is important to send a follow-up letter to candidates, thanking them for their time visiting your school and informing them of your plan to be in contact with them in the near future. A quick follow-up is important, especially for those candidates for whom you will be sending offer letters, as there is heavy competition for well-qualified faculty. Use the follow-up time to reinforce the exciting vision of how their coming on board with your institution will be a win–win for both sides.

Melnyk, B. M. (2011). Creating a vision: Motivating a change to evidence-based practice in individuals and organizations. In B. Melnyk & E. Fineout-Overholt (Eds.), *Evidence-based practice in nursing & healthcare: A guide to best practice* (2nd ed.). Philadelphia, PA: Wolters Kluwer/Lippincott, Williams & Wilkins.

Melnyk, B. M., & Davidson, S. (2009). Creating a culture of innovation in nursing education through shared vision, leadership, interdisciplinary partnerships, and positive deviance. *Nursing Administration Quarterly, 33*(4), 288–295.

Shirey, M. (2006). Stress and burnout in nursing faculty. *Nurse Educator, 31*(3), 95–97.

Bernadette Mazurek Melnyk

Faculty Retention

The U.S. faculty nursing shortage, according to the American Association of Colleges of Nursing (AACN), is driven by a number of factors, including noncompetitive salaries and the inability to compete with practice salaries; insufficient, doctorally prepared faculty; prospective faculty who do not have the right specialty mix who are unable or unwilling to teach clinical courses; and high faculty workload. Even schools reporting no vacancies in the AACN survey indicate a pressing need to increase the number of faculty positions given enrollment increases and demand (Fang & Tracy, 2009–2010). Finally, there is an increase in faculty resignations, not only for retirement but also for reasons such as dissatisfaction and burnout.

A national survey of nursing faculty by the National League for Nursing (NLN) and the Carnegie Foundation indicates that the workload of full-time nursing faculty on average is 56 hours per week compared to 45 to 55 hours per week for other American academics. One fourth of nurse educators in the NLN–Carnegie study, who reported a desire to leave their current positions, cited high workload as the driving factor (NLN, 2007). The Bureau of Labor Statistics (2010–2011) projects that positions for nurses of all types and levels are expected to increase by 581,500 or 22% by 2018.

Therefore, the demand for nursing faculty will continue to rise. In light of this demand, every nursing program should have a nursing faculty retention program addressing the primary drivers of faculty retention: cultural integration, compensation/workload, and career development and advancement.

CULTURAL INTEGRATION

For new faculty, retention begins with a substantive, formal orientation to the nursing program and the parent institution. Faculty need to understand the nature of the curriculum, academic policies and procedures, the organization of the program, the school, and how it aligns with the college or university, as well as appropriate channels of communication and opportunities for faculty to serve on program or college/university committees. Novice faculty often need organization and time management skills that will work to their advantage in the freedom of the academic setting and include lesson planning, preparation and revision time, and reasonable service to committees. Involving veteran faculty in new faculty orientation programs facilitates collegial relationships and may lead naturally to mentorship relationships, which can be most effective in improving faculty retention (Dunham-Taylor, Lynn, Moore, McDaniel, & Walker, 2008). Orientation of new faculty should also include an overview of student-driven issues such as dealing with students with disabilities or other challenges. Faculty should have the tools necessary to do their work, such as a suitable office, technology and learning spaces, and staff to support the teaching–learning effort. Periodic feedback from new and veteran faculty should be elicited to determine how best to improve the resources and environment. An engaged faculty will significantly contribute to the future of the profession and ultimately to patient care.

COMPENSATION AND WORKLOAD

It is a common occurrence in practice professions, such as law, medicine, and nursing that those who work in the practice arena earn much more than their counterparts in academia. Despite the fact that advanced degrees and years of experience are necessary prerequisites to a teaching career, compensation remains relatively low for nursing faculty compared to nurses in practice. It is especially disheartening to nursing faculty when the salaries of new nursing graduates in their first positions are higher than faculty salaries. As a rule of thumb, the starting salary of a new, master's prepared faculty member with clinical but little teaching experience should be 20% to 25% higher than the base salary of a new registered nurse. Compensation rates are most often driven by supply and demand factors. However, even though demand for faculty may be high, colleges and universities are increasingly engaging in significant belt-tightening because of legislative cutbacks or the vagaries of the economy. Faculty are increasingly required to teach heavier loads with fewer instructional resources and such demands can drive more nursing faculty back to practice as national surveys have indicated.

Workload and compensation are intimately intertwined. For example, a normal faculty load for a 9-month, 2-semester appointment may be 12 credits each semester for a total of 24 credits. The credit load, however, is not the whole story. The faculty member is also responsible for advisement hours, committee work (which can be substantive given the range of regulation to which nursing programs are subjected), scholarship, and/or research and other citizenship duties such as attending program, school, and university ceremonies. Although some schools may offer the opportunity to teach "overload" credits in the summer or during regular terms, this strategy could work against retention strategy and accelerate burnout. All elements of workload should be documented annually, analyzed, and interpreted to university administration given that "real-time"

workload in academic clinical programs is greater than in nonclinical programs.

CAREER DEVELOPMENT AND ADVANCEMENT

Both new and veteran faculty need clear guidelines on career development and advancement. Criteria for promotion should be published and understood. The administrator of the unit needs to create a culture in which faculty can identify and achieve their goals, including periodic review of faculty activities, such as teaching, advising, research, publications, and contributions to the unit or college/university. Celebrations of faculty success should be formalized. For example, some schools have a monthly e-newsletter or kudos list that publishes and distributes the accomplishments of faculty to all school constituencies.

Advancing through the professorial ranks validates a teacher's contributions not only to student learning but also to advancing the profession and nursing knowledge. Promoting the development, reward and recognition of both new and veteran faculty will result in a high level of faculty retention.

See also Nursing Shortage in the United States; Shortage of Nursing Faculty; Staff Retention

American Association of Colleges of Nursing; Faculty Shortages in Registered Nurses Preparatory Programs; National League for Nursing Carnegie Foundation: *National Study of Nurse Educators: Compensation, Workload and Teaching Practices.*

Bureau of Labor Statistics. *Occupational outlook handbook, 2010–11. Registered Nurses.* Retrieved October 3, 2010, from http://www.bls.gov/oco/ocos083.htm

Dunham-Taylor, J., Lynn, C. W., Moore, P., McDaniel, S., & Walker, J. K. (2008). What goes around comes around: Improving faculty retention through more effective mentoring. *Journal of Professional Nursing, 24*(6), 337–346.

Fang, D., & Tracy, C. (2009–2010). *Special survey on vacant faculty positions for academic year 2009–10*. Washington, DC: American Association of Colleges of Nursing. Retrieved September 24, 2010, from http://www.aacn.nche.edu/IDS/pdf/vacancy09/pdf

National League for Nursing. (2007). *Nationwide NLN-Carnegie Foundation Study examines nurse faculty workload*. Retrieved September 24, 2010, from http://www.nln.org/newsreleases/carnegie_092007.htm

Gloria F. Donnelly

FAILURE TO RESCUE

Failure to rescue is defined as a situation in which hospitalized patients die following hospital-acquired complications, specifically those situations in which a decline in a patient's condition is not identified and treated in a timely manner. Failure to rescue is based on the theory that the likelihood of patients being "rescued" from complications relates to the quality of patient surveillance by staff, the speed of recognition of causes of clinical deterioration, and the availability and timeliness of interventions to reverse it. Both the concept of failure to rescue and the original strategy for measuring rates of unsuccessful rescues using administrative data sources (specifically, hospital discharge abstracts) were developed by Dr. Jeffrey Silber, a physician and health services researcher at the University of Pennsylvania (Silber, Williams, Krakauer, & Schwartz, 1992), and were first applied to nursing research by the Center for Health Outcomes and Policy Research at the University of Pennsylvania School of Nursing (Aiken, Clarke, Sloane, Sochalski, & Silber, 2002). A number of different definitions and approaches to

calculating failure-to-rescue rates appear in the literature (Silber et al., 2007); current research is aimed at refining the measure and identifying new ways to apply the concept to clinical practice.

As a quality-of-care measure, failure to rescue has been endorsed nationally as a nursing sensitive measure of hospital performance. Guidelines and computer codes for calculating failure to rescue rates from patient discharge abstract data are available through the Agency for Healthcare Research and Quality (2006), the National Quality Forum (2008), and the Centers for Medicare and Medicaid Services (Medicare Program; Changes to the Hospital Inpatient Prospective Payment Systems for Acute Care Hospital and Fiscal Year 2010 Rates; and Changes to the Long-Term Care Hospital Prospective Payment System and Rate Years 2010 and 2009 Rates, 2009). Although failure to rescue was initially validated in general surgical patients, the broader concept clearly has applications in other patient populations (Beaulieu, 2009; Friese, Earle, Silber, & Aiken, 2010; Kutney-Lee & Aiken, 2008).

It has been argued that failure-to-rescue rates may measure quality of care as much or perhaps more than the occurrence of complications themselves, which tend to be closely linked to patients' underlying conditions. Links between failure to rescue and nursing are felt to relate to nurses' central role in patient surveillance and mobilizing health care teams to implement rescues (Bader et al., 2009; Kutney-Lee, Lake, & Aiken, 2009). Organizational context as set by managers and other health care leaders in the form of staffing levels and elements such as relationships between nurses and physicians, continuing education and other resources, and support of clinicians' decisions by administrators is believed to be key to successful rescues

F

(Aiken et al., 2010; Aiken, Clarke, Sloane, Lake, & Cheney, 2008). Failure-to-rescue rates appear to be lower in hospitals with higher ratios of nurses to patients and in those with more nurses holding higher educational credentials (Aiken et al., 2010; Aiken, Clarke, Cheung, Sloane, & Silber, 2003; Harless & Mark, 2010; Kutney-Lee & Aiken, 2008) as well as in teaching hospitals and those with high-technology facilities (Ghaferi, Osborne, Birkmeyer, & Dimick, 2010; Silber et al., 2008).

The use of failure to rescue as a quality measure and the identification and treatment of complications have become a priority of the patient safety movement. The Joint Commission has endorsed a National Patient Safety Goal (No. 16) to "improve recognition and response to changes in a patient's condition" (The Joint Commission on the Accreditation of Healthcare Organizations, 2008), which has aided in the emergence of rapid response teams (mobile teams of well-trained nurses, physicians, and others who can quickly troubleshoot and intervene at the earliest signs of trouble to favor rescues). The concept of rapid response teams has been further promoted through the Institute for Healthcare Improvement (2010), which provides an intervention package on implementing and deploying rapid response teams as part of their Protecting 5 Million Lives from Harm campaign.

See also Agency for Healthcare Research and Quality (AHRQ); Institute for Healthcare Improvement; Rapid Response Teams

Agency for Healthcare Research and Quality. (2006). *Patient safety indicators overview.* Retrieved from http://www.qualityindicators.ahrq.gov/psi_overview.htm

Aiken, L. H., Clarke, S. P., Cheung, R. B., Sloane, D. M., & Silber, J. H. (2003). Education levels of hospital nurses and surgical patient mortality. *Journal of the American Medical Association, 290*, 1617–1623.

Aiken, L.H., Clarke, S. P., Sloane, D. M., Lake, E. T., & Cheney, T. (2008). Effects of hospital care environment on patient mortality and nurse outcomes. *Journal of Nursing Administration, 38*(5), 223–229.

Aiken, L. H., Clarke, S. P., Sloane, D. M., Sochalski, J., & Silber, J. H. (2002). Hospital nurse staffing and patient mortality, nurse burnout, and job dissatisfaction. *Journal of the American Medical Association, 288*, 1987–1993.

Aiken, L. H., Sloane, D. M., Cimiotti, J. P., Clarke, S. P., Flynn, L., Seago, J. A., et al. (2010). Implications of the California nurse staffing mandates for other states. *Health Services Research, 45*(4), 904–921.

Bader, M. K., Neal, B., Johnson, L., Pyle, K., Brewer, J., Luna, M., et al. (2009). Rescue me: Saving the vulnerable non-ICU patient population. *Joint Commission Journal on Quality and Patient Safety, 35*(4), 199–205.

Beaulieu, M. J. (2009). Failure to rescue as a process measure to evaluate fetal safety during labor. *American Journal of Maternal Child Nursing, 34*(1), 18–23.

Friese, C. R., Earle, C. C., Silber, J. H., & Aiken, L. H. (2010). Hospital characteristics, clinical severity, and outcomes for surgical oncology patients. *Surgery, 147*(5), 602–609.

Ghaferi, A. A., Osborne, N. H., Birkmeyer, J. D., & Dimick, J. B. (2010). Hospital characteristics associated with failure to rescue from complications after pancreatectomy. *Journal of the American College of Surgeons, 211*(3), 325–330.

Harless, D. W., & Mark, B. A. (2010). Nurse staffing and quality of care with direct measurement of inpatient staffing. *Medical Care, 48*(7), 659–663.

Institute for Healthcare Improvement. (2010). *Protecting 5 million lives from harm.* Retrieved from http://www.ihi.org/IHI/Programs/Campaign/Campaign.htm?TabId=2&player=wmp#GENERALIMPROVEMENTSTRATEGIES

Kutney-Lee, A., & Aiken, L. H. (2008). Effects of nurse staffing and education on the outcomes of surgical patients with comorbid serious mental illness. *Psychiatric Services, 59*(12), 1466–1469.

Kutney-Lee, A., Lake, E.T., & Aiken, L. H. (2009). Development of the Hospital Nurse Surveillance Capacity Profile. *Research in Nursing & Health, 32*, 217–228.

Medicare Program; Changes to the Hospital Inpatient Prospective Payment Systems for

Acute Care Hospital and Fiscal Year 2010 Rates; and Changes to the Long-Term Care Hospital Prospective Payment System and Rate Years 2010 and 2009 Rates, 74 Fed. Reg. 43,754 (2009, August 27) (to be codified at 42 C.R.F pt. 413).

National Quality Forum. (2008). *NQF-Endorsed Standards*. Retrieved from http://www.qualityforum.org/Measures_List.aspx#k=failure&e=1&st=&sd=&s=&p=1

Silber, J. H., Romano, P. S., Rosen, A. K, Wang, Y., Even-Shoshan, O., & Volpp, K. G. (2007). Failure to rescue: Comparing definitions to measure quality of care. *Medical Care, 45*(10), 918–925.

Silber, J.H., Rosenbaum, P. R., Romano, P. S., Rosen, A. K, Wang, Y., Teng, Y., et al. (2008). Hospital teaching intensity, patient race, and surgical outcomes. *Archives of Surgery, 144*(2), 113–120.

Silber, J. H., Williams, S. V., Krakauer, H., & Schwartz, J. S. (1992). Hospital and patient characteristics associated with death after surgery. A study of adverse occurrence and failure to rescue. *Medical Care, 30*(7), 615–629.

The Joint Commission on the Accreditation of Healthcare Organizations. (2008). 2009 National Patient Safety Goals. *Joint Commission Perspectives, 28*(7), 11–14.

Jeannie P. Cimiotti
Sean P. Clarke
Linda H. Aiken

FAMILY EDUCATIONAL RIGHTS AND PRIVACY ACT OF 1974 (THE BUCKLEY AMENDMENT)

The Family Educational Rights and Privacy Act (FERPA) of 1974, also known as the Buckley Amendment, is a federal law that gives students rights to privacy regarding their academic and financial records. The complete document may be accessed within the Code of Federal Regulations as follows: 34 CFR Part 99.1–99.8 (Code of Federal Regulations, 2010). Within the Code of Federal Regulations, FERPA is divided into five subparts. Subpart A is further divided into eight additional categories that describe which educational institutions are regulated by this act, the purpose and definition, the rights of students and parents, and notification procedures and legal concerns. Subpart B covers three areas regarding the parental rights of inspection of records, the fees for photocopying of records, and the specific limitations regarding record viewing. Subpart C outlines three sections related to amending academic records, requirements, and rights to a hearing. Subpart D covers 10 areas related to consent for disclosing information including record keeping, limitations, emergency or medical issues, directories, and legal concerns. Last, Subpart E identifies eight areas related to enforcement concerns including complaints, involvement of the Secretary of Education, and potential conflicts with state or local laws (Family Educational Right and Privacy Act Regulations, 2009). It is essential for academic faculty and administrators to understand the nuances of this federal law as it covers student's records that may include grades, advisement, clinical and theory assessments and evaluations, and potential concerns regarding unsafe clinical practice. This act provides students with access to information that is placed in their files. It also explicitly defines that only select educational personnel may access their files. The student's permission must be received in writing for any other person or party to see or read their file. If a student is financially dependent on their parents while pursuing a degree, the parents have access to these records without consent (FERPA, 2010).

Code of Federal Regulations Title 34. (2006). Retrieved September 20, 2010, from http://www.access.gpo.gov/nara/cfr/waisidx_10/34cfr99_10.html

F

Family Educational Rights and Privacy Act. (2010). Retrieved September 20, 2010, from http://www2.ed.gov/policy/gen/guid/fpco/ferpa/index.html

Family Educational Rights and Privacy Act Regulations. (2009). Retrieved September 20, 2010, from http://www2.ed.gov/policy/gen/guid/fpco/pdf/ferparegs.pdf

Ronda Mintz-Binder

FINANCING HEALTH CARE

The financing of health care in the United States has progressed from charitable enterprise to big business. Technological developments in the late 19th and 20th centuries, including anesthesia, understanding the germ theory through science, surgery, and medical education, along with the rapid evolution of the nursing profession, created a need and use for modern hospitals, the foci of American health care delivery. Religious groups, ethnic organizations, philanthropists, women's associations, and civic bodies among others began and staffed hospitals in large and small communities. Among the earliest principles established for these institutions was that patients could or would pay for hospital services in the same way medical care was paid for: by fees for services (Stevens, 1999). From this principle evolved a role for insurance and public payments for hospital and medical care for enrolled or eligible patients; charity was displaced.

Beginning in 1929, nonprofit Blue Cross and Blue Shield Associations were established by hospital associations to ensure payment and by the 1950s became the largest private insurance plans for financing health care for workers. Soon life insurance companies expanded to sell health insurance products in a growing for-profit industry. Employers paid for health insurance as a benefit for employees in lieu of wage increases. Medicare and Medicaid programs followed in 1966 with payments for hospitals and doctors on behalf of the elderly and the poor. Today, patients are asked by hospitals and doctors to "assign" the health insurance benefits to them; thus, patients see little (except for co-payments and deductibles) of the financial transactions performed by these "third parties" on their behalf. Nearly all the provisions of the governmental programs were based on the fee-for-service model that the Blue Cross used for hospitals and Blue Shield employed to pay physicians. The "Blues" were managed by hospitals and doctors in arrangements that ensured that costs of providing services were covered in the charges made by the hospitals to the insurance companies.

Ensuring a revenue stream for hospitals and doctors, especially when the poor and elderly were covered, guaranteed growth and prosperity for all involved in providing health services. As the health services sector was not dependent on investors, much of the excess revenue was devoted to providing more and better services. Few, if any, births or deaths occurred in hospitals a hundred years ago, and now most take place there, for example. Escalation in service provision over the course of the century led to investments in health services that were once a negligible part of the gross domestic product and grew to 17.3% or $2.4 trillion of the 2008 GDP (Truffler et al., 2010).

The tension between the use of public and private monies for health services surfaced soon after the 1966 beginning of the public Medicare and Medicaid programs and reflected political currents that went from liberal to conservative to liberal and back again. Neither philosophy, however, had any demonstrable effect on reducing the provider-induced escalation in services and their costs. Health care cost control has shifted from public to private initiatives and back, but neither had sufficient support to do more than to make the shift back and forth from public to private anything more than temporary. The United States continues to spend more on health services than any other industrialized country. The government and employers shifted some costs to users, but even this has not yet slowed growth. Gaps in public and private financing for health care have resulted in 50 or so million people without health care coverage, more than 16% of the population, many members of working families (Kaiser Family Foundation, 2010).

Regarding the costs of medical care, the committee issued a 1932 report promoting the bundling of medical and hospitals costs and offering these services for a prepaid monthly premium (Ross, 2002). The few health maintenance organizations that followed were successful, mostly on the West Coast (the Kaiser Family Foundation and the Group Health of Puget Sound principally among them). These prepaid group plans and other so-called managed care programs were given a boost when Yale scientists found the diagnosis-related groups.[1] Diagnosis-related groups facilitated the clinical interpretation of hospitals costs, melding financial and medical data and enabling the setting of all inclusive rates. Even in many prepaid plans, physicians continue to receive fees for services. Hospitals now receive flat-rate payments for specified patient conditions either through Medicare or negotiations with managed care and insurance carriers.

The 2008 cost of registered nurses, principally as employee hourly wage costs, is a significant but small fraction of health care costs (6% of National Health Expenditures [NHE] or $141 billion),[2] but since Medicare, they have been declining as a proportion of the total NHE. The costs of nurses and nursing, as a proportion of NHE, began to decline in 1966 when as much as half of a hospital's expenses were for nurses, including nursing education. Nurse education expenses were shifted from hospitals to community colleges in the first decade after Medicare. Although more nurses were educated and employed, growth in health care expenses for administration, drugs, construction and equipment, and advertising, among others, far exceeded growth in the cost of nurses.

Concern for unchecked growth in NHE occupied the attention of state and federal policy makers until President Obama and the 111th Congress acted on health care reform legislation. The Patient Protection and Affordable Care Act of 2010 comprehensively addresses health care and reform with provisions that started in 2010 and phased in more than 4 years. Greater emphasis on prevention and quality is one of the elements of the Affordable Care Act, which include an individual mandate to purchase health insurance shared with employers, a comprehensive benefit designed to cover 70% of costs to individuals, new insurance rules that eliminate preexisting condition, and cancellation clauses. A number of new initiatives are

---

[1] John D. Thompson, RN, and Robert Fetter were the Yale scientists. Thompson says he found the diagnosis-related group in Florence Nightingale's 1863, *Notes on Hospitals*, third edition, which argued that hospital mortality could only be compared by comparing the mortality of like cases among hospitals; Yale researchers substituted cost for mortality in their comparisons.

[2] Calculated using information from HRSA (2010) for numbers and salary data and the National Center for Health Statistics (2008) Health, United States—2008, Centers for Medicare and Medicaid Services, Office of the Actuary, Washington, DC, for NHE.

introduced including a Community Living Assistance Services and Supports Act and incentives to establish a specific nurse service called the Nurse–Family Partnership (Olds et al., 1997, 2002).

Although the British Medical Association advocates for patients to see nurses before they see physicians (many of the patient needs can be handled by nurses and, further, physicians in the British National Health Service are not paid more for seeing more patients), time will tell if the Affordable Care Act (ACA) will develop incentives that transform American nursing (*British Medical Journal*, 2002). Nurses in primary care, using the International Council of Nurses concept, *Basic Principles of Nursing Care*, where nurses support, encourage, and teach, are indeed the services many need to prevent and manage chronic illnesses (Halloran, 2009; Henderson, 1997). Thorpe (2005) promoted such disease prevention and health promotion as keys to the efficient and effective reform of the U.S. health care system. Some of the most significant recent nursing research has demonstrated the capacity of nurses in keeping selected vulnerable sick people away from doctors and hospitals with greater patient satisfaction (Brooten et al., 1986; Harrell, Pearce, & Hayman, 2003; Mishel et al., 2002; Naylor et al., 1999; Olds et al., 1997, 2002). These studies get much less application than they could in part because the results have run counter to the financial interests of doctors and hospitals, the predominant employers of nurses.

Provisions of the Patient Protection and Affordable Care Act may well produce incentives for nurses to more actively manage patient care and prevention. Among the provisions of the ACA are incentives for doctors and hospitals to group services into accountable care organizations that tie reimbursements to quality measures and reductions in the cost of care. Noting the need for strengthened primary care within the ACA, pay incentives were created for establishing "medical homes" or organizations of primary care providers where enrolled patients care is coordinated, not unlike the health maintenance organizations like Kaiser-Permanente, which is a demonstration site for the effectiveness of medical homes.

The ACA has created opportunities for advanced practice nurses that may place more emphasis on graduate education for clinical nurses who would complement medical services in a comprehensive health care system. A planned health system would seek out nurses to provide primary care for the chronically ill to diminish the need for delayed, more expensive institutional care.

Leadership is needed to see that patients have access to the services of nurses in primary care in more than token numbers. The Institute of Medicine (2010) report on the future of nursing recommends nurses lead change to advance health. Nurses can contribute to the solution of health care financing by collaborating in the provision of primary care, as is done in health management organizations (HMOs) or even by competing with doctors and hospitals for access to patients. As it is now, costs for nurses are seen as part of the problem of financing health care in the United States, yet their hopeful future in an efficient and effective reformed health care system is promising.

The ACA is a dynamic law. The 4-year implementation plan will be modified through negotiations between elected officials and those who provide them financial support. The 1966 Medicare legislation originally contained incentives for post hospital care modeled on the Loeb Center for Nursing and Rehabilitation where registered nurses fostered patient independence. The nursing home lobby successfully convinced legislators they could provide Loeb-like services without the expense of nurses and foisted a for-profit, dependence-oriented nursing home industry on the public at great expense in efficiency and effectiveness. A basis for nurses' participation in any of the ACA provisions is required; nurses' unique contributions should be made explicit as a guide to consistent and constructive action. One universally recognized concept of nursing authored by Virginia Henderson for the International Council of Nurses says: "Nurses help people, sick or well, in the performance of those activities contributing to health or its recovery (or to a peaceful death) that they would perform unaided if they had the necessary strength, will or knowledge. It is likewise the function of nurses to help people gain independence as rapidly as possible" (Henderson & Nite, 1978).

Financing health care, long based on fee-for-service principles and the adoption of business practices used in for-profit enterprises, has produced phenomenal growth in provider-induced medical services. Noting deficiencies in American health care, the ACA will precipitate changes that may well improve care quality and reduce cost. A well-educated nursing workforce, basing its services on valid concepts, tested through research, promises to become an integral component of financing reform.

British Medical Journal. (2002). News roundup: BMA suggests nurses could become gate-keepers of the NHS. *BMJ, 324,* 565. Retrieved March 18, 2002, from http://bmj.com/cgi/eletters/324/7337/565

Brooten, D., Kumar, S., Brown, L. P., Butts, P., Finkler, S. A., Bakewell-Sachs, S., et al. (1986). A randomized clinical trial of early hospital discharge and home follow-up of very-low-birth-weight infants. *New England Journal of Medicine, 315*(15), 934–939.

Halloran, E. (2009). The International Council of Nurses Virginia Henderson Lecture: Women hold up half the sky. *International Nursing Review, 56*(4), 410–415.

Harrell, J. S., Pearce P. F., & Hayman, L. L. (2003). Fostering prevention in the pediatric population. *Journal of Cardiovascular Nursing,* 18(2), 144–149.

Henderson, V. (1997). *ICN's basic principles of nursing care.* Geneva, Switzerland: International Council of Nurses.

Henderson, V., & Nite, G. (1978). *Principles and practice of nursing* (6th ed.). New York, NY: Macmillan. (Reprinted by the ICN in 1997). The opening paragraph of this seminal book informs the reader of the necessity for describing the function of the nurse—"If the concept is clear and valid, it can guide them [nurses] to consistent and constructive action; if it is confused and uninformed it can lead to inconsistent, ineffective, or even harmful action."

HRSA. (2010). *Preliminary findings: The registered nurse population—national sample survey of RNs—2008.* Rockville, MD: HRSA, HHS.

Institute of Medicine. (2010). *The future of nursing: Leading change, advancing health.* Committee on the Robert Wood Johnson Foundation Initiative on the Future of Nursing at the Institute of Medicine. Washington, DC: National Academies Press.

Kaiser Family Foundation. (2010, September). *Five facts about the uninsured* (Newsletter). Washington, DC: The Henry J. Kaiser Family Foundation.

Mishel, M., Belyea, M., Germino, B., Stewart, J., Bailey, D., Robertson, C., et al. (2002). Helping patients with localized prostate carcinoma manage uncertainty and treatment side-effects: Nurse-delivered psychoeducational intervention over the telephone. *Cancer, 94*(6), 1854–1866.

Naylor, M. D., Brooten, D., Campbell, R., Jacobsen, B. S., Mezey, M. D., Pauly, M. V., et al. (1999). Comprehensive discharge planning and home follow-up of hospitalized elders: A randomized clinical trial. *Journal of the American Medical Association, 281*(7), 613–620.

Olds, D., Eckenrode, J., Henderson, C., Kitzman, H., Powers, J., Cole, R., et al. (1997). Long-term effects of home visitation on maternal life course and child abuse and neglect: Fifteen year follow up of a randomized clinical trial. *Journal of the American Medical Association, 278*(8), 637–643.

Olds, D., Robinson, J., O'Brian, R., Luckey, D., Pettitt, L., Henderson, C., et al. (2002). Home visiting by paraprofessionals and by nurses: A randomized, controlled trial. *Pediatrics, 110*(3), 486–496.

Ross, J. S. (2002). Committee on the costs of medical care and the history of health insurance in the US. *Einstein Quarterly Journal of Biology and Medicine, 19*, 129–134.

Stevens, R. (1999). *In sickness and in wealth* (pp. 30–39). Baltimore, MD: Johns Hopkins University Press.

Thorpe, K. E. (2005). The rise in health care spending and what to do about it. *Health Affairs, 24*(6), 1436–1445.

Truffler, C. J., Keehan, S., Smith, S., Cylus, J., Sisko, A., Poisal, J. A., et al. (2010). Health spending projections through 2019: The recession's impact continues. *Health Affairs, 29*(3), 522–529.

Edward J. Halloran

FLEXTIME

Flextime is a system used in employee staffing and scheduling to retain employees, allowing employees to select time schedules that meet both work responsibilities and personal needs. Key features include variable start times, such as working longer or shorter than the 8-hour shift, arriving on or leaving a unit at different times, for example, five nurses arrive at 0700 and work until 1500 or one nurse arrives at 1100 and works until 1900, and weekend programs. Leader-manager pitfalls of flextime can include disruption in continuity of patient care and communication, particularly in situations with families, over- or understaffing, and difficulty in coordinating appropriate coverage by staff.

Additional information is available from the following sources:

American Nurses Association. (2002). *Background information and legislative maps: Nurse staffing plans and ratios.* Retrieved September 5, 2007, from http://www.nursing-world.org/HiddenDocumentVault/GOVA/Federal/2004StaffingPlansandRatios.aspx

Kelly, P. (2008). *Nursing leadership & management.* Clifton Park, NY: Thomson/Delmar.

Marquis, B. L., & Huston, C. J. (2009). *Leadership roles and management functions in nursing: Theory and application* (6th ed.). Philadelphia, PA: Lippincott Williams & Wilkins.

Martha J. Greenberg

FOUNDATION FUNDING OF HEALTH CARE AND NURSING

Foundations are defined as organizations or entities that exist for the sole purpose of supporting charitable works. Foundations are often supported by the generous, philanthropic donations of individuals or families with the intention of supporting a particular mission that is of importance. For example, the John A. Hartford Foundation was developed to support health care for older Americans, an issue that was of great importance to the founders and that continues to be carried out today. Other foundations are supported by an endowment, which is defined as a stable account housed within a particular *institution*, such as a hospital, university, or foundation, to be used for a defined purpose. Still other foundations are supported through the collective charitable donations of a group of people with common interests, such as the Alzheimer Disease Foundation. Foundations may be privately owned and operated or public and housed within a public charity such as the National Philanthropic Trust. Whether private or public, foundations are excellent vehicles in which a life meaning or purpose may be fulfilled and offer private tax benefits for the donating person, family, or institution. From a health care and nursing perspective, foundations provide a growing and exciting source of funding for specific health care issues.

One of the first foundations set up exclusively to support nursing was the Helene Fuld Health Trust, established in 1935. The Robert Wood Johnson Foundation has supported nursing programs since its inception and over the years has dedicated more than $140 million to nursing projects. Other major foundations that have supported nursing and health care include the W. K. Kellogg Foundation, the Pew Charitable Trusts, the Rockefeller Foundation, the Commonwealth Fund, the Josiah Macy Foundation, and more recently, the Bill and Melinda Gates Foundation. In addition, there are hundreds of small local, regional, and national foundations that support nursing and health care initiatives, for example, the New York–based Donald and Barbara Jonas Center for Nursing Excellence.

Key foundations that have supported nursing work include that of the Robert Wood Johnson Foundation and the Pew Charitable Trusts, which in 1988 jointly supported a multimillion dollar national project titled "Strengthening Hospital Nursing: A Program to Improve Patient Care" to provide better patient care through innovative, hospital-wide restructuring; the John A. Hartford Foundation support of geriatric nursing initiatives through several education and research projects; and the Independence Foundation, which funded endowed professorships at 10 private schools of nursing.

Foundations that support health care and nursing generally are organizations with a particular purpose, such as enhancing research about a particular disease or promoting a certain type of care. The missions may be broad, such as that of the Robert Wood Johnson Foundation to improve the health and health care of all Americans, or more specific such as the Lance Armstrong Foundation, which aims to educate and empower cancer survivors. Thus, it is important in seeking foundation funding that health care and nursing professionals target foundations with similar missions. In this way, relationships may be built that provide a continued source of support for important research and work in health care. In developing such relationships and grant applications, it is also important to be aware that although these foundations often fund health care, they may not have nurses and health care providers on the review board for applications. Consequently, it is important that nursing and health care jargon be avoided and the project under review explained in a manner that all populations will understand. Finally, from an ethical perspective, the researcher may have greater experience in identifying consent and approval issues than the foundation. Thus, great attention must be made to adhering to ethical nursing standards for research, regardless of foundation requirements.

See also Philanthropy/Fund Raising

Additional information is available from the following Web sites:

Association of Small Foundations. Retrieved from www.smallfoundations.org

Council on Foundations. Retrieved from www.cof.org

Foundations.org. Retrieved from www.foundations.org

Foundation Center. Retrieved from www.fdn-center.org

Grantmakers in Health. Retrieved from www.gih.or

National Philanthropic Trust. Retrieved from http://www.nptrust.org

Network Solutions. Retrieved from www.nnh.org/NewNNH/foundations.htm

Meredith Wallace Kazer
Joyce J. Fitzpatrick

FUNDING FOR NURSING RESEARCH

Funding for nursing research is generated from multiple sources that are public and private in nature. Funding is important because it allows for generating and testing knowledge that guides professional practice and health policy. Without funding, research ideas can be generated but not tested sufficiently. From a scientific perspective, extramural funding, especially, provides credibility for the research ideas being studied. It means that the ideas have been peer reviewed and deemed worth of investment.

INTRAMURAL FUNDING OF NURSING RESEARCH

Research can be funded intramurally or extramurally. Intramural funds are provided in university and research institute environments by the parent organization. These funds are invested in scientists whose ideas show strong potential for long-term contributions to a discipline and can be expected to be funded by extramural sources. Intramural funding usually requires application and review process just as extramural funding, so merit and potential contribution judgments can be made. For nursing, faculty in university or other educational settings are usually able to compete for intramural funding from the office within the university charged with reviewing grant proposals and awarding funds, for example, the Vice President for Research office.

Some schools of nursing also provide small pilot monies for research. Clinical nurse researchers are able to compete for specific hospital investigator awards. These are examples of research funds that are intramural and the source is the parent organization.

EXTRAMURAL FUNDING OF NURSING RESEARCH

There are numerous extramural sources for funding nursing research, for example, federal agencies, private foundations, and professional associations. Several common practices exist across the different sources. First, each entity has a focus for its research funding, broad or narrow, and generally has a set of priorities or areas of emphasis for funding. It is important to systematically match the research interests of the investigator with the priority areas of the funding body. Second, almost all of the funding entities have a structured application and review process. The investigator seeking funds needs to be conversant with such processes and if possible be communicating with an individual who has been funded by the entity and can provide "helpful hints" in terms of the application.

Multiple opportunities are provided for funding of research through the federal government, especially in the area of health. The Department of Health and Human Services houses the National Institutes of Health (NIH), the Agency for Healthcare Research and Quality, the Centers for Disease Control and Prevention, and the Centers for Medicare and Medicaid Services (CMS), and others. Nurse researchers can be and have been funded through each of these entities.

The NIH provides the majority of funding for nursing research. NIH is composed of 27 institutes, centers, and offices that have extramural funding for biomedical and behavioral health research. One of the institutes is the National Institute of Nursing Research, which has the largest concentration of resources for funding nursing research in the United States. However, nursing research can also be funded in any of the other NIH entities as well. Each of the institutes and centers has formal extramural programs that offer funding opportunities through a variety of mechanisms. Each institute and center will have a different array of funding mechanisms, and only the larger institutes have the full set of them. However, all the institutes and centers have the funding mechanisms for the investigator-initiated grants (RO1), the small grant mechanism (RO3), the Academic Research Enhancement Award (AREA), the Small Business Innovative Research (SBIR), and Small Business Technology Transfer award (STTR), and the NIH Pathway to Independence Award (K99/R00) as well as the Program and Center Awards, for example, Research Program Project grant (PO1) and Center Core Grants (P30). In addition to the routine awards, there are special requests for proposals and applications that offer opportunities for funding research. The NIH and especially the National Institute of Nursing Research offer research training fellowships either to individuals for predoctoral and postdoctoral education (F31, F32) or to institutions (T32). Career development awards of several kinds are available (K awards) as well as senior fellowships (F33). Funding of research can be obtained through completion for cooperative agreements and contracts. With these two mechanisms, the institute or center is more involved with the planning and implementation of the science.

The research focus for the Agency for Healthcare Research and Quality is to improve the quality, safety, efficiency, and effectiveness of health care. The research tends to involve organization systems in terms of patient safety as well as comparative effectiveness studies of alternative therapeutic interventions. The extramural program grant mechanisms are similar to those used at NIH. Grants, cooperative agreements, and contracts are funding opportunities.

As the name implies, the Centers for Disease Control and Prevention focuses on research on health promotion for individuals and populations. Approximately 85% of the agency's funding is for extramural grants and contracts that promote health and quality of life by preventing and controlling disease, injury, and disability. This agency also provides funding opportunities for emergency preparedness and response, environmental health issues, life stages, and populations as well as injury, violence, and safety.

The CMS is primarily a service agency for the programs and regulation of Medicare and Medicaid. However, the agency offers request for proposals and applications for demonstration projects. The Health Care Recovery Act placed funds with the CMS for demonstration projects on alternative models for delivering health care. Such projects are funded through the grants and contracts mechanism.

There are a multitude of private foundations that offer opportunities for funding research. Because the major areas of funding activity include health education, arts, and culture plus human services, nursing research is well received in these competitive arenas. The foundation center provides up to date facts and figures on such foundations and is an important source of information. The critical factor in applying for foundation monies is achieving a strong match between the investigator's research interest and the funding focus and priorities of the foundation. There

F

are a number of articles written about the importance of this match and how to assess it (www.foundationcenter.org). In addition, it is important to talk with the staff at the foundation once a possible match has been assessed. Foundation staff often wish to be collaborative in tailoring grant applications to match a particular priority. There are several examples of foundations that historically have funded nursing research and demonstration programs.

The Robert Wood Johnson Foundation is the nation's largest philanthropy devoted to the public's health. Their focus is on both the health of the American people and the health care system. This funding includes programs that influence professional practice and health policy. The latest well-known funding of a nursing policy issue was the collaboration with the Institute of Medicine (IOM) to produce the study panel report on *The Future of Nursing: Leading Change, Advancing Health.*

The W. K. Kellogg Foundation has redefined its mission to focus on "children, families and communities as they strengthen and create conditions that propel vulnerable children to achieve success as individuals and as contributors to the larger community and society" (www.foundationcenter.org). The funding usually involves community health care programs that increase access and quality of care to vulnerable populations.

The Josiah Macy, Jr. Foundation often provides opportunities for the funding of innovative health professional education. It is particularly interested in interdisciplinary education and teamwork. For example, the Macy foundation has funded a number of workshops with physicians and nurses focused on interdisciplinary primary care and community access to care. This foundation also funds demonstration projects for new educational programs; for example, Macy funded the early pilots of BSN

to PhD programs. Two of the priorities for funding include career development of underserved minorities and education for the care of underserved populations.

The Commonwealth Fund is a private foundation originally started by a woman philanthropist. The Commonwealth Fund promotes high-performing health care systems that achieve better access, improved quality, and greater efficiency, especially for society's vulnerable populations. The topics of interest include health insurance, Medicare services, health system performance, health care quality, health disparities, and patient-centered care.

The PEW Charitable Trusts foundation focuses on shaping health policy at multiple levels. Currently, the priorities include public health and human service policy, family financial security issues, and science and technology. Like other foundations, PEW is interested in evaluating innovative models for health care in the new health care reform era.

PROFESSIONAL ASSOCIATIONS

A number of health professional associations provide limited funding for pilot studies for either new investigators, researchers changing scientific direction, and/or innovative higher risk ideas that traditional funders may not consider without early data suggesting successful trends. Several nursing associations provide small grants or career development awards for nursing research. The American Nurses Foundation is the funding arm of the American Nurses Association. They provide awards for both beginning and experienced researchers. In addition, the American Nurses Foundation collaborates with different professional association partners to sponsor career development opportunities such as working with the American Academy of Nursing and the IOM to fund the Distinguished Nurse Scholar program at the IOM. Sigma Theta Tau International also funds a number of research awards and collaborates with other organizations to enhance the funding amounts. The Web site for Sigma Theta Tau International lists more than 60 professional nursing associations that promote research through funding awards (www.nursingsociety.org). Many of the professional associations are organized according to a specific disease or a particular body organ, for example, the American Heart Association, the American Cancer Society, or the American Lung Association. These organizations fund investigators from multiple health professions.

In summary, there are numerous opportunities for the funding of nursing research. Funding that supports long-term research programs primarily comes from the federal government. Private foundations have more limited funding with clearly stated specific priorities. These funds tend not to be recurring but expect the investigator to apply for future monies from another source, generally the federal government. Professional associations are excellent sources for limited amounts of funding for evaluation of innovative scientific endeavors.

www.DHHS.gov
www.NIH.gov
www.ninr.nih.gov
www.AHRQ.gov
www.CDC.gov
www.VMS.gov
www.foundationcenter.org
www.rwjf.org
www.josiahmacyfoundation.org
www.commonwealthfund.org
www.pewtrusts.org
www.nursingsociety.org
www.anfonline.org
www.iom.edu
www.heart.org
www.cancer.org

Ada Sue Hinshaw

G

GENDER AND LEADERSHIP

Tomorrow belongs to women forecasts Tom Peters in one of his latest works on leadership. Peters realizes, as others have, that women's talents are much better suited to the new service economy of the 21st century than men's. Because of gender differences in the way they process the world around them, many experts believe that women are better at a lot of the skills that matter in leadership (Peters, 2005). For instance, relationship skills are vital to the new breed of transformational leaders. Leaders have an uncanny ability to "connect" with followers and, often, other leaders. Trust is a crucial ingredient, as are empathy and emotional intelligence. These are areas in which women excel. Women have a talent with relationships and often can read all the guideposts and relationship barometers that tell you whether you're on the right track (Peters, 2005). Women have a greater capacity to read body language or nonverbal cues (Peters, 2005). They generally have greater emotional sensitivity, intuition, and empathy and generally are more patient and have the ability to do many things simultaneously. Undoubtedly, many of us have noticed that emotionally sensitive traits like these are more prevalent—in general—in women than men. Now there is science to back up this claim.

Fairly dramatic differences in the reactions of the brains of the men and women have been found (Gur et al., 1999). Female brains show reactions that span eight times greater an area in the brain than that of male subjects in the limbic or emotional seat of the brain. Findings have led to the same conclusion: The thoughts and emotional processes of men and women are fundamentally different in a number of ways. Men's thinking is more compartmentalized, whereas women's thinking is more integrated.

Research on feminine cognition reveals the ability to move more gracefully from intellect to intuition and from linear to nonlinear thought than men. This is the reason why women—our wives and our mothers and the female leaders—are so good at multitasking, the ability to do many different things at once. Their male counterparts, brilliant though they may be in their fields, are not as able to juggle many activities simultaneously.

UNBROKEN WHOLENESS: IT'S BECOMING A "WOMAN'S WORLD"

These new scientific findings are very significant for leadership when you consider new findings in physics that herald a fundamental shift in our scientific worldview. The shift changes our perspective from a mechanical, compartmentalized

Cartesian view to a worldview of unbroken wholeness in which everything is linked and interrelated. Just as Newtonian science and its dependence on mechanical force has produced a "masculine world," the new physics and its dependence on the power inherent in relationship and connection herald the advent of a world that values things that are "feminine" in essence. We have long favored the separateness of the individual self over connection to others, leaning more toward an autonomous life of work than toward the interdependence of love and connection toward each other. In addition, all that is slowly changing. Somehow through interaction, subatomic particles are briefly summoned out of a world of potentiality and possibility into the solid world of tangible things and events. At this level, all is interconnected. How we subjectively experience events, interactions, and our inner self is "observer created"—created by us (Hawkens, 2003).

The exploitation of nature has gone hand in hand with the exploitation of women, who have been identified with nature throughout the ages. Francis Bacon, the father of the scientific method, was predisposed to leave women out of the picture. Bacon said of science that it is like a "woman to be brought into submission and bound and conquered as a slave," leaving an indelible black mark on female ways of knowing (Shearer, 1997). The objective reality that we were all brought up to believe in has proven to be illusive. Space and time are relative. People do not perceive distance and time in exactly the same way. In fact, relative space and time have been shown to be quite subjective; everyone has a different opinion about what they see. In the meantime, the thinking of men like Bacon has created a world that is preoccupied with control and obsessed with carving things into pieces and maintaining boundaries to achieve control. As

a result, the high values we place on separation, independence, and autonomy have always been taken as fact and not simply the views of the thought leaders of science at the time.

As Harvard psychologist Carol Gilligan (1993)—known for discovering that female development centers around connection, not separation—states, "The dissociation between thoughts and feelings, suppressing what one knows, the use of one's voice to cover rather than convey one's inner world, so that relationships no longer provide channels for exploring the connections between one's inner life and the world of others," is characteristic of our masculine-minded culture. As the new millennium becomes a more feminine world, our interdependence will create a new understanding of the power of relationships. Gilligan said, "You cannot take a life out of history," as she discovered that Erik Erikson's (1963) well-known theory of *human* development was really a conception of *male* development. His well-known stages of development were centered on separation and autonomy because the study of the male as well as mechanistic worldviews was the norm in science. Scientific discoveries do not exist in a vacuum either but reflect the beliefs and values of the people in a society, including men like Erikson.

It is no accident that as a new scientific paradigm reveals a world with a new respect for the feminine, the sheer demographic power of baby boomer women in society gives them unprecedented influence. Baby Boomer women have ushered in major social reforms including childbearing, reproductive choice, and reforms in women's health, such as the inclusion of women in clinical trials. They represent nearly 25% of the population, and they are the most educated cohort of women in society that there have ever been. Currently,

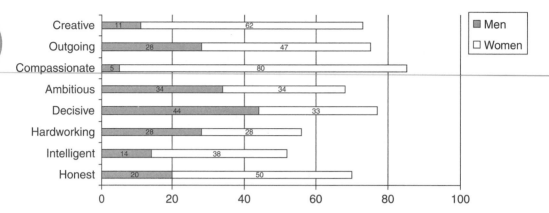

FIGURE 2: Leadership Traits: Percent saying this trait is more true of men or women.

there are one million perimenopausal Baby Boomer women who have brought menopause and reproductive rights out of the closet.

Pew conducted a study in 2008 to examine gender and leadership. The results indicated that women outpaced men in the certain leadership traits (Pew Social Trends Staff, 2008) (see Figure 2).

It has been a task for women to provide leadership throughout history and "Go on believing in life when there was almost no hope," in the words of Margaret Meade. Now science is emerging as the powerful context for a new age of women leaders. Women have always shown love and compassion. The movement in science and the urge toward the feminine are bound to make female leadership the tsunami of the millennium.

Erikson, E. H. (1963). *Childhood and society*. New York, NY: W. W. Norton & Company.

Gilligan, C. (1993). *In a different voice*. Cambridge, MA: Harvard University Press.

Gur, R. C., Turetsky, B. I., Matsui, M., Yan, M., Bilker, W., Hugett, P., et al. (1999). Sex differences in brain gray and white matter in healthy young adults: Correlations with cognitive performance. *Journal of Neuroscience, 19*(10), 4065–4072.

Hawkens, D. R. (2003). *Reality and subjectivity*. Sedona, AZ: Veritas Publishing.

Peters, T. (2005). *Excerpt from "Re-imagine."* Retrieved August 20, 2006, from http://www.usatoday.com/money/books/2003-12-05-reimagineexcerpt_x.htm

Pew Social Trends Staff. (2008, August 25). *Men or women: Who's the better leader?* Retrieved February 16, 2011, from Pew Research Center: http://pewsocialtrends.org/2008/08/25/men-or-women-whos-the-better-leader

Shearer, A. (1997). *Athene*. New York, NY: Penguin Books.

Pam Maraldo
Mary Samost

GENERATIONAL DIFFERENCES IN LEADERSHIP AND MENTORING

When it comes to understanding organizational behavior, including leadership and mentoring preferences, there is a growing awareness that generational differences matter. Depending on when you were born, you have been shaped by events that make you predisposed to certain ways of looking at the world. Those born before 1940 are often described as traditionalists, with those born between 1934 and 1945 are referred to more specifically as the Silent Generation. Shaped by the aftermath of World War II, they tend to prefer well-defined situations, have respect for hierarchy and authority, and are loyal, hardworking, and rule followers. Members of the Baby Boomer Generation, beginning postwar and ending 1960–1964, were shaped by major societal changes—the Vietnam War, the civil rights movement, various assassinations, and the women's movement. Those experiences left them independent, ambitious, process oriented, seeking rewards and recognition, inclined to think they are entitled, and workaholics; they prefer a collegiate and consensual style of relationships.

Members of Generation X, beginning in the early 1960s and ending 1975–1982, knew financial, family, and/or social insecurity growing up. Those experiences left them less respectful of authority and cynical but able to take uncertainty, diversity, and change in stride. They value honesty, fairness, competence, and straightforwardness; are technically competent and practical in their approach to problem solving, favoring an outcomes orientation; crave mentors; and value family. Members of Generation Y (also known as the Net Generation or Millennials), beginning after 1980 and going through the turn of the century, expect to have a polite relationship with authority because many of them grew up closer to their parents than the previous generation did. They value diversity and change, meaningful work, lifelong learning, intellectual stimulation, more structure, and see family as the key to happiness; they take technology for granted, and prefer collective action and leaders who pull people together (Sessa, Kabacoff, Deal, & Brown, 2007).

Bickel and Brown (2005) have written about the often overlooked generational differences that shape the mentor–mentee relationship, causing both sides to have different and somewhat conflicting expectations about how they wish to be treated and what it means to be an effective leader. Boomers respect authority and believe in paying their dues, but Generation Xers question authority and do not think that paying dues is relevant. The former may still view mentoring as a kindness, whereas the latter regard mentoring as a right not a privilege. Boomers may be uncomfortable providing the frequent, frank feedback that Generation Xers prefer. This can lead older professionals to go on about how unappreciative the younger generation is—"they don't make them like they used to"—with mutual withdrawal as the consequence instead of a generative relationship.

It is important to target your mentoring and leadership style, so that you bring out the strengths of someone not of your generation. For example, the younger generation generally wants to work *with* you as opposed to *for* you. Boomer leaders may still have difficulty with some issues—diversity, change, and technology—that the subsequent generations find relatively unproblematic. For example, Generation Xers accept diversity and use technology, and their successors, the Millennium Generation, celebrate diversity and assume technology (Thiefoldt & Scheef, 2004), so the savvy leader will take advantage of how comfortable these generations are with negotiating differences and virtualities. The Boomer leader who "lives to work" may have difficulty understanding and dealing with the younger generations who believe that you "work to live." So the former may think a flexible work schedule is unreasonable when the latter will switch positions if such needs are not met.

G

It is, however, important to remember that the differences across generations are smaller than the similarities. All generations value mutual respect in relationships and want a supportive work environment, even if the older generations think more in terms of job security, whereas the younger generations think more in terms of career security, making them more interested in portable pension benefits and their professional advancement than their predecessors (Lavoie-Tremblay et al., 2010). What is important is that leaders/mentors acknowledge differences, understand the dissimilarities in expectation that may exist across the generations, and build on the strengths of individuals and their generations (Keepnews, Brewer, Kovner, & Shin, 2010).

In addition, it is not always a case of the older trying to understand the younger. With multigenerational workforces, leaders may be managing their parents' or even their grandparents' generation who value considerate feedback, when the leaders prefer immediate feedback, making this a situation that requires particular tact because the younger generation's quickness to respond can feel abrupt and rude when that is not the intention. Being sensitive to generational differences in leadership and mentoring, however, has the added advantage of making the professional sensitive to all of the other generational differences that shape the health experience of patients and their families, for example, differences in health-seeking behaviors, from one generation to another.

See also Constructive Feedback; Leadership Development; Mentoring

Bickel, J., & Brown, A. J. (2005). Generation X: Implications for faculty recruitment and development in academic health centers. *Academic Medicine, 80,* 205–210.

Keepnews, D. M., Brewer, C. S., Kovner, C. T., & Shin, J. H. (2010). Generational differences among newly licensed registered nurses. *Nursing Outlook, 58,* 155–163.

Lavoie-Tremblay, M., Paquet, M., Duchesne, M. A., Santo, A., Gaurancic, A., Courcy, F., et al. (2010). Retaining nurses and other hospital workers: An intergenerational perspective of the work climate. *Journal of Nursing Scholarship, 42,* 414–422.

Sessa, V., Kabacoff, R. I., Deal, J., & Brown, H. (2007). Generational differences in leader values and leadership behaviors. *Psychologist-Manager Journal, 10*(1), 47–74.

Thiefoldt, D., & Scheef, D. (2004, August). Generation X and the Millennials: Mentoring the new generations. *Law Practice Today.* Retrieved February 18, 2011, from http://www.abanet.org/lpm/lpt/articles/mgt08044.html

Angela Barron McBride

GLOBAL NURSING SHORTAGE

The global nursing shortage has affected nearly every country and spawned both competition and cooperation among countries desperate for nursing care provided at the level of registered nurses. The recruitment reaction by the international community has led to an increase in both the migration and existing shortage of nurses (Thobaben et al., 2005). The reasons for the shortage are complex and multifaceted. In the United States, they emanate primarily from high-stress academic and practice environments, an aging nursing workforce as well as an aging population, changes in nursing school enrollments, an increase in both attractive and more lucrative educational and career opportunities for women, the devalued image of nursing, and a constantly increasing demand for sophisticated nursing care by those with advanced degrees.

Not all of these issues, however, are specific to the United States. The International Council of Nurses (ICN) issued *The Global Shortage of Registered Nurses: An Overview of Issues and Actions* (2004) and suggested, among other things, that all countries must address the issue of the ratio of nurses to patients. International recruitment, especially from low-income countries that have inadequate nurse-to-patient ratios, has nevertheless significantly increased. The practice of high-income countries recruiting nurses from less-developed countries that are in need of nurses to address their own health care shortages has not only complicated the shortage, but has created serious ethical dilemmas. For example, this practice challenges the principles of nonmaleficence or "do no harm," autonomy and justice. As a result, recruitment from low-income countries is being increasingly scrutinized.

International health care leaders are questioning whether it is ever justified to recruit foreign-educated nurses from developing countries that are sorely in need of health care providers. However, nurses have the right to make their own decisions, and to pursue economic and professional career options in more advantaged countries such as the United States, the United Kingdom, Ireland, Norway, and Australia, also called "destination countries" by the World Health Organization (WHO) (Buchan & Sochalski, 2004, pp. 587). With outward migration, however, less-advantaged countries experience a decrease in their own supply of available nurses. By pursuing advanced education in the United States and other countries, where there is greater technology, research, and highly sophisticated nursing care, nurses have the opportunity to return to their countries with new knowledge and skills that they can invest in their residential health care systems and enhance the quality of life of patients and families (Bannon & Roodman, 2004). However, the reality is that there is no guarantee that they will return to their home countries, and data that track their migration, adjustment, and length of stay in destination countries are sparse (Buchan & Sochalski, 2004).

This conundrum generates additional questions and concerns that nurse administrators and leaders need to address when they embark on programs of international recruitment. Founded in 2005 as a joint endeavor between Council of Graduates of Foreign Nursing Schools (CGFNS) International and the International Council of Nurses, the International Centre on Nurse Migration (ICNM) serves as a global resource for the development, promotion and dissemination of research, policy and information on global nurse migration (ICN-ICNM, n.d.). Yet, global migration is commonplace with an estimated 214 million international migrants worldwide, constituting the equivalent of the fifth most populous country in the world (UN, 2009).

Should foreign-educated nurses be encouraged to stay in the United States, or should they return to their own countries when their recruitment contracts have ended? If their employment in a high-income country contributes to their families' incomes at home, should they be required to return home after their employment contract is over? Which country has the priority and what are the implications for the migrating nurse in these situations? Additionally, foreign-educated nurses may have difficulty with the new culture, language, and legal requirements, which can place strains on them, their families, and even their employers. They must understand the jargon, culture, values, nursing practice (Ea, Itzhaki, Ehrenfeld, & Fitzpatrick, 2010), and people of their new country, and may become disillusioned by their new lives (Ea, 2007). In

G

response, hospitals, in particular, need to provide enculturation programs to assist these nurses with their adjustment, as well as with the patient care they provide, the language, and their social interactions. The ethical considerations in these situations need to be addressed directly, and more importantly; the time has arrived for nurse recruitment to be within the domain of hospital ethics committees.

A study on international nurse mobility (WHO/ICN/RCL, 2003) sponsored by the WHO, ICN, and the Royal College of Nursing suggests that inadequate working conditions and aggressive recruiting have created "push-pull" forces (Ea, 2007; WHO/ICN/ RCL, 2003) that foster unhealthy international nurse migration patterns. On the one hand, nurses are needed in the country sponsoring the recruitment; on the other hand, nurses are needed in the countries from which they are being recruited. Although migrating nurses worsen the "brain-drain" (Institute of Medicine [IOM], 2010) and health care shortage in their own countries when they practice abroad, their incomes often subsidize their families, and indirectly, improve the economy of their communities, as well as contribute to a better quality of life. In response, the WHO has been developing global evidence-based, ethical policies for recruiting, managing, and retaining the health workforce in varied labor markets (Rosenkoetter, 2005). In 2006, in *The Global Nursing Shortage: Priority Areas for Intervention*, the ICN/FNIF released an extensive report on global nursing shortages, trends, and proposed interventional solutions to address the many challenges. The report states that the three most critical challenges are the impact of HIV/AIDS, internal and international migration, and the need for effective health sector reform and reorganization.

In the United States, the American Academy of Nursing's expert panel on global health and nursing has studied the complex interrelated factors involved in the shortage, and in 2005 issued a *White Paper on Global Nursing and Health* (Rosenkoetter, 2005). Recognizing that a global problem calls for global collaboration in creating solutions, the panel's 13 recommended actions focus on the Academy's key role in fostering dialogue, sharing ideas, and disseminating viable solutions among nurse leaders internationally.

The challenge now for "resourced-countries" is to develop national policies on self-sufficiency. Nurse leaders in health care systems and professional organizations can meet this challenge by participating in the development of policies on the ethical recruitment, retention, and enculturation of foreign nurses, while developing strategies that support their return to their homelands with new practice skills and advanced education. One such strategy is the agreement between the United Kingdom and South Africa, allowing health care professionals to work in each other's countries for only a specified length of time before they must return home. These nurses return home, then, with new skills and resources that benefit their own country and its health system (Sheer, 2006). Another strategy to manage outward migration is the regional collaboration of the Pan American Health Organization (PAHO), nursing organizations, businesses, universities, and governmental agencies in the Caribbean to prevent the ad hoc recruitment of nurses in a region where the average nurse vacancy rate is now approximately 40%. These managed migration models call for regulated recruitment, a structured process, incentives to encourage return migration in an agreed-upon time frame, and ongoing dialogue between destination and source countries to ensure a more beneficial process (Salmon & Yan, 2005).

Recruiting nurses from other countries today involves not just seeking out those nurses but the obligation to understand and adequately appreciate the legal and financial implications of migration to the United States and other countries. These nurses must now complete the VisaScreen™ but have the more recent advantage of taking the NCLEX-RN® in international locations, including Hong Kong, London (UK), and Seoul, (Korea). The process is expensive, especially for nurses who come from low-income countries, and can easily exceed US $2500 and take years to complete. In addition, there are the costs for relocation, including international travel, language courses, courses to upgrade nursing knowledge and skills, housing, and insurance. The nurse administrator or the recruiter may decide to assume the responsibility for all or some of these costs. This increases the financial burden of recruitment considerably and may not always be a fiscally responsible decision. Yet, it is the incentive and rewards that play a key role in the decision of nurses to migrate (Kingma, 2008).

Finding solutions to the global nursing shortage requires a multidimensional approach not only to the global need for nurses and skilled health care providers but to solving the problems that have caused the shortage. To that end, nurse leaders can, and should, play a pivotal role in decisive strategy and policy development, and in advocating for the regulation and monitoring of international recruitment. After all, migration is a fundamental right (Xu, Zaikina-Montgomery, & Shen, 2010; Kingma, 2008). By promoting integrated transnational investigations of the causes for the global shortage and facilitating the development of multinational solutions, nurse leaders are at the forefront of addressing a critical issue in global health care.

Bannon, A., & Roodman, D. (2004). Partners for development? *Perspectives in Health, 9*(2), 14–21.

Buchan, J., & Sochalski, J. (2004). The migration of nurses: Trends and policies. *Bulletin of the World Health Organization, 82*(8), 587–594.

Ea, E. (2007). Facilitating Acculturation of foreign-educated nurses. *OJIN: Online Journal of Issues in Nursing, 13*(1). Retrieved November 19, 2010, from http://www.nursingworld.org/mainmenucategories/anamarketplace/ana-periodicals/ojin/tableofcontents/vol132008/no1jan08/articleprevioustopic/foreign educatednurses.aspx

Ea, E., Itzhaki, M., Ehrenfeld, M., & Fitzpatrick, J. (2010). Acculturation among immigrant nurses in Israel and the United States of America. *International Nursing Review, 57*(4).

Kingma, M. (2007). Nurses on the move: A global overview. *HSR: Health Services Research 42*(3), Part II. Retrieved November 19, 2010, from http://www.ncbi.nlm.nih.gov/pmc/articles/PMC1955376/pdf/hesr0042–1281.pdf

Kingma, M. (2008). Nurses on the move: Historical perspective and current issues. *OJIN: Online Journal of Issues in Nursing, 13*(2). Retrieved November 19, 2010, from http://www.medscape.com/viewarticle/577527

ICN-ICNM. (n.d.). *International Center on Nurse Migration.* Retrieved November 18, 2010, from http://www.intlnursemigration.org

ICN. (2001). Position statement: Ethical nurse recruitment. *International Council of Nurses.* Retrieved November 19, 2010, from http://www.icn.ch/images/stories/documents/publications/position_statements/C03_Ethical_Nurse_Recruitment.pdf

ICN. (2004). The global shortage of registered nurses: An overview of issues and action. *International Council of Nurses,* Geneva, Switzerland.

ICN/FNIF. (2006). The Global Nursing Shortage: Priority Areas for Intervention. *International Council of Nursing and Florence Nightingale International Foundation.* Retrieved November 18, 2010, from http://ners.unair.ac.id/materikuliah/report2006.pdf

G

G

IOM. (2010). Highly-skilled migration and the "brain drain" debate. *CARIM—Consortium for Applied Research on International Migration.* Retrieved November 19, 2010, from http://www.carim.org/index.php?callContent=544

Rosenkoetter, M. (2005). White paper on global nursing and health, *American Academy of Nursing, Expert Panel on Global Nursing and Health.* Retrieved August 5, 2007, from http://www.aannet.org/files/public/white_paper.pdf

Salmon, M., & Yan, J. (2005). The Caribbean context: Prelude to regional strategies. Paper presented at the *International Nurse Migration: Bellagio Conference.* Retrieved November 19, 2010, from http://www.authorstream.com/Presentation/Michelangelo-43183-salmon-Caribbean-Context-Prelude-Regional-Strategies-Purpose-region-unit-analysis-Common-as-Education-ppt-powerpoint

Sheer, B. (2006). *Highlights of the 4th ICN International Nurse Practitioner/Advanced Practice Nursing Network conference.* Retrieved August 5, 2007, from http://www.medscape.com/viewarticle/540557

Thobaben, M., Roberts, D., Badir, A., Wang, H., Murayama, H., Murashima, S., et al. (2005). Exploring nursing education in the People's Republic of China, Japan, and Turkey. *Contemporary Nurse, 19*(1–2), 5–16.

UN. (Revised, 2009). *United Nations' World Population Prospects: The 2008 Revision, Highlights.* Retrieved November 19, 2010, from http://esa.un.org/unpp/index.asp?panel=4

WHO/ICN/RCL. (2003). International nurse mobility: Trends and policy implications. *World Health Organization.* Retrieved November 19, 2010, from http://whqlibdoc.who.int/hq/2003/WHO_EIP_OSD_2003.3.pdf

Xu, Y., Zaikina-Montgomery, H., & Shen, J. (2010). Characteristics of internationally educated nurses in the United States: An update from the 2004 national sample survey of registered nurses. *Nursing Economics, 28*(1).

Marlene M. Rosenkoetter
Deena A. Nardi

Hartford Geriatric Nursing Initiative (HGNI)

Since 1996, when the Hartford Foundation, henceforth referred to as the Foundation, established the Hartford Institute of Geriatric Nursing (HGNI) at New York University, the Foundation has supported the development of leaders in gerontological nursing, with the ultimate goal of improving the health care of older Americans. The Foundation has focused on two strategies to prepare nurses to care for our aging society: (1) advancing faculty development through the Predoctoral Scholars and Postdoctoral Fellows Program of Building Academic Geriatric Nursing Capacity (BAGNC, see the separate entry on this program) and the nine Hartford Centers of Geriatric Nursing Excellence (CGNEs) at Schools of Nursing and (2) promoting aging-infused curricular efforts with grants to nursing organizations (the American Academy of Nursing, the American Association of Colleges of Nursing, and the National League for Nursing). The Foundation's aim is to ensure that expert geriatric nursing faculty and curricular champions prepare all nursing students to be competent to care for older adults.

By 2030, 72 million or one in five Americans will be older than 65 years (Administration on Aging, 2010). Nurses are the largest provider of health care services to older adults, yet the number of nurses with expertise in geriatric nursing is inadequate; for example, only 1.7% of the 290,000 advanced practice nurses specialize in aging (J. Stanley, personal communication, October 2010).

Leaders of HGNI programs and the Foundation recognized how, as a field, nursing is not ready to meet the needs of an aging society, the dearth of gerontological nurse leaders, and the magnitude of effort that will be needed for the future. Although HGNI projects tackled these issues individually, when provided a forum for collaboration, program leaders agreed that their collective efforts would be more powerful than what they could accomplish alone. The Hartford Foundation, therefore, supported forums that fostered new partnerships and provided new monies for collaborative projects.

Below are three examples of projects that grew from collaboration among leaders in the HGNI. They illustrate the power of assembling diverse leaders and key stakeholders to collectively advance geriatric nursing.

NURSING HOME COLLABORATIVE

The Nursing Home Collaborative began in 2006 as a plan for action by the CGNEs in Arkansas, California, Iowa, Oregon,

H

and Pennsylvania and their partners—nurses in nursing home settings, industry leaders and operators, regulators, consumers, advocates, and policy makers. Their collective vision was to improve the quality of care provided in nursing homes. Papers summarizing the collaborative's initial work were published in a special issue of *Research in Gerontological Nursing* in July 2008. With support from the Hartford Foundation and The Atlantic Philanthropies and under the direction of Dr. Cornelia Beck, the Collaborative developed into the Center for Nursing Excellence in Long Term Care at Sigma Theta Tau (www.nursingsociety.org/Media/Pages/CenterforNursingExcellence.aspx).

GEROPSYCHIATRIC NURSING INITIATIVE

In 2005, Drs. Cornelia Beck, Kathleen Buckwalter, and Lois Evans, leaders in geropsychiatric nursing, organized the Geropsychiatric Nursing: State of the Future conference. To respond to conference recommendations, the leadership team obtained funding from the Hartford Foundation to "improve the quality of mental health care provided to older adults by enhancing the knowledge and skills of nurses." A grant to the American Academy of Nursing supported three CGNEs in developing core geropsychiatric nursing enhancements for competencies for all levels of nursing education and disseminating geropsychiatric nursing curriculum content (www.aannet.org/i4a/pages/index.cfm?pageid=3833).

ADULT-GERONTOLOGY PRIMARY CARE NURSE PRACTITIONER COMPETENCIES

The Hartford Foundation supported the American Association of Colleges of Nursing and the Hartford Institute of Geriatric Nursing to develop adult-gerontology primary care nurse practitioner competencies in response to the new national model of regulation for advanced practice nurses. Panels of experts—representing stakeholders from the world of nursing licensure, accreditation, certification, and education—developed and validated the 2010 competencies (www.aacn.nche.edu/Education/curriculum/adultgeroprimcareNPcomp.pdf). The new competencies will serve as the foundation for curricular efforts and changes to certification exams. Because of this work, more nurses will be better educated to provide care to older adults.

CONCLUSION

Collaborations of nursing leaders such as these described are both exciting and complicated to bring to fruition. HGNI leaders have taken risks, managed conflict and tension, shared credit, and acted for the long-term good to improve care for elders. Furthermore, they have modeled behavior for nursing leaders to come.

Their philosophy was embraced by BAGNC alums who, in 2009, formed a BAGNC alumni organization—developing goals, objectives, and organizational structure. Under the leadership of Drs. Adriana Perez (Fellow–2009) and Amy Silva-Smith (Fellow–2009), alums worked together across institutional settings to organize symposia for the Gerontological Society of America and regional nursing research organizations and a special issue of *Research in Gerontological Nursing* highlighting 10 years of research by BAGNC alums. Valuing collaboration has been passed down to the next generation.

See also Building Academic Geriatric Nursing Capacity

H

Administration on Aging. (2010). *Aging Statistics.* Retrieved October 25, 2010, from http://www. aoa.gov/AoARoot/Aging_Statistics/index. aspx

Patricia G. Archbold
Rachael Watman

HEALTH CARE REFORM

After failed attempts by many presidents and decades of bitter debate, the nation's first comprehensive health care reform law was enacted in March 2010. The legislation actually has two parts: the Patient Protection and Affordable Care Act was signed into law on March 23 and was amended by the Health Care and Education Reconciliation Act on March 30. The name Affordable Care Act is used by the government to refer to the final, amended version of the law. It does not guarantee health care as a human right, cover undocumented individuals living in the United States, or include a single-payer reimbursement system. While the Affordable Care Act is currently being challenged in state and federal courts, the federal government is proceeding with implementing the timeline as outlined on its Web site: www.healthcare.gov.

The top 10 provisions of the law include the following:

1. People cannot lose their insurance coverage when they get sick; insurance companies are prohibited from dropping coverage.

2. Individuals with preexisting health problems will be able to access insurance. Children with preexisting conditions cannot be denied coverage by insurance companies. Adults with preexisting conditions can enroll in the preexisting insurance plan.

3. Consumers will not be at risk of losing benefits because of costly treatments; lifetime caps on insurance coverage are banned; and annual caps on coverage are restricted.

4. Children up to age 26 years can be covered on their parents' insurance plans.

5. Consumers will not have to share the costs for preventive services. Individuals who join new plans will have greater access to preventive care services such as breast cancer screenings, immunizations, and colonoscopies; co-pays for these services will be eliminated.

6. Women may receive obstetric or gynecological care from any primary care provider and insurance companies will treat their authorizations the same; primary care providers include physicians, nurse practitioners, and certified nurse-midwives.

7. Consumers will have greater access to emergency services; insurers must provide covered emergency services regardless of whether the provider is in network.

8. Patients will have a greater choice of primary care providers, including nurse practitioners and certified nurse midwives. New plans will allow patients the choice of any primary care provider available.

9. Consumers will have stronger rights to appeal insurers' decisions they feel are unfair or discriminatory.

10. Seniors who reach the "donut hole" gap in their Medicare prescription drug coverage benefit will receive a rebate and extended coverage until the "hole" is eliminated in 2014.

Informational Web sites for consumers include www.healthcare.gov and www. healthcareandyou.org.

Halverson, G. (2009). *Health care will not reform itself: A user's guide to refocusing and reforming American health care.* New York, NY: Productivity Press.

Jacobs, L.R., & Skocpol, T. (2010). *Health care reform and American politics: What everyone needs to know.* New York, NY: Oxford University Press.

Staff of the Washington Post. (2010). *Landmark: The inside story of America's new health care law and what it means for us all.* Philadelphia, PA: The Washington Post.

Karen A. Ballard

HEALTH CARE SYSTEMS

In the broadest sense, "health care systems" reflect the totality of the health care industry and delivery system—from the patients who receive care, to the providers who manage the care of patients, to the suppliers of equipment and pharmaceuticals used in caring for patients, to the insurers who pay for care, to the decision makers who set local, state, and national policies that guide the delivery of health care (Finkler, Kovner, & Jones, 2007). When viewed in this macrolevel manner, health care systems encompass the structures and processes for delivery and financing of care as well as the outcomes of care delivery. Important considerations at this macrolevel are the economic, political, social, and regulatory environments. These considerations influence the structural aspects of health care systems financing, and the financing of health care systems (including public and private sources) influences the structures and processes of care delivery and, ultimately, the outcomes of care delivered.

"Health care systems" also can be viewed at a microlevel to reflect a single organizational entity—which may include one or more organizations—that provides an array of health care services (Bazzoli, Shortell, Dubbs, Chan, & Kralovec, 1999; Dubbs, Bazzoli, Shortell, & Kralovec, 2004). Bazzoli and colleagues distinguish health *systems* from health *networks*, primarily on the basis of the issue of ownership: Health care systems have a single owner and represent a tightly connected organizational arrangement, whereas networks have two or more owners and organizations within the network are loosely connected. The authors also use the term "health systems" versus "health care systems," yet "health systems" necessarily implies that care is delivered within the organizational arrangement. The macrolevel health care systems described here influence the microlevel health care systems through policymaking and financing, which in turn influence specific organizational arrangements.

"Health care systems" is also a specific area of study in business, nursing, and health care leadership. For example, in the Wharton School of Business at the University of Pennsylvania (2011), the Department of Health Care Management and Policy offers a course on Comparative Health Care Systems, which prepares master's of business administration students with knowledge of global issues that pertain to health care economics and financing, managing health care organizations and resources, the cost, quality, efficiency, and equity of care delivery, and health policy to enable them to provide leadership in health care systems, in health care–related fields, and in the global health care. The faculty in this department also conduct research that supports this area of study, such as examining health care payment systems, health care management strategies, and health care policymaking in the United States and worldwide (Wharton School of Business at the University of Pennsylvania, 2007).

Schools of nursing also offer graduate programs in "health care systems." The development of these programs reflects a comprehensive view of potential nursing leadership roles that expands beyond the traditional nursing administration programs. For example, since 2004, the University of Rochester School of Nursing (2011) has offered a program of graduate study in "leadership in health care systems" that focuses on preparing graduates for health care organization and management and clinical research coordination and as clinical nurse leaders. The University of North Carolina at Chapel Hill School of Nursing (2011) also offers a health care systems program of graduate study focusing on nursing administration, education, informatics, quality improvement, and the clinical nurse leader role. Other similar programs are offered in schools of nursing across the United States (see, e.g., the Johns Hopkins University School of Nursing [2011], and the Loyola University Chicago Marcella Niehoff School of Nursing [2011], the University of Minnesota School of Nursing [2011]). These programs have the shared characteristics of preparing nursing leaders with advanced knowledge of the structures, processes, and outcomes of health care systems and particularly the environments within which nursing and health care is delivered. Faculty who teach in these programs conduct research to support this area of study, such as examining models of nursing and health care delivery, nursing workforce issues, and the organization and delivery of nursing and health care—all of which affect and are affected by the health care systems described earlier and within which nursing and health care services are provided.

Health care systems have relevance for nursing leaders because they must distinguish between the various usages to appreciate the associated points of reference and the characteristics of each; however, there are more practical reasons for nursing leaders to possess a clear understanding of the differing usages of the term health care systems. Nurses are increasingly called on to fill leadership roles in both micro- and macrolevel health care systems. These nursing leaders must first possess a solid understanding of the intricate relationships among key participants at the macrolevel of health care systems. Understanding these relationships provides a context for positioning nursing and nursing leadership roles and opportunities within health care systems around the world.

Second, nursing leaders must understand health care systems at the microlevel to appreciate important characteristics of the system, such as its structure, processes, and outcomes as well as its culture, resilience, and weaknesses or vulnerabilities in the health care system (Carthey, de Leval, & Reason, 2001). This level of understanding also allows nursing leaders to promote learning within health care systems (Reason, Carthey, & de Leval, 2001). Third, an understanding of the health care system at both the macro- and microlevels is necessary to understand how the systems and individuals within them behave. For example, microlevel health care systems may take certain actions that influence the practices of individuals within them because of health care systems decision making at the macrolevel (Finkler et al., 2007).

Finally, given that health care systems is fast becoming recognized as an area of study within nursing, business, and health care, nursing leaders must understand this area of study to successfully deploy and manage nurses and other health professionals who possess this level and type of training. Today's nursing leaders are challenged to think broadly about health care systems locally and globally, and the provision of high-quality, safe, and fiscally

H

H

sound nursing and health care to the diverse populations served within them. This more comprehensive educational view encompasses critical economic, political, regulatory, social, and management aspects of health care systems and holds great promise for preparing nursing leaders with the knowledge, skills, and abilities to bring change, innovation, and transformation to health care systems and care environments worldwide and to be leaders in providing better care for patients in the future.

Bazzoli, G. J., Shortell, S. M., Dubbs, N., Chan, C., & Kralovec, P. (1999). A taxonomy of health networks and systems: Bringing order out of chaos. *Health Services Research*, *33*(6), 1683–1717.

Carthey, J., de Leval, M. R., & Reason, J. T. (2001). Institutional resilience in health care systems. *Quality and Safety in Health Care*, *10*(1), 29–32.

Dubbs, N. L., Bazzoli, G. J., Shortell, S. M., & Kralovec, P. D. (2004). Reexamining organizational configurations: An update, validation, and expansion of the taxonomy of health networks and systems. *Health Services Research*, *39*(1), 207–220.

Finkler, S. A., Kovner, C. T., & Jones, C. B. (2007). *Financial management for nurse managers and executives*. St. Louis, MO: W. B. Saunders.

Johns Hopkins University School of Nursing. (2011). *Health systems management*. Retrieved May 11, 2011, from http://www.son.jhmi.edu/academics/academic_programs/masters/healthsystems

Loyola University Chicago Marcella Niehoff School of Nursing. (2011). *Health systems management advanced practice nursing*. Retrieved May 11, 2011, from http://www.luc.edu/nursing/graduate_hsm.shtml

Reason, J. T., Carthey, J., & de Leval, M. R. (2001). Diagnosing "vulnerable system syndrome": An essential prerequisite to effective risk management. *Quality in Health Care*, *10*(4, Suppl. II), 21–25.

University of Minnesota School of Nursing. (2005). *Health innovation and leadership*. Retrieved May 11, 2011, from http://www.nursing.umn.edu/DNP/Specialties/HealthInnovationandLeadership/home.html

University of North Carolina at Chapel Hill School of Nursing. (2011). *MSN: Health care systems*. Retrieved May 11, 2011, from http://nursing.unc.edu/degree/msn/hcs.html

University of Rochester School of Nursing. (2011). *Leadership programs*. Retrieved May 13, 2011, from http://www.son.rochester.edu/programs/leadership/index.html

Wharton School of Business at the University of Pennsylvania. (2007). *Health care management*. Retrieved May 11, 2011, from http://www.wharton.upenn.edu/mbaresource/curriculum/hcmg

Cheryl Bland Jones

HEALTH INFORMATION MANAGEMENT SYSTEMS SOCIETY

The Health Information Management Systems Society (HIMSS) was created in 1961 under the name of the Hospital Management Systems Society. It was a professional organization that supported management engineers who worked in hospital settings doing optimization, workflow, and time–motion studies before the introduction of electronic health record technologies and the automation of the clinical work environment. This emphasis on the hospital work environment by management engineers is reflected in their seeking and attaining professional affiliation with the American Hospital Association as a personal member group in 1966. In those early decades, membership grew from 50 to 2,000 members, representing practicing hospital management engineers, hospital administrators, consultants, and academicians.

With the introduction of patient information systems, medical devices, and monitoring systems in the late 1980s, the

"Society," as the Hospital Management Systems Society referred to itself, morphed to include "information" in its name and extended its membership to information technology professionals, clinical informaticists, and health care administrators. The Health Information Management Services Society has been known as HIMSS since that transition. In the 1990s, the annual HIMSS' meeting grew to be the major source for bringing together the health care suppliers of software, devices, and hardware systems for health care systems in the United States. The educational side of the annual meeting featured presentations from organizations in different stages of using information technology (IT), specific systems in given settings beyond just acute care wards, implementation methodologies, and approaches for capturing return on investment. Nurses were members of HIMSS in the 1990s but served in generalists' positions within their organizations' IT departments or vendor employers.

In the late 1990s and into the early 2000s, two drivers again transformed HIMSS into a mega-professional technology organization with global extensions. These two drivers were massive technology innovation around the Internet and communication technologies and a global push for the use of electronic health records in health care. By 2004, under President's Bush's push for all Americans to have an electronic health record that would go from birth to the grave, there was explosive growth in the health care information technology industry. HIMSS invested in nursing leadership within its professional salaried staff with the purpose of creating an active nursing community.

HIMSS describes itself as "a cause-based, not-for-profit organization exclusively focused on providing global leadership for the optimal use of information technology (IT) and management

systems for the betterment of healthcare" and cites as its mission "transforming healthcare through the effective use of information technology and management systems"(HIMSS, 2010). Today, HIMSS has expanded its operations to include Europe and Southeast Asia, with offices in Chicago, Washington, DC, Brussels, Singapore, and Leipzig. In 2010, HIMSS cites having more than 30,000 individual members, of which two thirds work in health care providers and governmental and not-for-profit organizations. HIMSS also has organizational memberships and claim having more than 470 corporate members and more than 85 not-for-profit organizations that share as of late 2010.

As of 2010, nurse membership was approximately 2,500, and the sense of community is fostered by two committee structures—the Nursing Informatics Committee and the Nursing Informatics Task Force. These entities, along with the HIMSS support staff, organize numerous educational events throughout the year. These continuing education events are dedicated to the needs of applied nursing informaticists that hold positions within health care organizations, vendor companies, consulting groups, and academia. HIMSS's creation of a vice president level position for a nurse leader on its staff at the beginning of the decade provided the needed leadership to develop, foster, and grow the nursing informaticist community within HIMSS. Importantly, under this nursing staff leadership, HIMSS in collaboration with nursing informatics leaders and the American Medical Informatics Association formed the Alliance for Nursing Informatics, an organization of 27 distinct nursing informatics organizations to provide a single voice for nursing into public policy.

Over the past decade, HIMSS has developed its staff and focus to allow it

H

to take an active role in framing and leading health care practices and public policy. They have inserted themselves into the public policy stage through their content expertise, professional development, and research initiatives.

See also Electronic Health Record

HIMSS. (2010). Retrieved November 22, 2010, from http://www.himss.org/ASP/about HimssHome.asp

Charlotte Weaver

HEALTH POLICY

Florence Nightingale spent much of her career in the halls of the British Parliament promoting policy change to improve quality, dignity, and equity, first for the Crimean War soldiers and later for the poor of London. Her 3 years of clinical practice gave her clinical expertise and credibility to assume the role of policy maker. She embraced that role because of her high degree of internal distress and concern about needless suffering and premature death of her patients. Empowered by her clinical practice, she used data she collected systematically to persuade Parliament to make the needed military and civic law reforms that promoted health. In 1858, Nightingale became the first woman elected as a member of the Royal Statistical Society (Gill & Gill, 2005). Her work and prestige were Victorian-era validations of the core role that nursing has in the policy sphere and the importance of using evidence to inform policy. Nightingale's activism presaged the modern nursing role as patient advocate and policy shaper.

Policy involves decisions that influence the life of citizens on a daily basis.

Longest (2006) defined health policy as the authorative decisions pertaining to health or health care, made in the legislative, executive, or judicial branches of government that are intended to direct or influence the actions, behaviors, or decisions of citizens. Although there are many definitions of "policy" and "politics," according to Longest, policy generally refers to "decisions resulting in a law or regulation"; however, increasingly the actions of some private groups, such as large health plans and private accrediting organization, also have an important impact on health care delivery (p. 7).

It is the responsibility of a multitude of policymakers, whether mayors, county supervisors, government employees, legislators, governors, and presidents, to make health policy. Overall responsibility generally places authority with the legislative branch to craft laws, the executive branch crafts rules to implement the laws, and the judicial branch interprets conflicts between the states, the spheres of government, the citizens, or the private entities. The U.S. government plays a substantial role in setting health policy, although to a far lesser degree than nations with centralized, government-run health care systems. American health care is largely under private sector control, making U.S. health policy development incremental, fragmented, and decentralized.

Longest (2006) has conceptualized policymaking as an interdependent process, with an agenda-setting phase, a policy formulation phase, an implementation phase, and a modification phase. This has immense utility for nursing because it amplifies the incremental and cyclical nature of policymaking, two of the most important features of the U.S. health policy making process. Essentially, all health policy decisions are subject to modification because policymaking in the United States involves making decisions that are revisited when circumstances shift. Our system is not designed for big, bold reform. Rather, it considers intended or unintended consequences of existing policy and tweaks changes (Longest, 2006).

POLITICS

Politics refers to power relationships and introduces nonrational, divisive, and self-interested approaches to policymaking, often along ideological lines. Any political maneuvering to enhance one's power or status within a group may be described as "politics." Politics is largely associated with a struggle for ascendancy among groups having different priorities and power relationships. Preferences and interests of stakeholders and political bargaining (favor swapping) are extremely influential political factors that overlie the policymaking process. Ideally, the self-interest paradigm does not apply to elected officials who seek office to serve the public interest, not their own. However, to be successful in the electoral process, they need financial contributions, rendering them beholden to fundraising (Feldstein, 2006). Highly politicized decisions may often create outcomes that have little to do with efficient use of scarce resources and what is best for the general public. These forces, which may not be based on evidence, contribute to the lack of coordination among health policies in the United States, making policy formulation highly complex.

FEDERALISM VERSUS STATE'S RIGHTS

To effectively influence policy, nurse leaders must be aware of the broader societal issues that influence health policy decisions, including the tensions between the states and the federal government. The locus of responsibility between the states and the federal government is shared in programs such as Medicaid, S-CHIP, and the creation of an interoperable health information technology system. Federalism is the allocation of "governing" responsibility between the states and the federal government. The states and the federal government have a complex relationship regarding health policy, which explains a large part of our chaotic and fragmented approach to health care in place today.

Nurse leaders must deepen their commitment to and become masterful at critiquing, formulating and influencing policies that interfere with human wholeness and health. All nurse leaders in practice today have experienced the effects of ill-conceived polices that lead to poor health and care delivery. Policy competency has been historically core to nursing beginning with the work of Florence Nightingale during the Crimean War. She fought for equity, dignity, and equality, advocating for the needs of the soldiers and later for the needs of the poor (Gill & Gill, 2005).

Although the policymaking process is a continuous, interrelated cycle, most efforts to change policy stem from the negative effects of an existing policy. The modification phase creates a feedback loop to the agenda-setting process. This concept of continuous, often modest modification of existing polices is known as *incrementalism*. Minor changes of existing policies play out slowly over time and are more predictable; therefore, incrementalism promotes stability and stakeholder compromise.

POLITICAL COMPETENCE

Powerful nursing clinical experiences, when effectively communicated by nurse leaders, serve to deepen policymakers'

H

understanding of the issues. Nurse leader's professional experiences provide poignant stories that bring the evidence base alive, clarify policy issues by providing a human context, and bring nursing's value to the health policy arena (O'Grady & Johnson, 2008). This experience, coupled with the ability to analyze the policy process, provides a strong foundation to propel nurse leaders into politically competent action. At every stage of the policymaking process, nurse leaders have the capacity to shape health policy.

Another essential responsibility for nurse leaders is to inform and contribute to the public discourse on important health policy issues because nurse's interests and public interests are not at odds. Gaining public support and influencing public opinion can help get the attention of policymakers or propel issues onto the policy agenda. Submitting opinion editorials to major news outlets is one powerful way to do this. This requires writing that links the issues to the community, uses poignant stories to bring the problem to life, and incorporates evidence to build a strong case as to why a policy change is needed. Nurse leaders must use their professional credentials and expertise with this sense of responsibility toward educating the public and not be hesitant to be active advocates based on their knowledge and experience.

Feldstein, P. (2006). *The politics of health legislation: An economic perspective* (3rd ed.). Chicago, IL: Health Administration Press.

Gill, C., & Gill, G. (2005). Nightingale in Scutari: Her legend re-examined. *Clinical Infectious Diseases, 40,* 1799–1805.

Longest, B. (2006). *Health policymaking in the United States* (4th ed.). Washington, DC: Health Administration Press.

O'Grady, E. T., & Johnson, J. (2008). Health policy issues in changing environments. In A. Hamric, J. Spross, & C. Hanson (Eds.), *Advanced practice nursing: An integrative approach* (4th ed.). St. Louis, MO: Elsevier-Saunders.

Eileen T. O'Grady

HEALTH RESOURCES AND SERVICES ADMINISTRATION

The Health Resources and Services Administration (HRSA) was created in 1982 when two parent agencies, the Health Resources Administration and the Health Services Administration, combined. The HRSA is an agency within the U.S. Department of Health and Human Services and is the principal federal division aimed at improving health care access to vulnerable and special needs populations (HRSA, 2010a). Six bureaus and 13 offices are coordinated through HRSA, thereby offering specialized grants to medical and nursing professionals across the United States and to U.S. territories. Examples include the HIV/AIDS Bureau, which houses the Ryan White HIV/AIDS Program that gives core medical treatment and support programs to roughly 530,000 low-income Americans (HRSA, 2010b). The Bureau of Primary Health Care financially supports 7,900 health clinics that provide health care services to 19 million low-income and uninsured Americans (HRSA, 2010c).

Known as the nation's access division, HRSA has seven broad goals that underscore their focus on the underserved and medically vulnerable: (a) to offer better medical care access, (b) to improve health related outcomes, (c) to enhance the quality of medical care, (d) to eradicate health related inequalities, (e) to enhance community health, (f) to increase the response to health-related emergencies, and (g) to attain superior management styles (HRSA, 2010a).

The HRSA grant availability is announced two ways: (a) HRSA Preview through the HRSA Web site and (b) the Grants.gov Web site. Through these online resources, the program title and number, related governing agency, purpose, top funding priorities, review criteria, available monies, application deadline, and project timeline are published for each funding option (HRSA, 2010d). As of 2010, the required grant submission procedure for this agency is through the Grants.gov online system.

Health Resources and Services Administration. (2010a). *About HRSA*. Retrieved September 6, 2010, from http://www.hrsa.gov/about/index.html

Health Resources and Services Administration. (20010b). *HIV/AIDS bureau*. Retrieved September 6, 2010, from http://www.hrsa.gov/about/organization/bureaus/hab/index.html

Health Resources and Services Administration (2010c). *Primary health care*. Retrieved September 6, 2010, from http://www.hrsa.gov/about/organization/bureaus/bphc/bphc.pdf

Health Resources and Services Administration. (2010d). *Apply for a grant*. Retrieved September 6, 2010, from http://www.hrsa.gov/grants/apply/index.html

Ronda Mintz-Binder

HORIZONTAL VIOLENCE

Horizontal violence, also known as horizontal hostility, lateral violence, or bullying, can be described as interpersonal conflict that is perpetrated by one nurse toward another nurse. Horizontal violence comprises a range of covert and overt harassment behaviors such as raised eyebrows, sarcastic comments, withholding important information (sabotage), verbal or emotional abuse, intimidation, humiliation, unjust or excessive criticism, denial of access to opportunity, and being given too much responsibility without sufficient support (Farrell, 1997; Lewis, 2006; McKenna, Smith, Poole, & Coverdale, 2003).

The existence of horizontal violence in nursing is often explained through the lens of oppression theory. Oppression theory argues that because "nurses are dominated (and by implication oppressed) by a patriarchal system headed by doctors, male administrators, and marginalized nurse leaders, nurses lower down the hierarchy of power resort to aggression amongst themselves" (Farrell, 1997, p. 502). The expression that nurses "eat their young" is consistent with the phenomenon of horizontal violence.

Horizontal violence has significant negative effects on nurses, patients, and the health care organization. The psychological and physical sequelae of horizontal violence on the individual nurse includes anxiety, increased stress, diminished confidence, depression, and decreased job satisfaction. Newly registered nurses may be the most vulnerable to the effects of horizontal violence. Adjusting to the demands of the professional role is stressful and the new graduate's relative lack of knowledge, experience, and confidence leaves their work open to scrutiny (Griffin, 2004; McKenna et al., 2003).

The effect of horizontal violence on the health care organization and the patients it serves can be devastating and costly. Horizontal violence negatively effects staff morale and productivity, recruitment and retention, sick time, and quality patient care (Griffin, 2004; McKenna et al., 2003). The Joint Commission (2008) identified unresolved conflict and disruptive behavior as a significant issue that hinders the

H

organization's ability to achieve and maintain an environment of patient safety and quality.

Nursing leaders can take steps to change organizational structures and processes that inadvertently reinforce a culture of horizontal violence and allow it to persist (Jackson, Clare, & Mannix, 2002). In some cases, horizontal violence is so embedded in the organizational culture that people do not recognize it. However unintentional, health care organizations that ignore horizontal violence or deny its existence indirectly reinforce and perpetuate the culture. One of the first steps to changing the culture is to raise consciousness through educational programs to increase awareness of horizontal violence and its devastating effects and strategies for reporting and effectively responding to it. The literature calls for the development of primary prevention programs that empower nurses to cope with interpersonal conflict (McKenna et al., 2003).

Griffin (2004) found that newly licensed registered nurses who were taught about lateral (horizontal) violence and practiced cognitive rehearsal to confront the behavior were able to effectively cope with and confront the lateral violence offender. Griffin further reported that among the perpetrators who were confronted, horizontally violent behaviors ceased.

Clearly, nursing must work to eliminate horizontal violence. Porter O'Grady and Malloch (2011, p. 377) recommend 10 principles leaders should implement to minimize toxic behaviors in their organization:

1. Know thyself
2. Walk the talk
3. Be willing to listen
4. Value the truth of the whole
5. Empower employees
6. Build relationships on respect
7. Act as an agent of transformation
8. Screen job candidates for dysfunction
9. Expect accountability
10. Reward value-adding behaviors

Nursing leaders play a key role in establishing a healthy workplace climate and are uniquely positioned to transform the culture to one where professional and civil behavior is the norm, members are supported, and new members are nurtured. Simply put, nurse leaders have a responsibility to "return humanity to the workplace" (Porter O'Grady & Malloch, 2011, p. 387).

Farrell, G. A. (1997). Aggression in clinical settings: Nurses' views. *Journal of Advanced Nursing, 25,* 501–508.

Griffin, M. (2004). Teaching cognitive rehearsal as a shield for lateral violence: An intervention for newly registered nurses. *Journal of Continuing Education in Nursing, 35*(6), 257–263.

Jackson, D., Clare, J., & Mannix, J. (2002). Who would want to be a nurse? Violence in the workplace—A factor in recruitment and retention. *Journal of Nursing Management, 10,* 13–20.

Lewis, M. A. (2006). Nurse bullying: Organizational considerations in the maintenance and perpetration of health care bullying cultures. *Journal of Nursing Management, 14,* 52–58.

McKenna, B.G., Smith, N.A., Poole, S. J., & Coverdale, J.H. (2003). Horizontal violence: Experiences of registered nurses in their first year of practice. *Journal of Advanced Nursing, 42*(1), 90–96.

Porter O'Grady, T., & Malloch, K. (2011). *Quantum leadership: Advancing information, transforming healthcare* (3rd ed.). Sudbury, MA: Jones and Bartlett.

The Joint Commission. (2008, July 2). *Behaviors that undermine a culture of safety.* Retrieved 2010 from http://www.jointcommission.org/SentinelEvents

Darlene Del Prato

HUMAN DIGNITY AND ETHICAL DECISION MAKING IN NURSING

Ethical dilemmas in health care today present new and complex issues for the profession of nursing. Since the early Christian era, nursing has a long and illustrious history in responding to the forces of cultures and societies that threaten the dignity of the human person be it related to illness, health care inequities, discrimination, privileged allocation of resources, limited access to health services, or the application of unjust social policies. Defending and protecting the dignity, freedom, and autonomy of the human person is nursing's intrinsic, indelible, and irrefutable commitment to caring for persons living in a world order where the intrinsic dignity of all persons may be at risk.

THE DOCTRINE OF HUMAN DIGNITY

Through the doctrine of intrinsic human dignity, the central moral principle in health care, we can come to a fuller understanding of the ethical issues in the multiple domains of nursing and how our response to them protects and affirms the dignity and freedom of the human person.

Kant, a German philosopher, has been credited with providing our current understanding of human dignity. In his *Metaphysics of Morals,* Kant (Gregor, 1996) states,

A human being is regarded as a person, that is, as the subject of a morally practical reason, and is exalted above any price; for as a person he is not to be valued merely as a means to the ends of others or even to his own ends, but as an end in himself, that is, he possesses a dignity (an absolute inner worth) by which he exacts respect

for himself from all other rational beings in the world. (p. 186)

This absolute inner worth is intrinsic dignity; that exalted level of value that is present in every person who has even been born simply because the person is human. No authority of any kind, of any nation, of any laws, or organization, or any illness, or station in life can ever obliterate intrinsic dignity from the character of the human person.

A MODEL FOR MAKING ETHICAL DECISIONS IN NURSING

Philosophical and theological frameworks, models for ethical decision making, and professional codes of ethics are well established in the professional literature and are readily applied in nursing practice. Although the nursing profession does not advocate for one distinctive framework, the American Nurses Association's Code of Ethics (2001) is the most frequently cited. Its very first article states,

The nurse, in all professional relationships, practices with compassion and respect for the inherent dignity, worth and uniqueness of every individual, unrestricted by considerations of social or economic status, personal attributes, or the nature of health problems. (p. 7)

Complimenting an ethical framework and its methodological application in nursing is the nursing process, which provides a systematic method for identifying health care and nursing needs of patients bringing some resolution to them. The examination of actual and potential ethical issues in health care and nursing that affect the patient, family, community, organization, or society benefits from the same rigorous investigation and analysis found in the nursing process. Commitment to evidence-based practice and to caring for the whole

H

person (and not the disease alone) requires that the identification and analysis of ethical issues in patient care be systematically integrated into every step of the nursing process.

The following protocol, designed by the ethicists at the Center for Clinical Bioethics at Georgetown University (1991), focuses on the protection and affirmation of the dignity of the patient and the clinician as ethical issues in health care are examined and resolved. The steps of the protocol, applicable as well to the analysis and resolution of organizational ethical issues, are briefly outlined below:

1. *What are the facts with this patient?* Diagnosis, prognosis, therapeutic options, chronology of the occurrence of clinical events, biography of the patient (age, gender, family, ethnicity, culture, career, etc.), decisional capacity and informed consent, who is the decision maker (i.e., the patient or the health care proxy), current clinical setting, time constraints (health status; identification of decision makers), and existence of a some form of advance directive and a health care proxy who is readily available, competent, and understands the responsibilities of the role.

2. *What are the issues with this patient?* Are the issues ethical in nature? Are there problems in communication or differences in clinical opinions and treatment protocols? Are there resource allocation issues that may interfere with treatment and care, that is, absence of health insurance? Are there limitations on third-party reimbursements? Are there conflicts among the moral values and ethical principles of the patient, the family, the nurse, the attending physician, and the health care facility?

3. *What is the good to be achieved for this patient?* (a) The patient's biomedical good—the technically good act according to standards of medical and nursing practices

identified by clinicians and decided by patient or health care surrogate; (b) the patient's perception and informed understanding of his or her own good at the time and in the particular circumstances of the clinical issues and impending decisions; (c) the good of the patient as a human person capable of reasoned choices (freedom, dignity, autonomy, and self-determination); (d) the patient's ultimate good (human flourishing, value and meaning of life, suffering, God, family, and society).

4. *What are the goods and interests of other parties?* (a) Family, (b) community, (c) society, (d) the law, (e) policies of health care institutions/clinical settings, and (f) members of the health care team.

5. *How do the issues stand vis-à-vis the issues in comparable cases?* (a) Is this case analogous to others? (b) Has some moral consensus been achieved in the analogous cases? (c) Are there ethical and legal precedents? (d) How well does this particular case fit paradigmatic cases in terms of the facts, the issues, and the framing of the issues?

6. *The prudential question—what to decide?* In synthesizing the data from these questions and moving toward a proposed intervention two critical questions emerge: (a) What can be done for this patient? (b) What should be done for this patient?

7. Health science, clinical research, innovative technology, and evidence-based clinical practice continue to evolve at a phenomenal pace. Today, the lives of persons with chronic illnesses can be extended and the quality of life enhanced. Certain forms of cancer once considered fatal now successfully respond to treatment. Treatment of neurological diseases, once causing permanent disability, has given new life to millions. With advanced technology, much *can be done* to treat specific illness. The question that is paramount in analyzing the needs and resolving ethical dilemmas of the whole person is what *should*

be done for this patient—what is both the technically good and morally right action for *this patient.* The answer to this question requires a careful review of all of the data accumulated in the course of the clinical analysis. Critical to this analysis is the centrality of the dignity, freedom and autonomy of the human person, and the good that he or she identifies as important as a person with intrinsic dignity and worth.

8. *Evaluation*: Once decisions are made and treatments implemented, an assessment of the integrity of the process should be carefully reviewed throughout the clinical experience. This evaluation is a continuous process that requires reconsideration of decisions and interventions as the patient progresses toward healing or toward death.

CHALLENGES IN MAKING ETHICAL DECISIONS IN NURSING

As administrators, clinicians, researchers, and educators, nurses are in a strategic position to protect and defend the dignity and the freedom of the patient and health care proxy who often must make difficult treatment decisions. To be unwilling to enter into the experience of the suffering and healing of the patient moves the nurse to the position of a technician and abandons the person as patient at a time when he or she is most vulnerable and in need of support. With an increase in the vulnerability of the patient, the dignity of the person is once again at great risk.

There are times, however, when the choices of the patient, family, nurse, physician, health care organization, or managed care group are in conflict. Clinical ethics consultations that are grounded in protecting and defending human dignity can often resolve conflicts in a satisfactory manner.

Today, we are confronted with threats to human dignity through euthanasia; physician-assisted suicide; malnutrition and assisted nutrition and hydration; persistent vegetative states and post-coma unresponsiveness in the terminally ill; the mentally and physically challenged; those stigmatized by cancer, AIDS, and substance use; those who have had abortions, women, children and the elderly, persons of color, the homeless, minorities, single parents; those who have limited or no access to health services; legislation that is unresponsive to human need; a national health care system that is driven by the commodification of the human person; and a growing culture where moral relativism is the ethical paradigm of choice.

Regardless of the reason for the illness or the person's decisional capacity, a living person is never less than fully human. The application of the doctrine of human dignity requires nurses and all others caring for the sick and who participate in ethical decisions to continually reexamine the direction of their moral compass and focus on the question "What should be done for this patient?" How this challenge is embraced and applied in light of caring for persons diminished in any way by reason of illness will speak loudly about the clinician's self-understanding of intrinsic human dignity and faithfulness to nursing's intrinsic, indelible, and irrefutable commitment in protecting and affirming human dignity of every person who has ever been born.

American Nurses Association. (2001). *Code of ethics for nurses with interpretative statements.* Washington, DC: Author

Center for Clinical Bioethics. (1991). *The ethics workup.* Washington, DC: Center for Clinical Bioethics, Georgetown University Medical Center

Gregor, M. (Ed.). (1996). *Immanuel Kant: The metaphysics of morals.* New York, NY: Cambridge University Press.

Ignatius Perkins

H

HUMAN RESOURCE MANAGEMENT

One of the most important roles of the nurse leader is that of a human resource manager. Understanding key concepts of recruitment, selection, credentialing, assignment, retention, developing, promoting, and terminating are core competencies of the nurse leader. Challenges to human resource management in the 21st century include managing a culturally diverse workforce, shifting demographics, and focusing on personnel productivity. The way an organization manages and develops its human resources is increasingly recognized as centrally important to the execution of its strategy (Hambrick, Frederickson, Korn, & Ferry, 1989; Roussel, Swansburg, & Swansburg, 2006). In addition to strategic implications, Lado and Wilson (1994) concluded that human resource strategies may be an especially important source of sustained competitive advantage.

NURSE RECRUITMENT

A formal nurse recruitment plan should be developed and reviewed at least annually by the nurse leader. According to Pattan (1992), the following elements should be included in a nurse recruitment plan:

1. A supply and demand analysis.
2. Clear objectives for the plan.
3. Strategies to accomplish the objectives.
4. An annual recruitment budget.
5. Operational plans to implement strategies.
6. A feedback process to take corrective action.

In addition to a solid recruitment plan, the nurse leader should implement marketing strategies to increase the pool of qualified nursing applicants. Typically, marketing to nurses is focused on many things, such as job profile, organizational culture, working locations and conditions, the reputation of the institution, and compensation (Pattan, 1991). One of the best methods for recruiting is the use of existing employees. Word-of-mouth recruiting supplemented with incentive programs for employee referrals is a cost-effective and highly successful means of recruiting staff.

CANDIDATE SELECTION

The typical selection process includes the interview, an offer by the employer, the acceptance by the employee, and, in some cases, the execution of an employment contract. Before scheduling the interview, the nurse leader should review an applicant's resume and application. On verifying that the applicant meets the minimum requirements of the role, such as licensure and certification, careful attention should be given to the applicant's employment history. Be aware of gaps in employment and be sure to question about gaps during the interview process. After carefully reviewing the application, the nurse leader should begin preparing for the interview. Hiring managers should elicit the input of those with whom the candidate will be working on a daily basis, including support staff and physicians. Many organizations have implemented structured peer interview processes and include the peer interview as a key component of employee selection. Before implementing this process, the nurse leader should work with human resource professionals to provide adequate training to staff on the appropriate methods for conducting interviews. It is critically important that frontline staff who participate in peer interviews understand the laws related to interviews and especially what is appropriate to ask a candidate.

Following the interview, the nurse leader should prepare a formal offer for the prospective employee. In some organizations, the offer is managed by the human resources representative. Either way, it is always a good practice to consult with human resource professionals before making final offers of employment. The formal offer is best provided face to face or over the phone and then immediately followed up in writing. At minimum, the offer should include the job title, the shift the employee will be working, the details about compensation and benefits, any preemployment requirements such as employee health screening, and a start date. It is good management practice to ask the applicant to acknowledge and accept the offer by signing a copy of the offer letter and returning it to the hiring nurse leader. A copy of the signed offer letter should be placed in the employee's permanent human resource file. Finally, as hospitals have increased the number of new graduate training programs, it is becoming more common to have new graduate nurses execute employment contracts. Typical contracts include a sliding scale repayment program in the event the new graduate leaves the organization before the end of an agreed-on time frame, generally 1 to 2 years, for example, in the case where the nurse completes an internship program.

EMPLOYEE RETENTION

The retention of competent nurses is a major problem of the health care system in the United States. A study by Spitzer-Lehmann (1990) indicated that nurses stayed in their jobs when they received peer support, participated in professional practice activities, received tuition reimbursement, and had input into decision

making; when communication was open; and when medical staff was supportive. In 1983, an American Academy of Nursing study described both nurse administrators and staff nurses as agreeing on which factors attracted nurses to become and remain employees of the hospital. These hospitals were labeled Magnet hospitals (American Academy of Nursing Task Force on Nursing Practice in Hospitals, 1983). Today, Magnet hospitals are national leaders not only in nurse retention but also in nurse sensitive patient outcomes. Jones-Schenk (2001) and Kramer and Schmalenberg (2002) cited the essentials factors of Magnet organizations, known as the 14 forces of magnetism:

1. Quality of nursing leadership
2. Organizational structure
3. Management style
4. Personnel policies and programs
5. Quality of care
6. Professional models of care
7. Level of autonomy
8. Quality assurance
9. Consultation and resources
10. Community and the hospital
11. Nurses as teachers
12. Image of nursing
13. Nurse–physician relationships
14. Professional career development

These variables should be considered in any well-developed retention program. It is important to remember that retention begins with the initial contact with the organization and is rooted in a solid orientation program.

DEVELOPING AND PROMOTING EMPLOYEES

Professional career development and coaching are integral parts of the nurse

H

leader's role. The first step in developing and promoting is assisting the nurse in assessing his or her interests, skills, and values. Next, the nurse compares the results of this assessment with open and available positions. Although it is always preferable to keep great employees in one's own organization, appropriate opportunities may only be available outside the organization and the nurse leader should support nurses who wish to advance in this manner.

In addition to a traditional promotion, many organizations have reinstituted clinical ladder programs. A clinical ladder is a horizontal development system based on specific criteria used to develop, evaluate, and promote nurses who are in direct care providing roles. Furthermore, clinical ladder programs in larger organizations are tending toward specialized tracks for clinical practice, education, administration, and research. The clinical ladder framework provides a solid model for the development and promotion of staff. The model can be adapted to other types of development, such as management promotions. The most important factor in establishing a solid promotion and development program is proactive succession planning. Succession planning is a formal process where senior leaders look at current and potential vacancies and assess the internal talent pool for potential development and/ or promotion opportunities.

TERMINATING EMPLOYEES

Firing an employee is an unpleasant but sometimes necessary part of the nurse leader's job. Before considering termination, frontline managers should consult with superiors and human resource professionals to ensure all policies and procedures have been consistently followed. Clear documentation should exist

demonstrating that a progressive discipline process, moving from coaching, to written, to suspension or final written warning has taken place. In rare instances, an employee's conduct may be so egregious that progressive discipline may not be appropriate and termination is the first and only step in the disciplinary process.

Planning is key to a successful termination session. The nurse leader should plan well ahead of the session and take the following steps:

1. Discuss the termination with human resources, superiors, and union representatives if applicable.

2. Plan the session at a time when a witness is available. Never terminate an employee without a witness. The witness should be a human resources representative or another manager in the organization. This person should cosign the termination document to indicate his or her presence in the meeting.

3. Prepare detailed documentation in accordance with your organization's policies.

4. Be open, honest, and direct in your communication with the employee. If you are nervous about the meeting, practice with another manager before the session.

5. Be prepared for any reaction (Dumville [1993] identified four stages of employee reaction to termination: shock with physical symptoms, rejection, emotion, and withdrawal).

6. Provide the employee with a signed copy of the termination documentation and your organization's grievance policy.

In the United States, employees are protected by a variety of federal policies such as the National Labor Relations Act, the Civil Rights Act of 1964, the Age Discrimination in Employment Act, the Vocational Rehabilitation Act, the

Occupational Safety and Health Act, and laws that protect whistle-blowers.

SUMMARY

Managing human resources is a key core competency for the nurse leader and can be one of the most rewarding aspects of the role. Not only is the function important in creating a positive culture for employees, recent studies show a link between the management of human resources and patient mortality in acute care hospitals. A study by West et al. (2002) demonstrated this link. Specifically, their work noted that the sophistication and extensiveness of appraisal and training for hospital employees and the percentage of employees working in teams in the hospital were all significantly associated with measures of patient mortality.

See also Clinical Ladder; Conflict Management; Credentialing; Cultural Competence; Cultural Diversity; Magnet Hospitals; Orientation and Staff Development

American Academy of Nursing Task Force on Nursing Practice in Hospitals. (1983). *Magnet hospitals: Attraction and retention of professional nurses*. Kansas City, MO: American Nurses Association.

Dumville, J. C. (1993). Delivering the mortal blow. *Supervision, 54*(4), 6–7.

Hambrick, D. C., Frederickson, L. B., Korn, B., & Ferry, R. M. (1989). Preparing today's leaders for tomorrow's realities. *Personnel, 8*, 23–26.

Jones-Schenk, J. (2001). How magnets attract nurses. *Nursing Management, 33*(1), 41–44.

Kramer, M., & Schmalenberg, C. (2002). Essentials of magnetism. In M. McClure & A. Hinshaw (Eds.), *Magnet hospitals revisited: Attraction and retention of professional nurses*. Kansas City, MO: American Nurses Publishing.

Lado, A., & Wilson, M. (1994). Human resource systems and sustained competitive advantage: A competency-based perspective. *Academy of Management Review, 19*, 699–727.

Pattan, J. E. (1991). Nurse recruitment: From selling to marketing. *Journal of Nursing Administration, 21*(9), 16–20.

Pattan, J. E. (1992). Developing a nurse recruitment plan. *Journal of Nursing Administration, 22*(1), 33–39.

Roussel, L., Swansburg, R. C., & Swansburg, R. J. (2006). *Management and leadership for nurse administrators* (4th ed.). Salisbury, MA: Jones and Bartlett.

Spitzer-Lehmann, R. (1990). Recruitment and retention of our greatest asset. *Nursing Administration Quarterly, 14*(4), 66–69.

West, M., Borrill, C., Dawson, J., Scully, J., Carter, M., Anelay, S., et al. (2002). The link between the management of employees and patient mortality in acute hospitals. *International Journal of Human Resource Management, 13*(8), 1299–1310.

Martha J. Greenberg

HUMAN RIGHTS

The Universal Declaration of Human Rights, adopted by the United Nations in 1948, was based on a universal recognition of the inherent dignity and equal and inalienable rights of all members of the human family. This document set forth what has now become a widely accepted summary of basic human rights (United Nations, 2010a, 2010b). Human rights can be thought of as those rights that are inherent to all human beings, whatever their nationality, place of residence, gender, national or ethnic origin, race, ethnicity, religion, language, or any other status by which groups can be differentiated. These are the rights to which all are equally entitled, without discrimination.

Health is universally recognized as a fundamental human right. The enjoyment

H

of the highest attainable standard of health as a right of every human being is a guiding principle of the World Health Organization. Health and human rights are inextricably linked. Violations or lack of attention to human rights can result in serious health consequences for individuals throughout the world; health policies and programs have the power to either promote or violate human rights through their design or implementation; and vulnerability and the impact of ill health can be reduced by taking steps to respect, protect, and promote human rights (World Health Organization, 2010a).

International nursing organizations have acknowledged and supported the fundamental link between health and human rights. The International Council of Nurses (2001) views health care as a right of all individuals, regardless of financial, political, geographic, racial, or religious considerations. This right includes "the right to choose or decline care, including the right to accept or refuse treatment or nourishment; informed consent; confidentiality; and dignity, including the right to die with dignity" (p. 272).

In keeping with this philosophy, the American Nurses Association has indicated that members of the profession of nursing have a societal mandate to safeguard the health rights of all persons at all times and in all places. "The nurse, in all professional relationships, practices with compassion and respect for the inherent dignity, worth and uniqueness of every individual, unrestricted by considerations of social or economic status, personal attributes, or the nature of health problems" (American Nurses Association, 2001, p. 4).

The Transcultural Nursing Society, established in 1975 by Dr. Madeleine Leininger, is an international nursing organization committed to the rights of all peoples to enjoy their full human potential, including the highest attainable standard of health (Miller et al., 2008). Among the human rights championed by the Transcultural Nursing Society are access to quality care and access to culturally and linguistically competent health care providers.

The right to health is closely related to and dependent on the realization of other human rights, including the right to food, housing, employment, and education. Therefore, these rights can be seen as the social determinants of health. Social determinants of health are the economic, social, and health system conditions into which people are born, grow, live, work, and age, which determine their health (World Health Organization, 2010b). Because all human rights are considered interdependent and indivisible (Braveman & Gruskin, 2003), nurses should not only promote human rights through delivery of care, but they must also expand their involvement in advocacy and policy efforts targeting any of the social determinants that may impede the realization of the right to health.

Professional nurses have an important role to play in supporting a human rights-based approach to the design and implementation of health care services that meet the diverse needs of a global society. Actions suggested for these nurse leaders include supporting the participation of affected groups, especially vulnerable groups, in all efforts that concern them and working to ensure discrimination does not occur in the delivery of services or in the health outcomes experienced among different population groups (Gruskin & Ferguson, 2009).

See also World Health Organization (WHO)

American Nurses Association. (2001). *Code of ethics for nurses with interpretive statements.* Washington, DC: American Nurses Publishing.

Braveman, P., & Gruskin, S. (2003). Poverty, equity, human rights and health. *Bulletin of the World Health Organization, 81*(7), 539–545.

Gruskin, S., & Ferguson, L. (2009). Using indicators to determine the contribution of human rights to public health efforts. *Bulletin of the World Health Organization, 87,* 714–719.

International Council of Nurses. (2001). Codes and declarations. *Nursing Ethics, 8*(3), 272–282.

Miller, J. E., Leininger, M., Leuning, C., Pacquiao, D., Andrews, M., Ludwig-Beymer, P., et al. (2008). Transcultural Nursing Society position statement on human rights. *Journal of Transcultural Nursing, 19,* 5–7.

United Nations. (2010a). Human rights. *Office of the High Commissioner for Human Rights.* Retrieved from http://www.ohchr.org/EN/Issues/Pages/WhatareHumanRights.aspx

United Nations. (2010b). *Universal declaration of human rights.* Retrieved from http://www.un.org/Overview/rights.html

World Health Organization. (2010a). *Human rights.* Retrieved from http://www.who.int/topics/human_rights/en

World Health Organization. (2010b). *Social determinants of health.* Retrieved from http://www.who.int/social_determinants/en

Rebecca C. Lee

H

I

IMAGE OF NURSING

Nurses are critical to the health care system. They act in numerous roles to improve health for patients, families, and communities. They are clinicians, educators, administrators, and researchers. Two government reports, one by the U.S. Bureau of Labor Statistics (2001) and the other by the U.S. Department of Health and Human Services (2000) titled "National Sample Survey," shed light on the image of nursing. They found that nursing is an ethical, trustworthy, and caring profession. These reports were released to present a positive image of the nursing profession, but they did not reflect the true public image of nursing (Murray, 2002). The various ways nurses are portrayed in the popular media, film, literature, and theater does not reflect the value of the profession in our society. In fact, nurses are portrayed as not smart enough to be physicians; nice, kind, compassionate, and trustworthy girls, and if they are men, they must be gay.

According to Turow and Gans (2002), fictional TV significantly influences the state of our health care system and policy options for improving the delivery of care. In some instances, physicians are depicted on TV as controlling and providing care that nurses or other health professionals actually do in reality (Buresh & Gordon, 2001). This disastrously impacts the image of accurate care giving. Nurses have limited meaningful impact in Hollywood and have endured regressive, inaccurate images for decades (Kalisch & Kalisch, 1983, 1984; Kalisch & Kalisch, 1982, 1985, 1987). In 2001, the Center for Nursing Advocacy (www.nursingadvocacy.org) was formed as a watchdog group to "increase public understanding of the central, frontline role nurses play in modern health care." The center has changed ownership but has kept the same mission as the Center for Nursing Advocacy, and since 2008, it has been called, The Truth About Nursing (www.thetruthaboutnursing.org). The focus of each of these organizations is to promote more accurate, balanced, and frequent media portrayals of nurses and increase the media's use of nurses as expert sources" (Center for Nursing Advocacy, 2006; The Truth About Nursing, 2008). According to the mission statements of both organizations, the focus is in "its efforts on improving the portrayal of nurses in the media, especially Hollywood, since television and films are so influential" (Center for Nursing Advocacy, 2006; Truth About Nursing, 2008).

The media image of nurses as portrayed on popular medical television shows depicts nurses as handmaidens to physicians. The nurses on such programs are retrieving charts and laboratory data for the powerful and confident physicians. This portrayal is detrimental to recruitment efforts and will not attract young adults on their quest for a career (Murray, 2002). In a study of primary and secondary school students, most respondents wrongly described nursing as a girl's job, a technical job "like shop," and an inappropriate career for private school students (JWT Communications, 2000).

Although some physicians have a good sense of nursing, many do not. A physician's actions seem to reflect a self-absorbed culture of medicine. This culture equates medicine with health care and rarely questions society's traditional assumptions. Nurses cannot be expected to be immune to the effect of the media. The ill treatment of nurses in the media leads to decreased morale and pride, which in turns encourages cynicism and creates a world where nurses tend not to stand up for themselves or their patients (Gordon, 2005).

When members of the public seek out health care, the general term used for any female caring for their needs is "nurse," whether it is an individual who bathes patients, draws their blood, or delivers their meals. Actually, the nurse is the lifeline to the whole professional team. The recognition of men in nursing needs to be voiced by all nurses. Nurses must do a better job of educating the public to preserve their professional status. This can be done in a sensitive way by ensuring that nurses are known as nurses through their attire, demeanor, and their words (Zwerdling, 2003).

Although images of nursing in media are generally inaccurate, the future holds suggestions for changing that image. The Future of Nursing (2010) campaign sponsored by the Robert Wood Johnson Foundation has presented positive images of men and women in nursing in a variety of roles and from different racial and ethnic backgrounds and ages (thefutureofnursing.or).

According to Raymond (2004), "chuck the cartoon jackets unless you're in pediatrics," and develop a uniform of "solid well-tailored scrubs" with a "starched white lab coat," "nursing pins and honors," and a "name badge with last name and degrees." "Nursing image equals nursing power" (Buresh & Gordon, 2001). These small steps can change the face of the image of nursing.

Bureau of Labor Statistics, U.S. Department of Labor. (2001). *Occupational outlook handbook, 2006–07 edition, registered nurses.* Retrieved June 26, 2006, from http://stats.bls.gov/oco/ocos083.htm

Buresh, B., & Gordon, S. (2001). *From silence to voice.* Retrieved from, http://www.nursingadvocacy.org/news/2001_silence_to_voice.html

Center for Nursing Advocacy. (2006). *How does the media affect how people think?* Retrieved June 26, 2006, from http://www.nursingadvocacy.org

Gordon, S. (2005). *Nursing against the odds.* Ithaca, NY: Cornell University Press.

JWT Communications. (2000). *Memo to nurses for a healthier tomorrow on focus group studies of 1,800 school children in 10 cities.* Retrieved October 14, 2006, from http://www.nursingadvocacy.org/research/lit/jwt_memo1.html

Kalisch, B. J., & Kalisch, P. A. (1983). Heroine out of focus: Media images of Florence Nightingale: Part II. Film, radio, and television dramatizations. *Nursing & Health Care, 4*(5), 270–278.

Kalisch, B. J., & Kalisch, P. A. (1984). The Dionne quintuplets legacy: Establishing the "good doctor and his loyal nurse" image in American culture. *Nursing & Health Care, 5*(5), 242–251.

Kalisch, P. A., & Kalisch, B. J. (1982). The image of the nurse in motion pictures. *American Journal of Nursing, 82*(4), 605–611.

Kalisch, P. A., & Kalisch, B. J. (1985). When Americans called for Dr. Kildare: Images of physicians and nurses in the Dr. Kildare and Dr. Gillespie movie 1937–1947. *Medical Heritage, 1*(5), 348–363.

Kalisch, P. A., & Kalisch, B. J. (1987). *The changing image of the nurse.* Menlo Park, CA: Addison-Wesley.

Murray, M. K. (2002). The nursing shortage. *Journal of Nursing Administration, 32*(2), 79–84.

Raymond, P. (2004, June 1). Nursing image = nursing power [Special issue]. *The Sacramento Bee.* Retrieved from http://www.reallife-healthcare.com

The Future of Nursing: Campaign for Action. (2010). *Robert Wood Johnson Foundation.* Retrieved April 11, 2011, from http://thefu-tureofnursing.org

The Truth about Nursing. (2008). Retrieved April 11, 2011, from http://www.thetruthabout-nursing.org

Turow, J., & Gans, R. (2002, July). *As seen on TV: Health policy issues in TV's media dramas* (Report No. 3231). Kaiser Family Foundation. Retrieved from http://www.kff.org/ent media/3231-index.cfm

U.S. Department of Health and Human Services. (2000). *National sample survey.* Washington, DC: Bureau of Health Professions Division of Nursing.

Zwerdling, M. (2003). *Postcards of nursing: A worldwide tribute.* Philadelphia, PA: Lippincott.

Marilyn Jaffe-Ruiz

INDIVIDUAL DEVELOPMENT PLAN

As mentoring has evolved in importance, there has been increasing emphasis on linking it to the individual development plan (IDP), also known as the personal development plan (PDP), as a way of getting both mentor and mentee focusing on the same questions: What are the mentee's goals for the next year or two with regard to teaching, research, practice, service, and/or leadership? What specific actions will have to be taken to achieve these goals? What resources—consulting, networking, grant support and the like—are needed to move the goals forward? What is the time frame for completion of various activities? What are the expected outcomes and how will they be measured?

The assumption behind the IDP is that professionals must be prepared for lifelong learning. Even after they have obtained needed degrees, licensure, or certification, they must be committed to career development—preparing themselves for where their institutions are going, their next career stage, and/or leadership opportunities. Increasingly, institutions are regarding the IDP as an important component of their mentoring programs.

The IDP has been used broadly to promote leadership in universities (University of California, San Francisco Academic Affairs, 2006), practice settings (University of Virginia Health System Professional Nursing Staff Organization, 2011), government (Jacobson, 2002–2010), and professional programs like the John A. Hartford Foundation's Building Academic Geriatric Nursing Capacity Program and the Robert Wood Johnson Foundation's Nurse Faculty Scholars Program (McBride, 2009).

The IDP is also an important component of leadership development internationally. One of the signature programs of the International Council of Nurses (2010) is titled Leadership for Change™, and the use of the IDP is a major strategy. In the United Kingdom, all professionals are required to have PDPs, and they have been found to work best when appraisal of learning needs is linked to additional development that is actually implemented (Berridge, Kelly, & Gould, 2007). Not surprisingly, PDPs do not work as well if time is not allocated for either the appraisal or the developmental follow-through.

Whether programs or institutions formally require an IDP as part of their organizational commitment to professional development or not, the IDP can be a useful heuristic in getting clear about where a nurse is headed professionally and how he or she plans to proceed. Writing out what one wants to do makes one's goals more real: listing what must be done first, second and third provide an opportunity to inject a note of practicality into one's dreams; setting a time frame provides a way to be realistic about what can be reasonably accomplished in a given period; and spelling out the metrics of success means the work will be outcome oriented.

See also Career Stages; Hartford Geriatric Nursing Initiative; Leadership Development; Mentoring; Robert Wood Johnson Foundation Nurse Faculty Scholars Program

Berridge, E.-J., Kelly, D., & Gould, D. (2007). Staff appraisal and continuing professional development. *Journal of Research in Nursing*, 12(1), 57–70.

International Council of Nurses. (2010, April 12). *Leading for change. Individual development plans.* Retrieved February 18, 2011, from http://icn.ch/pillarsprograms/methodology-and-key-strategies

Jacobson, D. (2002–2010). *Using IDPs to leverage strengths*. Retrieved February 18, 2011, from http://govleaders.org/idp.htm

McBride, A. B. (2009). *Individual development plan*. Retrieved February 18, 2011, from http://www.geriatricnursing.org/leadership/docs/IDPworksheet.pdf

University of California, San Francisco Academic Affairs. (2006). *Faculty mentoring program*. Retrieved February 18, 2011, from http://acpers.ucsf.edu/mentoring

University of Virginia Health System Professional Nursing Staff Organization. (2011). *Ongoing staff and manager development.*

Retrieved February 18, 2011, from http://healthsystem.virginia.edu/internet/pnso/new/ProfDev/StaffDevelopment.cfm

Angela Barron McBride

INFORMED CONSENT (RESEARCH)

Informed consent is an essential requirement for all research that involves human subjects. It is an individual's voluntary consent to participate in a research study and is given after receiving and understanding essential information about the research.

REGULATIONS FOR THE PROTECTION OF HUMAN SUBJECTS

The Nuremberg Code was developed in 1949 and was the first international standard for the conduction of research. This set of directives details 10 conditions that must be met to research to be deemed ethically permissible. The first directive is that voluntary consent by the potential participant is absolutely essential (U.S. Department of Health and Human Services [HHS], 2005). The Nuremberg Code served as the basis for the Declaration of Helsinki, which was adopted in 1964, by the World Medical Association. The Declaration of Helsinki details ethical principles related to the protection of the life, privacy, health, and dignity of the human subject. Similar to the Nuremberg Code, the Declaration of Helsinki makes informed consent a central requirement for ethical research (National Institutes of Health Office of Human Subjects Research, 2004).

In 1973, the Department of Health, Education, and Welfare developed regulations for the protection of human subjects, including special protections for persons with limited capacity to give consent. In 1979, the National Commission for the Protection of Human Subjects of Biomedical and Behavioral Research was formed. The commission prepared and submitted the Belmont Report to the Department of HHS. This is the cornerstone document of ethical principles and HHS regulations for the protection of research subjects. The Belmont Report identified three principles essential to the ethical conduct of research with humans: respect for persons, beneficence, and justice. These three principles serve as the foundation for the current HHS guidelines for the ethical conduct of research with human subjects.

Following submission of the Belmont Report, HHS developed a set of regulations, Code of Federal Regulations Title 45, Part 46 Protection of Human Subjects, which is referred to as "The Common Rule." The Common Rule describes the required protections for all human subjects (U.S. Department of HHS, 2009). The Office for Human Research Protection is responsible for interpreting and overseeing the implementation of these regulations.

VULNERABLE INDIVIDUALS

The Common Rule defines specific groups of participants who are considered vulnerable. These include pregnant women, human fetuses, neonates, prisoners, and children. There are additional requirements for informed consent for these vulnerable populations and additional responsibilities for the Institutional Review Board (IRB) when reviewing and approving research (U.S. Department of HHS, 2009).

Children (minors) are deemed legally and mentally incompetent to give informed consent. They lack the ability to understand information about a research study and are unable therefore to make informed decisions about participating in or withdrawing from such a study. The involvement of a child in the informed consent process varies depending on the age of the child. Usually children up to the age of 7 years are not involved in the consent process; the parents or guardians give consent. When the child is 7 years of age, the child can usually assent to participate in the research study. Assent means that the child gives affirmative agreement to participate in the research. Older children should be more involved in decisions regarding their participation in research studies. The HHS guidelines recommend getting the assent of the child, if the child is capable, along with the consent of the parent or guardian (U.S. Department of HHS, 2009).

Prisoners who are confined to institutions are designated as a vulnerable population under Federal Law. They might feel coerced to participate because they fear negative consequences if they refuse to participate in the research. There are specific requirements in the Common Rule for inclusion of prisoners in research (U.S. Department of HHS, 2009).

Hospitalized patients may also be a vulnerable population because of their illness and being confined to a health care setting. They may feel obliged to participate in the research as they fear their care may be otherwise compromised. Other vulnerable individuals include employees, students, illiterate subjects, and those who do not speak English.

HHS also specifies that additional protections may be required for other vulnerable populations, which include mentally disabled individuals and those who are economically or educationally disadvantaged. The HHS regulations, however, do not specify what additional protections are required for these groups.

There are adults who because of mental illness, cognitive impairment, or being in a comatose state are incapable of giving consent. In these circumstances, the researcher must get consent from the individual's family and his or her legal representative to give consent on behalf of the person to be a participant in the research study. The inclusion of individuals with diminished autonomy in a research study is more acceptable if the research is therapeutic rather than nontherapeutic, and both vulnerable and nonvulnerable groups are included in the research study. In addition, it is expected that all aspects of the consent process are strictly followed to ensure the participant's rights.

Conducting Research With Older Adults

Although age alone does not make an individual more vulnerable, there are many normal age-related changes that may make the older adult more vulnerable (Tabloski, 2010). Age-related changes in vision and hearing may make standard methods of describing research and obtaining consent more of a challenge. The researcher may have to adjust the size and color of print on written documents and consent forms. The process of obtaining consent might need to be altered as well. Environmental modifications such as increased light and decreased ambient noise may be the needed as well. The researcher may also have to allow for more time to obtain consent because of a slower speed of cognitive processing. Chronic disease conditions, which might make the older adult more easily fatigued, may also warrant modifications in the manner in which informed consent is obtained.

A further consideration is in relation to weighing the risks and benefits of the research. What is not a burden for a younger person, for example, answering a long questionnaire, might tax an older adult considerably. A blood draw might not be a big burden for a younger person but may be for an older adult where blood drawing is more difficult.

Older Adults With Cognitive Impairment

Federal regulations do not detail special considerations required when conducting research with individuals with cognitive impairment. In addition, there is little consensus for definitive guidelines. IRBs often incorporate similar requirements as those used for other vulnerable populations (Romanchuck, 2008).

A diagnosis of dementia does not mean that an individual is unable to consent to participate in research. According to the Alzheimer's Association, decision-making capacity is task specific. Therefore, some cognitively impaired individuals retain the ability to make informed decisions about participating in research (Alzheimer's Association National Board of Directors, 1997). When a cognitively impaired individual does not have the capacity to consent to participate in research, a legally authorized representative is often approached for consent. The regulations also permit consent by a legally authorized representative. The federal regulations, however, do not specify who can fulfill this role; it is retained by individual states. Few states have defined who the legally authorized representative for research purposes would be. Similar to children, assent is obtained from the cognitively impaired individual (Aselage, Conner, & Carnevale, 2009).

THE INFORMED CONSENT DOCUMENT

Informed consent documents must include the eight basic elements of

I

informed consent provided in the Code of Federal Regulations Title 45, Part 46 Protection of Human Subjects (U.S. Department of HHS, 2009). There are six additional elements of informed consent that may be required depending on the research (U.S. Department of HHS, 2009). These elements provide an excellent framework for informed consent documents for all human subjects' research. The detailed information on the elements for the consent document in this section is taken from the Code of Federal Regulations Title 45, Part 46 Protection of Human Subjects (U.S. Department of HHS, 2009).

Each subject must be given information related to each of the eight basic elements of informed consent (http://www.hhs.gov/ohrp/humansubjects/guidance/45cfr46.html#46.116). In addition, there are the six additional elements of informed consent that may be required in the consent document. Additional information that will have an impact on a subject's willingness to voluntarily participate in the research and protects the subject's rights and welfare in a meaningful way should be included. The six additional elements may be found at http://www.hhs.gov/ohrp/humansubjects/guidance/45cfr46.html#46.116.

LANGUAGE OF THE INFORMED CONSENT DOCUMENT

The informed consent document must be in a language understandable to the participant or his or her legally authorized representative (U.S. Department of HHS, 2009). It must be written in a language that is at the appropriate reading and comprehension level for the targeted population. It must be in lay language and should not include technical language that would not be understandable to all potential subjects.

OBTAINING INFORMED CONSENT FOR RESEARCH

Individuals must be given detailed information about the research to decide whether or not they wish to participate or continue to participate in a research study. This includes information on all aspects of the study, including the risks and benefits. The informed consent process should include opportunities to allow potential subjects to ask questions. During the course of the study, subjects must be kept informed of any new information that may affect their willingness to remain in the study. Subjects can discontinue their participation at any point in time.

The HHS regulations require that informed consent be documented using a written form that either contains all of the required elements or a short form that states that all of the required elements have been presented verbally. The informed consent form must be signed by the participant or the participant's legally authorized representative (U.S. Department of HHS, 2009). A copy of the signed informed consent documents must be given to the subject or his or her legally authorized representative.

The principal investigator for an IRB-approved study is ultimately responsible for the conduct of the research study including all aspects of the informed consent process. All persons who will be obtaining consent must have a certificate in human subjects' protections. The IRB requires that documentation of informed consent be obtained from all subjects unless alternate procedures are approved by the IRB.

Alzheimer's Association National Board of Directors. (1997). Ethical issues in dementia research (with special emphasis on "informed consent"). Retrieved May 16, 2011, from http://www.alz.org/national/documents/statements_ethicalissues.pdf

Aselage, M. B., Conner, B., & Carnevale, T. (2009). Ethical issues in conducting research with persons with dementia. *Southern Online Journal of Nursing Research, 9*(4), 11.

Code of Federal Regulations, Title 45. Public Welfare, Part 46. Retrieved May 23, 2011, from http://www.hhs.gov/ohrp/humansubjects/guidance/45cfr46.html#46.116

National Commission for the Protection of Human Subjects of Biomedical and Behavioral Research. (1979). *The Belmont Report: Ethical principles and guidelines for the protection of human subjects of resarch.* Retrieved May 16, 2011, from http://ohsr.od.nih.gov/guidelines/belmont.html

National Insitutes of Health Office of Human Subjects Research. (2004). *World Medical Association Declaration of Helsinki.* Retrieved May 16, 2011, from http://ohsr.nih.gov/guidelines/helsinki.html

Romanchuck, R. (2008). Identification and accommodation of vulnerable populations in human research. *Research Practitioner, 9*(5), 158–173.

Tabloski, P. (2010). *Gerontologic nursing* (2nd ed.). Upper Saddle River, NJ: Pearson Health Science.

U.S. Department of Health and Human Services. (2005). *The Nuremberg Code.* Retrieved May 15, 2011, from http://www.hhs.gov/ohrp/archive/nurcode.html

U.S. Department of Health and Human Services. (2009). *Code of Federal Regulations.* Retrieved May 15, 2011, from http://www.hhs.gov/ohrp/humansubjects/guidance/45cfr46.html#46.111

Sharon Stahl Wexler

INSTITUTE FOR HEALTHCARE IMPROVEMENT

Founded in 1991, the Institute for Healthcare Improvement (IHI) is a not-for-profit organization located in Cambridge, Massachusetts, whose primary aim is to "improve the lives of patients, the health of communities, and the joy of the health care workforce" (IHI, 2011a). To achieve this mission, IHI focuses on a set of goals adapted from the Institute of Medicine's six improvement aims for the health care system: safety, effectiveness, patient centeredness, timeliness, efficiency, and equity (Committee on the Quality of Healthcare in America, 2001). IHI identifies this set of goals as the "no needless list": no needless death, no needless pain or suffering, no helplessness in those served or serving, no unwanted waiting, no waste, and no one left out (IHI, 2011a).

Appointed in 2010, the current president and CEO is Maureen Bisognano, who leads an IHI workforce of more than 100 individuals. Cofounder and former CEO is Donald M. Berwick, an international expert on health care performance improvement and since 2010 the Administrator of the Centers for Medicare and Medicaid Services of the United States Department of Health and Human Services.

One of Berwick's influential publications, *Escape Fire: Lessons for the Future of Healthcare* (Berwick, 2002), is an essay that describes gaps in the safety and quality of U.S. health care. In this publication he exhorts the public and clinicians to create a sense of urgency for fundamental health care reform. Berwick names the reform approach "escape fire," a metaphor that is drawn from a term that firefighters use for a deliberately burned piece of land, which, in an emergency, can create a safe haven from an oncoming blaze. The platform of "escape fire" has defined the work of IHI for more than 20 years, calling for the fundamental redesign of health care processes.

In 2008, IHI broadened its vision and defined an approach for total system performance in health care called the "Triple Aim": better care, better health, at lower cost (IHI, 2011b). The pursuit of the Triple Aim is one of IHI's leading frameworks to

I

improve the individual patient experience of care and the health of entire communities through exploring new designs for health care delivery.

IHI offers programs on a variety of health care topics in formats that include conference calls, live Web-based knowledge exchange programs, professional development seminars, workshops and conferences, collaborative innovation and learning communities, and on-demand Web-based events. It also publishes a series of monographs and "white papers" on innovation and performance improvement topics, many of which are available without charge. Organizational membership in a program called Passport includes access to practical performance improvement tools and ongoing expert support needed to achieve exceptional hospital care. In addition, IHI annually hosts a National Forum on Quality Improvement in Healthcare that draws health care leaders from around the world who participate in plenary sessions and more than 100 workshops.

IHI has also established the IHI Open School for Health Professions, a "virtual" interdisciplinary educational community that offers online courses, resources, and opportunities to connect with students, faculty, and professionals throughout the world. More than 40,000 students in 35 countries have registered in the IHI Open School, providing enrollees with the knowledge and skills to become change agents and champions for health care improvement.

IHI's history includes seven phases of events that have shaped their quality improvement journey: awareness, education, collaborative improvement, redesign, movement, full scale, and care for populations (IHI, 2010). The current phase of "care for populations" involves using the framework of Triple Aim to foster better care for individuals, improve health for populations, and reduce per capita costs.

Two IHI campaigns from the full-scale phase of IHI's history have significantly influenced patient safety initiatives in the United States. The first was the 100,000 Lives Campaign, which disseminated improvement tools throughout the American health care system. This campaign aimed to enlist thousands of U.S. hospitals in a commitment to deploy interventions that had been proven to prevent unnecessary death. These interventions included the following:

1. Deploy rapid response teams
2. Deliver reliable, evidence-based care for acute myocardial infarction
3. Prevent adverse drug events
4. Prevent central line infections
5. Prevent surgical site infections
6. Prevent ventilator-associated pneumonia

From 2006 to 2008, IHI sponsored the 5 Million Lives Campaign. The goal of this effort was to engage 4,000 U.S. hospitals to implement 12 interventions intended to prevent five million incidents of patient harm over a 24-month period. In addition to the six interventions from the 100,000 Lives Campaign, six new strategies were identified:

1. Prevent harm from high-alert medications
2. Reduce surgical complications
3. Prevent pressure ulcers
4. Reduce Methicillin-resistant *Staphlococcus aureus* infection
5. Deliver reliable, evidence-based care for congestive heart failure
6. Get boards on board by defining and spreading the best-known leveraged processes for hospital boards of directors

Another example of an IHI initiative that focused on nursing care and nursing practice is a partnership developed in 2003 with the Robert Wood Johnson Foundation. This program, Transforming Care at the Bedside, sought to empower nurses to redesign work processes on hospital adult medical-surgical units to improve the reliability of patient care. In 2011, the American Organization of Nurse Executives launched the Center for Care Innovation and Transformation whose foundation uses the basic tenets of Transforming Care at the Bedside but also includes an additional focus on nurse manager development, culture change, and implementation of national health care reform as defined in the Affordable Care Act of 2010 (American Organization of Nurse Executives, 2011).

Since the 1990s, an increasing focus on quality and safety in nursing and health care has been led by several national commissions that documented concerns with the U.S. health care system (Committee on the Quality of Healthcare in America, 2001; Institute of Medicine, 2003; Institute of Medicine, Board on Healthcare Services, 2004; Kohn, Corrigan, & Donaldson, 2000). The IHI has established a visible international profile and reputation for setting standards that have transformed knowledge and reformed systems for improved performance and results for patients, families, communities, and populations.

See also Transforming Care at the Bedside

American Organization of Nurse Executives. (2011). *Announcing the new AONE Center for Care Innovation and Transformation*. Retrieved May 26, 2011, from http://www.aone.org/aone/resource/CCIT/CCIT.html

Berwick, D. M. (2002). *Escape fire: Lessons for the future of healthcare*. New York, NY: The Commonwealth Fund.

Committee on the Quality of Healthcare in America. (2001). *Crossing the quality chasm: A new health system for the 21st century*. Washington, DC: National Academies Press.

Institute for Healthcare Improvement. (2011a). *IHI vision and values*. Retrieved May 26, 2011, from http://www.ihi.org/IHI/About/VisionValues

Institute for Healthcare Improvement. (2011b). The evolution of IHI's work and strategy. Retrieved May 26, 2011, from http://www.ihi.org/IHI/About/EvolutionIHIWorkStrategy.htm

Institute for Healthcare Improvement. (2010). Accelerating improvement worldwide: A history of IHI 1986–2010. Cambridge, MA: Author.

Institute of Medicine. (2003). *Health professions education: A bridge to quality*. Washington, DC: National Academies Press.

Institute of Medicine, Board on Health Care Services. (2004). *Committee on the work environment for nurses and patient safety*. Washington, DC: National Academies Press.

Kohn, L. T., Corrigan, J. M., & Donaldson, M. S. (Eds.). (2000). *To err is human: Building a safer health system*. Washington, DC: National Academies Press.

Thomas D. Smith

INSTITUTE OF MEDICINE

The National Academy of Sciences was created by President Abraham Lincoln on March 3, 1863, to "investigate, examine, experiment, and report upon any subject of science or art" whenever called upon by the government. That institution was expanded to include the National Research Council (1916), the National Academy of Engineering (1964), and the Institute of Medicine (IOM, 1970), and those four entities are now collectively known as the National Academies. The IOM is the body specifically charged by Congress with providing advice on the scientific and technological matters that help shape health policy. Committed to the improvement of health, the IOM has adopted processes that ensure the provision of unbiased, evidence-based, and authoritative information. Reports that synthesize and analyze the state of the science are regularly issued by expert committees peopled by member and nonmember experts. IOM is an honorific membership organization, more than 1,700 strong in 2010. Though most members are physicians, an interdisciplinary perspective is valued and approximately 60 members are nurses.

The IOM is important to nursing leadership because it is a venue through which nurse experts can join other health care professionals in evaluating what is known on a particular topic and what next steps need to be taken to improve practice, to fund additional research, and/or to develop new policy guidelines. The resulting reports provide excellent summaries of the state of the science on various topics; see the reports section of IOM's Web site for a complete listing (http://www.iom.edu). For example, the IOM (2003) issued a report on the five core competencies that all health care professionals will need in the 21st century and another one on the importance of nursing leadership in creating environments that keep patients safe (IOM, 2004), both of which have had profound implications for nursing education and practice (Finkelman & Kenner, 2009). The IOM (2011) report on the future of nursing, which was funded by the Robert Wood Johnson Foundation, makes recommendations likely to shape the destiny of current and future nurses, most dramatically by urging them to pursue higher levels of education and to seek a partner role with physicians in the redesign of health care.

The IOM's Board on Health Policy Educational Programs and Fellowships sponsors career-building opportunities that are available to nurses. The Robert Wood Johnson Health Policy Fellowship Program enables mid-career health professionals to gain an understanding of how health policy is developed, to contribute to the formulation of policies, and then to apply that learning as they exert leadership in a broad array of venues. The IOM Distinguished Nurse Scholar Program, co-sponsored with the American Nurses Foundation and the American Academy of Nursing, is designed to enable an accomplished nurse leader to play a more prominent role in health policy at the national level. For details about these opportunities, go to http://www.iom.edu/About-IOM/Leadership-Staff/Boards/Health-Policy-Educational-Programs-and-Fellowships.aspx.

Finkelman, A., & Kenner, C. (Eds.) (2009). *Teaching IOM: Implications of the Institute of Medicine reports for nursing* (2nd ed.). Silver Spring, MD: nursesbooks.org.

Institute of Medicine. (2003). The core competencies needed for health care professionals. In A. C. Greiner, & E. Knebel(Eds.), *Health professions education: A bridge to quality* (pp. 45–74). Washington, DC: The National Academies Press.

Institute of Medicine. (2004). Transformational leadership and evidence-based management. In A. Page (Ed.), *Keeping patients safe: Transforming the work environment of nurses* (pp. 108–161). Washington, DC: The National Academies Press.

Institute of Medicine. (2011). The future of nursing: Leading change, advancing health. Washington, DC: The National Academies Press.

Angela Barron McBride

INTERNATIONAL COUNCIL OF NURSES (ICN)

The International Council of Nurses (ICN) was founded in 1899 as an organization to represent nurses and their interests worldwide. ICN goals are as follows: (a) align nurses on a global level, (b) continue to internationally advance the profession of nursing, and (c) maintain a strong influence within health policy (ICN, 2010b). Within the ICN federation, more than 130 national nurse organizations represent their respective countries and thereby millions of nurses around the world.

ICN is the international voice of nurses through global efforts focused on three primary programs: professional practice, regulation, and social economic welfare (ICN, 2010a). Professional practice includes leadership development, the International Classification of Nursing Practice, and linkages to national and international organizations, such as the World Health Organization, the UNICEF, and the International Red Cross (ICN, 2010c). Within the leadership component, ICN offers a *Leadership for Change* focus consisting of five modules presented to course participants over a 2-year period of time. The regulation focus ensures high standards for education and practice globally. ICN works with the World Health Organization to promote regulatory standards for nursing (ICN, 2010d). The social economic welfare focus is targeted toward equitable and reasonable compensation with appropriate work benefits for nurses. ICN also represents nursing within the International Labour Organization to consistently protect nursing and nurses' workplace issues including the eradication of workplace violence (ICN, 2010e).

For the last 5 years, ICN has been supportive of a United Nations Agency for Women that would directly address gender equality with a specific focus on women's rights related to domestic violence, HIV/AIDS, and poverty. In July 2010, the United Nations General Assembly voted the approval of the creation of the United Nations Entity for Gender Equality and the Empowerment of Women (United Nations, 2010). A collection of ICN biennial reports, bulletins, and newsletters are published in the official ICN languages (English, French, and Spanish) and are available on the ICN Web site (www.icn.ch/). These publications cover leadership, regulations, research, socioeconomic news, nurse practitioner/advanced practice issues, and International Classification of Nursing Practice.

International Council of Nurses. (2010a). *Frequently asked questions.* Retrieved September 9, 2010, from http://www.icn.ch/about-icn/faq

International Council of Nurses. (2010b). *How can I join ICN's?* Retrieved September 9, 2010, from http://www.icn.ch/about-icn/how-can-i-join-icn-please-send-me-membership-information

International Council of Nurses. (2010c). *ICN professional practice.* Retrieved September 9, 2010, from http://www.icn.ch/pillarsprograms/professional-practice

International Council of Nurses. (2010d). *ICN regulation.* Retrieved September 9, 2010, from http://www.icn.ch/pillarsprograms/regulation

International Council of Nurses. (2010e). *ICN socio-economic welfare.* Retrieved September 9, 2010, from http://www.icn.ch/pillarsprograms/socio-economic-welfare

United Nations. (2010). *UN creates new structure for empowerment of women.* Press Release. Retrieved September 9, 2010, from http://www.unwomen.org/2010/07/un-creates-new-structure-for-empowerment-of-women

Ronda Mintz-Binder
Joyce J. Fitzpatrick

INTERNATIONAL LEADERSHIP IN NURSING

Effective leaders in nursing demonstrate an understanding of health care systems, are visionary, think strategically, plan effectively, contribute to policy development, manage change, and work effectively in teams. The effective nurse leader understands resource management, marketing, and media skills, communicates effectively, negotiates, and motivates and influences others (International Council of Nurses [ICN], 2010). With the increases of health reform in various parts of the world, it is essential that nurses with leadership training and background assist and support these efforts. Nurses who use their leadership and management skills to effect change across national boundaries are international leaders.

Nurse leadership efforts that are coordinated through international nursing organizations, such as ICN, assist in bringing forth global health concerns and engaging in united efforts to combat these issues. International leaders in nursing focus on health planning and decision making, professional development of nurses, promoting the contributions of nurses in health care, promoting nurse entrepreneurship, defining nursing roles and scope of practice, and promoting the legislative involvement of nurses in their home countries. They seek to increase nursing influence globally by building cooperative coalitions to effect change in local communities. Significant and ongoing issues of concern among global nursing groups have been gender disparity and working conditions for women.

Global issues facing nurse leaders are of wide scope and are being approached and critically evaluated in a cohesive and structured manner. The ICN has a vision statement that encourages nurses from across the world speak in unison with one voice (ICN, 2007). The ICN operates under three core areas that lead an international approach in creating change-based programs. These "pillars" are as follows: professional practice, regulation,

and socioeconomic welfare (ICN, 2010). Each of these pillars provide opportunities for uniting a global effort in causes such as strengthening leadership in nursing, providing a means for sharing new regulations for a better global approach to patient care, and securing a safe physical and emotional work environment for health care workers.

Five significant international issues of concern have been the global shortage of nurses, international migration of nurses, conquering multi-drug-resistant tuberculosis (MDR-TB), AIDS relief in Uganda, and creating positive workplaces for nurses. To address the issue of a global nursing shortage, The International Centre for Human Resources in Nursing was created in 2006 in association with the Florence Nightingale International Foundation and the Burdett Trust for Nursing. The goals of this Centre include being a resource for data collection and dissemination related to policies and health-related management and secondly to house an international holding of human resource materials related to nursing for analysis and assimilation at the national and global level (International Centre for Human Resources in Nursing, 2006).

As part of the global nursing shortage, critical challenges that affect world regions have been identified. The HIV/AIDS challenge, most prominent in sub-Saharan Africa, is one example. HIV/AIDS creates an increasing demand for health services yet reduces health team availability and functioning as mortality rates and absenteeism among health care workers increase. Because of the HIV/AIDS crisis, the nursing workforce challenge in sub-Saharan Africa is by far the most serious in comparison to any other geographical zone in the world (ICN, 2010). In addition, the rise noted in MDR-TB has been a second international area of concern. The ICN has unfolded a TB training project in 14 countries with high rates of TB to assure state-of-the-art materials, assessment skills, and appropriate treatment options for those with TB or MDR-TB.

To assure the best and most conscientious practice of all nurses, it is essential that workplaces are positive and violence free. From an international perspective, high-quality and safe work environments have become another major area of interest to the ICN in combination with a variety of other International Organizations such as the International Hospital Federation, the Global Health Workforce Alliance, and a number of other allied health world federations. Continued focused efforts to ensure a global view of safe nursing practice include: the International Centre on Nurse Migration and the Quality Workplaces for Quality Care Campaign (ICN, 2010).

See also Health Policy; International Council of Nurses (ICN)

International Centre for Human Resources in Nursing. (2006). *Introduction*. Retrieved September 9, 2010, from http://www.ichrn.org

International Council of Nurses. (2010). *ICN report 2007–2009. Health systems strengthening: Working together to achieve more*. Retrieved September 9, 2010, from http://www.icn.ch/images/stories/documents/publications/biennial_reports/ICN_Report_2007-2009.pdf

International Council of Nurses. (2007). *Vision for the future of nursing*. Retrieved September 8, 2010, from http://www.icn.ch/about-icn/icns-vision-for-the-future-of-nursing

Ronda Mintz-Binder
Kim L. Carnahan Lewis
Joyce J. Fitzpatrick

INTERNSHIPS

Internship refers to a supervised, practical experience that relates to a student's field of study. Internships are customarily completed concurrently with academic work, and may be paid or unpaid. The experience provides vital socialization and networking, mentoring and instruction, as well as practical experience in the area of study.

Entry to the workforce can be an awkward and uncertain time for the newly graduated nurse. Rising patient acuity levels and heavy workloads add a level of stress that detracts from successful transition into practice. New nurses can become disorientated and discouraged with their chosen profession quickly, and some studies report turnover rates of 50% after one year of clinical practice (Duchscher, 2008).

Theoretical models have been applied in some instances to guide internship progression. The stages of transition theory is one such framework that highlights the learner moving across the continuum from simple to complex tasks. Skill and knowledge development are broken into phases known as Doing, Being, and Knowing. Duchscher (2008) describes the application of this theory to new graduate transition as the "process of becoming."

Internships, or transition to practice programs, have proven to yield positive results regarding improved job satisfaction and retention of the new nurse graduate (Goode, Lynn, Krsek, & Bednash, 2009; Pine & Tart, 2007). Internship programs provide a controlled and methodical approach for the new graduate nurse to acquire information, assimilate into a new environment, provide for patient safety and quality during the learning process, and allow for the development of skill, comfort, and confidence in the new nurse (Winfield, Melo, & Myrick, 2009).

The opportunity to participate in a nursing internship provides a framework for a smoother transition into clinical practice. Adaptation to the hospital setting combined with mentoring relationships that evolve establishes a strong foundation for the new nurse graduate and is also an integral part of recruitment efforts utilized by health care organizations (Poynton, Madden, Bowers, & Keefe, 2007).

See also Entry Into Practice

Duchscher, J. B. (2008). A process of becoming: The stages of new nursing graduate professional role transition. *Journal of Continuing Education in Nursing, 39*(10), 441–450.

Goode, C. J., Lynn, M. R., Krsek, C., & Bednash, G. D. (2009). Nurse residency programs: An essential requirement for nursing. *Nursing Economics, 27*(3),142–147.

Pine, R., & Tart, K. (2007). Return on investment; benefits and challenges of baccalaureate nurse residency program. *Nursing Economics, 25*(1), 13–18.

Poynton, M. R., Madden, C., Bowers, R., & Keefe, M. (2007). Nurse residency program implementation: The Utah experience. *Journal of Healthcare Management, 52*(6), 385–396.

Winfield, C., Melo, K. & Myrick, F. (2009). Meeting the challenge of new graduate role transition: clinical nurse educators leading the change. *Journal of Nursing Staff Development, 25*(2), 7–13.

Kimberly B. Hall

INTERPROFESSIONAL COLLABORATION IN NURSING

Expert reports and commissions have identified interprofessional education, research, and practice as one of the keystones of providing the highest quality of health care to the nation. The Pew Health Professions Commission (1998) noted that an interdisciplinary model of care could best manage the care of both acutely and chronically ill patients because "…the expertise and instincts of a number of trained health practitioners are brought to bear in an environment that values brainstorming, consultation, and collaboration." Five years later, the Institute of Medicine (IOM; Greiner & Knebel, 2003) convened more than 150 health care leaders and experts to develop strategies for restructuring clinical education for the 21st century and recommended that future students and working professionals have experience "working as part of interdisciplinary teams" (Greiner & Knebel). The President's New Freedom Commission on Mental Health (2003) also suggested that a solution to the current fragmentation of mental health care in the United States is the expanded use of collaborative care models that promote interdisciplinary partnerships. Most recently, Benner, Sutphen, Leonard, and Day (2010) stated in *Educating Nurses: A Call for Radical Transformation*, that the more complex health care settings "…make clear communication and coordination between nursing and medicine imperative."

Over the past decade, several foundations have also promoted the development of interprofessional collaboration by providing valuable support to interprofessional training programs. For example, the John A. Hartford Foundation in New York funded the Geriatric Interdisciplinary Team Training Program to encourage interdisciplinary training among health professionals. Data from this program indicate that knowledge and attitudes related to interdisciplinary roles can be improved through such training, thereby promoting quality and cost-effective clinical outcomes (Fulmer et al., 2005). There is also evidence to support the idea that expanding screening and interdisciplinary care models, such as the Collaborative Care Model for treating late-life depression in primary care settings, reduces the prevalence and severity of depression symptoms or results in complete remission, leading to higher satisfaction with depression treatment (Unutzer et al., 2002). Further, the Josiah Macy, Jr. Foundation and the Carnegie Foundation for the Advancement of Teaching joined together to sponsor a conference, "Educating Nurses and Physicians: Toward New Horizons" in June 2010 to explore how to strengthen educational collaboration. The Macy Foundation has funded numerous grants that focus on both the development of curricula and strategies to foster interprofessional education in health professional schools.

The Robert Wood Johnson Foundation has been a leader among foundations in strengthening nursing and nursing's leadership in the health care system through its grants, convening health care leaders and partnering with the IOM and other national organizations such as the AARP. The AARP Foundation focuses on nursing's future. Most recently, the IOM's (2011) report, *The Future of Nursing: Leading Change, Advancing Health*, which was supported by the Robert Wood Johnson Foundation, highlights the importance of nurses as full partners with physicians and other health professionals in redesigning health care in the United States. Embedded in that key message of the report is the challenge for nurses to develop the leadership competencies linked with the responsibility and accountability associated with effective collaborative relationships with other health professionals.

The essence of interdisciplinary leadership is predicated upon expertise in some area of knowledge that is valued by and valuable to a range of disciplines. Nursing leadership has long recognized interdisciplinary practice, education, and research as both necessary and beneficial to good patient care. The American Nursing Association's Social Policy Statement (Ervin & McNamara, 2003) identifies nursing's scope of practice as one that "... overlaps those of other professions involved in health care...and members of various professions cooperate by sharing knowledge, techniques, and ideas about how to deliver quality health care." Virtually every major document that guides professional practice at the registered nurse and advanced practice levels promotes the importance of interdisciplinary leadership in improving patient outcomes, including the American Association of Colleges of Nursing's publications of the Essentials of Baccalaureate and Master's Education (www.aacn.nche.edu), the National Organization of Nurse Practitioner Facilities Competencies (www.nonpf.com), and the American Nursing Association Scope and Standards of Clinical Nursing Practice (www.nursingworld.org). The American Association of Colleges of Nursing's (2008) *The Essentials of Baccalaureate Education for Professional Nursing Practice* includes interprofessional communication and collaboration for improving patient health outcomes as one of its essentials for preparing the generalist nurse.

In recent years, interdisciplinary leadership by the nursing profession has gained visibility with, for example, a nurse-president of the American Heart Association, a nurse-president of the American Diabetes Association, a nurse-president of the American Public Health Association, a nurse-president of the Society of Behavioral Medicine, and a nurse-president of the Gerontological Society of America. These leadership inroads recognize the importance of nursing in promoting and sustaining national initiatives. Nurse leaders are voted into leadership positions because they are demonstrated experts in the specialty areas addressed by the organizations noted. The IOM (2011) report of the future of nursing suggests that such national leadership platforms provide excellent venues

I

for shaping health policy and implementation initiatives.

There are, however, barriers to sustaining interdisciplinary leadership, among these the inadequate commitment to interdisciplinary education by professional schools. Although this is changing with help from the Macy and Carnegie Foundations, as described above, without incentives from regulatory agencies, accrediting bodies or funders of health professional education to encourage professional schools to redesign curriculum requirements, schools may not emphasize or even provide room for interdisciplinary courses or activities. Therefore, professional educational silos will continue, and students will not have the opportunity to understand the history and theory of practice spheres of other professions, to develop interprofessional communication skills, or to gain experience with how interprofessional practice improves patient safety and outcomes.

The hierarchical nature of health delivery settings also serves to reinforce and replicate the professional separateness. Although there are, in most settings, daily incidences of collaboration and teamwork among professions, it usually is more due to individual preferences and style rather than to institutional policy. The teamwork that may exist at senior management levels of nursing and medicine is not always replicated at the point of patient care delivery. At the patient care level, nurses and physicians more commonly meet, make rounds, and have clinical conferences separately. Traditions related to how each profession organizes daily practice and the schedules and routines of the service delivery setting make it impossible to have, for example, one interdisciplinary conference to start the day.

As entrenched as these barriers to interdisciplinary education, research,

and practice seem, the nursing leadership in universities and colleges has unique opportunities to develop models of interdisciplinary collaboration and circumvent if not overcome them. For example, academic nursing leaders can agree to new models by pointing to the shared goals of academia—to produce new knowledge, to test new ideas and models, to translate them into practice, and to transfer a commitment to collaboration to the next generation of health professionals. Realistic action plans can gain support for (a) collaborative teaching within existing professional curricula using equitable revenue sharing models, (b) collaborative research in areas of shared clinical interests that capitalize on "low lying fruit," those areas of similar expertise and interest that reflect synergy across disciplines, and (c) collaborative faculty practices that demonstrate how multiple health professions contribute to quality and cost-effective patient outcomes.

One example of a new model is the interprofessional curriculum that is being developed by New York University's (NYU's) College of Nursing and School of Medicine, a project funded by the Josiah Macy, Jr. Foundation. This project, NYU3T (Teaching, Technology, and Teamwork), includes Web-based modules in the concepts of professional roles, communication and conflict resolution, health care safety, use of virtual patients, interprofessional simulation scenarios, and clinical crossover experiences. A strong commitment from the leadership of both programs is seeking to overcome the traditional barriers to interprofessional education such as aligning student and faculty schedules, different levels of learners, and limited access to patients in clinical settings due to patient safety concerns.

It is important in developing the new models of collaboration that academic nursing leaders communicate the values, expertise, and knowledge base of nursing throughout the university to increase the visibility and create an understanding of how nursing makes value-added contributions to the health care team. Academic nursing leaders also must convince the general university leadership that support for strong interdisciplinary collaboration in the health professions strengthens each profession's educational program and thus raises the visibility and status of the entire academic health science endeavor.

Beyond academics, our practice leaders can do much to influence interprofessional collaboration. Chief nurse officers can and do lead important interdisciplinary committees across an array of health care settings and should do all that is possible to learn essential leadership lessons from their experiences to advance the development of leadership competencies in the next generation of nurse leaders. For example, leadership development using a mentor–mentee model can be a powerful influence for advancing the interdisciplinary leadership skill set for these future academic, practice, and research leaders in their settings.

In the health policy arena, nurses who are experts have led interdisciplinary programs with major foundations and government agencies. For example, Mary Wakefield, PhD, RN, was appointed by President Obama as the Administrator of the Health Resources and Services Administration in the U.S. Department of Health and Human Services, which is the primary federal agency for improving access to health care services for people who are uninsured, isolated, or medically vulnerable. Also, there has been leadership in previous administrations. Dr. Shirley Chater headed the Social Security Administration during President William Jefferson Clinton's first

term, Sheila Burke was Chief of Staff to then Senator Robert Dole, Virginia Trotter Betts was an Undersecretary of Health and Human Services and is currently the Commissioner of TennCare, and Vice Admiral Richard H. Carmona, the former Surgeon General, started his health care career as a nurse. Each time examples of nurses who are leaders in health policy arenas are noted, the scope of their interdisciplinary influence must be recognized and new lessons must be learned from the exercise of their content expertise and political savvy and skill.

With the passage of the Patient Protection and Affordable Care Act in March 2010, there is even a more urgent need to develop interprofessional leadership in nursing. This legislation introduces provisions to expand health insurance coverage, to control health care costs, and to improve the health care delivery system. Under this law, the current health care delivery system will require more interprofessional collaboration and, consequently, present new challenges and opportunities for nursing practice and education. Nursing leadership can respond by taking immediate and aggressive steps to reinforce and expand existing interprofessional efforts and to develop new models. The nursing profession is strategically positioned to lead interprofessional efforts in education, practice, and research in the new health care environment. Indeed, it is imperative to do so to improve patient care and to meet the population's health needs in the coming decades.

American Association of Colleges of Nursing. (2008). *The essentials of baccalaureate education for professional nursing practice*. Washington, DC: Author.

Benner, P., Sutphen, M., Leonard, V., & Day, L. (2010). *Educating nurses: A call for radical transformation*. San Francisco, CA: Jossey-Bass.

Ervin, N. E., & McNamara, A. M. (2003). Nursing's social policy statement 2003. In *Nursing's social policy statement revision task force, 2001–2003*. Silver Spring, MD: The Publishing Program of American Nurses Association.

Fulmer, T., Hyer, K., Flaherty, E., Mezey, M., Whitelaw, N., Jacobs, M. O., et al. (2005). Geriatric Interdisciplinary Team Training Program: Evaluation results. *Journal of Aging and Health, 17*(4), 525–534.

Greiner, A., & Knebel, E. (Eds.). (2003). *Health professions education: A bridge to quality*. Washington, DC: National Academies Press.

Institute of Medicine. (2011). *The future of nursing: Leading change, advancing health*. Washington, DC: National Academies Press.

New Freedom Commission on Mental Health. (2003). *Achieving the promise: Transforming mental health care in America. Final report* (DHHS Publication No. SMA-03-3832). Rockville, MD: Author.

Pew Health Professions Commission. (1998). *Recreating health professional practice for a new century. The fourth report of the Pew Health Professions Commission*. Retrieved September 20, 2006, from http://www.futurehealth.ucsf.edu/pdf_files/rept4.pdf

Unutzer, J., Katon, W., Callahan, C. M., Williams, J. W., Jr., Hunkeler, E., Harpole, L., et al. (2002). Collaborative care management of late-life depression in the primary care setting: A randomized controlled trial. *Journal of American Medical Association, 288*, 2836–2845.

Hila Richardson
Judith Haber
Terry Fulmer

Interprofessional Leadership in Nursing

Interprofessional leadership (IPL) is a concept that is best described as a collaborative process that occurs at a management or decision-making level of an organization or work group, across disciplines and professions. The use of an interprofessional leadership model serves to promote understanding of varying perspectives, facilitate dialogue and debate, enhance teamwork and collaboration among a diverse group of leaders, and improve the overall quality of outcomes generated from the group.

Interprofessional leadership has been utilized within industry, public administration, and academia. The application of interprofessional leadership within health care, however, is a relatively new approach to navigating care demands and operational challenges. The primary goal for an interprofessional leadership approach in the context of health care is to achieve higher levels of patient safety because of effective communication and optimized clinical decision making between health care providers, as well as to achieve better patient outcomes (Baker, Egan-Lee, Martimianakis, & Reeves 2010).

The complex and dynamic nature of the current health care environment necessitates that health care professionals work together in order to effect improvements in the care that is delivered as well as the outcomes experienced by patients. The interprofessional approach demonstrates an historical shift, however. The disciplines represented within health care have traditionally been educated separately and functioned in silos, independent of one another, which created a lack of knowledge and understanding between disciplines. This lack of understanding has contributed to communication barriers, such as an absence of dialogue, resistance to new ideas, and an avoidance of things that exist beyond one's comfort zone. This gap between providers creates an opportunity for poor planning and decision making, unsafe patient care, and untoward patient events (Hammick, Freeth, Koppel, Reeves, & Barr, 2007).

There is a growing interest in the use of interprofessional leadership. Interprofessional leadership models have been utilized within health care administration and health care education for over a decade. An active and growing body of research is now available for review. Current studies are evaluating various models to identify participant perceptions of IPL, effects of IPL on collaboration, and the impact of IPL on operational and patient outcomes.

IPL is a concept that has demonstrated its worth because its goals are grounded in improving patient safety and overall patient outcomes. Through the process of program evaluation and curriculum revision, gold standard models for IPL will evolve and emerge to serve as guide tools for less developed programs (Reeves, Zwarenstein, Goldman, Barr, Freeth, Hammick, & Koppel, 2008).

Baker, L., Egan-Lee, E., Martimianakis, T., & Reeves, S. (2010). Relationships of power: Implications for interprofessional education. *Journal of Interprofessional Care, 25* (2), 98–104.

Hammick, M., Freeth, D., Koppel, I., Reeves, S., & Barr, H. (2007). A best evidence systematic review of interprofessional education: BEME guide no. 9. *Medicine Teaching, 29* (8), 735–51.

Reeves, S., Zwarenstein, M., Goldman, J., Barr, H., Freeth, D., Hammick, M., & Koppel, I. (2008). Interprofessional education: effects on professional practice and health care outcomes. *Cochrane Database Systematic Review, 23* (1).

Kimberly B. Hall

I

J

JOHNSON & JOHNSON WHARTON FELLOWS PROGRAM IN MANAGEMENT FOR NURSE EXECUTIVES

This program, commonly referred to as "The Wharton Fellows Program" (executiveeducation.wharton.upenn.edu/open-enrollment/health-care-programs/Fellows-Program-Management-Nurse-Executives.cfm) was established in 1983 at the Wharton School of Business at the University of Pennsylvania. It was the first program to offer health care management and leadership education for senior nursing executives in a business school setting. Chief Nursing Officers compete for admittance to each year's class. An application is required, and although tuition is waived, participants must pay for their own travel and living expenses during the program.

The program is three weeks long, admitting 40 participants a year. Current content areas include such topics as finance, value-driven decision making, emotional intelligence, business simulations, scenario planning, systems thinking, and managing complexity. Content and teaching methodologies are kept up to date with annual reviews from subject experts in business, health care and academics.

The goal of the program is to prepare chief nursing officers to act as full strategic partners with other organizational health care executives and members of governance boards. The anticipated outcome is that chief nursing officers will develop strong clinical voices in the senior management of the health care organization and can then serve as clinical advocates for quality patient care.

The program concludes with a 3-day executive forum that includes the chief nursing officer and his or her respective CEO/COO. The goal of this final session is for the pair to consider and plan ways to apply the learned management concepts in their home organization.

The Wharton Fellows program is internationally known as the leading program of its kind. Fellows develop a lifelong network of colleagues as well as friendships that continue throughout their career.

Pamela Austin Thompson

LEADERSHIP DEVELOPMENT

Leadership development implies learning experiences, processes, and devices that enable individuals to influence the thoughts or actions of another or others toward some specified purpose or goals. This means that leadership development is an aspect of human maturation that is essential for competent and effective leadership. Therefore, it is heralded as a key priority for enhancing the performance and achievements of individuals, groups, and organizations. In recent years, there has been a rapid emergence of leadership development programs and related training initiatives within academic institutions, health services systems, professional associations, and a wide array of freestanding groups and organizations (www.leadershipdevelopment.com).

The curriculum of most nursing schools and colleges provides content on leadership. There are master of science in nursing programs that offer a minor or concentration in leadership. In some cases, there are programs leading to a master of science degree in nursing leadership focused on such areas as public health, long-term care, complex health care organizations, and advanced practice. National nursing professional organizations and nursing service organizations in health care systems offer short-term training courses, workshops or institutes to advance the leadership development of nurse executives, educators, and clinical practitioners. Business schools around the country offer a wide range of leadership development opportunities and resources (Aroian & Dienemann 2005; Feldman & Greenberg, 2005). Many offer regularly scheduled seminars, courses, or workshops for middle and senior managers from private, public, and nonprofit sectors. In addition, leadership development programs are offered by numerous other enterprises that profess to strengthen the capacity of individuals and organizations. In several cases, the programs are based on specific models of leadership. Popular among them are Servant Leadership (www.greenleaf.org) and Transformational Leadership (www.tcslearning.com).

The perspectives of leadership development evolve from conceptions of the meaning and nature of leadership. Very often, leadership is conceived as the function of a single individual (i.e., a leader) within a group or organization. In numerous cases, this narrow conception of leadership is apparent in the descriptions of courses, programs, and other initiatives intended to enhance leadership capabilities. This reflects a limited perspective of what leadership development entails. In these cases, efforts are focused on preparing individuals for effective performance as *a leader*—absent comparable attention to their preparation for effective performance as a *follower*. Also missing are indications of the interactive and mutually dependent relationship between leaders and followers, which can enhance or undermine effective performance in these leadership roles. Furthermore, the principles and model approaches in these cases are inattentive to the impact of social, political, collective, and other contexts on the performance, achievement, and productivity of leaders and followers.

This tendency to equate *leader* development with *leadership* development compromises efforts to build the leadership capacity of groups and organizations. It is suggested that support for programs or other training initiatives that reflect this tendency has been a misallocation of resources (Iles & Preece, 2006). The most enlightening and productive leadership development approaches are those in which a broad conception of leadership is apparent. For example, the term "leadership" is used to refer to a mechanism, process, or modality for achieving some specified purpose or goals—not to refer to the purpose or goals, per se. The program or special initiative purports to prepare individuals for competent and effective performance in leadership roles—not merely to prepare leaders. Special attention is given to the interactive and mutually dependent relationships of leaders and followers; the nature and significance of authority, power, and related issues or problems that are ubiquitous in human groups and organizations; and the nature and significance of contextual factors that can enhance or inhibit effective leadership.

Comprehensive models for leadership development display the features described above (Bessent, 2006). There are no apparent indications of the tendency to equate *leader* development with *leadership* development or to confuse leadership with management. They give due attention to the play of group dynamics, interpersonal relationships, and intrapersonal processes on the performance of leaders and followers. They are purported to offer opportunities for individuals to obtain the kind of learning that attends the personal qualities, knowledge, and capabilities deemed essential for effective performance in leadership roles. The objectives are to promote the kind of learning that comes from direct experience of fact and situation, reflective and abstract thinking, and integrative and reflective practice (Bolden, 2004). They have been described as "learning *for* leadership," "learning *about* leadership," and "learning *to succeed* in leadership roles," respectively (Dumas, 2006). The modes of instruction are necessarily experiential as well as didactic. Although it is difficult to find all these features in a single leadership development program, close approximations are apparent in the offerings of such organizations as the A. K. Rice Institute (www.uvm.edu/~mkessler/akrice/index.html), the Center for Creative Leadership (www.ccl.org), the National Training Laboratories (www.ntl.org), the James MacGregor Burns Academy of Leadership (www.academy.umd.edu), the Grubb Institute (www.grubb.org.uk), the International Forum for Social Innovation (www.continents.com/FIIS.htm), and T-Consult (www.t-consult.biz).

MENTORING

Another aspect of leadership development is mentoring. Depending on the mentors' knowledge of leadership roles and style, this aspect, as described by Dumas (2008), has the capacity to capture the relationship between the leader and the follower, the ability to understand the role and system in which the leadership is possible, and the experiential development of leadership over a period of time.

Mentoring can be described as a dynamic, reciprocal, intense personal relationship in which a more experienced person acts as a guide, a role model, a teacher, and a sponsor of a less experienced person (Johnson & Ridley, 2008). It is also usually identified as an act of generativity, passing on a professional legacy or intentionally facilitating the career development of another. "Men Toring" is frequently associated with men, and nursing, being predominantly a female profession, has been late in grasping the power of this concept and process.

The term *mentor* originated from Greek mythology (Malone, 1998). Mentor was an Ithacan noble and a trusted friend of Odysseus. He was charged with caring for Odysseus's son, Telemachus, when Odysseus departed for the Trojan War. The goddess Athena assumed Mentor's form to serve as a coach, a teacher, a guardian, and a protector. It is interesting that the female Athena had to assume the form of a man to Men Tor the young man, perhaps a future warrior. In Athena's female form, she may have been identified as inadequately "nursing" Telemachus into his role. This contrast between the male mentor and the female nurse is challenging because both provide support and facilitate the growth and development of the individual. Yet, the gender difference may play a part as to the shortage of mentors and mentoring in the nursing profession.

There is also the question of the totally positive nature of mentoring. It could be described as a slightly narcissistic process reminiscent of Narcissus who drowned in a pool mesmerized by his own image. The mentor usually chooses the protégé based on a sense of resonance with the individual; that is, the less experienced nurse may remind the more experienced one of himself or herself at an earlier time in life. This attraction to resonating characteristics or qualities in the other provides a life line for the mentor who yearns for immortality and seeks it by choosing a protégé, who may be an idealistic representation of self. The protégé in turn, resonating to the mentor's role and abilities, yearns for the success, position, and wisdom of the mentor.

More recently, the traditional approach of a single mentor has lost favor in comparison with a network of mentors (DeLong, Gabarro, & Lees, 2007; Kram & Higgins, 2008). The idea is for the young, less experienced nurse to establish mentoring networks that include peers as well as more than one traditional mentor. This grouping has been described as one's own personal board of directors.

See also Mentoring

Aroian, J., & Dienemann, J. A. (2005). Practice oriented leadership education. In H. R. Feldman & M. Greenberg (Eds.), *Educating nurses for leadership*. New York, NY: Springer Publishing.

Bessent, H. (2006). *The soul of leadership*. Battle Creek, MI: The W. K. Kellogg Foundation.

Bolden, R. (2004). Leadership and performance. In *What is leadership? Southwest research report*. Exeter, UK: Centre for Leadership Studies, Exeter University. Retrieved June 2, 2006, from www.leadershipsouthwest.com

DeLong, T., Gabarro, J., & Lees, R. (2007). *When professionals Have to Lead*. Cambridge, MA: Harvard Business School Press.

Dumas, R. G. (2006). *Leadership: An enlightened perspective*. Unpublished manuscript. University of Michigan, School of Nursing.

Dumas, R.G. (2008). Leadership development. In H. R. Feldman, (Ed.). *Nursing leadership: A concise encyclopedia*. New York, NY: Springer Publishing.

Feldman, H. R., & Greenberg, M. J. (Eds.). (2005). *Educating nurses for leadership*. New York, NY: Springer Publishing.

L

Iles, P., & Preece, D. (2006). Developing leaders or developing leadership? *Leadership*, 2(3), 317–340.

Johnson, W. B., & Ridley, C. (2008). *The elements of mentoring.* New York, NY: McMillan.

Kram, K., & Higgins, M. (2008, September 22). A new approach to mentoring. *Wall Street Journal*.

Malone, B. (1998). A song of power. In C. Vance & R. Olson (Eds.), *The mentor connection in nursing*. New York, NY: Springer Publishing.

Beverly Louise Malone

LEADERSHIP IN PRACTICE SETTINGS

Leadership in practice settings refers to the skill sets that facilitate care delivery, or to the roles of leadership in various positions that informally or formally constitute an agency's leadership structure. Leadership skill sets are best described by primary sources, such as Kouzes and Posner (1997) in their text on evidence-based practice. In brief, the best practices of leadership are characterized by (1) challenging the process, (2) inspiring a shared vision, (3) enabling others to act, (4) modeling the way, and (5) encouraging the heart. A writer and speaker whose work has greatly influenced organizational development in nursing is Tim Porter-O'Grady (Kruger, Wilson, & O'Grady, 1999). Leadership, using these concepts, ultimately is embodied in shared governance structures that may be as formalized as elected bodies of staff who determine practice.

In patient care settings, leadership has several roles, ranging from clinical leadership at the bedside to the leadership/management of the chief nursing officer (CNO). Leadership principles must be exercised by the nurse providing direct care that both delivers and integrates the plan of care with the patient and family, by the charge nurse coordinating the activities of the unit during a shift, and by the formal leader of a division of patient care units. An emerging role is that of the Clinical Nurse Leader® (www.aacn.nche.edu), a nurse whose leadership focuses on care coordination of a distinct group of patients while also providing direct care in complex situations. This role is delivered and implemented in various settings.

Novice leadership skills are expected of new graduates, with mutual understanding that an organization provides support and development of the following skills: prioritization, time management, communication, interdisciplinary collaboration, patient/family education, and delegation, and follow-up with ancillary care staff. Recognition of the need to further develop the leadership role of new graduates is evidenced in the growth of nurse internship or residency programs.

Leadership of a group of nurses during a shift involves the ability to facilitate patient flow, to allocate human resources (nursing staff) that match patient needs based on acuity and goals of care, and to effectively communicate the "hand off" to the next leader. The nurse manager position, as the 24-hour leader, is the single most critical position in most organizations. This formal leader is responsible for the hiring, development, and termination of nursing staff, the fiscal performance of the unit, and the quality and safety outcomes of patients and staff. The development and engagement of nurse managers is a national priority (Mackoff, 2011). A breadth of resources is available on this topic (American Organization of Nurse Executives, 2007; www.aone.org). Additional nursing leaders essential to patient safety, staff support, and agency operations are supervisors or nurse administrators who are both nursing and hospital/facility representatives on evenings, nights, and weekends. These unsung nursing leaders form the arms around the living delivery system of patient care.

The chief nurse executive or the CNO in an excellent organization is a transformational leader who communicates expectations, develops leaders, and evolves the organization to meet current/anticipated needs and strategic priorities (ANCC, 2008). The CNO is optimally positioned in the organization to influence change operationally and strategically via vision, mission, advocacy, and resources as outlined in the nursing strategic plan, aligned with the organization's plan. This role is complex, demanding, and requires a portfolio of both leadership and management skills. The CNO must possess and demonstrate an understanding of the discipline of nursing practice, financial, change, performance and outcomes management, quality drivers, information technology, regulatory compliance, the value of evidence-based practice and research, cultural diversity, ethics, interdisciplinary collaboration, and governance. The CNO of an excellent organization inspires passion about nursing, care delivery, healthy work environments, and culture of quality and patient safety by exemplifying transformational leadership (a component of the revised Magnet Recognition Model© that sets the standard for excellence in practice).

See also American Organization of Nurse Executives; Clinical Nurse Leader (CNL®); Shared Governance Is Structure Not Process; Staff Retention

Kouzes, J. M., & Posner, B. Z. (1997). *The leadership challenge*. San Francisco, CA: Jossey-Bass.

Krueger Wilson, C., & Porter-O'Grady, T. (1999). *Leading the revolution in healthcare*. Gaithersburg, MD: Aspen Publications.

Mackoff, B. (2011). *Nurse manager engagement: Strategies for excellence and commitment*. Salisbury, MD: Jones & Bartlett Publishers.

Additional information is available at the following Web sites:

American Association of Colleges of Nursing. Retrieved from http://www.aacn.nche.edu/CNL/faq.htm

American Nurses Association. Retrieved from http://www.ana.org

American Nurses Association. (2009). *Scope & standards of nurse administrators*. Washington, DC: Author.

American Nurses Credentialing Center. Retrieved from http://www.nursecredentialing.org

American Nurses Credentialing Center. (2008). *Magnet recognition program*. Silver Spring, MD: Author.

American Organization of Nurse Executives. (2007). *Nurse manager leadership partnership*. Retrieved September 28, 2010, from http://www.aone.org/aone/resource/NMLP/nmlp.html

Executive Fellows.net. Retrieved from http://www.executivefellows.net

Susan Bowar-Ferres

L

LEADERSHIP TRAITS

In his classic book *On Becoming a Leader*, Dr. Warren Bennis (1994) stated that "managers are people who do things right, while leaders are people who do the right thing." Being a leader, as distinct from a manager, requires certain attributes or leadership traits. Controversy has existed as to whether these traits are inborn or are acquired. The main categories of useful leadership characteristics are moral and ethical values, technical competence, knowledge and conceptual skill, a desire to be a leader, personality, and people skills. These traits encompass an intellectual and emotional ability to envision and to communicate that vision, an ability to establish successful interpersonal relationships, and the ability to use power to influence.

Leaders must have in-depth knowledge in the field in which they lead, an ability for abstract thinking, a history of achieving results, an ability to communicate, motivate, and delegate, and an ability to cultivate talent in others, good judgment, and good character. Leaders are able to motivate others, use highly developed knowledge and technical skill, and lead change. Some are inspirational, or charismatic; all need to be clear communicators who show commitment and compassion. A leader must be willing, trustworthy, and just. Moral leadership is critical; one must do *good*, in as honest and courageous a way as possible. Leadership means to be vulnerable, to take risks, and to be willing to accept mistakes.

Many different descriptions of leadership abound, including relational, servant, transactional, transformational, directive, supportive, participative, achievement oriented, charismatic, and quantum. Quantum leadership is based on the concepts inherent in chaos theory, which states that the environment is constantly shifting and becoming more complex, everything is interconnected, and that roles are fluid and outcome-oriented (Malloch & Porter-O'Grady, 2009, p. 4).

The current thinking of what constitutes a good leader is a departure from the past when the focus was on control and command. Today's leader, who is transformational, needs to have a healthy quotient of emotional intelligence and the desire and confidence to empower others. Persons who are successful leaders have self-awareness, capacity to self-reflect, insight, and empathy. The importance of these traits was emphasized in the late 1990s when "emotional intelligence" was identified by Goleman (1998) in the book *Working with Emotional Intelligence*, as a critical skill necessary for effective leadership. These characteristics have been historically true for nurses.

The term "transformational leadership" was first coined by Burns (1978), in his seminal work, *Leadership*. Transformational leadership builds on complexity theory, and these leaders are described as having vision, self-confidence, self-direction, honesty, energy, loyalty, commitment, and ability to develop and implement a vision while empowering followers (Barker, Sullivan, & Emery, 2006; Finkelman, 2006). Burns drew these conclusions after looking at the leadership styles of famous political leaders such as Mahatma Gandhi, Franklin Delano Roosevelt, and John Fitzgerald Kennedy. Leaders must have purposes that are positive and productive and followers whose needs are met and satisfied and thus motivated to high levels of performance (Barker et al., 2006).

To be successful and transformative, one needs to be in a transformational culture where working with change becomes the norm, a way of life, and the expectation is that the transformational leader will enable others to develop their leadership potential. Transformation can only happen in the context of an interactive relationship.

Nursing leadership in today's world, with its rapidly changing health care environment, requires talent and skills necessary to keep up with and stay ahead of the curve. The Institute of Medicine (2003) report, *Keeping Patients Safe: Transforming the Work Environment of Nurses*, underscores this belief as a way to increase safety and reduce errors. Transformational leadership that recognizes the interdependence between a chaotic environment and a visionary leader is required to be successful. The multiplicity of demands and the rapidity of change require the successful leader to have the necessary traits to know how to manage effectively in a chaotic environment.

See also Change; Complex Adaptive Systems (Chaos Theory); Emotional Intelligence; Power and Leadership

Barker, A. M., Sullivan, D. T., & Emery, M. J. (2006). *Leadership competencies for clinical managers*. Boston: Jones and Bartlett.

Bass, B., & Avalio, B. (1994). *Improving organizational effectiveness through transformational leadership*. Thousand Oaks, CA: Sage.

Bennis, W. (1994). *On becoming a leader*. Reading, MA: Perseus Books.

Burns, J. M. (1978). *Leadership*. New York: Harper and Row.

Emmerling, R.J., Shanval, V.K., & Mandal, M.K. (Eds.) (2008). *Emotional intelligence: Theoretical and cultural perspectives*. Hauppauge, NY: Nova Science Publishers.

Finkelman, A. (2006). *Leadership and management in nursing*. Upper Saddle River, NJ: Prentice Hall.

Goleman, D. (1998). *Working with emotional intelligence*. New York: Bantam Books.

Institute of Medicine. (2003). *Keeping patients safe: Transforming the work environment for nurses*. Washington, DC: Author.

Malloch, K., & Porter-O'Grady, T. (2009). *The quantum leader: Applications for the new world of work* (2nd ed.). Sudbury, MA: Jones and Bartlett.

Marilyn Jaffe-Ruiz

LEAPFROG GROUP

The Leapfrog Group was officially launched in November 2000 amid discussions sparked by the 1999 Institute of Medicine's report, *To Err Is Human: Building a Safer Health System*. The report brought to light serious concerns regarding errors in U.S. hospitals, which may account for as many as 98,000 deaths annually. The report went on to recommend many potential solutions, one of which is for large employers to use their purchasing power to exert market pressures on hospitals to pay more attention to quality standards (Kohn, Corrigan, & Donaldson, 1999). According to the organization's Web site, the Leapfrog Group is "a member supported program aimed at mobilizing employer purchasing power to alert America's health industry that big leaps in health care safety, quality and customer value will be recognized and rewarded" (Leapfrog Group, n.d.-a, para. 1). The foundation of the Leapfrog Group was made possible through funding from the Business Roundtable, and the members constitute several Fortune 500 companies representing more than 37 million Americans in 50 states (Leapfrog Group, n.d.-a).

The data collected by the Leapfrog Group are based on hospitals' self-reporting and is completely voluntary. The Leapfrog Group Hospital Quality and Safety Survey is the tool used, and it is most applicable to urban acute care hospitals, although any hospital is invited to participate. The data are then posted on a monthly basis for the public and employers to view when making decisions regarding care (Leapfrog Group, n.d.-b). More than 1,960 hospitals that participate in the survey encompass 31 regions of the United States (Leapfrog Group, n.d.-b). According to Leapfrog Group 2009 survey, less than 50% of hospitals met Leapfrog's outcome, volume, and process standards for six high-risk procedures and conditions. Research suggests that following evidence-based guidelines for these procedures and conditions is known to save lives (Danforth, 2010). See Table 1.

L

Table 1
EVIDENCE-BASED GUIDELINES

High-risk surgery	Reporting hospitals that fully met Leapfrog's standard in 2009 (%)
Aortic valve replacement	11.8
Abdominal aortic aneurism repair	36.1
Pancreatic resection	33.5
Esophageal resection	31.5
Weight-loss (bariatric) surgery	36.6
High-risk deliveries	29.9

The use of informational technology is critical to leveraging and advancing patient safety and quality. The Obama administration included Computerized Physician Order Entry (CPOE) as part of the final Meaningful Use regulations, which was published March 2010 in the Federal Register. By including CPOE, the nation has acknowledged that technology can be lifesaving and is critical step to move quality care forward. However, regardless of committing as much as $30 billion to informatics technological upgrades, the regulations do not require hospitals to reassure taxpayers that the technology is safe. To demonstrate "meaningful use" of health information technology and receive federal money, hospitals are not required to substantiate that their system actually works as intended and improves patient outcomes. The Leapfrog Group believes the regulations should require this additional protection for Americans (Danforth, 2010).

The Leapfrog Hospital Rewards Program is "a pay-for-performance program to recognize and reward hospitals for their performance in both the quality and efficiency of inpatient care" (Leapfrog Group, n.d.-c, para. 1). The rewards may be in the form of a bonus payment, higher reimbursement rates, public recognition, or increased patient market share. According to a study by the Center for Studying Health System Change (HSC) in Washington, DC, however, most hospital executives report difficulty implementing the safety practices because of financial constraints and limited financial incentives after implementation (Few Hospitals are Close to Filling Leapfrog Goals, 2004). The Leapfrog Group creates guidelines and tools to determine appropriate incentives, yet it remains up to the employers or insurance companies to be willing to provide these financial incentives.

The impact of implementing the safety initiatives outlined by the Leapfrog Group is subject to varying support in the literature. Although some of the initiatives, such as the standards of care for the patient suffering acute myocardial infarction, are supported by a great deal of research and backed by the American Heart Association, others have less reliable data supporting their implementation. A study found in *Critical Care Medicine* created a model to analyze the financial implications of staffing intensive care units with intensivists. The findings indicate an average cost savings of $510,000 to $3.3 million for a 6- to 18-bed intensive care unit. However, a limitation of this study is its partial funding by the Business Roundtable, which also sponsors the Leapfrog Group (Pronovost et al., 2006). In addition, issues are at play with the operations of initiatives such as CPOE. There is very little known about the impacts of verbal orders and RNs entering orders into CPOE as a courtesy to physicians. The health care industry needs to ensure its practices and improvement initiatives are founded on evidence-based care.

Another key component when discussing the Leapfrog Group initiatives is the consideration of nurses' impact on patient safety and quality standards. The goals currently outlined by the Leapfrog Group have very little to do with direct nursing care. Nursing leaders voice the need to look at the nursing shortage and quantify its impact on patient safety and outcomes (Wynd, 2002). Several studies are finding that "a number of medical, cardiac, and respiratory complications and length of stay [are] directly related to nursing care" (Hudon, 2003, p. 236). How nursing contributes to patient safety is not clearly understood by the public or by the members of the Leapfrog Group. A great deal of this is a result of limited nursing research indicating clear, measurable impacts on patient safety.

The Leapfrog Group has certainly been successful in heightening the awareness of patient safety issues in hospitals for both consumers and providers; however, the implementation is lagging mainly as a result of fiscal barriers and some uncertainty regarding patient safety and outcomes estimates. The Leapfrog Group safety initiatives would benefit from more research to quantify the impacts of their implementation. The nursing profession needs to clearly define and measure its impact on patient safety to be become a larger part of the equation. Only then will the Leapfrog Group, consumers, and employers be able to grasp the significance of nursing on patient safety and outcomes.

See also Evidence-Based Practice; Institute for Healthcare Improvement

Danforth, M. (2010). *Statement by the Leapfrog Group on the final meaningful use rule: Good first step, but grave concerns*. Retrieved January 28, 2011, from Leapfrog Group: http://www.leapfroggroup.org/news/leapfrog_news/4779269

Few hospitals are close to filling Leapfrog goals. (2004, April 1). *Healthcare Risk Management*, 45.

Hudon, P. S. (2003). Leapfrog standards: Implications for nursing practice. *Nursing Economic$*, 21, 233–236.

Kohn, L. T., Corrigan, J., & Donaldson, M. S. (1999). *To err is human: Building a safer healthcare system*. Washington, DC: National Academies Press.

Leapfrog Group. (n.d.-a). *Leapfrog Group fact sheet*. Retrieved September 28, 2006, from http://www.leapfroggroup.org/about_us/leapfrog-factsheet

Leapfrog Group. (n.d.-b). *How Leapfrog works*. Retrieved September 28, 2006, from http://www.leapfroggroup.org/about_us/how_leapfrog_works

Leapfrog Group. (n.d.-c). *Leapfrog hospital rewards program*. Retrieved September 28, 2006, from https://leapfrog.medstat.com/hrp/index.asp

Leapfrog Group. (2010). *Time to recommit to preventing "never events."* Retrieved January 28, 2011, from Leapfrog: http://www.leapfroggroup.org/news/leapfrog_news/4783929

Pronovost, P. J., Needham, D. M., Waters, H., Birkmeyer, C. M., Calinawan, R. B., Birkmeyer, J. D., et al. (2006). Intensive care unit physician staffing: Financial modeling of the Leapfrog standard. *Critical Care Medicine*, 34(2), S18–S24.

Wynd, C. (2002). AONE's leadership exchange: Leapfrog Group jumps over nursing. *Nursing Management*, 33(12), 20.

Stacy Hutton Johnson

LEGAL NURSE CONSULTING

A legal nurse consultant combines nursing expertise with specialized training to assist attorneys with medical-related cases. Legal nurse consultants come from every nursing specialty and apply their nursing knowledge and skills to all kinds of health care and nursing issues. The legal nurse consultant is a full-fledged professional member of the attorney's litigation team. While the attorney is the expert on legal issues, the legal nurse consultant is the expert on nursing, the health care system, and medical record documentation. Few attorneys know how to review medical records or understand the health care issues important to medical malpractice and personal injury lawsuits.

Consulting with a legal nurse consultant is far more cost-effective for the attorney than using an MD expert, and legal nurse consultants have a better grasp of the medical records. Because nurses spend more time than doctors educating patients, legal nurse consultants are also superbly qualified to educate attorneys on medical terminology, disease processes, and the health care system in general. This expertise saves the attorney time and money and benefits the legal system by promoting fair and just resolution of medical-related cases.

TYPES OF CASES ON WHICH LEGAL NURSE CONSULTANTS CONSULT

Legal nurse consultants consult on a myriad of cases, from simple back injuries caused by auto accidents, to complex cases, such as brain injuries in newborns.

Medical and Nursing Malpractice Cases

Medical and nursing malpractice cases involve alleged professional negligence of a health care provider or facility. Every year, 98,000–195,000 people in hospitals die from medical negligence. On average, hospitals experience one medication error per patient every day (see Web reference reports and synopses listed below). Medical malpractice litigation pervades practically every nursing specialty. A legal nurse consultant's role in these types of cases is to research standards of care that apply and point out any deviations from or adherences to the applicable standards.

General Negligence Cases

General negligence cases are nonprofessional negligence cases, such as auto accidents, falls in grocery stores, amusement park–ride deaths, and so on. The legal nurse consultant helps the attorney understand the extent of the injuries and examine whether or not they were caused by that particular incident.

Product Liability Cases

Product liability cases involve allegedly defective products, such as medical devices, pharmaceuticals, and nonmedical devices, such as defective automobiles, washing machines, or hair dryers. Legal nurse consultants have worked on many headline cases in the news, for example, FenPhen, Vioxx®, Fosamax, and implantable defibrillators. The legal nurse consultant's role in these instances is to identify whether or not the defective product caused the alleged injuries.

Toxics Torts and Environmental Cases

Toxics torts and environmental cases involve injuries as a result of exposure to toxins and chemicals, such as dumping of toxic sludge into a residential community and contamination of groundwater by a manufacturing plant. The role of the legal nurse consultant is to help identify whether or not the toxins caused the injuries or deaths.

Workers' Compensation and Workplace Injury Cases

Workers' compensation and workplace injury cases include any job-related injury, for example, cumulative trauma disorders, back injury, and body part amputations.

Criminal Cases

A crime is any act that society has deemed contrary to the public good. Legal nurse consultants work on criminal cases ranging from driving under the influence of alcohol or other drugs to homicide to other types of physical abuse.

Any Case in Which Health, Illness, and Injury Is an Issue

Probate or Medicare fraud and custody battles are examples of other types of cases where legal nurse consultants provide a variety of services to attorneys, for example, they may:

- identify, locate, review, and interpret relevant medical records, hospital policies and procedures, and other essential documents and tangible items;
- search and summarize medical and nursing literature and integrate results of the search into case analysis;
- identify adherences to and deviations from the applicable standards of care;
- assist with discovery and preparing for court;
- identify issues of tampering with the medical records;
- identify causation issues, assess damages/injuries, and identify contributing factors;
- identify and recommend potential defendants;
- identify, locate, and interface with testifying experts needed for the case;

- interview plaintiff and defense clients, key witnesses, and experts;
- prepare questions for deposition or trial examination (direct or cross);
- assist with exhibit preparation and other demonstrative evidence.

Legal nurse consultants may consult with attorneys behind the scenes or testify as expert witnesses. In addition to working with plaintiff and defense attorneys, legal nurse consultants work with insurance companies, utilization review firms, government agencies, private corporations, and hospitals, both as staff members and as independent consultants.

THE LEGAL NURSE CONSULTANT'S IMPACT ON THE LEGAL SYSTEM

As representatives of the nursing profession, legal nurse consultants uphold the standards of care for the entire health care community. By giving their objective opinions on the merits of cases and deviations from recognized standards, they help to improve the quality of nursing practice. Legal nurse consultant's opinions also contribute to the effectiveness of the legal system and are often critical in reaching a fair and just outcome for all parties. As a result, the legal nurse consultant plays an invaluable role on the litigation team. Another contribution legal nurse consultants make is identifying fraudulent and non-meritorious claims, thus helping to defend against such claims or keep them out of the system. By making all parties aware of the documented facts and research connected with a case, legal nurse consultants help to ensure that the legal system uses this information properly and without distortion.

L

LEGAL NURSE CONSULTING CERTIFICATION AND CAREER OPTIONS

Nurses wishing to enter the field of legal nurse consulting must undergo training and certification. The Certified Legal Nurse Consultant^{CM} certification is the official certification of the National Alliance of Certified Legal Nurse Consultants (NACLNC®). With 5,000 members, the NACLNC is the largest and most recognized association of legal nurse consultants.

The legal nurse consulting profession affords nurses of all ages and experience levels an option for establishing a satisfying and profitable part-time or full-time career. Registered nurses are best prepared to enter the specialty when they have had at least 3 to 5 years of clinical experience. Certified Legal Nurse Consultants typically earn fees of $150 per hour by using their nursing expertise in new and exciting ways. The field of legal nurse consulting is rapidly growing in popularity with attorneys as well as with registered nurses and was voted one of the 10 hottest jobs for 2007 by CareerBuilder.com.

See also Malpractice

Additional information is available at these Web sites:

Core Curriculum for Legal Nurse Consulting® textbook. Retrieved from Amazon.com

Vickie's Legal Nurse Consulting Blog. Retrieved from LegalNurse.com/VickiesBlog

CLNC® Success Stories, Fourth Edition. Retrieved from Amazon.com

Preview Your New Life as a CLNC® Consultant DVD. Retrieved from LegalNurse.com

National Alliance of Certified Legal Nurse Consultants. Retrieved from LegalNurse.com

Report. Retrieved from http://www.nap.edu/catalog.php?record_id=11623

Press release/synopsis. Retrieved from http://www8.nationalacademies.org/onpinews/newsitem.aspx?RecordID=11623

Vickie L. Milazzo

LETTERS OF RECOMMENDATION

Letters of recommendation are important throughout the career of a nurse. They are needed to apply for admission to a university or a new position, for review of promotion or tenure application, and for consideration for a fellowship, grant or honor. The person writing the letter of recommendation, often a mentor, speaks to your abilities, strengths, and promise; that evaluation complements other available sources of information, for example, a curriculum vitae, undergraduate or graduate transcripts, test scores, reviews, publication reprints, and the like. Both the person requesting a letter and the person writing the letter need to keep certain things in mind for maximum effectiveness.

The person soliciting the reference should choose someone who is accomplished, at the level to which the applicant aspires (e.g., an assistant professor seeking promotion would ask an associate professor or full professor to serve as reference), and likely to write a convincing letter by the required deadline. If applying for a national position, the applicant would not want all references to come from her or his home institution because it would look as if he or she is held in high regard solely by day-to-day colleagues. If applying for a new position, however, it would look suspect if you did not ask someone who is currently in the same workplace to serve as a reference. If applying for an honor, someone who is a coauthor of several articles may seem too disposed in your direction to be objective so that person should not be the primary or sole supporter; if the honor being applied for is interdisciplinary, then the sponsors should be interdisciplinary too. Unless he or she knows the person very well and that individual has already agreed to serve as a reference as needed, at the time of the search the person should be asked to serve in that capacity before being listed as such. The requester should make sure the sponsor has a copy of everything needed to write a comprehensive letter, for example, guidelines specifying what the reference should speak to (guidelines for promotion and tenure at a particular university, etc.), the requester's latest curriculum vitae, or an outline of career highlights that relate to the grant or honor.

When it comes to writing letters of recommendation, there are some that are written for the sake of the profession, for example, when you are asked to evaluate someone you do not know for promotion or tenure, and some that are helpful to a specific person. Regarding the latter, there may be times when it is appropriate to say "I don't think I would be the best person to write a letter of support," particularly if the person is not well known to the recommender or if the person is not held in high regard. The writer should be clear about what background materials are needed to complete the task and be prepared to meet the deadline. A good letter of recommendation adds greater depth of understanding about the applicant, makes clear from the onset the purpose of the letter, does not replicate the information already available in the curriculum vitae (providing concrete examples of how the person responded to challenges or demonstrated important qualities), makes useful comparisons with others to provide needed context ("I have supervised 25 dissertations and she is one of the top two I have worked with"), and ends with a summary statement that reaffirms key points made (McBride & Lovejoy, 1995). The writer should end the letter listing title(s) and credentials to reaffirm the authority behind the words and check to make sure the spelling and grammar are correct because mistakes (using principle investigator instead of principal investigator) can reduce one's perceived authority.

Vague words and trite phrases (nice, good, solid performance, relates well to others) are to be avoided because they may be construed as negative in certain situations, or, at the very least, do not convey much added understanding of the candidate. Because there is evidence that men are described more using standout adjectives—superb, outstanding, remarkable—and that using communal characteristics to describe women—kind, sympathetic, sensitive, nurturing—may mean that they are judged stereotypically as less capable of leadership, it is important that letter writers review what they say for unintended consequences (Madera, Hebl, & Martin, 2009). This caution also holds for ambiguous statements: "This person should be well qualified to achieve tenure at your institution." "I am pleased to say this applicant is a former colleague of mine."

The biggest criticism of narrative letters is that they tend to be overly positive. To counteract that possibility, some admission processes and grant applications are making use of standardized letters of reference with demonstrated validity and reliability. The person being evaluated is typically judged in terms of a set list of qualities or abilities, with the rater forced to make judgments comparing that individual to others in the same situation. For a review of available tools, read Megginson (2009). However, even when standardized letters of reference are used, they often are coupled with space for narrative comments because the judgment of those who have worked closely with the person remains important information in deciding whether that individual is worthy of an opportunity.

See also Career Stages; Gender and Leadership; Mentoring

Madera, J. M., Hebl, M. R., & Martin, R. C. (2009). Gender and letters of recommendation for academia: Agentic and communal differences. *Journal of Applied Psychology, 94,* 1591–1599.

McBride, A. B., & Lovejoy, K. B. (1995). Requesting and writing effective letters of recommendation: Some guidelines for candidates and sponsors. *Journal of Nursing Education, 34,* 95–96.

Megginson, L. (2009). Noncognitive constructs in graduate admissions: An integrative review of available instruments. *Nurse Educator, 34,* 254–261.

Angela Barron McBride

LEVERAGING

Leveraging is best defined within the context of a discipline or intent. The word "leveraging" brings to mind a variety of motive or outcome—gain, advantage, enhance, power, improve, and expand. The concept has been shown to be relevant in nursing practice, education, research, administration, and policy. For example, in clinical nursing practice, Arora, Johnson, Lovinger, Humphrey, and Meltzer (2005) studied the power of leveraging to improve patient safety by minimizing communication failures in patient sign-outs. Kitt, Kreider, Leonard, Szekendi, and Lewis (2008) analyzed the advantage of leveraging technology for nursing hand-offs. Jeffs, MacMillan, and Malone (2009) described the advantage of leveraging safer nursing care in near misses. Potempa, Phancharoenworakul, Glass, Chasombat, and Cody (2009) described managing HIV/AIDS through leveraging the role of public health nursing. The outcomes achieved by a national collaboration strategy expanded the role of public health nurses and the initiation of a nurse practitioner's role in the prevention and treatment of HIV/AIDS. They found that with these changes, the capacity of the health care system in Thailand was more effective in meeting the challenges posed by all infectious diseases, particularly HIV/AIDS.

The advantage of leveraging multimedia for learning and social media to enhance relationships and business pervades the literature (Leveraging Multimedia for Learning, 2010). Leveraging organizational knowledge to deliver long-term advantage involves knowledge management, that is, engineering various knowledge-centric processes and developing organizational structures to support those that in turn require technology to capture, codify, store, disseminate, and reuse the knowledge (Alavi & Leidner, 2001). Nursing research to transform the healthcare system is also empowered through leveraging (Edwards, 2008). In addition, nursing academic administration benefits by using leveraging to lead (Yucha & Witt, 2009).

Expanded organizational influence results from use of leveraging. For example, the Alliance for Nursing Informatics (2010) is a clear illustration of a national organizational partnership to empower over 25 organizations and 5,000 informatics professionals toward a unitary voice in nursing informatics. The Technology Informatics Guiding Educational Reform (2010) initiative is an example of how broad informatics needs are addressed across practice, education, administration, research, and policy. The idea is to catalyze a dynamic, sustainable, and productive relationship between the Alliance for Nursing Informatics with its 25 nursing informatics professional societies and major nursing organizations, including the American Nurses Association, the American Organization of Nurse Executives, the American Association of Colleges of Nursing, and others, which collectively represent more than 2 million nurses.

These examples demonstrate the applicability of "leveraging" across practice, education, administration, research, and policy. In addition, there is evidence of leveraging with respect to the diffusion of common finance characteristics within nursing and health care. For example, according to finance literature, leverage is a general term for any technique to multiply gains and minimize losses (Brigham & Houston, 2009). The concept of considering liabilities and affect on total assets is considered (Weston, Brigham, & Brigham, 1969). The use of "leveraging" is expected to provide positional advantage, power to act effectively, and improvement in one's speculative capacity with an increased rate of return from an investment to supplement, improve, or enhance (*The American Heritage Dictionary*, 2009). In short, engaging "leveraging" is fundamentally grounded in principles of holism and synergy, that is, the sum is greater than the parts.

In summary, leveraging as a concept is core to moving beyond a leadership that is based on physical or personality strength to one based on team and interprofessional values. Leveraging is core to creative, dynamic, and innovative leadership applicable to this century and beyond.

Alavi, M., & Leidner, D. (2001). Review: Knowledge management and knowledge management systems: Conceptual foundations and research issue. *MIS Quarterly*, (1), 107–136.

Alliance for Nursing Informatics. (2010). Retrieved October 3, 2010, from http://www.allianceni.org

Arora, V., Johnson, T., Lovinger, D., Humphrey, H., & Meltzer, D. (2005). Communication failures in patient sign-out and suggestions for improvement: A critical incident analysis. *Quality and Safety in Health Care*, *14*, 401–407.

Brigham, E., & J.F. Houston (2009). *Fundamentals of financial management*. Stamford, CT: Thomson One.

Edwards, N. (2008). Leveraging nursing research to transform healthcare systems. *Nursing Inquiry, 15*, 81–82.

Jeffs, L., MacMillan, K., & Maione, M. (2009, April/June). Leveraging safer nursing care by conceptualizing near misses as recovery processes. *Journal of Nursing Care Quality, 24*(2), 166–117.

Kitt, S., Kreider, N., Leonard, K., Szekendi, M., & Lewis, D. (2008, September/October). Leveraging technology for nursing handoffs. *CIN: Computers, Informatics, Nursing, 26*(5), 304–305.

Leveraging Multimedia for Learning. (2010). Retrieved October 2, 2010, from http://www.adobe.com/products/captivate/pdfs/captivate_leveraging_multimedia.pdf

Potempa, K., Phancharoenworakul, K., Glass, N., Chasombat, S., & Cody, B.J. (2009). Leveraging the role of public health nursing in managing HIV/AIDS in Thailand: A journey of international collaboration. *Collegian, 16*(2), 49–53.

Technology Informatics Guiding Educational Reform. (2011). Retrieved October 3, 2010, from http://www.tigersummit.com/About_Us.html

The American Heritage Dictionary of the English Language, Fourth Edition. (2009). Boston, MA: Houghton Mifflin Company.

Weston, J., Brigham, F., & Brigham, E. (1969). *Managerial finance*. New York, NY: Holt, Rinehart and Winston Publisher.

Yucha, C., & Witt, R. (2009). Leveraging higher salaries for nursing faculty. *Journal of Professional Nursing, 25*(3), 151–155.

Connie White Delaney

LICENSURE

In the United States, the legal authorization to practice certain professions is a state's right and controlled by each state's relevant statutes (laws), rules, and regulations. The privilege to practice the profession of nursing as a registered professional nurse (RN) (independent licensure) or a licensed practical nurse (LPN) or licensed vocational nurse (LVN) (dependent licensure requiring supervision of practice) and, in some states, as an advanced practice registered nurse (APRN) is separately authorized by each state, territory, and commonwealth. In 1903, the first statutes (registration laws) governing the practice of nursing were passed in North Carolina, New Jersey, New York, and Virginia. It would be the mid-1930s before some states began to pass Nurse Practice Acts requiring licensure by the state of all those who would practice the profession of nursing (Driscoll, 1976).

Once licensed as an RN or LPN/LVN, one is "never not a nurse," and it is a privilege granted by the state to practice the profession of nursing, not a right of ownership. Nurses who in their personal lives are charged or convicted of tax evasion, driving while under the influence or intoxicated, committing acts of civil disobedience, or who are convicted of other types of misdemeanors or felonies are usually reported to the state oversight agency. Depending on the state's laws and regulations, this may result in an interruption of practice privileges by either temporary or permanent loss of licensure.

Licensure is a state's legal mechanism for protecting the public from harm and ensuring that an individual has the basic competence to practice nursing (RN or LPN/LVN). Only those so authorized can use the credentials (title protection). Most states require that an applicant for licensure have completed a course of study from an approved school of nursing or, if from a foreign country, can demonstrate equivalency of education. States also require successful passage of the National Council Licensure Examination for Registered Nurses (NCLEX-RN) or

NCLEX-PN for licensure; there is a single national pass rate, and the examinations are electronically administered unless an applicant requests a modification based upon a recognized disability. States may have additional state-specific qualifying criteria such as child abuse, domestic violence, HIV/AIDS, and pain management education; compliance with social laws such as payment of student loans, alimony, or state fines; and being of "good moral character" with no outstanding felony or misdemeanor charges/convictions (Daly, Sandra, Jackson, Lambert, & Lambert, 2005). Once licensed, the state expects that a nurse will remain professionally committed to meeting any new educational requirements, maintaining appropriate competence in practice and refraining from acts of professional misconduct.

When moving to a new state, an RN or LPN must apply for licensure to practice in that state; this process is known as "endorsement" and can differ among states. One may hold licensure in as many states or territories that one wants as long as the nurse meets the requirements to maintain the license or places it on inactive status according to the regulations of the particular state. The nurse who is licensed in multiple states is required to know the different state nurse practice acts and any variations in scope of practice among the states of licensure. Most states have an ongoing registration process (2 or 3 years) that requires nurses practicing in the state to register their licenses by paying a fee and bringing personal information up to date with the state's oversight agency. Some states require that RNs, who are also APRNs—specializing as nurse anesthetists, nurse midwives, nurse practitioners, or clinical nurse specialists, obtain a second license from the state to practice in such a role. The uniformity that exists in RN and LPN licensure does not exist with regard to APRNs, and therefore some states strictly regulate the authorization to practice whereas other states require no separate permission to practice in these roles. In the past, the National Council of State Boards of Nursing (2007, 2008) has addressed the differences in state licensure laws for RNs, LPNs, and APRNs by promoting two types of voluntary licensure compacts for the states (similar in theory to the national driver's license compact). These are known as the Multi-state RN/LPN Licensure Compact and the APRN Licensure Compact (http://www.ncsbn.org). These compacts have not been passed in all states because of issues such as negative opinions from state attorneys general on legality, loss of revenue streams to the state and oversight agency, concerns about discipline issues, and public's ability to have recourse when dissatisfied with a nurse's practice. In addition, various professional and regulatory nursing organizations have developed a consensus document on the licensure, accreditation, certification, and education of APRNs (https://www.ncsbn.org/170.htm).

See also Advanced Practice Registered Nurses; National Council of State Boards of Nursing, Inc.

Daly, J., Sandra, S., Jackson, D., Lambert, V., & Lambert, C. E. (2005). *Professional issues: Concepts, issues and challenges.* New York, NY: Springer Publishing.

Driscoll, V. M. (1976). *Legitimizing the profession of nursing: The distinct mission of the New York State Nurses Association.* Schenectady, NY: The Foundation of the New York State Nurses Association.

National Council of State Boards of Nursing. (2007). *Nurse licensure compact—About.* Retrieved September 2, 2006, from www.ncsbn.org/156.htm

National Council of State Boards of Nursing. (2008). The consensus model for APRN regulation: Licensure, accreditation, certification and education. Retrieved January 20, 2011, from https://www.ncsbn.org/170.htm

Karen A. Ballard

LIVING LEGENDS

In 1994, the board of directors of the American Academy of Nursing (AAN) created the "Living Legend" Program to honor fellows who were leaders among leaders. Not only was there a perceived need for such a senior-level recognition program, but there were organizational problems that this initiative was expected to address: many of the most distinguished (and older) fellows were no longer attending meetings because they did not know the younger fellows who also did not know them. Thus, the Living Legend Program was meant to serve as a history lesson and to strengthen intergenerational understanding by highlighting the achievements of pioneering role models.

To be eligible for this recognition, fellows must have been active in the AAN for 15 or more years, must have made extraordinary and sustained contributions to nursing and health, and must continue to influence the profession. The first two cohorts (1994 and 1995) honored legendary figures in all aspects of the profession: Faye Abdellah, Myrtle Aydelotte, Mary Elizabeth Carnegie, Luther Christman, Rheba de Tornyay, Ildaura Murrillo-Rohde, Virginia Ohlson, Hildegard Peplau, Rozella Schlotfeldt, Jessie Scott, and Harriet Werley. By the end of 2010, 66 additional leaders had been awarded that distinction. For additional information about this designation and the names of those awarded this distinction, refer to the AAN Web site (www.aannet.org).

L

The AAN has made use of these living legends in various ways. A leadership conference is held annually as part of the "Building Academic Geriatric Nursing Capacity" Program, which the AAN manages in partnership with the John A. Hartford Foundation (Conn, 2006). One popular feature has been an interview with living legends, for example, Mary Starke Harper, Florence Wald, Luther Christman, Claire Fagin, Loretta Ford, Shirley Chater, and Gloria Smith, during which the individual reminisces about her or his career trajectory. To listen to some of these conversations, go to www.geriatricnursing.org/leadership/msh-lectureship.asp. At its 2004 annual meeting, the AAN instituted an "Emerging Leader" Program, and one aspect of that programming was breakfast discussions with living legends. The commitment to fostering leadership is particularly important if we are to develop future legends in nursing.

See also American Academy of Nursing

Conn, V. S. (2006). Innovative model for building academic nursing. *Western Journal of Nursing Research, 28,* 367–368.

Angela Barron McBride

LOBBYING

Activities designed to shape public policy by influencing the outcomes of federal, state, or local legislative action are often referred to as *lobbying*. Lobbying is carried out by a broad range of organizations and is an important aspect of advocacy. Many professional and trade organizations in health care employ professional lobbyists to advocate on behalf of the organization by meeting with legislators and other elected officials explaining the organization's positions on legislation, often to urge support or opposition to specific legislative proposals. These lobbyists also generally help to analyze and explain proposed legislation to the organization's leadership and membership.

The American Nurses Association (ANA) first established a legislative office with a full-time lobbyist in 1951 (Thompson, 1972). For several years, it was the only national nursing organization with a lobbying program. Today, dozens of national nursing organizations engage in lobbying activities, as do a large number of state organizations.

Lobbying activities are regulated by federal and state laws. These laws typically require lobbyists (and/or their employing organizations) to register and to file regular reports of their lobbying activities. Federal lobbyists register and file reports with both the House of Representatives and the Senate (Honest Leadership and Open Government Act of 2007). State laws differ in terms of registration and reporting requirements. Generally, these requirements at both the federal and state levels are designed to maintain transparency and to avoid illegal or unethical tactics to gain favor with policymakers.

Some organizations, especially larger ones, directly employ lobbyists as members of their professional staff. For example, the ANA, the American Hospital Association, and the American Medical Association each employ several staff lobbyists. Many organizations contract with a lobbyist or lobbying firm, who typically also contracts with several other clients to provide advocacy services. Some organizations do both—maintaining a lobbying staff and contracting with a lobbying firm to help with one or more high-priority legislative issues. Some professional lobbyists are former legislative staff members; some are themselves former members of Congress or state legislators.

Although professional lobbyists play a major role in carrying out organizations' policy agendas, nursing organizations have increasingly emphasized the importance of involving their members in legislative advocacy—a practice often referred to as *grassroots lobbying*. Grassroots lobbying is "the attempt to influence legislation by affecting the opinions of the general public or any segment of the public" (Internal Revenue Service, 1999). It is based on the idea that elected officials are likely to be most responsive to their own constituents. Such activities generally seek to have members contact their members of Congress or state legislatures to urge support for or opposition to proposed legislation. This is an important leadership role for all nurses. For example, ANA, the National League for Nursing, the American Association of Colleges of Nursing, or the American Organization of Nurse Executives might send an e-mail to its members to call or write to their members of Congress to urge them to vote in favor of increased federal funding for nursing education. As electronic communication has become more sophisticated, organizations have been increasingly capable of targeting their messages—for example, contacting members whose federal or state representatives are key "swing" votes on priority legislation to encourage a vote for or against that legislation.

Many organizations also seek to involve their members in advocacy activities by holding an annual meeting in Washington, DC, while Congress is in session in order to visit their representatives' offices in person to urge them to vote for or against specific legislation. Many state affiliates of national organizations hold similar meetings in state capitals to involve their members in lobbying their state representatives. Nurses have an important place in this process because of their fundamental knowledge of health care and health care systems.

Honest Leadership and Open Government Act of 2007, Pub. L. No. 110-81.

Internal Revenue Service. (1999). Attempting to influence legislation. *Internal Revenue Manual* (Pt. 7, chap. 25, Section 3.17). Retrieved from http://www.irs.ustreas.gov/irm/part7/irm_07-025-003-cont03.html#d0e5223

Thompson, J. (1972). *The ANA in Washington.* Kansas City, MO: American Nurses Association.

David M. Keepnews

LONG-TERM QUALITY ALLIANCE

For years, strategies to increase the quality of care and decrease costs have focused mostly on reducing hospitalizations for people with chronic disease who are not disabled and live in their own homes. They have not focused on frail elderly people and adults with disabilities who receive long-term care in community settings or in institutions like nursing homes. Despite significant growth in the home- and community-based sector, there are very few measures available to assess the quality of care in those settings. In response to these challenges, the Long-Term Quality Alliance (LTQA; www.ltqa.org) was formed in January 2010. The LTQA, which is comprised of the nation's leading health, nursing, consumer, and aging advocates, is a first of its kind, convening voice working to make sure that the 10 million people needing long-term services and supports (LTSS) in the United States receive the highest quality of care regardless of the setting in which it is delivered. The mission statement of the LTQA is "to improve the effectiveness and efficiency of care and the quality of life of people receiving LTSS by fostering person- and family-centered measurement and advancing innovative best practices."

LTQA is needed because current practices for measuring long-term care quality focus too much on clinical services delivered in nursing homes, and they ignore the perspectives of consumers and their family caregivers. The LTQA hopes to spur development and advancement of a set of measures that reflect what is important to consumers and families and apply those across settings. In addition, the LTQA is working to give nurses and other health professionals access to evidence-based practices that accurately assess and improve the quality of life and the quality of care of the people they treat.

The LTQA aims to achieve these goals by fostering "person-centered" (a focus on individual experiences versus purely clinical data) quality measures. The LTQA's strategic plan for the next 2 years are as follows: (a) to advance the use of key person- and family-centered quality indicators specific to adults who require LTSS that are focused on improvement in care transitions and health-related qualify of life and reductions in potential avoidable hospitalizations, re-hospitalizations, and total health care costs; (b) to achieve wider dissemination and adoption of person- and family-centered, effective transitional care practices; and (c) to achieve engagement and "buy-in" for policies and mechanisms that advance high-quality, person- and family-centered transitional care (Lipson, Simon, Wenzlow, Brown, & Stone, 2009).

Priority goals, outlined by the LTQA board, determined to make tangible differences are achieving agreement among stakeholders on key definitions of transitional care and by creating a framework to accelerate quality improvement; providing meaningful regulatory input to the federal government on how provisions of the Affordable Care Act relate to promoting quality person- and family-centered care; advancing meaningful measures to accelerate quality improvement; achieving adoption of effective transitional care practices that contribute to demonstrable improvements in quality for people who need LTSS; and promoting engagement and buy in for policies and mechanisms that advance high-quality person- and family centered transitional care.

Implementation of the LTQA's priorities will have a direct impact on nurses in both long-term care settings and hospitals. Too often, long-term care recipients are admitted to hospitals for avoidable reasons and return to their previous setting (nursing home, HCBS setting, or home) in worse, more confused states than before. With the number of Americans needing LTSS set to double to 27 million by 2050 (U.S. Department of Health and Human Services and U.S. Department of Labor, 2003), an efficient and well-run long-term care system is critical. By focusing on "person-centered" quality measures, the LTQA seeks to provide nurses and other providers with the best tools and resources to improve care, reduce costs, and enhance quality of life.

By bringing a diverse group of leaders together that blends advocacy, research, and policy, the Alliance is in a position to create innovative, meaningful change. The LTQA board is comprised of 30 leaders from organizations representing caregivers, nurses, consumers, quality improvement, nursing homes, accreditation, aging issues, foundations, the federal government, private payers, and academia.

Board members include representatives from Agency for Healthcare Research and Quality, Centers for Medicare and Medicaid Services, Administration on Aging, American Association of Retired Persons, Brookings Institute, LeadingAge (there has been a formal name change of the American Association of Homes and Services for the Aging), National Alliance for Caregiving, Alzheimer's Association, and Visiting Nurse Service of New York.

Lipson, D. J., Simon, S., Wenzlow, A., Brown, R., & Stone, C. (2009, October 30). *A strategic plan for the Long Term Care Quality Alliance.* Recommendations of Mathematica Policy Research, Final Report. Princeton, NJ: Mathematica Policy Research Inc. Retrieved from http://www.mathematica-mpr.com

U.S. Department of Health and Human Services and U.S. Department of Labor. (2003). *The future supply of long-term care workers in relation to the aging baby boom generation: Report to Congress.* Washington, DC: Office of the Assistant Secretary for Planning and Evaluation. Retrieved December 1, 2009, from http://aspe.hhs.gov/daltcp/reports/ltcwork.htm

Mary D. Naylor

L

M

MAGNET HOSPITALS

In the early 1980s, the United States was experiencing a serious nursing shortage. In an effort to assist in solving the problems involved, the American Academy of Nursing appointed a Task Force on Hospital Nursing Practice. The members were Margaret L. McClure (chair), Muriel A. Poulin, Margaret D. Sovie, and Mable Wandelt.

During the course of their early deliberations, the task force observed that there were a small number of hospitals that, unlike others, were not having difficulty recruiting and retaining professional nurses. Moreover, it was clear that although there was a substantial body of literature related to turnover, virtually no studies had been done regarding the retention of nurses. As a result, the task force undertook a national study, specifically focused on identifying the critical factors that made selected hospitals highly attractive to registered nurses, even in a time of severe shortage. In addition, because of their ability to attract and retain their staff, the task force labeled them "Magnet Hospitals." Forty-one such facilities comprised the sample, and the data were collected through interviews conducted with nurse executives and staff nurses from each of the institutions. The results of the study were published in a monograph titled *Magnet Hospitals: Attraction and Retention of Professional Nurses* (McClure, Poulin, Sovie, & Wandelt, 1983).

After publication of the study, several nurse scholars, most notably Marlene Kramer and Linda Aiken, continued to conduct research involving the Magnet Hospitals. Their findings not only validated those of the original research but also demonstrated a link between the Magnet organizations and high-quality patient outcomes (McClure & Hinshaw, 2002)

In the early 1990s, the American Nurses Credentialing Center (ANCC) began a new program, designed to allow hospitals to apply to be designated as Magnet Hospitals. Using the 14 characteristics identified in the original research and expanding them further to include findings from other studies, as well as the American Nurses Association's *Standards for Organized Nursing Services*, the ANCC developed a rigorous methodology by which the applicant hospitals could be judged; today, this process involves the submission of extensive written materials as well as site visits conducted by specially trained appraisers. The outcomes are then reviewed by the Commission on Magnet Recognition, and that group makes the final determination regarding designation. It is important to emphasize that hospitals that receive the Magnet designation must repeat the application process every 4 years to maintain their standing.

Over the years, the Magnet Hospital designation has become a coveted award, one that is sought by many institutions in the United States and abroad. Early international Magnet Hospitals can be found in Australia, Lebanon, and Singapore.

A wealth of additional information regarding the Magnet Hospital Recognition program can be found in an ANCC publication titled, *Magnet: The Next Generation—Nurses Making the Difference* (Drenkard, Wolf, & Morgan, 2011). In addition, the reader is referred to the Web site www.nursecredentialing.org.

See also American Academy of Nursing; American Nurses Association; American Nurses Credentialing Center

Drenkard, K., Wolf, G., & Morgan, S. (2011). *Magnet: The next generation—Nurses making the difference.* Washington, DC: American Nurses Credentialing Center.

McClure, M. L., Poulin, M. A., Sovie, M. D., & Wandelt, M. (1983). *Magnet Hospitals: Attraction and retention of professional nurses.* Washington, DC: American Nurses Association.

McClure, M. L., & Hinshaw, A. S. (2002). *Magnet hospitals revisited: Attraction and retention of professional nurses.* Washington, DC: American Nurses Publishing.

Margaret L. McClure

MALCOLM BALDRIGE NATIONAL QUALITY AWARD

Malcolm Baldrige was the U.S. Secretary of Commerce from 1981 until his accidental death in 1987. Baldrige was a firm believer and supporter of quality management as a primary focus to enhance the strength and financial success of our country. He was extensively involved in the creation of the quality improvement act that was named after him. To recognize and honor his efforts, Congress named this award after him (National Institute of Standards and Technology, 2009).

The Malcolm Baldrige National Quality Award is given by the President of the United States to businesses as well as education and health care organizations on the basis of performance excellence as evaluated by independent board members. The seven areas that are judged are leadership; strategic planning; customer and market focus; measurement, analysis, and knowledge management; human resource focus; process management; and results (American Society for Quality, n.d.). The awards represent a successful partnership between the government and the private sector. The government commits approximately $5 million, which is then enhanced by $100 million in donations from the private sector and state and local organizations. The Board of Examiners is a collection of 550 industry, educational, government, and nonprofit organization volunteers who are responsible for reading the applications, visiting the nominated businesses, and issuing feedback regarding strengths and weaknesses (National Institute of Standards and Technology, 2010). The education and health care categories were established in 1999. In addition, a nonprofit and a government category were both added in 2007 (American Society for Quality, n.d.).

The following are a few of the recent health care organizations that have won this prestigious award in 2009: Honeywell Federal Manufacturing & Technologies, LLC, AtlantiCare, Midway USA, Heartland Health, and VA Cooperative Studies Program Clinical Research Pharmacy Coordinating Center. The criteria and the application process are available through the National Institute of Standards and Technology Web site located at www.nist. gov/baldrige/publications/criteria.cfm.

American Society for Quality. (n.d.). *Malcolm Baldrige National Quality Award.* Retrieved September 28, 2010, from http://asq.org/learn-about-quality/malcolm-baldrige-award/overview/overview.html

National Institute of Standards and Technology. (2009). *Frequently asked questions about the Malcolm Baldrige National Quality Award.* Retrieved September 28, 2010, from http://www.nist.gov/public_affairs/factsheet/bald-faqs.cfm

National Institute of Standards and Technology. (2010). *Why take the Baldrige journey?* Retrieved September 28, 2010, from http://www.nist.gov/baldrige/enter/index.cfm

Ronda Mintz-Binder

MALPRACTICE

Malpractice was defined many years ago as "…a limited class of negligent activities committed within the scope of performance by those pursuing a particular profession involving highly skilled and technical services" (Lesnick & Anderson, 1962). More recently, malpractice, now also called professional negligence, has been defined as "…the failure of a person with professional education and skills to act in a reasonable and prudent manner" (Wacker-Guido, 2007, p. 62). For malpractice to exist, certain elements must be present. First, there is a duty owed to a patient, and a breach of that duty occurs when the nurse does not follow the standard of care. For purposes here, "duty" is constituted by virtue of the fact that the nursing professional has entered into a contract with the patient, either written

or understood, to provide reasonable and safe nursing care. Forseeability refers to the nurse's knowledge that not following the standard of care may result in harm to the patient. Next, the nurse's action, or nonaction, must be the direct cause of some physical injury to the patient resulting in damages that have a financial impact (Wacker-Guido, 2007). Negligence, by contrast, is defined as "the omission of an act that a reasonable and prudent person would perform in a similar situation or the commission of something a reasonable person would not do in the situation" (Evans & Aiken, 2006, p. 164). With both negligence and malpractice, the resulting harm is unintentional, meaning the individual did not intend for the injury to occur (Wacker-Guido, 2007).

In prior decades, professional practitioners such as nurses and doctors in not-for-profit organizations were literally exempt from litigation. Thus, across the years, the incidence of litigation involving malpractice/negligence issues among health care organizations and professions was exceedingly low. This situation remained so until *Darling v. Charleston Memorial Hospital*, in the state of Illinois in 1965. Outcomes of this particular lawsuit dispelled the notion of charitable immunity, paving the way for litigation of heath care organizations and health care professionals. Since that time, the number of litigations involving hospitals and health care providers has escalated; however, health care litigation has led to the development and implementation of standards of practice and care specific to the various categories of health care practitioners and specific to given communities. In addition, personnel manuals, policy manuals, written job descriptions, quality improvement programs, and adherence to standards of accreditation are all part of the modus operandi of health care organizations and dictate the conditions of third-party reimbursement as well as participation in federal Medicare and Medicaid programs.

Nurse leaders need to be aware of the most common malpractice claims against professional nurses. These include staffing issues, failing to follow standards of care, improper use of equipment, lack of communication, poor documentation, and inappropriate delegation practices (Reising & Allen, 2007; Reynolds, Wheeler, & Iyer, 2001). For medical-surgical nurses, many of these problem areas stem from family perceptions of what should be done for their loved ones, the challenges of the aging population in relation to increased care needs and greater risk to fall status, and the use of resources during clinical emergencies in which nurses are pulled to care for one patient to the detriment of others (Reynolds et al., 2001). These areas provide nurse leaders a framework for the development of competencies intended for patient safety, patient satisfaction, and prevention of litigation for nursing students, nurse educators, and nursing practitioners.

Darling v. Charleston Memorial Hospital, 211 NE2d253 (IL 1965).

Lesnick, M. J., & Anderson, B. E. (1962). *Nursing practice and the law*. Philadelphia, PA: Lippincott.

Reising, D. L., & Allen, P. N. (2007). Protecting yourself from malpractice claims. *American Nurse Today*, 2(2), 39–44.

Reynolds, K.A., Wheeler, W.B., & Iyer, P. (2001). Medical-surgical nursing: Malpractice issues. In P. Iyer (Ed.). *Nursing malpractice* (pp. 375–415). Tucson, AZ: Lawyers and Judges Publishing Company, Inc.

Wacker-Guido, G. (2007). Legal and ethical issues. In P. Yoder-Wise (Ed.), *Leading and managing in nursing* (pp. 59–87). St. Louis, MO: Mosby.

Gina M. Myers
M. Janice Nelson

MANAGEMENT BY OBJECTIVES

M

In 1954, Peter Drucker first published his management concept called *management by objectives* (MBO) in his book *The Practice of Management*. Drucker, who died in November 2005 at the age of 95 years, was known as the father of modern corporate management as well as one of the world's most influential business theorists (Sullivan, 2005). During his life, Drucker published more than 36 books and in 30 languages. He believed that strong workers need to be empowered and that the goal of a manager was to prepare and then free their employees to perform at optimal levels (Sullivan, 2005). MBO is an objective-driven approach to performance evaluation that involves five major principles: (1) defined organization-based goals and objectives, (2) member-driven individualized objectives, (3) shared decision making, (4) specified time frame for evaluation, and (5) employee work–based evaluation and mutual feedback (12 Manage Rigor and Relevance, 2006).

Drucker's premise encourages a shared commitment and understanding between the employee and the employer and elicits employee acceptance of individualized objectives to be met in the time frame ahead. In assessing the quality of the objectives, the SMART technique was also introduced by Drucker (1992). Objectives need to be: specific, measurable, achievable, realistic, and time related. Objectives are best met when they are clearly written, easily understood, and appropriate to the situation. The principles of MBO were extrapolated into the more current value-based management techniques. In the 1990s, Drucker did state that MBO works well if the objectives are known; however, 90% of the time, employees do not know them (12 Manage Rigor and Relevance, 2006). Efficient and proactive nurse leaders use Drucker's theory in relation to employee evaluations when evaluation criteria are objective-focused and mutually understood. By assuring that employees are extremely clear on their evaluation criteria, nursing leaders can assure effective and comprehensive evaluations that are supportive, fair, and elicit meaningful shared dialogue toward accomplishment and advancement.

12 Manage Rigor and Relevance. (2006). *Management by objectives (Drucker) SMART.* Retrieved November 18, 2010, from http://www.12manage.com/methods_smart_management_by_objectives.html

Drucker, P. (1954). *The practice of management.* New York, NY: Harper and Row.

Drucker, P. (1992, September–October). The new society of organizations. *Harvard Business Review*, 95–105.

Sullivan, P. (2005). *Management visionary Peter Drucker dies.* Retrieved November 18, 2010, from http://www.washingtonpost.com/wp-dyn/content/article/2005/11/11/AR2005111101938.html

Ronda Mintz-Binder
Joyce J. Fitzpatrick

MANAGING ANGER/EMOTIONS

Negative emotions are like viruses; they are highly contagious in the hectic, stressful workplaces where health care is delivered. Effective leaders learn how to manage their own anger and other emotions. They also know how to gauge the "emotion titer" of the work unit, and to assist their staff with intelligent emotion management. The best leaders help staff to stay in a positive, optimistic emotional range, which is vital to staff retention.

However, the literature is replete with descriptions of mismanaged anger and conflict, along with dismal statistics about nurse burnout and the rapid exodus of new graduates (Casey, Fink, Krugman, & Probst, 2004; McKenna, Smith, Poole, & Coverdale, 2003; Thomas, 2009; Vessey, DeMarco, Gaffney, & Budin, 2009).

DIFFERENTIATING BETWEEN HEALTHY AND UNHEALTHY ANGER

It is important to differentiate between healthy and unhealthy anger. Anger is a normal emotional reaction to violations of values, rights, or beliefs (Thomas, 2009). Research shows that nurses become angry when they are (1) overloaded and overwhelmed, (2) treated disrespectfully, (3) blamed and scapegoated, (4) not listened to by management when voicing concerns, (5) morally distressed about the maltreatment of patients, (6) powerless to accomplish changes in the work unit, and/or (7) unsupported by peers and management (Thomas, 2009). Anger in such situations is legitimate and healthy. It can be used to assertively advocate for oneself or for one's patients. Healthy anger is expressed directly to the provocateur, when possible, or channeled into constructive action to resolve the problem. If no constructive action is possible at the time, the health-promoting strategy is to discharge the anger harmlessly via physical activity or a calming technique such as a breathing exercise or meditation.

Many nurses (especially female nurses) lack such strategies to manage the emotion of anger because they had no role models demonstrating healthy anger management while growing up. Many women (and some men) learned that anger is ugly, irrational, or even immoral. Therefore, anger often goes underground after arousal. When anger is suppressed, it leads to rumination and resentment because its cause remains unresolved. It also begins to leak out in unhealthy ways, such as fault finding, bickering, and backbiting. Horizontal and vertical violence are particularly destructive forms of mismanaged anger. Horizontal violence (also called lateral violence) is a term applied to hostile and sabotaging behaviors between peers at the same level in the institutional hierarchy. Vertical violence refers to emotionally abusive behavior exhibited by superiors (such as administrators or faculty) toward persons under their supervision (such as students) (Thomas & Burk, 2009). "Bullying" is sometimes used as an umbrella term for the interpersonal violence that is prevalent among nurses across the globe (Johnson, 2009; Stanley, Martin, Nemeth, Michel, & Welton, 2007; Vessey et al., 2009).

STRATEGIES TO PROMOTE HEALTHY ANGER MANAGEMENT IN YOUR TEAM

It is the responsibility of the work unit leader to be vigilant regarding negativism and disrespectful treatment. This means that team anger issues are dealt with promptly and honestly, as they arise. When anger is justifiable, the leader can acknowledge its legitimacy and assist the individual to consider options for constructive action. When anger is irrational (e.g., perceived unfairness), the leader can encourage a more rational view of the situation. Some staff anger and frustration may dissipate simply because management takes time to listen. If necessary, the leader acts as the third-party manager of conflict among staff members. The individuals are brought together and asked to assertively state their grievances. "Linguistic shading" (McNamee & Gergen, 1999) also can diminish strong emotion. For example, tension is a less inflammatory term than

anger. Individuals can learn to "shade" flaring tempers by saying "there is tension between us." In response, team members can be urged to commit to new goals. For example, everyone can agree that (1) good patient care is the priority and (2) a harmonious workplace is desirable. Asking staff at the end of each work day to tally the positive events that occurred that day is another tactic that a leader can use to deliberately generate positive emotions.

Firm limits must be set on bullying or subversive activities that are creating turmoil. A chronically angry individual should be referred to employee assistance programs or counseling. In complex situations of long-festering conflict, a psychiatric nurse specialist might be asked to lead weekly group meetings of the staff. Effective leadership depends on one's ability to identify these conflicts and act by finding the solutions that are specific to each situation.

Casey, K., Fink, R., Krugman, M., & Probst, J. (2004). The graduate nurse experience. *Journal of Nursing Administration, 34*, 303–311.

Johnson, S. L. (2009). International perspectives on workplace bullying among nurses: A review. *International Nursing Review, 56*, 34–40.

McKenna, B. G., Smith, N. A., Poole, S. J., & Coverdale, J. H. (2003). Horizontal violence: Experiences of registered nurses in their first year of practice. *Journal of Advanced Nursing, 42*, 90–96.

McNamee, S., & Gergen, K. (1999). *Relational responsibility*. Thousand Oaks, CA: Sage.

Stanley, K. M., Martin, M. M., Nemeth, L. S., Michel, Y., & Welton, J.M. (2007). Examining lateral violence in the nursing workforce. *Issues in Mental Health Nursing, 28*, 1247–1265.

Thomas, S. P. (2009). *Transforming nurses' stress and anger: Steps toward healing*. New York, NY: Springer Publishing.

Thomas, S. P., & Burk, R. (2009). Junior nursing students' experiences of vertical violence during clinical rotations. *Nursing Outlook, 57*, 226–231.

Vessey, J. A., DeMarco, R., Gaffney, D., & Budin, W. (2009). Bullying of staff registered nurses in the workplace: A preliminary study for developing personal and organizational strategies for the transformation of hostile to healthy workplace environments. *Journal of Professional Nursing, 25,* 299–306.

Sandra P. Thomas

MANAGING FINANCES IN NURSING PROGRAMS

Moving from a faculty or clinical position into a leadership or management position in a nursing program can be a rude awakening. Although being a brilliant teacher, researcher, or practitioner may have facilitated the move into leadership, it is not a guarantee of success. Managing and leading a nursing program or academic unit requires keen business skills such as human resource management, resource garnering and allocation, budgeting that includes an understanding of the relationship between revenue and expense, and managing through fiscally challenging times. Cultural, political, and communication savvy must complement the hard skills because fiscal management in any organization is a complex web of history, relationships, and values.

Three metaphorical ages capture the fiscal management development of a successful nursing academic leader: the Age of Innocence, the Age of Competence, and the Age of Sophistication.

THE AGE OF INNOCENCE

The new academic leader often has the preconceived belief that just because a nursing program exists, there is sufficient budget to underwrite operations and support growth. In addition, when the first fiscal bump in the road occurs, transparency is often not the administration's strong suit in explaining why resources are not being provided. Therefore, during the age of innocence, the new academic leader needs to gain a full understanding of the revenue generated by the nursing program, what is spent to operate the program both instructional and operating expenses, and what is left, sometimes called the margin or the program's contribution to the college or the university (Donnelly & Misener, 2005). Once this is discerned, the leader can develop a budget according to what should be a published process that occurs annually. In some institutions, the academic leader must submit an operating budget but may not be asked to calculate revenue. In other institutions, there may be a university or statewide formula that determines budget based on enrollment. Alternatively, responsibility-centered budgeting may be used, in which each academic unit develops a revenue and expense budget with the goal of contributing to the institution out of the margin that accrues (Whalen, 1991). Finding a finance mentor, one who has mastered the mechanics of budgeting in the institution as well as the nuances of negotiation, will help. Learning how to quantify and articulate the need for faculty, staff, equipment, and developmental resources and to negotiate nursing's needs compared to other units should bring an end to innocence in developing financial skills.

THE AGE OF COMPETENCE

Once the hard skills are mastered, the leader needs to seek a deep understanding of the position of nursing programs in the institution. For example, if there are historical or reputational flagship schools in the university that are maintained and supported despite their financial performance, nursing programs may be thought of as a contributor in support of these entities. Alternatively, if the nursing program is in a state institution with an allocation formula based on enrollment, research, or other measures, legacy may be less of an issue in garnering resources. Not every decision in a university is made objectively, so it is best to gain an understanding of the institution's valuing of nursing among the mix of all programs in the college or university. This understanding is best gained by finding trusted colleagues in the institution and informally exploring the historical and current image of nursing as a profession and program. For example, the administrator to whom the nursing chair or dean reports and who will make resource allocation decisions may be harboring "pillow fluffing" stereotypes of nurses. A leader knows that they are well entrenched in the age of competence when the case for resources can be made objectively and succinctly with comparative data and documentation that supports the request and when the response to such requests is considered and rational. Nursing academic leaders who are consistently put in a "make do" position, even in the face of growth, need to consider their options because a lack of human and operational resources can severely compromise the quality of any nursing program. Competence evolves to sophistication when the academic leader views financial management as the quantitative expression of how well the unit operates.

THE AGE OF SOPHISTICATION

Nursing academic leaders have reached the age of sophistication in financial management when they can talk the language of finances in their own institution, when they can comfortably explain fiscal decisions to faculty and staff, when they regularly publish updates on the unit's or program's fiscal performance, and when they look forward to budget development, review, and negotiation with senior administrators. Financial modeling is also a sign of sophistication, that is, looking at the balance between cost and quality as a function of different faculty staffing models and designing educational delivery methods to maximize both quality and revenue outcomes at the same time. For example, some nursing programs have learned that a blend of full-time faculty and clinically current adjunct faculty yields not only fiscal efficiency but also a higher level of student learning as evidenced by pass rates on the National Council of State Boards of Nursing Licensure Exam and other summative measures. A sophisticated nursing academic leader knows the business culture of the institution and the main players, be it the dean, the vice president for academic affairs, or the chief financial officer, asks reasonable questions, and responds rationally even to negative allocation decisions, "No mission, no money" and its corollary, "No money, no mission" is a simple philosophy for guiding financial management. Academic nursing leaders need a clear vision to design and operate high-quality, clinical education programs with great student outcomes; however, sophisticated financial management will be key to success.

Donnelly, G. F., & Misener T. (2005). Financial issues in nursing education (Editorial). *Nursing Leadership Forum, 9*(4), 135. Entire issue is on Nursing Education Finances.

Whalen, E. L. (1991). *Responsibility centered budgeting: An approach to decentralized management for institutions of higher learning.* Bloomington, IN: Indiana University Press.

Gloria F. Donnelly

M

MEANINGFUL USE RULE

The meaningful use rule is part of a coordinated set of regulations outlined in the 2009 federal economic stimulus package under a broad government effort, the Health Information Technology for Economic and Clinical Health Act (HITECH), to help create a private and secure 21st-century electronic health information system. HITECH's goal was not adoption alone but "meaningful use" of electronic health records (EHRs) by providers to achieve significant improvements in care. The legislation tied hospital qualifications for Medicare and Medicaid bonus payments specifically to the achievement of advances in health care processes and outcomes spurring adoption of health information technology. The HITECH legislation further requires that meaningful use include electronic reporting of data on the quality of care.

On June 18, 2010, the Department of Health and Human Services (DHHS) issued a rule that laid out a process for the certification of EHRs, so that providers can be assured they are capable of meaningful use. The department also issued another regulation that lays out the standards and criteria that EHRs must meet in order to be certified. Realizing that the privacy and security of EHRs are vital, the DHHS has been working hard to safeguard privacy and security by implementing new protections contained in the HITECH legislation.

The final meaningful use rule also defines a hospital-based eligible professional as someone who performs nearly all services in an inpatient hospital setting or emergency department, and it expands the definition of acute-care hospital to include designated Critical Access Hospitals for the Medicaid incentive program. States have discretion about who is considered to be an eligible provider as well as when they will pay out incentive money. States must also prove to the Centers for Medicare and Medicaid Services (CMS) that additional requirements do not add to the financial burden of providers. The Medicaid meaningful use eligibility from state to state will not vary, which is how Medicare works. The federal reporting standards apply nationwide.

Included in the final regulation are a set of core objectives that constitute an essential starting point for meaningful use of EHRs and a separate menu of additional important activities from which providers will choose several to implement in the first two years (healthpolicyandreform.nejm. org/?attachment_id=3742). Core objectives comprise basic functions that enable EHRs to support improved health care. As a start, these include the tasks essential to creating any medical record, including the entry of basic data: patients' vital signs and demographics, active medications and allergies, up-to-date problem lists of current and active diagnoses, and smoking status. Other core objectives include using several software applications that begin to realize the true potential of EHRs to improve the safety, quality, and efficiency of care. These features help clinicians to make better clinical decisions—and avoid preventable errors. To qualify for incentive payments, clinicians must start using such clinical decision support tools. They must also start using the capability that undergirds much of the value of EHRs: using records to enter clinical orders and, in particular, medication prescriptions. In addition, to begin extending the benefits of EHRs to patients themselves, the meaningful use requirements will include providing patients with electronic versions of their health information.

In addition to the core elements, the rule creates a second group: a menu of

10 additional tasks, from which providers can choose any five to implement in 2011–2012. This gives providers latitude to pick their own path toward full EHR implementation and meaningful use. For example, the menu includes capacities to perform drug-formulary checks, incorporate clinical laboratory results into EHRs, provide reminders to patients for needed care, identify and provide patient-specific health education resources, and employ EHRs to support the patient's transitions between care settings or personnel. For most of the core and menu items, the regulation also specifies the rates at which providers will have to use particular functions to be considered meaningful users. These rates reflect shared views and experiences of average practices and providers and therefore are achievable.

The standard calls for hospitals and physicians to use computerized physician order entry systems for at least 30% of their medication orders. One of the core objectives requires providers to handle at least 40% of prescriptions electronically. Clinicians will have to report data on three core quality measures in 2011 and 2012: blood pressure level, tobacco status, and adult weight screening and follow-up (or alternates if these do not apply). Clinicians must also choose three other measures from the lists of metrics that are ready for incorporation into electronic records. Providers will be informed about their own performance and will eventually inform the public as well.

See also Electronic Health Record

Blumenthal, D., & Tavenne, M. (2010). The "meaningful use" regulation for electronic health records. *New England Journal of Medicine, 363,* 501–504. Retrieved October 11, 2010, from http://www.nejm.org/doi/full/10.1056/NEJMp1006114?source=hcrc

Weinstock, M. (2010, February). *Defining meaningful use gatefold.* Hospitals and Health Networks. Washington, DC: Health Forum Inc.

G. *Rumay Alexander*

MENTORING

Formal education is essential in learning the fundamentals so necessary to exerting leadership, but socialization experiences are equally important. The mentoring relationship, whereby the expert provides guidance to the novice in responding to new role expectations and understanding contextual cues, is essential to the development of excellence. Mentoring is crucial to learning what is typically not taught in class, for example, managing time, networking, developing communication skills, deciding where and what to publish, leading teams, and understanding political pressures. The mentor provides the mentee or protégé with perspectives that can only be gained from experience, for example, thinking strategically about next steps and responding appropriately to criticism.

The mentoring relationship contributes to the mentor's leadership abilities too. It is personally and professionally gratifying to share what one has learned and to advance future generations of leaders. The mentor is likely to be energized by the mentee's enthusiasm, and the person being mentored may bring special skills to the mentor's projects. Mentees expect their mentors to be role models and to have the demeanor and expertise needed to provide guidance and support; mentors seek mentees who are motivated for success and leadership.

Historically, mentoring was seen as a single, sustained hierarchical relationship occurring during the school years, but that is no longer the prevailing opinion.

M

Over the course of a career, a person will have multiple relationships of varying lengths that are important to advancement (Chandler & Kram, 2007). Mentoring over the course of a career can take many forms. Modeling values and practices, helping set career goals, and encouraging problem solving are important in the preparation stage of career. Once they function independently either as a clinician or educator, nurses need help in navigating the inner workings of their work environment and in meeting institutional and professional benchmarks of success. Nurses who have assumed responsibility for the development of others and of the setting need mentors who can teach them how to mentor and to delegate, and nurses who are ready to shape the future of health care need help in thinking through strategy and trends. Even nurses about to retire need some mentoring in envisioning postretirement opportunities (McBride, 2011).

Good mentoring can be assessed (Lee, Dennis, & Campbell, 2007). Does the mentor appreciate individual differences? Is the person available to others? Does the person practice active questioning to lead a mentee toward a solution? In addition, there are beginning attempts to tackle the problem of measuring the effectiveness of institutional mentoring (Berk, Berg, Mortimer, Walton-Moss, & Yeo, 2005).

Effective mentoring has assumed even greater importance as professionals endeavor to function effectively in ever-changing environments, and it requires an array of learned competencies. For example, mentoring is essential in the development of research competence (Byrne & Keefe, 2002). The Institute for Clinical Research Education at the University of Pittsburgh (2011) has established a mentoring resources Web site that speaks about commonplace concerns with helpful suggestions. Gone are the days when institutions can assume experts will "be helpful" to novices without organizational supports in place to expedite mentoring, including expectations for best practices (Pfund, Pribbenow, Branchaw, Lauffer, & Handelsman, 2006). The more complicated new role expectations are, the more necessary mentoring becomes. The more nurses are diverse in backgrounds and the roles they play, the more important mentoring will be (Manson, 2009; Mkandawire-Valhmu, Penninah, & Stevens, 2010).

See also Career Stages

Berk, R. A., Berg, J., Mortimer, R., Walton-Moss, B., & Yeo, T. R. (2003). Measuring the effectiveness of faculty mentoring relationships. *Academic Medicine, 80,* 66–71.

Byrne, M. W., & Keefe, M. R. (2002). Building research competence in nursing through mentoring. *Journal of Nursing Scholarship, 34,* 391–396.

Chandler, D. E., & Kram, K. E. (2007). Mentoring and developmental networks in the new career context. In H. Gunz & M. Peiperl (Eds.), *Handbook of career studies* (pp. 241–267). Thousand Oaks, CA: Sage Publications.

Lee, A., Dennis, C., & Campbell, P. (2007). Nature's guide for mentors. *Nature, 447,* 791–797.

Manson, S. M. (2009). Personal journeys, professional paths: Persistence in navigating the crossroads of a research career. *American Journal of Public Health, 99,* S20–S25.

McBride, A. B. (2011). Career stages and mentoring needs. In *The growth and development of nurse leaders* (p. 55). New York, NY: Springer Publishing.

Mkandawire-Valhmu, L., Penninah, M. K., & Stevens, P. E. (2010). Mentoring women faculty of color in nursing academia: Creating an environment that supports scholarly growth and retention. *Nursing Outlook, 58,* 135–141.

Pfund, C., Pribbenow, C. M., Branchaw, J., Lauffer, S. M., & Handelsman, J. (2006). The merits of training mentors. *Science, 311,* 473–473.

University of Pittsburgh Institute for Clinical Research Education. (2011). *Welcome to the mentoring resources Web site.* Retrieved January

20, 2011, from http://www.icre.pitt.edu/mentoring/index.aspx

Angela Barron McBride

MILITARY NURSING

The demands of war provided the opportunity for Florence Nightingale to develop the skills and knowledge that were the origins of nursing as a profession; there she observed "What the horrors of war are, no one can imagine" (Nightingale, 1992). Nightingale's military experience provided the impetus for changes in the civilian health care system. Military nursing in America has an equally distinguishing heritage that is evident in the advancement of nursing as a profession in addition to providing women emancipating work outside of the home environment.

Military nursing in America began when General Washington established a hospital organization in the Continental Army. Through the 18th and 19th centuries, women continued to be employed intermittently and in small numbers as military nurses. The Civil War required an increase in the number of nurses to care for soldiers. Women with minimum formal nursing education and training applied to serve as Army contract nurses in addition to other women volunteers. A detailed chronology of the early decades of military nursing is described in *A History of the Army Nurse Corps* (Sarnecky, 1999).

Military nursing languished until 1898 when Dr. Anita Newcomb McGee, representing the Daughters of the American Revolution, volunteered to assist the Army Surgeon General to select the best candidates to become Army nurses in preparation for the Spanish-American War (1898). The skilled and compassionate care provided by contract nurses in the Spanish American War was the impetus for Dr. McGee and a committee from the Red Cross to draft legislation for Congress to create the Army Nurse Corps (female) as part of The Army Reorganization Act. On February 2, 1901, the Army Nurse Corps (female) was founded and was followed by the Navy Nurse Corps in 1908.

In between World War I and World War II, the several hundred nurses that were serving in the Army and Navy were not sufficient for a military that waxed and waned in response to national and world events. The Red Cross provided ongoing support to military nursing in terms of training and recruitment of qualified women. The survival of military nursing between wars can be attributed to the professionalism of military nurses and the organizational structure that fostered the education and training of nurses to function in the midst of battlefield hazards, extremes in the environment, and the unique demands of military life.

Although the need for nurses in the military was validated at the beginning of the 20th century with the creation of the Army Nurse Corps and the Navy Nurse Corps, the status of nurses in the military was ambiguous. Nurses had no military rank, equal pay, or other benefits, including retirement or veteran's benefits. In 1944 and later in 1948, Congress passed legislation to give women (mostly nurses) in the armed services full pay and privileges equivalent to what men were receiving; however, the treatment and management of women in the military services was not equal or fair when compared with their male colleagues. There were, for example, limitations on the number of women who could achieve rank and there was no opportunity for a woman to be selected for promotion to general or admiral.

M

On April 16, 1947, the Army–Navy Nurse Act of 1947 (Public Law No. 36–80C) provided permanent commissioned officer status for members of the Army Nurse Corps in the grades of second lieutenant through lieutenant colonel. In May of 1949, Secretary of Defense Louis Johnson directed the U.S. Air Force to assume responsibility for its own medical support, and on July 1, 1949, an independent Air Force Medical Service was established with the Air Force Nurse corps as an integral part.

At the outset, the military nursing corps was limited to female nurses. Allowing male nurses to serve as officers did not occur until 1955 when male nurses were authorized to hold reserve commissions in the Army Nurse Corps. In 1967, President Lyndon B. Johnson signed Public Law No. 90–130 "to amend titles 10, 32, and 27, United States Code, to remove restrictions on the careers of female officers in the Army, Navy, Air Force, and Marines, and for other purposes." Additional legislation was needed to remove restrictions on marital status and having children under the age of 16 years. In the 1970s, the segregation of women in separate corps was eliminated, and in 1976, women were allowed admission into the service academies and discussion began to allow women to serve on ships and military airplanes. It is clear that military nurses were on the leading edge for implementing change for the women's rights movement in the United States.

Military nurses (all nurses in the Army, Navy, and Air Force, regardless of whether they are in the active, reserve, or guard component) confront a range of health problems in ambulatory clinics, community hospitals, medical centers, hospital ships, field hospitals, ships, aircraft, and other sites (Smolenski, Smith, & Nanney, 2005; Sarnecky, 1999; Sterner, 1998). Patients vary in age from the neonate to the elderly and encompass those mortally wounded in combat and those who are chronically ill. The military nurse must have knowledge and skills that are transferable to a variety of challenging peacetime and wartime scenarios. The Army, the Navy, and the Air Force Nurse Corps all agree that the knowledge and skill sets of nurse officers must be research based.

In fiscal year 1992, Congress appropriated an initial funding of $1 million to establish the TriService Nursing Research Program (TSNRP; www.usuhs.mil/tsnrp) to support targeted research by military nurses. In 1995, the program's advisory group commissioned the Institute of Medicine to make recommendations for program management, areas for future research funding, and allocation of resources to program functions and to identify both short- and long-term objectives. TSNRP continues as the only program funding and supporting rigorous scientific research in the field of military nursing. Funded research focuses on enhancing health care delivery systems and processes to improve clinical outcomes, advancing the practice of military nursing in support of mission readiness and deployment, and contributing to the health status and quality of life of military personnel and their beneficiaries. From 1992 to 2010, Congress appropriated $89.4 million for the TSNRP providing support and funding for more than 300 military nursing research studies.

Legacies of military nursing include leadership and innovations in nursing practice. Military nurses are leaders at all levels of unit and hospital management, including the command of major medical units. Many prototypes for nursing practices had their origins in military nursing. These include ward management, team nursing, and advanced nursing practices roles, with the most prominent being, the nurse anesthetist and the flight nurse. Military nurses were among the first to use penicillin, renal dialysis, and Stryker frames. A new dimension was provided to nursing research when military nurses in Vietnam conducted research on malaria, shock, and body temperature. In the early 1970s, military nurses were in the vanguard of professional nursing when the services mandated the baccalaureate degree as the entry level requirement for career status as a military nurse.

In December 1989, an interim progress report on the Uniformed Services School of Nursing was presented to the Federal Nursing Chiefs. The task force evaluated various options for types and levels of programs, curriculum, and payback requirements. In November 1992, Congress approved $1 million to plan and implement the master's nurse practitioner program at the Uniformed Services University of the Health Sciences (USUHS), Bethesda, Maryland; in 1993, the USUHS created the Graduate School of Nursing. Graduate programs at the USUHS Graduate School of Nursing are designed to prepare advanced practice nurses and PhDs for the unique challenges of military medicine (www. usuhs.mil/gsn).

On July 13, 1970, Navy Captain Delores Cornelius, deputy director of the Navy Nurse Corps, requested authority to install a bronze plaque on the Nurses Monument in Arlington National Cemetery. The inscription on the plaque reads:

This monument was erected in 1938, and rededicated in 1971, to commemorate devoted service to country and humanity by Army, Navy, and Air Force Nurses.

During the Vietnam War, more than 265,000 women served in the armed forces of the United States; nearly 10,000 served in country during the conflict, many in combat areas. On November 11, 1993, the Vietnam Women's Memorial was dedicated as part of the Vietnam Veterans Memorial.

The Vietnam Women's Memorial was established not only to honor those women who served, but also for the families who lost loved ones in the war, so they would know about the women who provided comfort, care, and a human touch for those who were suffering and dying.

The Women in Military Service for America Memorial, dedicated October 18, 1997, is a unique, living memorial honoring all military women—past, present, and future—and is the only major national memorial honoring women who have served in our nation's defense during all eras and in all services.

On March 18, 2009, the Senate Appropriations Committee's defense subcommittee heard testimony from the Nurse Services' nursing chiefs: Army Maj. Gen. Patricia D. Horoho, Navy Rear Adm. Christine M. Bruzek-Kohler, and Air Force Maj. Gen. Kimberly A. Siniscalchi. Each reported to Congress on a health force that plays a vital role in maintaining the health of America's service members and saving lives on the battlefield. Maj. Gen. Kimberly A. Siniscalchi testified, "Our warriors and their families deserve the best possible care we can provide. It is the nurses' touch, compassion and care that often wills a patient to recover or soften the transition from life to death."

See also Florence Nightingale

Additional information is available from the following sources:

Committee on Military Nursing Research, Institute of Medicine (1996). The Program for

M

Research in Military Nursing: Progress and Future Direction. Washington, DC: National Academies Press.

Nightingale, F. (1992). *Notes on nursing: What it is, and what it is not*. Philadelphia, PA: J. B. Lippincott Company.

Sarnecky, M. T. (1999). *A history of the U.S. Army Nurse Corps*. Philadelphia, PA: University of Pennsylvania Press.

Smolenski, M. C., Smith, D. G., & Nanney, J. S. (2005). *A fit, fighting force. The Air Force Nursing Services chronology*. Washington, DC: Office of the Air Force Surgeon General.

Sterner, D. M. (1998). *In and out of harm's way: A history of the U.S. Navy Nurse Corps*. Seattle, WA: Peanut Butter.

Carol Ledbetter
John McDonough
Margaret Holder

N

NATIONAL BLACK NURSES ASSOCIATION

The National Black Nurses Association (NBNA) has become an incubator for nursing leadership. For example, with the October 2010 release of the Institute of Medicine/Robert Wood Johnson Future of Nursing Report, the work of Dr. Linda Burnes Bolton, former NBNA president, has been nationally and internationally recognized. Dr. Bolton served as co-chair of this historic transformational report along with Chair Dr. Donna Shalala former Secretary of Health during the Clinton administration. The NBNA produces leaders.

NBNA was organized in 1971 under the leadership of Dr. Lauranne Sams, former Dean and Professor of Nursing, Tuskegee University, in Alabama. The NBNA is a nonprofit organization representing 150,000 African American registered nurses, licensed vocational/practical nurses, nursing students, and retired nurses from the United States, Eastern Caribbean, and Africa, with 79 chartered chapters in 34 states.

The NBNA mission is "to provide a forum for collective action by black nurses to investigate, define and advocate for the health care needs of African Americans and to implement strategies that ensure access to health care, equal to, or above health care standards of the larger society." In leading this mission, the NBNA has had nine presidents in its 35-year history: Dr. Lauranne Sams, 1973–1977; Dr. Carrie Rogers Brown, 1977–1979; E. Lorraine Baugh, 1979–1983; Ms. Ophelia Long, 1983–1987; Dr. C. Alicia Georges, 1987–1991; Dr. Linda Burnes Bolton, 1991–1995; Dr. Betty Smith Williams, 1995–1999; Dr. Hilda Richards, 1999–2003; Dr. Bettye Davis Lewis, 2003–2007; and Dr. Debra Toney inaugurated in 2007 and currently serving (Gorham & Davis-Lewis, 2006).

The NBNA has developed and implemented strategies that facilitate the realization of the mission statement. These strategies include the areas of collaboration, scholarship, policy, and leadership. Practice is integrated into all four areas. The following is a summary that highlights these programmatic strategies.

COLLABORATIVE COMMUNITY HEALTH MODEL

Since its inception, improving the health of African Americans through the provision of culturally competent health care services in community-based health programs has been the cornerstone of the NBNA. The Collaborative Community Health Model developed by past presidents Bolton and

N

Georges is the basis for the collaborative partnerships and health programs that are the hallmark of the NBNA. Chapters are the primary mechanism through which the national, state, and local community-based programs are successfully implemented. African American nurses who are direct members (in cities where no chapters are established) also assume leadership roles in mounting community-based programs.

COLLABORATIVE PARTNERSHIPS

Working in partnership with community-based organizations, corporations, and other organizations, NBNA has sponsored health fairs and health education and outreach for national organizations, such as the National Urban League, the International Black Professional Firefighters, the One Hundred Black Men of America, and the National Council of Negro Women. The NBNA has collaborated with the Black Congress on Health, Law, and Economics, a 17-member, multi-professional organization, the Oncology Nursing Society, the American Cancer Society, the American Heart Association, the American Diabetes Association, the American Association of Nurses in AIDS Care, the National Coalition for Health Professional Education in Genetics, and the International Society for Hypertension in Blacks, among others.

As a founding organization of the National Coalition of Ethnic Minority Nurse Associations, Dr. Betty Smith Williams was the first National Coalition of Ethnic Minority Nurse Associations president and a past NBNA president. This collaboration gives voice to 350,000 minority nurses. For many years, NBNA has had a Memorandum of Understanding with the American Red Cross to help provide nursing services in times of natural and man-made disasters. In 2006, NBNA

representatives participated in several American Red Cross workshops on diversity. The purpose of the workshops was to craft curriculum that would help Red Cross volunteers to provide services in a culturally competent manner.

INVOLVEMENT IN POLICY

The National Black Nurses Day on Capitol Hill serves to educate the U.S. Congress on timely topics related to the nursing profession as well as health care disparities. Following the day on Capitol Hill, the National Black Nurses Foundation hosts continuing education unit sessions and an awards ceremony honoring public health advocates. In 2005, NBNA and five other organizations were awarded a $300,000 grant from the U.S. Office of Minority Health to provide services to Katrina survivors. In 2006, NBNA published a manual on surviving disasters that was distributed to 1,000 entities in Houston and along the Gulf states. Also, the NBNA holds membership on various national and federal advisory committees, including the National Advisory Committee for the Office of Minority Health, the National Advisory Council on Nursing Education and Practice, the FDA Nominating Group, the National African American Drug Policy Coalition, Inc., the Joint Commission of Healthcare Organizations Nursing Advisory Committee, the National Council of Negro Women, the Balm in Gilead Cervical Cancer Advisory Board, the Healthy Mothers, Healthy Babies Coalition, and the *Nursing Spectrum Magazine*.

SCHOLARSHIP

Published twice annually, the *Journal of the National Black Nurses Association* contains peer refereed health research based articles. Dr. Joyce Newman Giger, Professor and Lulu Wolf Hassenplug Endowed Chair, UCLA School of Nursing, has been the editor since 1997. The quarterly *NBNA Newsletter* includes information on membership and articles written by NBNA members, partners, and sponsors on a variety of nursing and health issues. Themes have included public policy, aging, and research. In 2005, NBNA published a special issue on "Surviving the Storms: Katrina, Wilma and Rita." The articles were written by NBNA members as survivors and caregivers. The NBNA Women's Health Research Program was established in 1999 for nurse researchers to enhance existing research or develop new research around women's health issues. Its goals include support for the development of a cadre of ethnic nurses reflecting the nation's diversity; advocacy for culturally competent, accessible, and affordable health care; promotion of the professional and educational advancement of ethnic nurses; education of consumers, health care professionals, and policy makers on health issues of ethnic minority populations; development of ethnic minority nurse leaders in areas of health policy, practice, education, and research; and endorsement of best practice models of nursing practice, education, and research for minority populations.

LEADERSHIP

At the 2006 Annual Conference, NBNA launched the Institute of Excellence, which is to honor African American nurses for their contributions in the areas of clinical skills, research, academia, and policy. Twenty-five nurses were inducted in the first class. NBNA president Toney chaired the launch of NBNA Founders Leadership Institute at the 2009 NBNA Conference. Twenty NBNA members were selected to enhance their leadership skills in moving to the next level of leadership in their

jobs, within the NBNA and as volunteers or paid advisory board members. In 2008 on Capitol Hill during the National Black Nurses Day and 29th anniversary, the National Obesity Initiative was launched to help stem the tide of chronic diseases caused by obesity and lack of exercise particularly in the African American Community. The 79 NBNA Chapters have been challenged to collectively lose 360 pounds each.

See also National Coalition of Ethnic Minority Nurse Associations

Gorham, M., & Davis-Lewis, B. (2006). *Nursing leadership: A concise encyclopedia* (1st ed.). New York, NY: Springer Publishing.

Additional information is available from the following Web sites:

Asian American/Pacific Islander Nurses Association. Retrieved from Aapina.org

National Coalition of Ethnic Minority Nurses Associations. Retrieved from Ncemna.org

National Alaska Native American Indian Nurses Association. Retrieved from nanainanurses.org

National Association of Hispanic Nurses. Retrieved from www.thehispanicnurses.com

Philippine Nurses Association of America, Inc. Retrieved from www.mypnaa.org

Beverly Louise Malone

NATIONAL COALITION OF ETHNIC MINORITY NURSE ASSOCIATIONS

Seismic shifts in the demographics of the populations in the United States have been well documented and so have the gaps in unequal health care outcomes for people of color. Increasing diversity in the nursing

N

workforce by increasing the nursing pipeline at all levels is thought to be of utmost importance if the existing gaps are to be closed.

In May 1997, the U.S. Department of Health and Human Services, Bureau of Health Professions, and the Division of Nursing held a conference on minority health issues, bringing together distinguished nursing leaders of color representing their respective organizations. The result was the development of a coalition that became a collective gives voice for 350,000 ethnic minority nurses and the lived health experience of a constituency marginalized from mainstream health delivery systems. The four founding member associations were the National Black Nurses Association (www.nbna.org), the National Association of Hispanic Nurses (www.thehispanicnurses.org), the National Alaska Native American Indian Nurses Association (www.nanaina.com), and the Asian American/Pacific Islander Nurses Association (www.aapina.org). A fifth member, the Philippine Nurses Association of America (www.pnaa03.org), joined shortly after the formation of the coalition. Individual nurses cannot join.

From its inception, the coalition has been a collaborative national force and powerful advocate for both the concerns of minority nurses and the health care needs of ethnic minority populations that continue to suffer disproportionately high rates of disease and mortality compared with the majority population. In the past 7 years, the National Coalition of Ethnic Minority Nurse Associations (NCEMNA; www.ncemna.org) has conducted workshops, prepared white papers on the health status and needs of particular ethnic communities, and made recommendations for nursing research to improve the health of these populations. Through a partnership with Aetna and a grant from the Aetna Foundation, a scholars program was initiated to support 10 minority nursing students, two from each NCEMNA member association.

A primary focus for NCEMNA is creating programs to increase the number of ethnic minority nurse scientists and researchers who can investigate the causes of minority health disparities and find solutions for eliminating them. The award of a $2.4 million grant from the National Institute of General Medical Sciences funded a 5-year landmark project designed to engage and cultivate the next generation of nurse scientists from racial and ethnic minority populations known as "NCEMNA: Nurse Stimulation Program." This initiative will create a database of minority nurse researchers and students and provide mentoring development. More information about NCEMNA and the founding members and their various approaches to decrease the gap of unequal health outcomes through the encouragement of minority nurse researchers can be obtained from their Web sites.

G. Rumay Alexander

NATIONAL COUNCIL OF STATE BOARDS OF NURSING, INC. (NCSBN)

The National Council of State Boards of Nursing, Inc. (NCSBN), is a not-for-profit organization whose members consist of nursing regulators from boards of nursing in the 50 states, the District of Columbia, and five U.S. territories—American Samoa, Guam, Northern Mariana Islands, Puerto Rico, and the Virgin Islands. Established in 1978, the purpose of NCSBN is to provide an organization through which state boards of nursing collaborate on matters related to regulation of the profession. A major function of the organization is to develop the National Council Licensing Examination for Registered Nurses (NCLEX-RN®) and the National Council Licensing Examination for Practical Nurses (NCLEX-PN®), which are used by all member boards as a requirement for licensure. In addition, NCSBN maintains a national data bank on disciplinary action taken against nurses' licenses, conducts regulatory research, promotes uniformity in the regulation of nursing practice, provides nurse licensure data, and serves as a venue for dialogue and information exchange for its members. The National Council of State Boards of Nursing provides a Web site (www.ncsbn.org), which includes information about its mission, programs, and services.

Barbara Zittel

NATIONAL INSTITUTE OF NURSING RESEARCH

The National Institute of Nursing Research (NINR; www.ninr.nih.gov) is one of 27 institutes, centers, and offices at the National Institutes of Health (NIH), which is an agency within the U.S. Department of Health and Human Services (DHHS). The mission of the NINR is consistent with that of the parent organization, NIH:

- The NIH mission is to generate basic and clinical knowledge about the nature and behavior of living systems and the application of that knowledge to enhance health, to lengthen life, and to reduce the burdens of illness and disability.
- The NINR mission is to promote/improve the health of individuals, families,

communities, and populations through supporting and conducting clinical and basic research to create a scientific base for the care of individuals across the life span.

The NIH is considered a premier research organization that has grown from a single laboratory founded in 1887 as an innovative scientific initiative of the Marine Hospital Service. The National Cancer Institute was established in 1937. As the leader of a multi-institute/center organization. NIH is world renowned for its scientific processes and discoveries and is considered a leader in the mainstream of biomedical and behavioral research for the United States. It is the largest funding source for health research in the world, with a multibillion-dollar budget that funds more than 300,000 research personnel at more than 3,000 universities and research focused institutions across the nation. Approximately 6,000 scientists conduct investigations within the NIH's intramural program at one of the world's largest research hospitals, the Clinical Center.

ESTABLISHMENT OF THE NINR

The NINR celebrated its 25th anniversary during the 2010–2011 year. The NINR was first created as a National Center for Nursing Research (NCNR) in 1985 by Public Law 99–158: the Health Research Extension Act. Legislative support for a nursing research presence at NIH was strong, as illustrated by the Congress overriding a Presidential veto for its creation. The NCNR was formally established on April 16, 1986, but was redesignated as an institute in 1993 under Public Law 103–43, the NIH Revitalization Act. Thus, nursing research formally returned to NIH after an absence of 31 years, having started in the Research Grants and Fellowship Branch of

N

the Division of Medical Sciences (currently known as the National Institute of General Medical Sciences) with the first nursing research extramural funding entity reviewed through the Nursing Research Study Section in 1955.

The highlights of the early years of the NCNR include developing the infrastructure for the new nursing research entity, focusing the research endeavors of the profession's scientists through the National Nursing Research Agenda, integrating the NCNR/NINR into the mainstream of NIH through collaboration with other institutes/centers, and encouraging interdisciplinary investigations. In addition, a major focus in the early years was educating both colleagues at NIH and congressional members on what nursing research entailed.

The first director (acting) of the NCNR was Dr. Doris H. Merritt who was a highly respected physician with strong NIH experience. She focused on developing the NCNR infrastructure, the extramural grant submission, review, and management processes and initiating collaboration with other NIH institutes and centers. Dr. Ada Sue Hinshaw was the first permanent director of the NCNR and the first director of the NINR, beginning her tenure in June 1987 and ending in July 1994. Her emphasis focused on evolving a national definition of nursing research, developing a National Nursing Research Agenda to build programs of research with nurse investigators that generated substantive bodies of knowledge, facilitating integration of nursing research into the NIH, educating congressional members and NIH colleagues about nursing research and, lastly, initiating the intramural program needed to allow the NCNR to be redesignated as an institute. Dr. Suzanne S. Hurd was the acting director of NINR from July 1994 to April 1995. Dr. Patricia A. Grady subsequently became the second permanent director of the NINR, assuming the

office in April 1995 to the present. Under her leadership, the science for nursing practice has grown rapidly, showing increasing scientific rigor and the integration of biobehavioral processes in nursing research as well as involving many disciplines. She has placed the NINR in leadership positions with several NIH scientific initiatives, for example, End of Life Science. The motto for the 25th anniversary, "Bringing Science to Life," addresses the current strong focus on the translation of research to practice and health policy.

ORGANIZATION OF THE NINR

The NINR has four divisions and four offices reporting to the director: the Division of Extramural Activities, the Division of Intramural Research, the Office of Administrative Management, the Office of Science Policy and Public Liaison, the Division of Extramural Activities has three components, the Office of Extramural Programs (OEP), the Office of Grants and Contracts Management, and the Office of Review. The OEP invites innovation research grant applications and counsels extramural investigators, whereas the Office of Grants and Contracts Management manages the business aspects of the grants/contracts program and the Office of Review maintains an independent review process for research training and special applications. The extramural investigator community is primarily in direct contact with the OEP. There are four sections in the OEP labeled for the major areas of research grant submissions: neuroscience, genetics, and symptom management; child and family health and health disparities; immunology, infectious disease, and chronic disorders; and acute and long-term care, end of life, and training. Investigators and potential trainees have access to the majority of the NIH mechanisms for grants, contracts, traineeships, and fellowships. The major grant mechanism is the individual investigator-initiated application (RO1), but other grant mechanisms are available, ranging from center grants (e.g., P30s) to small research grants (RO3s). For research training, both individual and institutional National Research Service awards are available; in addition, Career Development Fellowships are also awarded.

The Intramural Research Program (IRP) of the NINR focuses on underlying biological mechanisms of diverse symptoms and individuals' responses to nursing interventions. There are two sections in IRP: symptom management branch and research training. In the Symptom Management Branch, the research focuses on studies such as patient response to certain cancer treatments and exploring the molecular and genetic mechanisms that explain people's response to analgesic treatment for acute pain. The IRP also offers several trainee opportunities for postdoctoral research and dissertation research (Graduate Partnership Program).

All NIH Institutes are mandated to have a national advisory council. This council serves several purposes: council members provide the second level of review for grants and contracts submitted, especially as they relate to the priority and relevance to the institute's mission; in addition, council members bring diverse perspectives to the science and management of the institutes. Like other institutes, the NINR benefits from the expertise of 15 individuals with varied backgrounds, including nurse researchers, corporate executives, health policy specialists, and others from several related disciplines. By mandate, 10 members must be in the health science disciplines whereas the other five are drawn from the general public and may represent law, economics, business, and other fields. There are several ex-officio members, including the Secretary of DHHS, the NIH Director, the Chief Nursing Officer of the Department of Veterans Affairs, the Assistant Secretary for Health Affairs of the Department of Defense, and the Director of the Division of Nursing, Health Resources and Services Administration, DHHS.

NINR STRATEGIC PLANNING AND RESEARCH EMPHASIS

The programs and priorities of the NINR are consistently guided by a strategic plan developed by a joint effort of the community of nurse scholars and the NINR program staff and leaders. The 2006–2010 strategic plan consisted of two major components: strategies for building the science and areas of research emphasis.

Four strategies were outlined in the NINR strategic plan for enhancing the scientific rigor and relevance of nursing research:

- integrating biological and behavioral science for better health;
- adopting, adapting, and generating new techniques for better health care;
- improving methods for future scientific discoveries;
- developing scientists for today and tomorrow.

Under that strategic plan, there are four areas being emphasized for nursing research: (1) promoting health and preventing disease, (2) improving quality of life, (3) eliminating health disparities, and (3) setting directions for end-of-life research.

In terms of promoting health and preventing disease, the NINR's specified and varied interests include developing biomarkers to assess disease risk and response to treatment; improving biobehavioral methods, measures, and intervention strategies for optimizing health; and designing intervention studies using community-based

N

approaches to facilitate health promotion. Improving quality of life covers several areas of research, for example, self-management, symptom management, and caregiving.

Eliminating health disparities is of particular concern to NINR, with a focus primarily on elucidating mechanisms underlying disparities and developing interventions for their elimination, designing culturally appropriate interventions for testing, identifying strategies that reduce the long-term adverse consequences of poor maternal and reproductive health in minorities, and evaluating and modifying partnership and training programs to build capacity to address health disparities.

For end-of-life research, several foci are emphasized, for example, integrating biological behavioral mechanisms and interventions to address end-of-life care.

THE FUTURE

In 2011, the NINR unveiled a draft of the next stage of the strategic plan titled, "Bringing Science to Life." Once again, this was developed by an invited group of nurse investigators and is designed to guide the next several years of science generation for nursing and other disciplines. The draft document outlines the areas purposed for NINR investment for nursing research that fits the institute's mission.

In summary, the NINR motto of "Bringing Science to Life" has clearly directed the rapid advancement of nursing research in the first 25 years of the NINR's existence. Not only have they supported a rapidly evolving body of knowledge through their research programs, more important, there is evidence of the impact that this science is having on guiding professional practice and shaping health policy.

Ada Sue Hinshaw

NATIONAL LEAGUE FOR NURSING

Since its creation in 1893 as a society formed for "the establishment and maintenance of a universal standard of training" for nursing, the National League for Nursing (NLN; www.nln.org) has continued to be a leading professional association for nursing education. The mission of the NLN is to promote excellence in nursing education to build a strong and diverse nursing workforce to advance the nation's health. The NLN implements its mission guided by four dynamic and integrated core values that permeate the organization and are reflected in its work—caring, integrity, diversity, and excellence.

The NLN's strategic plan calls for the organization (1) to enhance the NLN's national and international impact as the recognized leader in nursing education; (2) to build a diverse, sustainable, member-led organization with the capacity to deliver our mission effectively, efficiently, and in accordance with our values; (3) to be the voice of nurse educators and champion their interests in political, academic, and professional arenas; and (4) to promote evidence-based nursing education and the scholarship of teaching.

Members of the NLN include nurse educators, schools of nursing, health care agencies, and interested members of the public. The NLN offers faculty development, networking opportunities, testing services, nursing research grants, and public policy initiatives to its 34,000 individual and 1,200 institutional members who represent all types of nursing education programs from doctoral to licensed practical nursing.

Beverly Louise Malone

National League for Nursing Accrediting Commission (NLNAC)

The American Society of Superintendents of Training Schools for Nurses (the "Society") was formed in 1893 to establish and maintain a universal standard for the training of nurses, becoming the first nursing organization of its type in the United States. It later became known as the National League for Nursing. Following the turn of the 20th century, the Society issued numerous publications addressing the standardization of curricula for schools of nursing and, eventually, through the collaborative efforts of faculty at Teachers College, Columbia University, issued the well-known *Goldmark Report*, which was the first survey of nursing and nursing education in the United States (Christy, 1969). In 1912, the Society became the League for Nursing Education. Ever concerned about the standardization and quality of the education of nurses, by 1938, the "league" initiated accrediting activities for schools of nursing. It was not until 1952, however, that the process of accreditation of nursing schools was brought under the aegis of the National League for Nursing.

In 1996, the National League for Nursing Board of Governors approved the recommendation for the establishment of an independent organization to be known as the National League for Nursing Accrediting Commission (NLNAC). The 15 commissioners consist of nine nurse educators, three executives, and three public members. These commissioners that oversee the organization assume full responsibility for the management, financial decisions, policymaking, and general administration of the NLNAC. The NLNAC is recognized by the U.S. Department of Education as the national accrediting body for all types of programs in nursing education. NLNAC is also recognized by the National Council of State Boards of Nursing, State Boards of Nurse Examiners, the U.S. Department of Health and Human Services, Bureau of Health Professions, Nursing, and the U.S. Uniformed Nursing Services, to name a few. As of December 2006, NLNAC assumed responsibility for the accreditation of nursing programs, ranging from licensed practical nursing through the master's degree level. In 2009, they accredited their first clinical doctorate program, with many more to follow (NLNAC, 2010). NLNAC accreditation offers to schools of nursing the following:

1. the national recognition that the program or school has been evaluated by a competent and respected independent group, which determines whether the program meets or exceeds predetermined criteria as set forth by the NLNAC for nursing programs within their respective categories (e.g., practical nursing, diploma granting, or degree granting);

2. the opportunity to demonstrate that the program or school fosters ongoing self-examination and reevaluation of nursing education programs for purposes of quality improvement; and

3. the assurance that the program or school demonstrates a quality educational offering and that students and graduates of the program are eligible for educational mobility, starting with the licensed practical nursing programs.

See also National Council of State Boards of Nursing, Inc.; National League for Nursing

N

Christy, T. E. (1969). *Cornerstone for nursing education*. New York, NY: Teachers College Press, Teachers College, Columbia University.

Additional information is available at these Web sites:

National League for Nursing Accrediting Commission. (n.d.). Retrieved December 30, 2010, from http://www.nlnac.org/home.htm

National League for Nursing Accrediting Commission. (2010). 2010 Report to Constituents. Retrieved December 30, 2010, from http://www.nlnac.org/reports/2010.pdf

Gina M. Myers
M. Janice Nelson

NATIONAL ORGANIZATION OF NURSE PRACTITIONER FACULTIES

The National Organization of Nurse Practitioner Faculties (NONPF) was established in 1974 "to promote national and international quality nurse practitioner education:...the NONPF domains and core competencies for nurse practitioner (NP) practice have provided guidance to curriculum development across NP programs. NONPF also has led the development of entry-level competencies for NP specialty practice and of national guidelines for NP educational programs. These seminal documents support the preparation of 'highly qualified health professionals'" (www.nonpf.com). NONPF is a resource to faculty and practitioners. The vision of this organization is to "elevate and foster the highest standards of nurse practitioner education and innovative instructional approaches" (www.nonpf.com/history&goals). In addition to the core competencies in primary and acute care, NONPF has published a number of statements on seminal topics in nursing education, including a response to the National Council of State Boards of Nursing's *Vision Paper: The Future Regulation of Advanced Practice Nursing*, recommendations on the practice doctorate in nursing, and a monograph on mentoring. Listed on the NONPF Web site are resource centers of the organization, namely, Practice Doctorate Resource Center, Community Health Resource Center, and Faculty Practice Resource Center. These are designed, in part, to convey the perspective of NONPF, the latest updates on committee work, and available resources for members, so that members are educated about the latest issues that may affect their practice in clinical and academic areas. NONPF represents more than 90% of all institutions in the United States, with NP programs as well as faculty programs in Canada, the United Kingdom, and other countries.

See also Advanced Practice Registered Nurses; National Council of State Boards of Nursing, Inc.; Regulatory Boards

Paule V. Joseph
Harriet R. Feldman

NATIONAL STUDENT NURSES' ASSOCIATION

Founded in 1952, the National Student Nurses' Association (NSNA) is a nonprofit organization for students enrolled in pre–registered nurse (RN) licensure programs and RN to Baccalaureate of Science in Nursing completion programs. It is dedicated to fostering the professional formation of nursing students. Over the years, hundreds of thousands of nursing students have carried the NSNA membership card as a tangible symbol of their early commitment to the nursing profession. As the only independent organization for nursing students, NSNA

- brings together and mentors students preparing for initial registered nurse licensure as well as those enrolled in baccalaureate completion programs;
- conveys the standards and ethics of the nursing profession;
- promotes development of the skills that students need as responsible and accountable members of the nursing profession;
- advocates for high-quality, evidence-based, affordable, and accessible health care;
- advocates for and contributes to advances in nursing education; and
- develops nursing students who are prepared to lead the profession in the future.

NSNA members participate in community health projects, legislation education, global education initiatives, and activities to recruit students into the profession. Special activities include the following:

- Breakthrough to Nursing Project®, designed to increase the number of registered nurses from underrepresented populations into the nursing profession;
- Community health projects offering opportunities to address the health needs of the public;
- Implementation of the Bill of Rights and Responsibilities for Students of Nursing and model Code of Ethics for students to adopt;
- Legislation Education program to encourage involvement in understanding the legislative process, voter registration, and get-out-the vote activities;
- Global Initiatives in Nursing Committee, established in 2010 to recognize the International Year of the Nurse, educates nursing students about global

opportunities in nursing, and encourages students with diverse experiences to share their special knowledge;
- NSNA Leadership University (www.nsna-leadershipu.org) encourages students to earn academic credit for participating in NSNA's many shared governance and leadership activities;
- Opportunity to build and maintain an electronic, Web-based professional portfolio.

Success in nursing school is an important focus for NSNA. Education programs at the Annual Convention and Annual Mid-Year Conference cover a wide range of topics that broaden a student's perspective as well as to help them pass the RN licensure examination and plan a successful nursing career. Approximately 5,000 nursing students attend educational programs and participate in leadership and professional development activities. Faculty who attend NSNA meetings are awarded continuing education credit for several programs designed to enhance their teaching skills.

NSNA is governed by a Board of Directors and House of Delegates. Ten nursing students who are elected to serve for 1 year comprise the Board of Directors. Two consultants appointed by the American Nurses Association and the National League for Nursing provide guidance to the Board (without vote). Four students are also elected to serve on the Nominating and Elections Committee. A House of Delegates meets annually to elect officers and to debate resolutions that focus on issues relevant to nursing education and practice. Delegates come from 700 school and state NSNA chapters. National staff provides administrative support. Scholarships, ranging from $1,000 to $5,000, are offered through the Foundation of the National Student Nurses' Association (FNSNA). In addition to the general scholarship program, the

N

N

Promise of Nursing Regional Scholarship Program, administered by the FNSNA, provides undergraduate and graduate nursing scholarships, fellowships, and school grants. Funds for the Promise of Nursing program are raised by regional events sponsored by Johnson & Johnson.

All NSNA members receive *Imprint* magazine, published five times during the academic year. Other publications include *NSNA e-News, Dean's Notes*, and several *Guidelines for Planning* booklets. A variety of programs produced by NSNA include DVDs and videos on the following: mentoring, recruitment into the nursing profession, career advancement (*Nursing—the Career of a Lifetime*), convention keynote addresses and plenary sessions, history of NSNA, history of the American Nurses Association, and NSNA membership recruitment. Membership and involvement in NSNA has grown over time. Nursing students with a desire to share their experiences and passion for nursing and to have a voice in the future of the profession comprise more than 56,000 members nationwide. Involvement in leadership activities as a student has inspired many NSNA alumni to become leaders of the nursing profession.

See also American Nurses Association; Mentoring; National League for Nursing

Diane Mancino

NURSE RESIDENCY

Residency programs, first reported in the literature in the 1980s, are of documented value in the successful transition of the graduate nurse into professional practice (Altier & Krsek, 2006). It has become increasingly more difficult for new graduates in acute care hospitals to transition to the staff nurse role. To meet the needs of hospitalized patients, today's graduates must have the knowledge and skills necessary to care for acutely ill patients presenting with complex needs (Goode & Williams, 2004). A well-designed residency program enables the nurse resident to progress from the comprehension of evidence-based practice to the actual application of learned knowledge and skill in the work setting (Krugman et al., 2006).

Various descriptions of nurse residency programs exist in the literature (Goode & Williams, 2004; Rosenfeld, Smith, Iervolino, & Bowar-Ferres, 2004). A residency program is a unique educational opportunity that allows the expansion of skills in a nurturing, supportive environment. Effort is acknowledged, the individual's importance is validated, and positive outcomes result. Collegial relationships established during the program continue to grow after residency completion (Altier & Krsek, 2006).

Residency programs generally include extended orientation time, relationship with a mentor, and structured educational/didactic sessions (Goode & Willliams, 2004; Herdrich & Lindsay, 2006; Rosenfeld et al., 2004).

Nurse residency programs have been acknowledged as a key strategy in the recruitment and retention of graduate nurses (Herdrich & Lindsay, 2006; Joint Commission on Accreditation of Healthcare Organizations, 2002; Nursing Executive Watch, 2002; Robert Wood Johnson Foundation, 2002).

In 2002, the University HealthSystem Consortium and the American Association of Colleges of Nursing (UHC/AACN) jointly developed the National Post-Baccalaureate Residency Program curriculum, addressing the needs identified by new graduates and hospitals that employ them. This standardized curriculum is based on a series of learning and practice experiences involving cohort relationships and clinical narratives. Core content is divided into three topic areas: leadership, patient outcomes, and professional role development. Critical thinking and communication threads are woven throughout the year-long program (Krugman et al., 2006). The AACN (2008) has adopted accreditation standards for these programs. A unique feature of the UHC/AACN residency model is the partnership between the academic hospital and the paired college of nursing. This collaboration affords an opportunity to share resources, strengthen the relationship between service and academe, and incorporate the cross-fertilization of knowledge between the clinical enterprise and the university (Goode & Williams, 2004). The desired outcomes of this project are the reduction of new graduate turnover, the enhanced job satisfaction and autonomy, the increased critical thinking skills, the increased support for the new graduate, and the attainment of the additional competencies needed to function as a staff nurse in a manner that promotes patient safety (Goode & Williams, 2004).

Evidence of nurse residency success within the acute care setting is available that supports their impact in increasing nurse retention (Altier & Krsek, 2006; Goode & Williams, 2004; Krugman et al., 2006; Rosenfeld et al., 2004), improving critical thinking skills (Herdrich & Lindsay, 2006), improving organizing and prioritizing abilities, and reducing graduate nurse stress (Krugman et al., 2006). Further evaluation of the need for nurse residency programs outside of acute care settings is necessary, particularly as patient care moves from hospital to community-based settings, and increasingly new graduates need to be prepared for their role in these settings.

Altier, M. E., & Krsek, C. A. (2006). Effects of a 1-year residency program on job satisfaction and retention of new graduate nurses. *Journal for Nurses in Staff Development, 22*(2), 70–77.

American Association of Colleges of Nursing. (2008). *The essentials of baccalaureate education for professional nursing practice.* Washington, DC: Author. Retrieved from http://www.aacn.nche.edu/education/pdf/BaccEssentials08.pdf

Goode, C. J., & Williams, C. A. (2004). Postbaccalaureate nurse residency program. *Journal of Nursing Administration, 34*(2), 71–77.

Goode, C. J., Lynn, M. R., Krsek, C. A., & Bednash, G. D. (2009). Nurse residency programs: An essential requirement for nursing. *Nursing Economics, 27*(3), 142–147, 159.

Herdrich, B., & Lindsay, A. (2006). Nurse residency programs: Redesigning the transition into practice. *Journal for Nurses in Staff Development, 22*(2), 55–62.

Joint Commission on Accreditation of Healthcare Organizations. (2002). *Health care at the crossroads: Strategies for addressing the evolving nursing crisis.* Retrieved from http://www.jcaho.org

Krugman, M., Bretschneider, J., Horn, P. B., Krsek, C. A., Moutafis, R. A., & Smith, M. O. (2006). The national post-baccalaureate graduate nurse residency program: A model for excellence in transition to practice. *Journal for Nurses in Staff Development, 22*(4), 196–205.

Nursing Executive Watch. (2002). *Hospitals exploring nurse residencies to improve retention.* Washington, DC: Healthcare Advisory Board.

Robert Wood Johnson Foundation. (2002). *Health care's human crisis: The American nursing shortage.* Princeton, NJ: Author. Retrieved from www.rwjf.org

Rosenfeld, P., Smith, M. O., Iervolino, L., & Bowar-Ferres, S. (2004). Nurse residency program: A 5-year evaluation from the participants' perspective. *Journal of Nursing Administration, 34*(4), 188–194.

Mary Ann McGinley

N

NURSE SATISFACTION IN THE PROFESSIONAL PRACTICE ENVIRONMENT

Over the years, renewed emphasis has been placed on the reorganization and redesign of the professional practice environment (PPE) of nurses and other health care providers (Champy, 1996). This emphasis continues, especially in light of the changes proposed by the Institute of Medicine's (2010) *Future of Nursing Report*, which places strong focus on nursing leadership, increased practice autonomy, and reduction of the barriers that compromise nursing's ability to provide care within its' full scope of practice. The effect of the changing economic trends, diminishing resources, and increasing demands on nurses in the workplace has affected the recruitment and retention of nurses, particularly within the acute care environment, which has focused increased attention on nurses' practice environments (Ebright, 2010; Lake, 2007). Although these factors can affect patient satisfaction and patient centric care, they also can affect the nurse practice environments and challenge the delivery of evidence-driven, cost-effective, quality, safe, and efficient patient care. Today, the consumer as well as the clinician seeks to work and be cared for in a setting that promotes patient/family-centered care and supports professional practice. As restructuring of health care environments continues, the evaluation of the patient's satisfaction with care keeps advancing. Equally important is the evaluation of the work setting that the clinician works in to deliver high-quality care each day. The organizational culture that creates the environment in which the care is delivered plays a very important role in affecting clinical practice and patient outcomes (Aiken, Sochalski, & Lake, 1997). The leadership provided by those responsible for implementing such an environment is critical to the recruitment and retention of professional care providers (Poghosyan, Clark, Finlayson, & Aiken, 2010). Measuring the effectiveness of the PPE remains both a challenge and an opportunity that fosters to be a challenge.

In the early 1980s, the work of McClure, Poulin, Sovie, and Wandelt (1983) initiated the American Academy of Nursing's Task Force on Nursing Practice in Hospitals. This initiative focused on the collection of data to identify successful work environments in the United States (McClure, Poulin, Sovie, & Wandelt, 2002). Data from this project indicated that hospital settings with characteristics such as high autonomy, control over practice, and collaborative nurse–physician relationships also reported increased nurse retention and low staff turnover and were places where nurses liked to work. These settings were characterized by the research team as Magnet Hospitals. This research was followed by a series of studies conducted by Kramer (1990) and Kramer and Schmalenberg (1993) that supported the findings from the original Magnet study. The elements of autonomy control over practice and effective communication among nurses and physicians continued to yield a positive work experience and supported a positive work environment for clinicians.

Future studies by Kramer and colleagues provided data that resulted in the first multidimensional measure of satisfaction with the PPE. The Nursing Work Index (NWI), developed by Kramer and Hafner (1989), consisted of 65 items designed to measure those organizational elements first identified by the Magnet Hospitals. Nurses were asked to evaluate their level of agreement with items measured on a 4-point Likert scale, indicating what elements were important for them to experience job satisfaction and be able to offer patients high-quality care. In 2000, Aiken and Patrician evaluated the NWI and reduced it to 55 items. The NWI-Revised (NWI-R) measured three conceptually derived elements that support an effective PPE: nurse autonomy, control over practice, and relationships with physicians. Specific scoring procedures for both the NWI and the NWI-R, have been developed and are available for use by other researchers. In 2002, Lake revised the NWI and created the Practice Environment Scale (PES), which contained 45 items from the original 65 items. Through research, Lake established the psychometric properties of the PES with five factors defined: nurse participation in hospital affairs, nursing foundations for quality care, nurse manager ability, support for nurses, and staffing and resource adequacy. The use of the PES–NWI continues to grow worldwide. Recent recommendations for use internationally include the reduction in tool length, consistency in scoring across testing sites, using the tool over time in similar sites, and increased attention to cultural variation (Warshawsky & Havens, 2010).

In 1998, the PPE scale was developed by a team from the Massachusetts General Hospital (MGH) to expand on the elements included in both the NWI-R and the PES. In addition to measuring the original Magnet constructs, the PPE was a new instrument developed to address the challenges of the current health care environments, including cultural diversity, responsiveness potential for workplace conflicts emerging in a fast-paced work setting, and motivation of the workforce in the face of limited resources and demands for cost effectiveness. The original PPE scale consisted of 35 items anchored on a 4-point Likert scale

that measured eight PPE characteristics, namely, leadership and autonomy over practice, clinician–physician relationships, control over practice, communications about patients, teamwork, conflict management, internal work motivation, and cultural sensitivity. The 35-item PPE scale was used between 1999 and 2001 with satisfactory internal consistency reliability estimates for the subscales (above .75). In 2004, a revised 40-item PPE scale was developed to clarify problem items identified by respondents. The scale was psychometrically evaluated with a sample of 849 respondents from within the professional practice staff (across disciplines) at the MGH. In the data analysis, all items, with two exceptions, met the minimum item-total correlation criterion of .30. The resulting 38-item scale, with a Cronbach's alpha of .93, produced an eight-component solution with Cronbach's alphas ranging from .78 to .88. These results established the instrument as a valid and reliable measure of staff perception of the professional practice work environment (Ives Erickson, Duffy, Gibbons, Fitzmaurice, Ditomassi, & Jones, 2004).

In 2006, MGH staff undertook more editorial revision on the PPE Scale that included making each item a complete declarative statement and adding two items to the Handling Disagreement/Conflict subscale. In addition, the now 40-item scale was developed for use online and called the Revised Professional Practice Environment (RPPE) Scale (Ives Erickson, Duffy, Ditomassi, & Jones, 2009) The RPPE-Online, which was distributed electronically too, yielded a 61% response rate ($n = 1,837$). The psychometric evaluation of the RPPE-Online was then undertaken on all nurses in the 2006 sample who had no missing data on the scale ($n = 1,550$). A random sample cross-validation procedure (Cudeck & Brown, 1983) was used to test whether the eight factors in the calibration sample ($n = 775$) could also be derived in a second, comparable validation sample ($n = 775$) drawn from the same population of MGH nurses. The two samples were comparable with no significant differences on demographic characteristics. Sample size for both samples was more than adequate to undertake principal components analyses with each sample having an approximate 20:1 case-to-variable ratio (Comrey, 1988; Tabachnick & Fidell, 2007).

Internal consistency for the 40-item RPPE–Online was .93 for the calibration sample and .92 for the validation sample. Principal components analysis was next undertaken on the calibration and validation samples with the original eight PPE scale components being demonstrated. In the calibration sample, 59.0% of total variance was explained by the eight components; in the validation sample, 59.5% was accounted for by the same eight components. Cronbach's alpha internal consistency reliabilities ranged from .76 to .87 in the calibration sample and from .76 to .88 in the validation sample. In both samples, the same three items were dropped because of low item-total correlations. Thus, findings from this cross-validation psychometric evaluation indicated that the 37-item RPPE-Online is reliable and valid for use in health outcomes research examining eight characteristics of the PPE of RN staff working in acute care settings.

Over the years, the PPE and RPPE have been used to evaluate nurses' perception of PPEs. Several researchers have translated the tool into other languages for testing within culturally diverse populations (Chang, 2009; Halcomb, Davidson, Caldwell, Salomonson, & Rolly, 2010). Study results support the RPPE as an effective measure of professional practice settings. Some sites have reduced the number of items, whereas others have added questions focusing on professional development (Chang, 2009).

Continuing work on the importance of creating a work environment has been reported in the literature. Those PPEs that celebrate professional autonomy, control over practice, and promote collaboration and team work also affect the recruitment and retention of staff and enhance the delivery of high-quality, safe, effective, efficient, patient centric patient care (Armstrong, Laschinger & Wong, 2009; Barden, 2005; Sherman &Prossm, 2010).

See also American Academy of Nursing; Consumer Satisfaction; Magnet Hospitals; Staff Recruitment; Staff Retention

Aiken, L. H., & Patrician, P. A. (2000). Measuring organizational traits of hospitals. The Revised Nursing Work Index. *Nursing Research, 49*(3), 146–153.

Aiken, L., Sochalski, J., & Lake, E. (1997). Studying outcomes of organizational change in health services. *Medical Care, 35*(Suppl. 11), NS6–NS18.

Armstrong, K., Laschinger, H., &Wong, C. (2009).Workplace empowerment and Magnet hospital characteristics as predictors of patient safety climate. *Journal Nursing Quality Care, 24,* 55–62.

Barden, C. (2005). AACN standards for establishing healthy work environment: a journey of excellence. Washington, DC: AACN.

Champy, J. (1996). *Reengineering management: The mandate for new leadership.* New York, NY: Harper Business.

Chang, C. C. (2009). *Psychometric properties of the translated Chinese version of the Professional Practice Environment tool.* Doctoral dissertation, University of Michigan.

Comrey, A. (1988). Factor analytic methods of scale development in personality and clinical psychology. *Journal of Consulting and Clinical Psychology, 56,* 754–761.

Cudeck, R., & Brown, M. (1983). Cross validation of covariance structures. *Multivariate Behavioral Research, 18,* 147–167.

Ebright, P. (2010). The complex work of the RN: Implications health work environment. *Online Journal of Issues in Nursing, 15.*

Halcomb, E. J., Davidson, P. M., Caldwell, B., Salamonson, Y., & Rolley, J. X. (2010). Validation of the Professional Practice Environment Scale in Australian practice. *Journal of Nursing Scholarship, 42*(2), 207–213.

Institute of Medicine. (2010). *The future of nursing leading the change in health care.* Washington, DC: National Academies Press.

Ives Erickson, J., Duffy, M., Gibbons, P., Fitzmaurice, J., Ditomassi, M., & Jones, D. (2004). Development and psychometric evaluation of the Professional Practice Environment (PPE) scale. *Journal of Nursing Scholarship, 36*(3), 279–284.

Ives Erickson, J., Duffy, M., Ditomassi, M., & Ives Erickson, J. M. (2009). Psychometric evaluation of the Revised Professional Practice Environment (RPPE) scale. *Journal of Nursing Administration, 29*(19)5, 236–243.

Kramer, M. (1990). The magnet hospitals: Excellence revisited. *Journal of Nursing Administration, 20*(9), 35–44.

Kramer, M., & Hafner, L. P. (1989). Shared values: Impact on staff nurse job satisfaction and perceived productivity. *Nursing Research, 38,* 172–177.

Kramer, M., & Schmalenberg, C. (1993). Learning from success: Autonomy and empowerment. *Nursing Management, 24*(5), 58–64.

Lake, E. (2002). Development of the Practice Environment Scale of the Nursing Work Index. *Research in Nursing & Health, 25,* 176–188.

Lake, E. (2007). The nursing practice environment: Measurement and evidence. *Medical Care Research and Review, 64*(2), 104S–122S.

McClure, M., Poulin, M., Sovie, M., & Wandelt, M. (1983). *Magnet hospitals: Attraction and retention of professional nurses.* Kansas City, MO: American Nurses Association.

McClure, M., Poulin, M., Sovie, M., & Wandelt, M. (2002). *Magnet hospitals: Attraction and retention of professional nurses (original study).* In M. McClure & A. Hinshaw (Eds.), *Magnet hospitals revisited: Attraction and retention of professional nurses* (pp. 1–24), Washington, DC: American Nurses Publishing.

Poghosyan, L., Clark, S. P., Finlayson, M., & Aiken, L. (2010). Nurse burnout and quality care: Cross-national investigation of six countries. *Research Nursing and Health, 33,* 288–298.

Sherman, R., & Pross, E. (2010). Growing future leaders to build and sustain healthy work environments at the unit level. *Online Journal of Issues in Nursing, 15.*

Tabachnick, B., & Fidell, L. (2007). *Using multivariate statistics* (5th ed.). Needham, MA: Allyn & Bacon.

Warshawsky, N. E., & Havens, D. S. (2010). Global use of the Practice Environment Scale of work index. *Nursing Research, 60*(1), 17–31.

Dorothy A. Jones
Jeanette Ives Erickson
Marianne Ditomassi

NURSES EDUCATIONAL FUNDS, INC.

Nurses Educational Funds, Inc. (NEF), is solely dedicated to providing scholarships for registered nurses to advance their education at the gradate level. Established in 1910, NEF has endowed 14 named scholarships as well as a general scholarship fund. Applicants must be registered nurses enrolled full time or part time in an accredited master's degree in nursing or in a doctoral degree program in nursing or a nursing-related field. Other eligibility requirements include membership in a professional nursing association and U.S. citizenship (or declaration of official intention of becoming a U.S. citizen). The criteria that are given the greatest consideration when selecting candidates include academic excellence and the potential for contributing to the nursing profession. NEF is a not-for-profit organization. Contributions to NEF are tax deductible. Application information is available on the NEF Web site (www.nef.org).

Diane Mancino

N

NURSES IMPROVING CARE FOR HEALTHSYSTEM ELDERS (NICHE)

Nurses Improving Care for Healthsystem Elders (NICHE) is the only national nursing program designed to address the specialized needs of the older adult patient. A program of the Hartford Institute for Geriatric Nursing at New York University College of Nursing, NICHE was founded by Dr. Terry Fulmer in 1992 and comprises a national network of hospitals and their affiliate health care organizations. The program provides initial and ongoing resources to assist hospitals to develop and strengthen both the individual nurse's geriatric expertise as well as a hospital's capacity to develop, use, and evaluate best-practice nursing care for older adults (Fulmer et al., 2002). This approach is consistent with the American Organization of Nurse Executives Guiding Principles for Creating Elder Friendly Hospitals (www. aone.org/aone/resource/elder.html).

The core components of NICHE include self-evaluation tools for the hospital; evidence-based clinical protocols and a resource-laden Web site and knowledge center, which offers geriatric curricula for nurses, patient care technicians, and other staff; and other E-learning educational materials (Bricoli, 2010). The Geriatric Institutional Assessment Profile is an instrument that helps NICHE-participating hospitals identify organizational attributes of the hospital relevant to geriatric care, including gaps in knowledge about geriatric care, attitudes, and perceptions that influence how staff work with older patients and specific practice issues and concerns (Abraham et al., 2002). Results are benchmarked against other NICHE hospitals and used to measure organizational readiness to provide quality care to older adults before implementing NICHE and to evaluate the effectiveness postimplementation of NICHE (Boltz, Capezuti, Kim, Fairchild, & Secic, 2009; Boltz, Capezuti, Kim, & Fairchild, 2010; Kim et al., 2007).

NICHE hospitals are linked through listserv, online discussion boards, ongoing conferences, and task forces that inform policy and resource development at the Hartford Institute for Geriatric Nursing at New York University College of Nursing. In addition, NICHE provides nursing practice models of care with consultation and guidelines provided for start-up and maintenance of the selected model.

PRACTICE MODELS

NICHE hospitals implement one or more geriatric practice models. The Geriatric Resource Nurse (GRN) Model is foundational to the NICHE program. The GRN model is based on the belief that primary nurses know the most about the daily patterns and needs of the older adults on their units and is associated with the institutional values of nurse autonomy and professional development (Fulmer, 2001). After receiving specialized education in nursing care of the older adult, the GRN receives ongoing mentorship and clinical support from an advance practice nurse. The GRN in turn provides consultation to staff nurse colleagues.

Many hospitals use NICHE principles and tools in their acute care environment (ACE) units. The ACE unit model provides a self-contained, specially prepared environment, nurse/geriatrician comanagement, and interdisciplinary collaboration. The program components include interdisciplinary team management, patient-centered nursing care, early discharge planning, and review of medical care for older adult patients (Mezey et al., 2004). ACE units provide elder-friendly furniture, sitting areas, low beds, sensory aids, such as hearing amplifiers, equipment to support activities of daily living (ADL) performance, and environmental design that is specialized to the needs of older adults (Siegler, Glick, & Lee, 2002). NICHE programs are also frequently aligned with other hospital initiatives, including a geriatric consultation service, the volunteer-intensive Hospital Elder Life Program, the Advanced Practice Nurse Transitional Care model, and the Care Transition Intervention program (Capezuti & Brush, 2009).

NICHE OUTCOMES

Hospitals have reported improved clinical outcomes, enhanced nurse knowledge and perceptions of quality, increased compliance with protocol application, and decreased length of stay upon implementing the NICHE program (Boltz, Capezuti, Bower-Ferres, Norman, Secic, et al., 2008; Guthrie, Edinger, & Schumacher, 2002; Lee & Fletcher, 2002; Lopez et al., 2002; Pfaff, 2002; Swauger & Tomlin, 2002). Also, NICHE programs are associated with improved Joint Commission performance and Magnet initiatives. The following key factors are instrumental in successfully implementing NICHE: a clear vision of geriatric care, an interdisciplinary collaboration, a process of including staff in relevant decision making, and mechanisms to address staff needs for education, equipment, and other geriatric specific resources (Boltz, Capezuti, Bowar-Ferres, Norman, Kim, et al., 2008). Thus, NICHE requires the commitment of nursing leadership to meet the requirement of ongoing NICHE designation, that is, the implementation of a geriatric model and the ongoing evaluation of its effectiveness.

See also American Organization of Nurse Executives; Evidence-Based Practice

Abraham, I. L., Bottrell, M. M., Dash, K. R., Fulmer, T., Mezey, M., O'Donnell, L., et al. (2002). Profiling care and benchmarking best practice in care of hospitalized elderly: The Geriatric Institutional Assessment Profile. *Nursing Clinics of North America, 34*(1), 237–255.

Boltz, M., Capezuti, E., Bowar-Ferres, S., Norman, R., Kim, H., Fairchild, S., et al. (2008). Hospital nurses' perceptions of the geriatric care environment. *Journal of Nursing Scholarship, 40*(3), 282–289.

Boltz, M., Capezuti, E., Bower- Ferres, S., Norman, R., Secic, M., Kim, H., et al. (2008). Changes in the geriatric care environment associated with NICHE. *Geriatric Nursing, 29* (3), 176–185.

Boltz, M., Capezuti, E., Kim, H., & Fairchild, S. (2010). Factor structure of the GIAP Professional Issues Scales. *Research in Gerontological Nursing, 3*(2), 126–134.

Boltz, M., Capezuti, E., Kim, H., Fairchild, S., & Secic, M. (2009). Test–retest reliability of the GIAP (Geriatric Institutional Assessment Profile). *Clinical Nursing Research, 18,* 242–252.

Bricoli, B. (2010). Evolution of a Web presence: NICHE launches new Web site to meet the quality imperative. *Geriatric Nursing, 31*(3), 236–238.

Capezuti, E., & Brush, B. (2009). Implementing geriatric care models: What are we waiting for? *Geriatric Nursing, 30*(3), 204–206.

Fulmer, T. (2001). The geriatric resource nurse: A model of caring for older patients. *American Journal of Nursing, 102,* 62.

Fulmer, T., Mezey, M., Bottrell, M., Abraham, I., Sazant, J., Grossman, C., et al. (2002). Nurses Improving Care for Healthsystem Elders (NICHE): Nursing outcomes and benchmarks for evidence-based practice. *Geriatric Nursing, 23*(3), 121–127.

Guthrie, P. F., Edinger, G., & Schumacher, S. (2002). TWICE: A NICHE program at North Memorial Health Center (CE). *Geriatric Nursing, 23*(2), 133–139.

Kim, H., Capezuti, E., Boltz, M., Fairchild, S., Fulmer, T., & Mezey, M. (2007). Factor structure of the geriatric care environment scale. *Nursing Research, 56*(5), 339–347.

N

Lee, V. K., & Fletcher, K. R. (2002). Sustaining the geriatric resource model at the University of Virginia. *Geriatric Nursing*, 23(3), 128–132.

Lopez, M., Delmore, B., Young, K., Golden, P., Bier, J., & Fulmer, Y. (2002). Implementing a geriatric resource model. *Journal of Nursing Administration*, 32(11), 577–585.

Mezey, M., Kobayashi, M., Grossman, S., Firpo, A., Fulmer, T., & Mitty, E. (2004). Nurses Improving Care to Healthsystem Elders (NICHE): Implementation of best practice models. *Journal of Nursing Administration*, 34(10), 451–457.

Pfaff, J. (2002). The Geriatric Resource Nurse Model: A culture change. *Geriatric Nursing*, 23(3), 140.

Siegler, E. L., Glick, D., & Lee, J. (2002). Optimal staffing for Acute Care of the Elderly (ACE) units. *Geriatric Nursing*, 23, 152.

Swauger, K., & Tomlin, K. (2002). Best care for the elderly at Forsyth Medical Center. *Geriatric Nursing*, 23(3), 145–150.

Marie Boltz
Elizabeth Capezuti

NURSING INFORMATICS

The American Nurses Association has recognized the specialty area of nursing informatics since 1992. The 2008 American Nurses Association's *Nursing Informatics: Scope and Standards of Practice* defines nursing informatics as "a specialty that integrates nursing science, computer science, and information science to manage and communicate data, information, knowledge and wisdom in nursing practice" (p. 1). Data are simply the numbers for example a pulse measured in beats per minute, respirations per minute, and an oral temperature. As these three data elements are viewed together, they become information and when interpreted by the nurse become knowledge. Using nursing knowledge to manage the care of patients

for the best possible outcome is wisdom. Nursing informatics combined with the application of complexity sciences provides the mechanism for improvement and transformation of health care.

Nurses working in informatics are known as nurse informaticists or nurse informaticians. Education in the field is obtained through on-the-job training, undergraduate, certificate programs, and graduate programs including the Doctor of Nursing Practice, where nursing informatics is both content and area of specialization. Nurse Informaticians bring use the nursing process to development, planning, implementation, education, and evaluation. The nurse informatician exhibits magnetic attraction, creating an energy field, with skills such as caring, educating, translating, negotiating, and even cheerleading, at the appropriate times with different people within organizations such as leaders, staff in information technology, and clinical information software vendors to achieve transformation of nursing practice with the electronic health record (EHR) (Swinderman, 2005).

The EHR is used interchangeably with electronic medical record (EMR). "Gradually, the informatics community has been adopting 'electronic health record' as a name more in keeping with modern perspectives on comprehensive health care, health maintenance, and multidisciplinary practice" (Hunter, 2001, p. 186). "Besides providing complete, accurate patient data, regardless of location of the patient, the system will provide decision support, contain clinical reminders and alerts, and provide links to related knowledge bases" (Thede, 2003, p. 320).

The past 50 years has seen the transition from the industrial age to the information age. In the past 25 years of nursing, "three elements have been instrumental in the increasing role and responsibility for thorough charting: changes in nursing practice and responsibility, regulatory agency requirements and the legal environments in which guidelines reflect the standard of care" (Meiner, 1999, p. 17). These include the Health Insurance Portability and Accountability Act for protection of health information privacy, the Systematized Nomenclature of Medicine–Clinical Term for standardization of terminology, and the National Healthcare Database established in conjunction with the Centers for Disease Control to ensure public health against the threat of bioterrorism. Included in the Systematized Nomenclature of Medicine–Clinical Term are standardize nursing classifications systems such as the North American Nursing Diagnosis Association (NANDA) and the Omaha System.

The documentation of nursing caring using an EMR is essential for obtaining the best possible patient outcomes. Historically, the recording of the nursing observation has been challenging. As the EMR emerges, it is imperative for nursing to participate in the transformation. Nursing Informatics is faced with the complexities of information systems and technology in all aspects of health care. Technology development is outpacing nursing research. There is no way of predicting which technologies will have a big impact on nursing and health care, nor is there a way to predict the affect of public policy and health care reform. Further, there is no way to know the direction in which nursing practice will transform with technology to meet future demands.

Currently, there are no shortages of oversight and regulatory agencies applying standards and deadlines to health care providers. The American Recovery and Reinvestment Act of 2009 contained the Health Information Technology for Economic and Clinical Health Act

and created the Office of the National Coordinator for Health Information Technology, which reports to the Secretary of Health and Human Services. The U.S. National Health Information Network is working toward a Health Information Exchange with the ultimate goal of establishing incentives for standardization and to facilitate electronic exchange of data by the year 2014 (American Recovery and Reinvestment Act, 2010). Health Level Seven is an example of a standardized messaging structure that facilitates interoperability or exchange of data between multiple systems.

Changes are occurring rapidly. The value of the nurse informaticians is vital in providing education to staff, patients, and communities. Understanding information systems and technology combined with an understanding of complexity science will prepare nurse informaticians with the skills needed for leadership in transforming health care. Nursing documentation is an important component of the EHR. Nursing research and practice benefits from the advances made with the EHR. Nursing is now in a unique position to contribute and advance nursing practice by articulating and documenting caring in nursing in the EHR.

See also Electronic Health Record

American Nurses Association. (2008). *Nursing Informatics: Scope and standards of nursing practice.* Silver Springs, MD: Nursebooks.org

American Recovery and Reinvestment Act (ARRA) Implementation Plan. (June 2010) U.S. Department of Health and Human Service. Retrieved September 27, 2010 from http://www.recovery.gov/Transparency/agency/Recovery%20Plans/HHS%20Recovery%20Act%20Plan%20-%20June%202010.pdf

Hunter, K. M. (2001). Nursing informatics theory. In V. K. Saba & K. A. McCormick (Eds.), *Essentials of computers for nurses* (3rd ed., pp. 179–190). New York, NY: McGraw-Hill.

N

Meiner, S. E. (1999). Current approaches in charting. In S. E. Meiner (Ed.), *Nursing documentation: Legal focus across practice settings* (pp. 15–27). Thousand Oaks, CA: Sage Publications.

Swinderman, T. D. (2005). *The magnetic appeal of nurse informaticians: Caring attractor for emergence.* Doctor of nursing science dissertation. Florida Atlantic University. Boca Raton, FL.

Thede, L. Q. (2003). *Informatics and nursing: Opportunities and challenges* (2nd ed.). Philadelphia, PA: Lippincott Williams & Wilkins.

U.S. Department of Health and Human Service. Retrieved September 27, 2010, from http://www.recovery.gov/Transparency/agency/Recovery%20Plans/HHS%20Recovery%20Act%20Plan%20-%20June%202010.pdf

Todd D. Swinderman

Nursing Organizations Alliance

The Nursing Organizations Alliance, also known as The Alliance, was created on November 17, 2001, with the merger of the National Federation for Specialty Nursing Organizations and the Nursing Organizations Liaison Forum. The decision to join forces was based on the desire of the members to provide a more unified and stronger solidarity for nurses (Nursing Organizations Alliance, 2010a). Any nursing organization with a strong national focus on current issues related to nursing and health care may become a member of The Alliance. The headquarters of The Alliance is located in Lexington, Kentucky, and in 2010, there were more than 65 member organizations, including the American Nurses Association, the Sigma Theta Tau International, the American Association of Colleges of Nursing, the National League for Nursing, the National Student Nurses'

Association, and a variety of specialty associations. Every November, a fall summit is held at a rotating location around the United States. The purpose of the summit is to provide opportunities for networking and sharing of new knowledge across all areas of education, research, advocacy, practice, and profession advancement among the top management of the membership (Nursing Organizations Alliance, 2010b). In addition, The Alliance offers an annual 4-day Nurse in Washington Internship Program, which teaches nurses or nursing students how to impact health care policy decision making through networking and participating within the legislative structure.

See also American Association of Colleges of Nursing; American Nurses Association; National League for Nursing; National Student Nurses' Association; Sigma Theta Tau International

Nursing Organizations Alliance. (2010a). *About us.* Retrieved November 18, 2010, from http://www.nursing-alliance.org/content.cfm/id/about_us

Nursing Organizations Alliance. (2010b). *Fall Summit.* Retrieved November 18, 2010, from http://www.nursing-alliance.org/content.cfm/id/fall_summit

Ronda Mintz-Binder

Nursing Shortage in the United States

The most recent national shortage of registered nurses (RNs) in the United States began in 1998 (Buerhaus, Staiger, & Auerbach, 2000). Most nursing shortages in this country have arisen from increases in the demand for RNs, but the most recent shortage began on the supply side of the nurse labor market. The shortage started when hospitals reported they could not find enough RNs to staff intensive care units (ICU) and operating rooms. At the time, a large proportion of ICU staff was composed of younger RNs aged less than 35. However, because of the growth of career opportunities for women outside of nursing, combined with a smaller pool of perspective nursing students compared with those in earlier decades, fewer younger people were becoming RNs by the mid to late 1990s. Consequently, hospitals began reporting a shortage of RNs in ICUs. With respect to the shortage of RNs in operating rooms, a different supply-side issue was at play. Because older RNs (over 50 years) dominated operating room and perioperative staffing, when these RNs began retiring in the late 1990s, hospitals reported shortages of operating room RNs. Thus, the shortage in 1998 began as a result of very few younger RNs to staff ICUs and too many older RNs retiring from operating room and perioperative positions. By 2000, in addition, hospital admissions were increasing, which led to increased demand for RNs in all clinical positions. The size of the hospital RN shortage increased quickly, and in 2001–2002, national hospital RN vacancy rates reached 13% with hospitals reporting 100,000 open RN positions (Buerhaus, Staiger, & Auerbach, 2008).

In 2001, the nation's economy slipped into a relatively short-lived recession. Although the recession lasted only 8 months and national unemployment rates increased to a high of 6.8%, it took an unusually long period for developing jobs recovery. As RN spouses either lost their jobs or feared they might (70% of RNs were married), many RNs rejoined the labor market while others increased their work hours. In total, during 2002 and 2003,

hospitals increased RN employment by an estimated 185,000 (Buerhaus, Auerbach, & Staiger, 2007). This RN supply response was reinforced by real (inflation-adjusted) wage increases of nearly 5% in 2002 and 2% in 2003. RN vacancy rates drifted down and by the end of 2006 stood at approximately 8%. The nursing shortage was perceived to have eased in many areas of the country.

In mid-2006, housing prices collapsed around the country and quickly led to the subprime crisis that resulted, in turn, in a crisis in financial markets around the world. By the end of 2007, the nation had slid into yet another recession and intensified to the point that during each of the last four months of 2008, hundreds of thousands of Americans lost their jobs. During 2009, the national unemployment rate increased sharply and spiked at 10.5% before falling below 10% in 2010. Not surprisingly, as unemployment rates increased, RNs returned to the workforce at all-time record levels: During 2007 and 2008, hospitals hired an estimated 243,000 RNs even though hospital real RN earnings decreased in both years (Buerhaus, Auerbach, & Staiger, 2009). Of this unprecedented increase in RN employment, more than 100,000 RNs hired were over the age of 50, and an estimated 50,000 RNs had left their jobs in nonhospital settings for high-income hospital positions, which offered richer benefits (particularly health insurance) and 12-hour shifts, thereby allowing some RNs to work two jobs and support their families during the lingering recession. By the end of 2008, the national nursing shortage that had begun in 1998 had all but ended.

NEAR- AND LONG-TERM UNCERTAINTIES

Once the economy strengthens and a strong jobs recovery ensues, many RNs' spouses

N

will return to work with the consequence that many, but not all, currently employed RNs could leave the workforce. The exit from the hospital workplace could be particularly strong among older RNs as many seek to resume or begin their retirement once their spouses rejoin the labor market; and just as fast as the current "great recession" unfolded, another nursing shortage could develop. Thus, in the near-term (through 2012), whether a new shortage develops will be driven by how soon a jobs recovery will unfold, whether the recovery will be a slow or fast, and how fast and intensely RNs will respond by withdrawing from the nursing workforce.

Over the next 15 years, it is reasonable to assume that demand for RNs will grow considerably because of the increasing size of the population, expansion of health insurance coverage, aging of the population, advances in technology, and the expected shortage of physicians that will shift more work onto nurses (Buerhaus, Staiger, & Auerbach, 2008). How much demand will grow is uncertain, but there is little doubt that it will outpace the growth rate in the size of the nursing workforce. Currently, nearly 900,000 RNs (out of an estimated 2.6 million working RNs) are over the age of 50, and large numbers of these RNs are expected to retire in the years ahead (independent of the pace and intensity of a jobs recovery). Thus, the long-term tasks before the profession are twofold: replace these aging Baby Boom RNs, and beyond that, increase the total supply of RNs to meet the increasing demand.

Buerhaus, P., Staiger, D., & Auerbach, D. (2000). Why are registered nurse shortages concentrated in hospital specialty care units? *Nursing Economic$*, 18(3), 111–116.

Buerhaus, P., Auerbach, D., & Staiger, D. (2007). Recent trends in the registered nurse labor market in the US: Short-run swings on top of long-term trends. *Nursing Economic$*, 25(2), 59–66.

Buerhaus, P., Auerbach, D., & Staiger, D. (2009). The recent surge in nurse employment: causes and implications. *Health Affairs*, (Web Exclusive, June 12, 2009) w657–668.

Buerhaus, P., Staiger, D., & Auerbach, D. (2008). *The nursing workforce in the United States: Data, trends, & implications*. Boston, MA: Jones-Bartlett, Inc.

Peter I. Buerhaus

O

Oregon Model: The Oregon Consortium for Nursing Education

The Oregon Model is a label loosely applied to several educational innovations that grew out of a 2001 workforce report warning of an imminent and severe shortage of registered nurses (Northwest Health Foundation, 2001) and a strategic plan to forestall this shortage (Oregon Nursing Leadership Council [ONLC], 2001). The ONLC plan called for doubling enrollment in nursing programs and for transforming nursing education to more closely align with emerging health care needs and a changing health care system (ONLC, 2001). Among the educational innovations developed in response to this plan were the Dedicated Education Unit, adopted by faculty at the University of Portland in partnership with Providence Portland Medical Center (Burke, Moscato, & Warner, 2009; Moscato, Miller, Logsdon, Weinberg, & Chorpenning, 2007), the Oregon Simulation Alliance (Seropian, Driggers, Taylor, Gubrud-Howe, & Brady, 2006), and the Oregon Consortium for Nursing Education (OCNE) (Gubrud et al., 2003; Tanner, 2010; Tanner, Gubrud-Howe, & Shores, 2008). Each of these innovations were designed to increase capacity in schools of nursing, and all shared as a core characteristic the development and/or strengthening of partnerships across institutional barriers. Both the Dedicated Education Unit and OCNE were showcased as promising innovations in the recent Institute of Medicine (2010) report.

OCNE is a partnership among eight community colleges and the multicampus state-supported university with the following goals:

1. expand capacity through efficient use of resources and innovative clinical education models;

2. improve access to baccalaureate nursing education, particularly in rural areas;

3. transform nursing education by

   - preparing graduates to provide nursing care to individual clients, families and communities, leading evidence-based, collaborative practice in health promotion, chronic illness management, acute care, and end-of-life care;

   - preparing graduates to practice in an environment characterized by a continuing severe shortage of nurses and continuous changes in health care delivery, requiring competence in clinical judgment, compassionate relationship-centered care, interprofessional team work, teaching and guiding others (licensed and unlicensed caregivers as well as families) in providing care, using health care technology and information management systems, and participating in system-wide efforts to improve quality of care and provide for patient safety; and

- using approaches to education based on advances in the science of learning and educational technology, including use of simulation, a learning objects repository, learning management systems, and other distance education technologies.

Major components of OCNE include the following:

1. A common shared curriculum, co-created and approved by faculty on all partner campuses and implemented beginning in 2006. The curriculum is identical on all campuses for the first 3 years (including a year of prerequisites). Students from community colleges are co-admitted to the university and enroll in courses offered by university faculty in the fourth year. The competency-based, integrated curriculum is organized around "foci of care": health promotion, chronic illness management, acute care and end-of-life care, with the final year devoted to population-based care and leadership and outcomes management.

2. A comprehensive faculty development program focusing on new approaches to curriculum development advances in the science of learning and new pedagogies. This program was first provided for the 40 faculty who participated most intensely during the 2-year process of developing the curriculum, then to the remaining faculty during summer workshops.

3. An infrastructure necessary to support a common curriculum and intercampus agreements to facilitate co-enrollment, seamless transfer of credit, and financial aid across institutional boundaries.

4. Efforts to increase clinical capacity, including the development and implementation of simulation laboratories on each campus. More recently, faculty and clinical partners collaborated to create a new clinical education model, which is being pilot tested on four OCNE campuses (Gubrud & Schoessler, 2009; Gubrud, Schoessler, & Tanner, in review).

Nursing faculty and their clinical partners in Oregon have engaged in a magnitude of change that is transformative in nature. Although other programs and systems have used components of the OCNE model (e.g., competency-based education, case-based instruction, articulation between associate degree and baccalaureate programs, clinical partnership to support clinical teacher), never has one explicitly combined best practices in curriculum and instruction, state-of-the-art educational technology, competencies based on assessment of emerging health care needs of a population, mechanisms to share faculty expertise in a consortia arrangement, co-admission of students to associate and baccalaureate degree programs, and collaborative efforts to create new clinical education approaches, all in an effort to better prepare graduates and to accommodate an increased number of students.

Three major studies are currently underway to evaluate outcomes of these efforts. Moscato et al. (2007) at the University of Portland are studying the impact of the Dedicated Education Unit on faculty capacity as well as learning outcomes.[1] OCNE faculty are completing an evaluation of the effectiveness of OCNE in preparing competent nurses, with greater

---

[1] Supported by a grant from the Robert Wood Johnson Foundation, Evaluating Innovations in Nursing Education.

numbers completing the bachelor's degree.[2] OCNE faculty are also studying the effectiveness of the new clinical education model on learning outcomes, staff nurse burden and use of student and faculty time.[3]

Burke, K., Moscato, S., & Warner, J. (2009). A primer on the politics of partnership between education and regulation. *Journal of Professional Nursing, 25*(6), 349–351.

Gubrud-Howe P., Shaver, K. S. Tanner, C. A., Bennett-Stillmaker, J., Davidson, S. B., Flaherty-Robb, M., et al. (2003, April). A challenge to meet the future: Nursing education in Oregon, 2010. *Journal of Nursing Education, 42*(4), 163–167.

Gubrud, P., & Schoessler, M. (2009). OCNE clinical education model. In N. Ard & T. Valiga (Eds.), *Clinical nursing education: Current reflections* (pp. 39–58). New York, NY: National League for Nursing.

Gubrud, P., Schoessler, M., & Tanner, C. (in review). A new model of clinical education. *Journal of Nursing Education.*

Institute of Medicine. (2010). The future of nursing: Leading change, advancing health. Washington, DC: National Academies Press. Retrieved from http://www.nap.edu/catalog.php?record_id=12956

Moscato, S. R., Miller, J., Logsdon, K., Weinberg, S., & Chorpenning, L. (2007). Dedicated education unit: An innovative clinical partner education model. *Nursing Outlook, 55*(1), 31–37.

Northwest Health Foundation. (2001). *Oregon's nursing shortage: A public health crisis in the making.* Portland, OR: Author.

Oregon Nursing Leadership Council. (2001). *Oregon Nursing Leadership Council strategic plan: Solutions to Oregon's nursing shortage.* Portland, OR: Author. Retrieved June 15, 2008, from http://www.oregon centerfornursing.org/documents/ONLCstrategicplan.pdf

Seropian, M. A., Driggers, B., Taylor, J., Gubrud-Howe, P., & Brady, G. (2006). The Oregon simulation experience: A statewide simulation network and alliance. *Simulation in Healthcare: Journal of the Society for Medical Simulation, 1*(1), 56–61.

Tanner, C. A. (2010). Transforming pre-licensure nursing education: Preparing the new nurse to meet emerging health care needs. *Nursing Education Perspectives,1*(6), 347.

Tanner, C. A., Gubrud-Howe, P., & Shores, L. (2008). The Oregon consortium for nursing education: A response to the nursing shortage. *Policy, Politics, & Nursing Practice, 9*(3), 203–209.

Christine A. Tanner

ORIENTATION AND STAFF DEVELOPMENT

Redefining orientation and staff development to promote professional development and to create a meaningful path for nursing practice to excel in the 21st century of health care is critical to the profession's contribution to discipline-specific education. The academic model of orientation and staff development has shifted in the workplace just as the health care industry has changed dramatically in the 21st century. The term "in service" has become an outdated approach to postgraduate learning for nurses. Mindful learning best captures the transition from the "stage" of learning from the classroom to the bedside. Nurse educators need to focus their clinical teaching to the process of clinical reasoning and immediacy as opposed to the passivity of learning knowledge and skills in a linear and isolated manner, such as in a classroom. Alternative approaches are advancing in education. Case-based learning combines the knowledge and skills with the practice of nursing and the patient's story—wherever that may be. Blended learning implies the addition of

[2] Supported by a grant from the Robert Wood Johnson Foundation.
[3] Supported by a grant from the U.S. Department of Education, Fund for Improvement of Postsecondary Education, Comprehensive Grant Program.

O

elearning to the mix and maintains the involvement of the "teacher" or now better termed "coach" and includes simulation, games, and online computer-mediated instruction. According to Stizmann and Ely (June 3, 2009), in a presentation on Web-based instruction, this blended approach has been shown to increase learning by an average of 11%. Many nurses have experience with a traditional learning model that is teaching centric. Today, a dynamic, learner centric model is critical to capture the attention of the "student"—a product of today's social network. According to Benner (2010), there are profound changes in science: technology, consumer activism, and a market-driven health care environment. Just as nursing practice is envisioned to transform according to the Institute of Medicine's (IOM) *Report on the Future of Nursing* (Stubenrauch, 2010), so will nursing education be positioned to make equivalent innovations. This is accomplished educationally by having educators and nurses engage in a more self-directed manner that can be adapted to the current state of practice. In education today, participation in virtual simulations incorporating experience as an avatar and/or social media that mirror the real world are becoming more standard processes rather than sitting passively listening to a lecture that is limited to the boundaries of the classroom.

Orientation can also be accomplished by using aspects of blended learning and innovative approaches within social media. The development of levels of orientation to meet individual needs of newly hired staff is encouraged with a focus on competency, practicing with confidence as well as the socialization into the practice of nursing. The IOM's, *Future of Nursing Report* recommends the implementation of nurse residency programs, which assume more coaching and preceptor development while preparing nurses to lead change

and advance health. Meeting together in a group learning environment interspersed within the orientation framework can provide rich and diverse learning exercises. When time is allotted to facilitate forums for critical discussions about patient care threaded with outcomes and metrics, practicing high-level technological skills in a safe simulated environment and creating online methods for dialogue about and interaction with new knowledge and skills, the transition to the "work world" is promoted. Meaningful connections, with the ability to continuously ask questions, obtain information quickly and develop a focus for the integration of outcomes in care delivery can be better realized using these teaching methodologies. Benner (2010) shares that new nurses must be prepared to practice safely, accurately and compassionately. An orientation must be developed with that goal in mind.

Team teaching is another valuable asset to any academic exercise in the workplace because it allows real-time interdisciplinary collaboration and role modeling of how an effective health care team works. Furthermore, staff development must take on the aspect of health care team and patient rounding and bedside teaching. The IOM's, *Future of Nursing Report* (2010) also states that nurses should be full partners with their physician colleagues and other members of the health care team to improve patient care. Interdisciplinary decision making is learned behavior. Nurses must also move beyond the collection of data and advance to the development of clinical reasoning abilities and achievement of outcomes and excel in the skills of involvement and perception. According to Benner (2006), astute clinical judgment and expert caring practices are more important than ever for quality health care outcomes. However, nurses need the space to reflect on their interpersonal engagement with patients as well as focusing on their technical expertise. Clinical reasoning gives nurses the ability to make a difference in their roles. Nurses who feel influential can look at the outcomes for their patients. This view goes beyond the practice of nursing to completing tasks but thinking "with the end in mind." According to Pesut and Herman (1999), education in the workplace must focus on getting nurses to helicopter above the forest and look down at it rather than through it. When nurses can effectively do this, they can develop a reflective and creative approach to patient care. Consequently, staff development today has to move beyond the boundaries of test taking and classroom techniques and complement with probing questions such as: "What is your plan?" "What are your outcomes for this patient?" "What are your metrics of success for your patient population such as nurse sensitive indicators, core measures and patient satisfaction?" Framing situations, according to Pesut and Herman, also guide perceptions and behaviors, not just develops tasks and skills. Education in the workplace can be very instrumental in promoting these higher levels of practice and meeting the challenges of health care reform and the future of nursing.

Benner, P. (2006). *Enhancing nursing excellence in a time of change and cost-containment: Benner Associates Brochure Statement*. (n.d.). Retrieved July 9, 2006, from http://home.earthlink.net/~bennerassoc/brochure.html

Benner, P. (2010). *Educating nurses: A call for radical transformation practice* (p. 1). San Francisco, CA: Jossey Bass.

Pesut, D., & Herman, J. (1999). *Clinical reasoning: The art and science of critical and creative thinking*. Albany, NY: Delmar Publishers.

Sitzmann, T., & Ely, K. (June 3, 2009) Presentation: *Web-based instruction—design and technical issues that influence training effectiveness*. Retrieved from http://in-the-middle-of-the-curve.blogspot.com/2009/06/ASTD09

Stubenrauch, J. (2010, December). IOM: Report on the Future of Nursing, *American Journal of Nursing, 110*(12), 21–22.

Maria L. Vezina

OUTCOMES MANAGEMENT

Outcomes management (OM) is the enhancement of physiologic, psychological, or socioeconomic results through the implementation of exemplary health practices and services driven by ongoing quantitative performance analyses (Wojner, 2001). The term *outcomes management* was first coined by Ellwood (1988) and defined as a "technology of patient experience designed to help patients, payers, and providers make rational medical care-related choices based on better insight into the effect of these choices on patient life." Ellwood suggested four essential principles for inclusion in an OM program:

1. an emphasis on standards that providers can use to select appropriate interventions;
2. the measurement of patient functional status and well-being, along with disease-specific clinical outcomes;
3. the pooling of outcome data on a massive scale; and
4. the analysis and dissemination of the database to appropriate decision makers.

Ellwood's theoretical vision of OM extends from earlier work proposed first by Codman in 1917 and later by Donabedian (1976). Codman pioneered the concept of OM by advocating for the measurement and publication of what he called physiologic and psychosocial "end results" as well as determination of the cause of all untoward outcomes. He radically suggested that hospitals use this information to improve the practice of their medical staff. Ironically, Codman's "end-result idea" was scoffed at by his peers, who viewed measurement and possible public knowledge of health outcomes as detrimental to the advancement of medical practice. In fact, he was labeled as an eccentric for recommending publicly that hospitals should know their results, compare their results with those of other hospitals, promote medical staff on the basis of their results, and commit to continuous improvement (Wojner, 2001).

In 1976, Donabedian proposed measurement and evaluation of the quality of health care services at three levels: structure, process, and outcome. Donabedian further proposed that foundational contributors such as manpower, technology, and other resources (structure), methods used to provide or access health care services (processes), and proximal and distal results (outcomes) must be assessed in a systematic manner given their interrelatedness to provide an understanding of quality and opportunities for improvement. Interestingly, despite Donabedian's well-crafted definitions and widespread adoption of his quality framework, it was not until Ellwood's vision for OM emerged that measurement of outcomes became apparent within most health care settings (Wojner, 2001). Even today, process measurement is common among health care providers, whereas outcomes measurement remains somewhat evasive, and many providers are unable to differentiate processes from outcomes.

In 1997, Wojner published an OM model that applied Ellwood's work to clinical measurement and management of patient outcomes. The model provided guidance to clinical application of OM techniques using a four-phase approach:

1. Phase 1: establishment of outcome targets, development of definitions and measurement systems, and capture of baseline performance.

2. Phase 2: comparison of baseline performance to results achieved from the implementation of evidence-based structures/ processes through review of related literature, networking, and dialogue with experts in the field; negotiation with practice stakeholders for adoption of best practices; and construction of structured care methods (e.g., pathways, algorithms, protocols, order sets) that standardize interdisciplinary care according to adopted evidence-based practices (EBPs).

3. Phase 3: implementation of structured care methods and practice change(s), including role modeling new practices and educating interdisciplinary team members, measurement of performance reliability, and collection of structure, process, and outcome data.

4. Phase 4: analysis of posttest data to determine if outcome target(s) have been achieved, widespread dissemination of results among interdisciplinary stakeholders and dialogue about additional opportunities for improvement, and return to Phase 2 as needed to identify further methods that may impact outcomes positively.

The OM model uniquely illustrates a cyclical approach to measurement and methodical management strategies based on Ellwood's (1988) work. A guiding premise for the OM model is the need to fully define at the start the goals/outcome targets that are desired, with emphasis on the need to capture and understand baseline performance contributors to substandard results before initiating changes in clinical practice. In addition, the model places an emphasis on the need to review the published literature for evidence of what was previously referred to as "best practices"

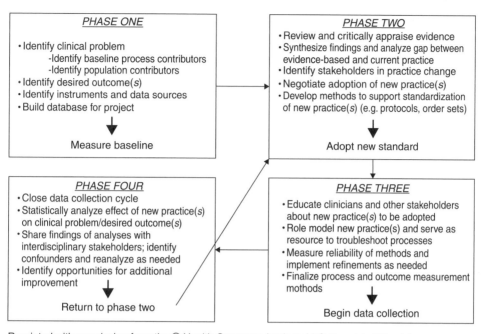

FIGURE 3: Outcomes management model.

but currently are referred to as EBPs. Figure 1 illustrates an updated version of the OM model using EBP terminology.

Today, many health care settings are embarking on a journey of implementing EBPs to support outcomes enhancement. It is important that this work be guided by a methodical approach to measurement of the impact of EBP on system, provider, and patient outcomes. Unfortunately, however, many institutions are immediately climbing aboard the EBP bandwagon without first establishing a clear understanding of baseline opportunities for improvement against which they can measure impact. OM provides a mechanism that in concert with EBP enables quantification of the effect of implementing evidence in practice. Using a wide lens for analyses of outcomes, providers that blend OM with EBP are capable of measuring a variety of results including: reduction in complications and

case severity; improved perception of the care experience, functional status, post-illness return to productivity, quality of life, and resource utilization; staff retention, workload, and satisfaction with the work environment; and cost and length of stay.

OM is not an easy process to establish, but its rewards are vast. It requires administrative and clinical support personnel with a background in research methods and statistics, an engaged interdisciplinary team, and technology to capture, manipulate, and analyze variables of interest. Many automated systems can be integrated in the process to reduce the workload associated with widespread OM; these range from electronic medical record systems to accounting and billing systems. Last, experience with the OM process is the best teacher of its widespread application. Experimentation with implementation should be encouraged, lessons

O

learned from the process, and continual refinements made to ensure optimal OM.

See also Consumer Satisfaction; Evidence-Based Practice; Staff Retention

Codman, E. A. (1917). The value of case records in hospitals. *Modern Hospitals, 9,* 426–428.

Donabedian, A. (1976). Measuring and evaluating hospital and medical care. *Bulletin of New York Academic Medicine, 52*(1), 51–59.

Ellwood, P. M. (1988). Outcomes management: A technology of patient experience. *New England Journal of Medicine, 318,* 1549–1556.

Wojner, A. W. (1997). Outcomes management: From theory to practice. *Critical Care Nursing Quarterly, 19*(4), 1–15.

Wojner, A. W. (2001). *Outcomes management: Application to clinical practice.* St. Louis, MO: Mosby.

Anne W. Alexandrov

P

PALLIATIVE CARE

Palliative care is both a philosophy of care and a system for delivering care for any patient and family, across the life span, experiencing serious, progressive, chronic, or life-threatening illness (National Consensus Project, 2009). Such illnesses include cancer, end-stage organ diseases, neurodegenerative disorders, dementias, HIV/AIDS, congenital anomalies, accidents, and other traumatic events. It is important for the nurse leader to understand this philosophy and the various environments in which palliative care is delivered.

The focus of palliative care is on the relief of suffering and promoting quality of life by addressing the physical, emotional, social, cultural, and spiritual needs of patients and families. Palliative care is offered from the time of diagnosis, throughout the course of the illness, including the death of the patient, and into the bereavement period for families. Given that palliative care is not dependent on prognosis, it can be delivered at the same time as curative, disease modifying, or life-prolonging treatments are being offered or as the main focus of care when solely comfort and supportive interventions are desired.

Palliative care involves the assessment and management of physical symptoms such as pain, dyspnea, nausea and vomiting, and constipation as well as the relief of psychological symptoms such as anxiety, agitation, and depression. Given that cultural and spiritual needs influence the illness experience of patients and families, palliative care practitioners recognize the importance of cultural and spiritual assessment and the value of offering culturally sensitive care and spiritual support (Matzo & Sherman, 2010).

Palliative care honors the wishes and preferences of patients and families and develops a comprehensive plan of care based on the best evidence available, and the clinical judgment and expertise of an interdisciplinary team of health professionals, including physicians, nurses, social workers, chaplains, psychologists, pharmacists, and others. Through the expertise of the interdisciplinary team, patients and families are offered guidance and support in making health-related decisions and matching treatments to the informed goals of patients and families (Meier, 2010).

Palliative care enhances the communication between patients, families, and members of the interdisciplinary team. Ethical concerns and preferences are addressed as it relates to patients' or families' decisions regarding resuscitation

P

and the use of life-sustaining therapies such as mechanical ventilation, hemodialysis, use of blood products or antibiotics, and nutrition and hydration within the context of life-threatening illness. Within the context of advanced care planning, palliative care professionals assist patients in identifying the goals of care and in the completion of advanced directives, including living wills or the appointment of a health care proxy. Other aspects of advanced care planning include identifying patients' values and discussing with patients their preferred location of death and related cultural or spiritual needs and rituals at the end of life. Palliative care promotes continuity of care as plans may be made for transitions to home or other settings. Consideration is also given to family burden, financial issues, and bereavement outcomes.

Hospice care is a form of palliative care that is offered enrollment in a hospice when the patient is expected to have six months or less to live. Today, many hospices are also providing palliative care so that patients who have greater than 6 months prognosis may also receive the holistic support needed to promote their quality of life. Therefore, the difference between palliative care and hospice care is the timing: palliative care may be offered at any point in time while hospice care is offered at the end of life (Jennings, Ryndes, D'Onofrio, & Baily, 2003). Palliative care and hospice care are based on the same key elements: the care of all patients with life-threatening illness of all ages, patient- and family-centered care, and comprehensive care (physical, emotional, social, and spiritual) offered by an interdisciplinary team of health professionals. When patients enroll in hospice, they have decided to forego curative treatments that are no longer beneficial or are causing more harm than good and decide to focus on achieving physical,

emotional, and spiritual comfort and support. Like palliative care, hospice is offered in the home, inpatient hospitals, nursing homes, assisted living facilities, and residential facilities.

Palliative care has been in increasing demand because of the aging of the population and longer life expectancies of patients with cancer, HIV/AIDS, and end-stage organ diseases. Palliative care is entering the mainstream of health care as it offers a universally available approach to meet the needs of the sickest and most vulnerable populations and is an important factor in improving health care in the United States (Meier, 2010). Palliative care outcomes include improvement of quality of life for patients and families by addressing physical, emotional, social, and spiritual needs; promoting the coordination and continuity of care; handling time-intensive family/patient/team meetings; assistance with determining goals of care; increase in patient, family, and staff satisfaction; and being associated with significant prolongation of life in certain patient populations (National Consensus Project, 2009; Temel et al., 2010).

Jennings, B., Ryndes, T., D'Onofrio, C., & Baily, M. (2003). Access to hospice care: Expanding boundaries, overcoming barriers. *Hastings Center Report*, S3-7, S9-13, S15-21.

Matzo, M., & Sherman, D. W. (2010). Palliative care nursing: Quality care to the end of life (3rd ed.). New York, NY: Springer Publishers.

Meier, D. (2010). The development, status and future of palliative car. In D. E. Meier, S. L. Isaacs, & R. Hughes. *Palliative care: Transforming the care of serious illness.* San Francisco: Jossey-Blass. Retrieved from http://www.rwjf.org/files/research/4558.pdf

National Consensus Project for Quality Palliative Care.(2009). *Clinical practice guidelines for quality palliative care.* Retrieved from http://nationalconsensusproject.org

Temel, J., Greer, J. Muzikansky, A., Gallagher, E., Admane, S., & Jackson, V. (2010). Early palliative care for patients with metastatic non-small-cell lung cancer. *New England Journal of Medicine*, 363(8), 733–742.

Deborah Witt Sherman

PARTICIPATIVE LEADERSHIP

Participative leadership, also known as democratic leadership, is a type of progressive leadership first described in the works of Kurt Lewin (1939). Lewin defined leadership in three distinct styles: autocratic (leaders have absolute power over workers and make decisions without input), democratic (leaders invite team members to contribute to the decision making process), and laissez-faire (leaders leave the team to work and make decisions on their own). In 1978, Burns identified participative leadership as a type of transformational leadership, accomplished by inspiring teams to take on greater ownership of their work. Bass (1995) further defined transformational leadership components as idealized influence, inspirational motivation, intellectual stimulation, and individualized consideration. In 2003, the Institute of Medicine's report *Keeping Patients Safe: Transforming the Work Environment of Nurses*, endorsed transformational leadership and evidence-based management practices as strategies that balance efficiency and safety, create and sustain trust, manage change, involve workers in decision making pertaining to work design and work flow, and establish the organization as a "learning organization."

The basic component of participative leadership style is the consideration of the thoughts and opinions of employees prior to decision making. At the highest level, the participative leader becomes a member of the team by acting as the team facilitator to implement new projects or solve problems. The participative leader supports the team's mission through collaborating with team members to develop a purpose, set goals, and establish norms for sharing opinions and thoughts. Team members are given the authority to make decisions and the responsibility to operationalize parts of the plan. Through this process, shared visions and values emerge, creating a cooperative and trusting work environment that is seen as fair and transparent. The efficiency of a participative process is the production of successful problem solving or execution of projects.

The characteristics of participative leaders include being available, approachable, caring, motivating, creative, innovative, and empowering. Participative leaders give constructive feedback, coach, mentor, promote teamwork and interprofessional collaboration, resolve conflicts through effective negotiation, and "walk the talk." They display emotional intelligence, give honest and complete information, and treat colleagues with respect and dignity in all interactions.

Shared governance, a foundational component of the Magnet framework, and the concept of healthy work environments are both rooted in participative processes of staff and leaders working together to produce outcomes (Kramer, Schmalenberg, & Maguire, 2010; Pearson et al., 2007; Tomey, 2009). The quality of care has been shown to improve through collaboration, autonomy, and shared decision making (Chiok Foong Loke, 2010; Germain & Cummings, 2010; Kramer, Maguire, Schmalenberg, et al., 2010). Current nursing literature attributes participative leadership as pivotal to achieving organizational outcomes, including effectiveness, increased job satisfaction, staff retention, productivity, organizational commitment, and productive nurse–leader relationships (Chiok Foong Loke, 2001; Cummings, Hayduk, & Estabrooks, 2005; Germain & Cummings, 2010; Kleinman, 2004; Kramer, Schmalenberg, & Maguire, 2010; Kramer, Maguire, Schmalenberg, et al., 2010). Improved patient care outcomes including patient satisfaction and decreased mortality and adverse events are also related to participative leadership (Squires, Tourangeau, Laschinger-Spence, & Doran, 2010; Wong & Cummings, 2007).

A significant challenge of participatory leadership style is often the increased demand on a leader's time, which is necessary to build a team and produce positive outcomes. Time must be provided for the management of power differences and conflicts between team members that emerge during the participatory process. It may also be time consuming to encourage and empower every team member to share ideas and opinions to capitalize on each individual's potential. This dedication of time and effort to use a participative leadership approach will likely be beneficial because current research and empirical evidence link staff involvement in decision making with improved patient safety outcomes.

Chiok Foong Loke, J. (2001). Leadership behaviors: Effects on job satisfaction, productivity and organizational commitment. *Journal of Nursing Management, 9*(4), 191–204.

Cummings, G., Hayduk, L., & Estabrooks, C. (2005). Mitigating the impact of hospital the responsibility of emotionally intelligent leadership. *Nursing Research, 54*(1), 2–12.

Germain, P. B., & Cummings, G. G. (2010). The influence of nursing leadership on nurse performance: A systematic literature review. *Journal of Nursing Management, 18*(4), 425–439.

Kleinman, C. (2004). The relationship between managerial leadership behaviors and staff nurse retention. *Hospital Topics: Research and Perspectives on Healthcare, 82*(4), 2–10.

Kramer, M., Maguire, P., Schmalenberg, C., Brewer, B., Burke, R., Chmielewski, L., et al. (2007). Nurse manager support: What is it? Structures and practices that promote it. *Nursing Administration Quarterly, 31*(4), 325–340.

Kramer, M., Schmalenberg, C., & Maguire, P. (2010). Nine structures and leadership practices essential for a magnetic (healthy) work environment. *Nursing Administration Quarterly, 34*(1), 4–17.

Pearson, A., Laschinger, H., Porritt, K., Jordan, Z., Tucker, D., & Long, L. (2007). Comprehensive systematic review of evidence on developing and sustaining nursing leadership that fosters a healthy work environment in healthcare. *International Journal of Evidence-Based Healthcare, 5*(2), 208–253.

Squires, M., Tourangeau, A., Laschinger-Spence, H., & Doran, D. (2010). The link between leadership and safety outcomes in hospitals. *Journal of Nursing Management, 18*, 914–925.

Tomey, A. M. (2009). Nursing leadership and management effects work environments. *Journal of Nursing Management, 17*(1), 15–25.

Wong, C. A., & Cummings, G. G. (2007). The relationship between nursing leadership and patient outcomes: A systematic review. *Journal of Nursing Management, 15*(5), 508–521.

Kelly Reilly

PATIENT CARE DELIVERY MODELS

It could be stated without argument that the first nursing care delivery model was initiated by Florence Nightingale (ca. 1859) during the Crimean War. It was Nightingale who differentiated between the "head" nurse (she who did the thinking, planning, and directing of patient care) and the "floor" nurse, who in essence was the provider of that care (Nightingale, 1859). Thus was born a hierarchical model for the delivery of patient care that prevailed for nearly a century in English and American health care facilities.

In the early years following the turn of the 20th century, professional nursing was dominated by private-duty nurses who were used through a "registry." These nurses cared for a single patient in the home or in the hospital (before the introduction of intensive care units). Oftentimes, the director of the nursing school also was the director of nursing in the hospital; nursing "pupils" provided the care of patients "on the wards," and nursing faculty provided the supervision of these students in their clinical rotations. After the stock market crash of 1929, when families could no longer afford private-duty nurses, hospitals began to staff the wards with graduate nurses (new graduates not yet licensed) using the original Nightingale hierarchical model.

In an effort to recruit and retain professional nurses, little by little, models such as team and primary nursing as well as all registered nurse (RN) staffs began to evolve in health care settings. Further, *advanced practice roles* such as the clinical nurse specialist and the nurse practitioner evolved, in an effort to impact the effective delivery of clinical nursing services, regardless of the setting. These models were popular in the second half of the 20th century.

Team nursing is undoubtedly one of the earliest models designed to replace the hierarchical structure of the Nightingale model. Within this context, each team is composed of a mix of RNs, licensed practical nurses (LPNs), and certified nursing assistants (aides) responsible for a single group of patients. The number of teams on a given patient unit is obviously determined by the size of the unit. The onset of the *advanced practice nurse*, such as the *clinical nurse specialist* and/or the *nurse practitioner*, has had a major impact on professional practice in the organizational setting while giving new meaning to the concept of team nursing. Although the nurse practitioner is generally thought of as providing primary care to a group of clients outside the hospital setting, many are employed within hospital-operated ambulatory care setting, or within the hospital itself, many times providing the initial physical assessments of patients required by regulating agencies such as the State Health Department and the Centers for Medicare and Medicaid Services. Primarily prepared at the master's level, these nurses in advanced practice roles serve as consultants to the nursing staff; they fill roles such as staff educator, researcher, administrator/manager, and, in many instances, as master clinician.

Primary nursing in its truest form assigns a "caseload" to the professional nurse, who is then responsible for each of his or her patients "around the clock," as it were. It is the responsibility of the primary nurse to make clinical rounds and to prescribe appropriate nursing interventions depending on client diagnosis. In the case of a hospital admission, the primary nurse maintains responsibility for the client(s) from admission to discharge; in a community health or long-term care, or home care setting, it is possible that the primary nurse maintains responsibility for the client over an extended period of time.

Like most of these other professional practice models, the *clinical ladder* concept was initiated as a retention mechanism for RNs. The concept was intended to provide an avenue for clinical advancement within the organization by way of achieving certain preset criteria intended for each level of performance. Each advanced step denotes a new level of clinical expertise and therefore also carries additional financial reimbursement.

An *all RN staff* is expensive but self-explanatory. Within this model, professional nurses provide all dimensions of direct patient care whereas ancillary personnel are responsible for those tasks not involved in direct patient care. With the tightening of fiscal belts, cutbacks in Medicare and Medicaid reimbursement, organizational mergers, changes in organizational philosophy, and the like, except for limited instances one might conclude that the all RN staff has largely become a phenomenon of the past.

In 2007, the Robert Wood Johnson Foundation funded an original research project to identify and profile new models of care that could be widely replicated throughout the United States. In collaboration with Health Workforce Solutions LLC and through a broad-based email inquiry, a literature search, and Internet research, 60 new care delivery models were selected for in depth research interviews.

The group was narrowed through a process of comparing the models to criteria developed by a select group of chief nursing officers and executives, nurse managers, and academics from a variety of nursing schools. Twenty-four models were further investigated and selected to be included in a white paper titled *Innovative Care Delivery Models: Identifying New Models that Effectively Leverage Nurses*, published in 2008 by the Health Workforce Solutions LLC. At the same time, the Robert Woods Johnson Foundation created a Web site that contains the complete profiles of each model described, including a detailed description, impetus for its development, results, consideration for implementation, and replication and selected tools (www.innovativecare models.com).

The models are divided into three categories: acute care models, models that bridge the continuum of care, and comprehensive care models. Within the acute care models, there are components of earlier care delivery models with a more comprehensive role for the professional nurse. Some incorporate team nursing: the medical-surgical unit team nursing, which is an RN-LPN team model, and the model RN line model. The nursing caring delivery model is a team-oriented primary nursing model for providing inpatient and outpatient care based on Watson's Theory on Human Caring. Other models in the acute care arena have elevated the RNs role to a care coordinator overseeing the patient care of several patients whose direct care is being provided by novice nurses, LPNs, or nursing assistants. A new role has been created from these models of care coordinator called the *clinical nurse leader* who is a master's prepared nurse who leads teams of caregivers. Examples of the care coordinator models include the patient-centered care, the primary care coordinator, the unit-based case manager model, and the 12-bed hospital developed at the Baptist Hospital of Miami.

The care transitions models are designed to bridge the continuum of care between acute care and home or outpatient services. This is a model that will meet the needs of the new health care reform initiatives. Even more critical to future health care models will be the comprehensive care models developed to focus on people lives from prevention and wellness through the entire continuum including social programs. (To learn more about each of these models go to www.innova-tivecaremodels.com.)

See also Advanced Practice Registered Nurses; Clinical Ladder; Florence Nightingale

Additional information is available from the following sources:

Bocchino, C. A. (1991). An interview with Joyce C. Clifford. *Nursing Economics, 9*(1), 7–17.

Forchuk, C., Mound, B., & Yamashita, M. (2005). Nurse case management: Negotiating care together with a developing relationship. *Perspectives in Psychiatric Care, 41*(2), 62.

Hall, L. E. (1969). The Loeb Center for Nursing and Rehabilitation. *International Journal of Nursing Studies, 6*, 81–95.

Joynt, J., & Kimball, B. (2008). *Innovative care delivery models: Identifying New Models that Effectively Leverage Nurses. A White Paper.* Washington, DC: The Robert Wood Johnson Foundation.

Kaiser Family Foundation. (2005). *Navigating Medicare and Medicaid.* Retrieved March 27, 2007, from http://www.kff.org/medicare/7240.cfm

Nightingale, F. (1859). *Notes on nursing: What it is, and what it is not.* Philadelphia, PA: J. B. Lippincott Company.

Connie A. Jastremski
M. Janice Nelson

Patient-Centered Medical Home

Primary care is the front line of the health care delivery system; providing preventive care, maintenance care for chronic illness, and ideally, coordinated transfers of care to other parts of the delivery system, including hospitals and specialty care. This core component of health care, however, is at risk for collapse because of the increased complexity of the health care system, the lack of care coordination, and the poor reimbursement for preventive care. The Patient-Centered Medical Home (PCMH) model of care addresses these concerns.

The PCMH concept was originally developed within the field of pediatrics in the 1960s as a care delivery model to support children with special needs. In the mid-2000s, several primary care professional organizations developed the "Joint Principles for PCMH."[1] Subsequently, the National Committee for Quality Assurance developed the PPC-PCMH program to recognize primary care practices as PCMHs.[2]

The Agency for Healthcare Research and Quality defines PCMH as patient-centered, comprehensive, coordinated, accessible, and continuously improved through a systems-based approach to quality and safety.[3] Developing a functional PCMH requires support for health information technology, expanded skills development for clinical and nonclinical staff, and payment systems that support delivery of high-performing primary care services. Nurse professionals are integral in providing leadership to drive the success of the PCMH model in many ways, most significantly by supporting effective management of people with chronic illness, providing leadership for practice redesign and providing professional leadership in health policy reform, nursing education, and participation of advance practice nurses in PCMH recognition programs.

The Centers for Disease Control reports that "7 out of 10 deaths among Americans each year are from chronic diseases with heart disease, cancer and stroke amounting to more than 50% of all deaths each year" (Kung, Hoyert, Xu, & Murphy, 2008). The prevalence of chronic disease accounts for a large portion of health care spending nationwide. Research shows that a PCMH model that partners an informed, activated patient with supportive, team-based care can improve the

---

[1] Retrieved September 27, 2010, from http://www.pcpcc.net/content/joint-principles-patient-centered-medical-home
[2] Retrieved September 27, 2010, from http://www.ncqa.org
[3] Retrieved September 27, 2010, from http://www.pcmh.ahrq.gov/portal/server.pt/community/pcmh__home/1483

P

quality of care and reduce costs related to care for people with prevalent chronic diseases (RAND Foundation, 2010). In addition, effective patient management requires a whole-person orientation that includes wellness, prevention, and behavioral health issues and addresses social determinants. The use of a population health registry further enhances a population-based approach to care that includes patient reminders, evidence-guided screening and care for chronic disease, and an ability to analyze practice data to note opportunities for improving care. Nurse leadership in wellness care and disease management drives patient-centered approaches to care that support value in health care delivery by providing high-quality, cost-effective care.

Most current primary care practices require added attention to systems and processes to enable implementation of the PCMH model. In particular, aligning screening and treatment with guidelines-based care and developing team-based care routines and systematic, data-driven quality improvement activities are key to transforming an average primary care practice into a high-performing, comprehensive PCMH. Nurses can support primary care practice transformational efforts by providing leadership and mentoring so that each member of the primary care team is supported to successfully help with and maintain the transformed practice.

Ensuring that the practice follows the most up-to-date evidence-based clinical guidelines ensures high-quality, outcomes-oriented care while reducing costs related to expensive diagnostic testing or unwarranted procedures. A nurse leader is able to identify best practices in clinical care and disseminate that information to clinicians through mini seminars and other multimedia methods. Combining best practices

and data-driven quality improvement interventions will optimize the quality of care for patients as well as proactively drive down costs of care.

Systematic, population-based, data-driven quality improvement activities are fundamental to improving the overall quality of care given to patients in the practice. Nurses can lead the effort to interpret data from the population health registry, identify potential concerns, and then lead staff in developing and implementing an intervention. A reevaluation of results after intervention shows whether these small tests of change had the desired outcome on patient care.

Finally, nurse leaders have the opportunity to drive support for the PCMH model by participating in health care policy discussions, assuring educational programs teach the appropriate skills to be effective in the PCMH model and by increasing the number of advanced practice nurses participating in national recognition programs.

Kung, H. C., Hoyert, D. L., Xu, J. Q., & Murphy, S. L. (2008). Deaths: final data for 2005. *National Vital Statistics Reports, 56*(10). Retrieved from http://www.cdc.gov/nchs/data/nvsr/nvsr56/nvsr56_10.pdf

RAND Foundation. (2010). *Improving chronic illness care evaluation: A RAND Health Project.* Retrieved September 25, 2010, from http://www.rand.org/health/projects/icice/findings.html

Julie Schilz
Lesley Reeder

PATIENT CLASSIFICATION SYSTEMS

Patient classification systems (PCSs) or taxonomies date back to the 1960s in the United States and were developed as *workload management* or *patient acuity* tools for staffing (Kelly, 2008; Marquis & Huston, 2009). Contemporaneously, PCSs are required for Medicare reimbursement and accreditation by the Joint Commission on Accreditation of Healthcare Organizations. These tools are used to determine the number and mix of staff needed to care for a group of patients, medical diagnosis, medical billing, and epidemiological study. The types of PCSs are the *critical indicator types*, also referred to as a prototype evaluation, and *summative* types, also referred to as a factor evaluation (Seago, 2002; Yoder-Wise, 2007). A critical indicator type categorizes patient activities using general factors of patient care activities, such as hygienic care, positioning, feeding, and medication administration. A relative intensity measure is one example based on the patient's diagnosis-related group. A summative type uses nursing care time per activity, for example, amount of time for teaching. The Nursing Intervention Classification system is a factor system. These systems may help leaders determine staffing mix on a daily basis; however, they are not a panacea. Reliability and validity issues related to nurses' self-reporting and legal issues related to inability to meet predicated staffing levels determined by the measures have caused some organizations to use other mechanisms to determine staffing needs. PCSs are also used to benchmark workload planning and outcomes monitoring particularly related to patient safety.

Other examples of PCSs are the *Physician's Current Procedural Terminology*, the *International Classification of Disease, Ninth Edition*, and the *Diagnostic and Statistical Manual of Mental Disorders, Fourth Edition* (Young, 2000). Some of these taxonomies, such as the *Diagnostic and Statistical Manual of Mental Disorders,* *Fourth Edition*, can be stored on PDAs for easy and accessible use for clinicians and students.

See also Accreditation in Nursing Practice

Kelly, P. (2008). *Nursing leadership & management.* Clifton Park, NY: Thomson/Delmar.

Marquis, B. L., & Huston, C. J. (2009). *Leadership roles and management functions in nursing: Theory and application* (6th ed.). Philadelphia, PA: Lippincott Williams & Wilkins.

Seago, J. (2002). A comparison of two patient classification instruments in an acute care hospital. *Journal of Nursing Administration,* 32(5), 243–249.

Yoder-Wise, P. S. (2007). *Leading and managing in nursing* (4th ed.). St. Louis, MO: Mosby/Elsevier.

Young, K. M. (2000). *Informatics for healthcare professionals.* Philadelphia, PA: F. A. Davis.

Martha J. Greenberg

PATIENT SAFETY

According to the Institute of Medicine (IOM; 2000), tens of thousands of Americans die each year from errors in medical care and hundreds of thousands are injured, or almost injured, during their care. In *Crossing the Quality Chasm: A New Health System for the 21st Century* (IOM, 2001), the IOM identified six dimensions in which health care systems were failing and where major gains would lead to improvement. According to the IOM, health care should be safe, effective, patient-centered, timely, efficient, and equitable. Although health care organizations have a long history of devoting resources to measuring contributing factors and outcomes related to quality of care, the IOM reports served as a wakeup call that more was needed to prevent harm to patients, and improve quality. Despite multiple efforts and millions of dollars directed toward improving safety in health care settings over the past ten years, no significant change in overall rate of harm has been achieved (Landrigan et al., 2010), with one researcher reporting only modest improvement in safety since 2004 (Wachter, 2010).

LOOKING TO OTHER INDUSTRIES FOR SOLUTIONS

An important and paradigm-changing reaction to the IOM reports was the search for solutions from industries other than health care for effective approaches to improving and sustaining safety. Patient safety health care leaders (e.g., Leape et al., 2000) called for adoption of strategies used by other industries (such as the airline industry) to prevent high stakes failures and reduce the harm surrounding error. As a result of turning to expert resources outside health care, a major change in thinking occurred as to why errors happen, the role of the individual in error generation, and the roles that health care providers and leaders play in increasing and sustaining patient safety.

Health care leaders learned that to make sustainable improvements in patient safety, their focus had to switch from individual health care providers and workers to the complex systems in which they work and to the complexity as well as limitations within individuals themselves. The new focus for understanding error turned from the traditional approach to patient safety that demanded perfect individual performance in imperfect situations to understanding the imperfect situations in which imperfect performers work. Reason's (1990) framework explained that the usual route to failure, or error, is the contribution of multiple latent failures and

gaps across multiple systems in an organization. Thus, although an individual makes a decision that may result in death, harm, or near harm to a patient, the complexity surrounding the event is what leads the individual to thinking it was the right decision given the circumstances (Cook & Woods, 1994).

A CHANGE IN ORGANIZATIONAL CULTURE REGARDING ERROR

The switch of health care to a focus on systems that contribute to error and away from the individual as the source of failure continues to be a challenge. Changing from a traditional health care culture of blaming individuals to a culture of non-blame surrounding error has been difficult at best. The tendency for those not associated with an error event to simplify the event after the fact, called hindsight bias, is a formidable hindrance in the search for details that explain how flawed systems are involved. And yet learning about the details of a situation and how systems as well as human factors contribute to error will provide the knowledge necessary to make improvements in and sustain patient safety.

The traditional accountability for health care providers involved performing perfectly without error. In the new approach to patient safety, the expectation for health care providers is to be open about their own errors and near misses, and to share and discuss the stories that surround error events. Furthermore, the new accountability for providers stipulates that they be open about extant system barriers that make it difficult to provide safe care, speak up about those barriers, and participate in planning to reduce or eliminate them. An effective safety culture is one where these behaviors are encouraged, facilitated and celebrated, reflective of characteristics demonstrated by high reliability organizations (Weich & Suttcliffe, 2007).

In this light, the new expectation for health care leaders is to facilitate a culture in which providers feel free to speak up about their errors and the barriers to providing safe and quality care. Rather than the weakest link in an otherwise unrealistic fail-proof system, this new approach positions the health care provider as the resilient component in the health care environment for learning about, making improvements in, and rescuing within the systems in which care is delivered. Although strategies for balancing a culture of nonblame with accountability have increased, lack of widespread adoption and embrace of these approaches for building an effective safety culture has limited the overall impact and sustainability of improvement efforts.

TOWARD A SAFER HEALTH CARE DELIVERY SYSTEM

Although ongoing efforts to change the culture surrounding error continue in health care across the Unites States, many other strategies have been developed to improve the safety of care. Design and production of equipment and information technology to support provider work and overcome human limitations has become a major industry as health care organizations search for effective interventions. As new products are implemented, leaders are learning the challenges related to implementing and sustaining any change in a complex system. Seemingly perfect solutions can cause unexpected changes that result in a more complicated environment and thus a higher risk for error.

And yet some approaches have galvanized health care providers and educators across the nation in organized efforts that show promise. Berwick's leadership of the Institute for Healthcare Improvement (http://www.ihi.org/ihi) has resulted in national patient safety improvement efforts to develop best-demonstrated practices in care delivery and adoption of care practices toward saving lives in health care. A new focus for research on understanding the actual work of health care providers and decision making in health care environments is increasing and will contribute to a knowledge base for redesign of health care environments for safe practice and health care provider education (Benner, Sutphen, Leonard & Day, 2010; Ebright, Patterson, Chalko & Render, 2003; Kalisch, 2006; Potter et al., 2005; Tucker, Singer, Hayes & Falwell, 2008;). Increasing evidence for the influence of communication and teamwork on safety and quality outcomes has directed new emphasis and efforts toward these aspects of provider relationships (Albolino, Cook, & O'Connor, 2007; Kahan, Klock & Cook, 2008). The National Patient Safety Foundation (http://www.npsf.org) and the Agency for Healthcare Research and Quality (http://ahrq.gov) fund research on patient safety and potential interventions for reaching patient safety outcomes.

Health care leaders continue to realize the enormous challenges to achieving major and sustainable improvements in patient safety (Leape & Berwick, 2005; Wachter, 2010; Landrigan et al, 2010). Strategies that incorporate culture change, new mechanisms for reporting and investigation of error and near-miss events, human factors limitations in design of environments, and new patient safety accountabilities related to communication and teambuilding for direct care providers and leaders are being used to address these challenges.

P

P

See also Agency for Healthcare Research and Quality (AHRQ); Institute for Healthcare Improvement

Agency for Healthcare Research and Quality (AHRQ), http://ahrq.gov/

Albolino, S., Cook, R., & O'Connor, M. (2007). Sensemaking, safety, and cooperative work in the intensive care unit. *Cognitive Technical Work,*. 9: 131–137.

Benner, P., Sutphen, M., Leonard, V., & Day, L. (2010). Educating nurses: A call for radical transformation. San Francisco, CA: Jossey-Bass.

Cook, R. I., & Woods, D. D. (1994). Operating at the "sharp end": The complexity of human error. In M. S. Bogner (Ed.), *Human error in medicine* (pp. 255–310). Hillsdale, NJ: Lawrence Erlbaum.

Ebright, P., Patterson, E., Chalko, B., & Render, M. (2003). Understanding the complexity of registered nurse work in acute care settings. *Journal of Nursing Administration, 33*(12), 630–638.

Institute for Healthcare Improvement (IHI), http://www.ihi.org/ihi

Institute of Medicine. (2000). *To err is human: Building a safer health system.* Washington, DC: National Academies Press.

Institute of Medicine, Committee on Quality of Healthcare in America. (2001). *Crossing the quality chasm: A new health system for the 21st century.* Washington, DC: National Academies Press.

Institute of Medicine. (2004). *Keeping patients safe: Transforming the work environment of nurses.* Washington, DC: National Academies Press.

Kahana, M, Klock, P.A, & Cook, R.I. (2008) Between shifts: Healthcare communication in the PICU In Nemeth CP (Ed.), *Improving Healthcare Team Communication.* Aldershot: Ashgate: 135–53.

Kalisch, B. (2006). Missed Nursing Care: A Qualitative Study. *Journal of Nursing Care Quality,* 21(4), 306 – 313

Landrigan, C.P., Parry, G.J., Bones, C.B., Hackbarth, M.P., Goldman, D.A., & Sharek, P.J. (2010). Temporal trends in rates of patient harm resulting from medical care. *New England Journal of Medicine, 363,* 2124–2134.

Leape, L. L., & Berwick, D. M. (2005). Five years after "To err is human." *Journal of the American Medical Association, 293*(19), 2384–2390.

Leape, L. L., Kabcenell, A. I., Gandhi, T. K., Carver, P., Nolan, T. W., & Berwick, D. M. (2000). Reducing adverse events: Lessons from a breakthrough series collaborative. *Joint Commission Journal of Quality Improvement, 26*(6), 321–331.

Morath, J., & Turnbull, J. (2005). *To do no harm: Ensuring patient safety in health care organizations.* San Francisco: Jossey-Bass.

National Patient Safety Foundation (NPSF), http://www.npsf.org

Potter, P., Wolf, L., Boxerman, S., Grayson, D., Sledge, J., Dunagan, C., et al. (2005). Understanding the cognitive work of nursing in the acute care environment. *Journal of Nursing Administration, 35*(78), 327–335.

Reason, J. (1990). *Human error.* Cambridge, UK: Cambridge University Press.

Tucker, A., Singer, S., Hayes, J. & Falwell, A. (2008). Front-line Staff Perspectives on Opportunities for Improving the Safety and Efficiency of Hospital Work Systems. *Health Services Research,* 43:5, Part II (October 2008).

Wachter, R.M. (2010). Patient safety at ten: Unmistakable progress, troubling gaps. *Health Affairs, 29*(1), doi: 10.1377/hlthaff.2009.0785

Weick K.E., & Suttcliffe KM. (2007). *Managing the unexpected: Resilient performance in an age of uncertainty.* San Francisco, CA: Jossey-Bass.

Patricia R. Ebright

PATIENT SELF-DETERMINATION ACT

The principle of autonomy, or the right to self-determination, is preserved in health care by ethical mandates and legislative rulings. The Patient Self-Determination Act (PSDA) is grounded in the principle of autonomy and empowers the patient to be an active and informed participant in health care. Patient autonomy moved to the forefront in health care during the latter half of the 20th century. Advances in technology expanded the boundaries of medical care. The potential to sustain a patient's life indefinitely was realized. These advancements, however, did not come without costs. Monetary considerations and quality of life issues were topics of debate in ethical, political, and social forums. As the physician's beneficiary role was questioned, courts were petitioned on behalf of the autonomous voice of the patient (Berg, Appelbaum, Lidz, & Parker, 2001; Duke, Yarbrough, & Pang, 2009; Kellum & Dacey, 2010; Watson, 2010). It was within this climate that the PSDA was passed and the concept of informed patient consent was meaningfully defined. The PSDA and informed patient consent promote patient autonomy.

The PSDA is a federal law that passed in 1990 and became effective on December 1, 1991. The PSDA sets forth regulations about the patient's role in treatment decisions. These apply to health care agencies receiving any federal funding. There are four provisions mandated by the PSDA: (a) provide written information to adults, upon admission, of their right under state law to make decisions about their medical care; (b) ask all adults if they have an advance directive and document the response accordingly in the medical record; (c) do not discriminate against any adult based upon whether the adult has an advance directive; and (d) educate the staff of the health care agency or program and the community at large about advance directives and any relevant institutional policies (Devettere, 2010; Watson, 2010).

Patients are empowered to make treatment decisions only if they are adequately informed.

Informed patient consent refers to a process of open communication between the patient and the health care professional through which information is shared, questions are raised, and values are clarified. Most legal, regulatory, medical, philosophical, and psychological sources identify the essential elements of this process as (a) competence, or decision-making capacity, (b) disclosure, (c) understanding, (d) voluntariness, and (e) consent (Beauchamp & Childress, 2009; Kellum & Dacey, 2010).

In language that the patient can understand, disclosure should include (1) information most patients would consider relevant, such as the risks, burdens, and benefits of all treatment options, (2) information the professional considers relevant, (3) the professional's recommendation, and (4) the purpose, nature, and limits of the consent (Beauchamp & Childress, 2009; Kellum & Dacey, 2010).

The courts judge adequacy of the disclosure by three standards: the *professional community standard* (what a typical physician would disclose), the *reasonable person standard* (what another person of sound reasoning would want to know), or the *subjective standard* (what the individual patient specifically needs to know) (Beauchamp & Childress, 2009; Berg et al., 2001).

The process of informed patient consent requires the patient to have decision-making capacity, and decision-making capacity assumes comprehension. Effort should be made to enhance the patient's understanding of the information disclosed as it relates to personal values and goals. If it is determined that the patient lacks decision-making capacity, the informed consent process should be initiated with an identified surrogate decision maker (Annas, 2004; Beauchamp & Childress, 2009). The actual consent must be voluntary. This implies that the patient consents freely, without controlling influences. Components of the informed consent process, and the patient's decision to consent or to refuse participation in the medical intervention, should be documented in the medical record (Beauchamp & Childress, 2009; Berg et al., 2001).

Some situations do not lend themselves to obtaining informed patient consent and are recognized as exceptions to the legal doctrine. These include circumstances of medical emergencies, legal or military directives, when the patient lacks decision-making capacity, when the patient waives his or her right to consent, and when therapeutic privilege is exercised (Beauchamp & Childress, 2009; Devettere, 2010).

Although the original intentions of the PSDA were to empower patients to make decisions about their own medical treatment, and to promote the use of advance directives, the means to achieve these goals were not well articulated. As a result, there has been limited success in meeting these intentions since its enactment.

One reason relates to ethnic influences. Autonomy and self-determination are core health care values within the United States. Not all cultures and ethnicities appeal to these values and prefer the family or physician to be the primary decision maker (Colclough & Young, 2007; Doolen & York, 2007; Duffy, Jackson, Schim, Ronis, & Fowler, 2006; Kring, 2007).

The implementation of advance directives themselves present challenges. The language of advance directives can be ambiguous and difficult to understand or interpret. When advance directives are completed by patients, they are often inaccessible. Family members who oppose a patient's advance directive can negatively influence a provider's decision to honor it (Kring, 2007; Watson, 2010).

Finally, providers and patients are hesitant to engage in meaningful discussions about death and dying. This is attributed to an awareness of medical uncertainties and other knowledge deficits, discomfort in addressing the topic, and the timing of such discussions (Duke, Yarbrough, & Pang, 2009; Kring, 2007; Watson, 2010).

Annas, G. J. (2004). *The rights of patients: The authoritative ACLU guide to the rights of patients* (3rd ed.). Carbondale, IL: Southern Illinois University Press.

Beauchamp, T. L., & Childress, J. F. (2009). *Principles of biomedical ethics* (6th ed.). New York, NY: Oxford University Press.

Berg, J. W., Appelbaum, P. S., Lidz, C. W., & Parker, L. S. (2001). *Informed consent: Legal theory and clinical practice* (2nd ed.). New York, NY: Oxford University Press.

Colclough, Y.Y., & Young, H.M. (2007). Decision-making at end of life among Japanese and American families. *Journal of Family Nursing, 13*(2), 201–225.

Devettere, R.J. (2010). *Practical decision making in health care ethics: Cases and concepts* (3rd ed.). Washington, DC: Georgetown University Press.

Doolen, J., & York, N. L. (2007). Cultural differences with end-of-life care in the critical care unit. *Dimensions of Critical Care Nursing, 26*(5), 194–198.

Duffy, S. A., Jackson, F. C., Schim, S. M., Ronis, D. L., & Fowler, K. E. (2006). Racial/ethnic preferences, sex preferences, and perceived discrimination related to end-of-life care. *Journal of the American Geriatrics Society, 54*, 150–157.

Duke, G., Yarbrough, S., & Pang, K. (2009). The patient self-determination act: 20 years revisited. *Journal of Nursing Law 13*(4), 114–123.

Kellum, J. A., & Dacey, M. J. (2010). *Ethics in the intensive care unit: Informed consent; withholding and withdrawal of life support; and requests for futile therapies.* Retrieved September 30, 2010, from http://uptodateonline.com

Kring, D. L. (2007). The patient self-determination act: Has it reached the end of its life? *JONA's Healthcare Law, Ethics, and Regulation 9*(4), 125–132.

Watson, E. (2010). Advance directives: Self-determination, legislation, and litigation issues. *Journal of Legal Nurse Consulting, 21*(1), 9–14.

Diane M. Gengo

PAY-FOR-PERFORMANCE AND VALUE-BASED PURCHASING

In recent years, there has been growing interest in the use of financial incentives to promote improvement in quality care, the underlying premise of which is that higher quality care will reduce expenses in the long run. However, survey and interview data obtained from providers to date yield a basis for concern as to whether financial incentives will motivate institutional and individual providers to invest in quality care improvements or whether financial incentives are even necessary to improve care. In addition, a comprehensive review of the most recent pay-for-performance (P4P) initiatives in the United States showed that the link between financial incentives to that of improvement is not clear (Christianson, Leatherman, & Sutherland, 2008). Congress, however, through the Centers for Medicare and Medicaid Services (CMS; www.cms.hhs.gov) is continuing to promote the use of financial incentives. Most recently, the CMS has released, for public comment, a proposed new ruling regarding a hospital value-based purchasing program that will reward hospitals for improving patients' experiences while making care safer by reducing medical mistakes (McKinney, 2011).

P4P was initiated in 2001 by the CMS, the largest purchaser of health care in the United States, when it launched several quality demonstration initiatives, such as the Hospital Quality Incentive Demonstration, because of the growing concern for the adequacy of care being received by patients as well as the rising cost of care (www.cms.hhs.gov). The intent of the P4P movement was to reward providers for providing quality care and

with this movement came the proliferation of metrics or preestablished measures for performance. It was a time when such reports as *To Err Is Human: Building a Safer Health System* (Institute of Medicine, 1999) and *Crossing the Quality Chasm* (Institute of Medicine, 2001) were released, questioning the quality of health care that Americans were receiving. Concurrently, there were also small experiments performed to reward physicians (in their offices or group practices) for improvements in preventive care; unfortunately, research findings were limited and only a few significant impacts on quality of care could be attributed to financial rewards (Christianson et al., 2008).

Today, the CMS continues to articulate a vision for health care quality—"the right care for every person every time." To achieve this vision, CMS is committed to care that is "safe, effective, timely, patient-centered, efficient, and equitable" (CMS Hospital Pay-for-Performance Workgroup, 2007). According to the Patient Protection and Affordable Care Act of 2010, a hospital value-based purchasing program is designed to provide incentive payments to hospitals that meet a specific set of quality measures (McKinney, 2011). This law shifts the requirement of hospitals from only having to report their quality data to now becoming more accountable for their outcomes. This creates a hospital payment system based on various methodologies aimed at the institutions' ability to demonstrate (1) the achievement of improved clinical quality, (2) the reduction of adverse or preventable medical errors, (3) the avoidance of unnecessary costs in the delivery of care, and (4) making these performance results transparent. The value-based purchasing program is designed to be budget neutral, which is to be achieved by the shifting of reimbursement through such strategies as penalties being imposed on

P

those hospitals that do not demonstrate an acceptable level of performance.

As Christianson et al. (2008) suggested, further study will be needed, as additional pay-for-performance initiatives are implemented, to determine the extent to which financial incentives actually serve to improve the quality of care in the nation.

Christianson, J. B., Leatherman, S., & Sutherland, K. (2008, December). Lessons from evaluations of purchaser pay-for-performance programs: A review of the evidence. *Medical Care Research and Review, 65*(Suppl. 6), 5S–35S.

CMS Hospital Pay-for-Performance Workgroup. (2007, January 17). *U.S. Department of Health and Human Services Medicare Hospital Value-Based Purchasing Plan Development: Issues Paper* (p. 1). Prepared in assistance with the RAND Corporation, Brandeis University, Booz Allen Hamilton, and Boston University.

Institute of Medicine. (1999, November). *To Err Is Human: Building a safer health care system.* Washington, DC: National Academies Press.

Institute of Medicine. (2001, March). *Crossing the Quality Chasm: A new health care system for the 21st century.* Washington, DC: National Academies Press.

McKinney, M. (2011, January 17). You get what you pay for. But double penalties, scoring issues in value-based purchasing proposal a wrinkle for some. *Modern Health Care, 41*, 6–7.

Laura Caramanica

Peer Review

Peer review is the process through which professional abstracts, proposals, grants, manuscripts, and practice are examined by a team of qualified reviewers who determine the quality of the work product in relation to current knowledge in that field (Smith, 2006; Southgate et al., 2001). This entry examines the process of peer review, identifies the criteria for the review team membership, and outlines the process of peer review from ethical and pragmatic perspectives.

Both the review of materials for publication or presentation and the review of professional practice for quality and safety are part of nursing leadership. In both cases, the practitioner whose work is being reviewed relies on the good intentions, ethical conduct, and expertise of those who make up the review team or panel. The work is reviewed using standards of the publication or organization as well as standards within the profession. Professionals who submit their work for review establish their reliability and character within the profession through the peer review process. They also are able to improve their writing or practice skills through participation in this review process. The professionals who serve on peer review panels demonstrate their professional leadership skills through the review process, the interaction with other reviewers and editors, and the helpful feedback they provide for the person whose work is under review. The outcome in both editorial and practice situations is similar—improvement of the discipline and patient care through quality assurance (Beyer et al., 2003). In these ways, leadership skills and abilities are displayed in the peer review process.

Peer review is considered to be at the core of the scientific method. It provides a structured approach to manuscript review (and job performance evaluation) that is reflective of this deductive process. Theory and conceptual development is presented in the first components of a research manuscript, while the methods and statistical analysis of the data are presented next. The reviewers collectively must, therefore, be knowledgeable in theory, methods, and statistics and in the logical interpretation of the results and conclusions. Similarly, in peer review of practice, the reviewer must be knowledgeable in the clinical care of specific types of patients, the protocols used in the profession and facility, and the quality measures applied in this specific case or group of cases.

The peer review process relies on the objectivity of the peer reviewers in evaluating the person's adherence to the scientific method and the quality of the work product. It is on this point that criticisms of the peer review process arise. The editor or peer review coordinator needs to assure the quality of the peer review process by examining the reviewer comments for bias, favoritism, or competition within a limited research or practice area. Leadership in the peer review process is a critical factor in maintaining quality and confidence in the process (Morby & Skalla, 2010). The key to the peer review process is the selection of appropriate professionals to serve as peer reviewers in sufficient numbers to allow for a good fit between the reviewers and the research topic or clinical area. As professional and governmental groups place increasing emphasis on quality and evidence-based practice, the value placed on the peer review process will no doubt increase. Leaders in education and practice will need to ensure the integrity of this process.

Beyer, M., Gerlach, F., Flies, U., Grol, R., Król, Z., Munck, A., Olesen, F., et al. (2003). The development of quality circles/peer review groups as a method of quality improvement in Europe. *Family Practice, 20*(4), 443–451. doi:10.1093/fampra/cmg420

http://grants.nih.gov/grants/peer/peer.htm

http://nature.com/nature/peerreview/debate/index.html

Morby, S. K., & Skalla, A. (2010). A human care approach to nursing peer review. *Nursing Science Quarterly, 23*(4), 297–300. doi:10.1177/0894318410380267

Smith, R. (2006). Peer review: A flawed process at the heart of science and journals. *Journal of the Royal Society of Medicine, 99*(4), 178–182.

Southgate, L., Cox, J., David, T., Hatch, D., Howes, A., Johnson, N., Jolly, B., et al. (2001). The General Medical Council's Performance Procedures: Peer review of performance in the workplace. *Medical Education, 35*(Suppl. 1), 9–19. doi:10.1046/j.1365-2923.2001.00002.x

Philip A. Greiner

PHILANTHROPY/FUND RAISING

Philanthropy—whether it takes the form of coalition building, mobilizing volunteers, fund raising, or board work—is steadily gaining in importance as a component of nursing leadership. Too often, however, the only overlap recognized between leadership and philanthropy is that successful leaders are expected to raise money for their organizations. That viewpoint grossly underestimates the profound relationship between the two. Both leadership and philanthropy require clarity regarding mission, values, and goals; ongoing strategic planning; making the "case" for why stakeholders should invest in the future; friend raising; image building; resource development; leveraging assets; and stewardship (McBride, 2000).

At the end of the 1980s, nursing's honor society Sigma Theta Tau International revamped its strategic plan—which had previously emphasized knowledge development, dissemination, and utilization—to add a fourth goal, resource development, to accomplish the other three. Having mounted the first major fund-raising campaign in nursing to build the International Center for Nursing Scholarship in Indianapolis, this organization recognized the importance of philanthropy in achieving nursing's preferred future and has since then created a Board Leadership Development Program

P

that prepares nurses to develop the afore-mentioned skills (www.nursingsociety.org/LeadershipInstitute/Omada/Pages/omada_resources.aspx).

Faced with mounting financial pressures globally, nonprofit organizations and the health care professionals employed by them have to be more creative in expanding the resource base through greater emphasis on gifts as investments (DeLellis, Kardos, & Langston, 1999). Scholarships are an investment in workforce development; endowed lectureships are a guaranteed means of bringing professionals together to discuss the issues of the day. Endowed chairs and professorships have grown significantly in the last two decades as a strategy for addressing the faculty shortage by attracting senior faculty capable of providing program leadership (Fitzpatrick, Fitzpatrick, & Dressler, 2005).

Rarely do nurses assume leadership positions with an interest in or knowledge about fund raising. To address this need, Fitzpatrick and Deller (2000) wrote a book on fund-raising skills for health care executives in which they confronted myths (no special skills are required; the primary responsibility for fund raising belongs to the development officer; gifts will naturally follow if programs are strong), articulated basic principles (people give to people; people give to vision not just need; if you do not ask, you're not likely to receive), and provided information regarding strategies and available resources.

Transitioning from individual to collective accountability, a nurse leader needs to be savvy philanthropically (Thompson, 2011). More and more leadership-development programs are, therefore, covering fund-raising fundamentals because of the demand for that material. For example, the John A. Hartford Foundation has created a Fundraising Toolkit for the directors of all the programs that they are supporting

as part of the Hartford Geriatric Nursing Initiative (www.hgni.org/fundraising) to promote program sustainability. Universities are developing centers to teach philanthropic principles to tomorrow's leaders and to expand the knowledge base; one of the largest of these in the world is the Center for Philanthropy at Indiana University, which can be accessed at www.philanthropy.iupui.edu.

Philanthropy is important to leadership because the dollars available can advance a nursing agenda and stimulate creativity (Wurmser, 2006). Funders, particularly foundations, typically support programs of a model-developing nature that can, once proven, be widely adopted and supported by other means (Maraldo, Fagin, & Keenan, 1988). Increasingly, funders want their dollars to be leveraged to attract additional resources—for example, encouraging partnerships across hospitals, local foundations, and state government—so no one organization or agency bears the full financial burden of the project (Henderson & Hassmiller, 2007).

Not only are nurses currying philanthropic support for their work, but they are increasingly playing a role in providing leadership to foundations, some as program officers—Helen Grace and Gloria Smith were legendary forces at the W. K. Kellogg Foundation; Sue Hassmiller is currently moving a nursing agenda at the Robert Wood Johnson Foundation. At the time of this writing, Rebecca Rimel is president and CEO of the Pew Charitable Trusts and Susan Sherman heads the Independence Foundation, and Marla Salmon is a member of the Robert Wood Johnson Foundation's board. This mounting level of philanthropic leadership bodes well for the future because the more nurses serve on boards and shape funding policies, the more likely it is that what is important to them will be front and center in funding inititatives.

See also Foundation Funding of Health Care and Nursing; Sigma Theta Tau International

DeLellis, A. J., Kardos, E. G., & Langston, N. F. (1999). Development in schools of nursing: Fund-raising to further long-range strategic plans. *Nurse Educator, 24*(3), 29–34.

Fitzpatrick, J. J., & Deller, S. S. (2000). *Fundraising skills for health care executives.* New York, NY: Springer Publishing.

Fitzpatrick, J. J., Fitzpatrick, M. L., & Dressler, M. B. (2005). Endowed chairs and professorships in schools of nursing: A 2004 update. *Journal of Professional Nursing, 21,* 244–252.

Henderson, T. M., & Hassmiller, S. B. (2007). Hospitals and philanthropy as partners in funding nursing education. *Nursing Economics, 25,* 95–100, 109.

Maraldo, P. J., Fagin, C., & Keenan, T. (1988). Nursing and private philanthropy. *Health Affairs, 7*(1), 130–136.

McBride, A. B. (Compiler) (2000). *Nursing & philanthropy. An energizing metaphor for the 21st century.* Indianapolis, IN: Center Nursing Press.

Thompson, C. (2011). Transitioning from a faculty to an administrative role: Part 1. Moving from individual to collective accountability. *Nurse Educator, 36*(1), 2–3.

Wurmser, T. (2006). Advance your nursing agenda with philanthropy and grant writing. *Nursing Management, 37*(3), 35–36, 38–39.

Angela Barron McBride

PLANETREE MODEL

The Planetree Model of patient care is "a patient-centered, holistic approach to healthcare, promoting mental, emotional, spiritual, social, and physical healing. It empowers patients and families through the exchange of information and encourages healing partnerships with caregivers. It seeks to maximize positive healthcare outcomes by integrating optimal medical therapies and incorporating art and nature into the healing environment" (Planetree.org). The concept model was developed by Angelica Thieriot in 1978 when she was hospitalized for a severe viral infection but disheartened by the environment. She envisioned an environment where patients would be partners in care and named the concept "Planetree," the tree that Hippocrates sat under as he taught some of the earliest medical students in ancient Greece (Planetree.org).

Planetree embodies several core beliefs that drive the model. They are, "we are human beings, caring for other human beings; we are all caregivers; care giving is best achieved through kindness and compassion; safe, accessible, high-quality care is fundamental to patient-centered care; in a holistic approach to meeting people's needs of body, mind and spirit; families, friends and loved ones are vital to the healing process; access to understandable health information can empower individuals to participate in their health care; the opportunity for individuals to make personal choices related to their care is essential; physical environments can enhance healing, health and wellbeing; illness can be a transformational experience for patients, families and caregivers" (Planetree.org).

The Planetree model and is implemented in acute and critical care departments, emergency departments, long-term care facilities, outpatient services, and ambulatory care and community health centers. For example, essential components of the model that facilitate healing in acute care settings are as follows: human interaction; family, friends, and social support; information and education; nutritional

P

and nurturing aspects of food; architectural and interior design that considers the patients' well-being and that engage the senses and break down barriers; arts and entertainment offer enjoyment to enhance the clinical environment; spirituality, from chaplains to meditation programs, which provide opportunities for reflection and support of spiritual needs; human touch reduces anxiety, pain, and stress, benefiting patients, families, and staff members; complementary therapies such as aroma and pet therapy, acupuncture, and Reiki are offered in addition to clinical modalities of care; and working with communities to partner toward health and wellness.

In 2008, Plantree expanded its score internationally and includes health care organizations in Canada, the Netherlands, Japan, and Brazil.

Martha J. Greenberg

Political Action Committees

Political action committees (PACs) are entities that are organized to contribute money to support or oppose candidates for political office. Federal election laws, administered by the Federal Election Commission, regulate the activity of PACs in supporting candidates for federal office. Further, state laws regulate PACs that are organized to support either state candidates or ballot measures. Nurse leaders should be familiar with PACs, what they do and how they function. Because PACs are a major focus of legislative advocacy for many nursing organizations, they often play a role in advancing those organizations' policy agendas and in shaping health policy. PACs may also thus be an important avenue for nurse

leaders themselves in becoming involved in political action and policy advocacy.

Many trade and professional associations have organized PACs as part of their overall advocacy strategies. Typically, these types of PACs are referred to as "connected PACs" that can receive and raise money from a "restricted class"— for example, nursing organizations can only raise money and receive contributions from their members, employees, and members' families. Those PACs are sometimes referred to as "Separate Segregated Funds" (Federal Election Commission, n.d.). Generally, such PACs contribute to candidates who are supportive of the organization's policy agenda and priorities. By electing candidates who are supportive (or supporting those with whom the organization seeks to maintain a good relationship), the organization seeks to advance its agenda. Of course, individuals are able to contribute to political candidates on their own. PACs, however, provide a means to pool individual contributions, providing the organization (and its members) with a more powerful voice.

The American Nurses Association (ANA) organized its PAC, first known as the Nurses Coalition for Action in Politics (N-CAP), in 1974. N-CAP subsequently changed its name to the ANA Political Action Committee (ANA-PAC). ANA-PAC is the oldest national nursing PAC. Some other national nursing organizations, including the American Association of Nurse Anesthetists, the American College of Nurse–Midwives, the American Academy of Nurse Practitioners, the American College of Nurse Practitioners, and the United American Nurses have subsequently established PACs. Many other health care organizations, including the American Hospital Association and the American Medical Association, have their own PACs. Since 1984, the ANA-PAC has endorsed and contributed to candidates for president and vice president in addition to endorsing and contributing to candidates for Congress (ANA-PAC Presidential Endorsement Process, 2008). Many other health care PACs choose not to endorse candidates for president.

In contrast to "connected PACs" such as those established by nursing organizations, nonconnected PACs may be formed by groups with an ideological mission, single-issue groups, and members of Congress and other political leaders. A 2010 U.S. Supreme Court decision, *Citizens United v. Federal Election Commission*, lifted restrictions on corporate spending in elections. One result has been the growth of independent expenditure-only committees, commonly known as "Super PACs." These committees spend money on efforts expressly advocating the election or defeat of clearly identified federal candidates. These expenditures may not be made in concert or cooperation with, or at the request or suggestion of, a candidate, a candidate's campaign or a political party (Federal Election Commission, 2010).

Citizens United and the growth of "Super PACs" have renewed debate about the influence of large donors in politics. PACs, such as those maintained by membership organizations, are likely to continue to be important as a means for these organizations' constituents to make their collective voices heard in election campaigns.

In addition to federal PACs, similar entities exist at the state level. Many health care organizations, including nursing organizations, have established state PACs. These state PACs are governed by state election laws, which differ from state to state.

"ANA-PAC Presidential Endorsement Process." (2008). *Capitol Update*, 6(8). Retrieved from http://www.rnaction.org/site/PageServer? pagename=CUP_Arch_103108_en3_pre sendorse

Federal Election Commission (2011). *Independent expenditure-only committees*. Retrieved from http://www.fec.gov/press/press2011/ ieoc_alpha.shtml

Federal Election Commission. (n.d.). Separate segregated funds and nonconnected PACs. Retrieved from www.fec.gov/pages/ brochures/ssfvnonconnected.shtml

David M. Keepnews

POWER AND LEADERSHIP

The root word of leadership is *lead* from the Anglo-Saxon Old English word *loedan*, the causal form of *lithan*—to travel. The *Oxford English Dictionary* defines *lead* as to guide with reference to action and opinion; to bring or take (a person or other) to a place, whereas the term *ship* indicates a state or condition (Grace, 2003). One could determine that leadership is the capacity (the state of being) to guide or take others to a place or an outcome.

The term power is ability or force to move an object or other from point A to point B. For example, when nurse faculty moves the minds of their students from point A to point B, it is called education. It is a powerful act. When a staff nurse moves the patient through the hospital system from entry to discharge, this activity while not often recognized as powerful is a vivid example of power and leadership.

Power provides the fuel for leadership. It sits under the umbrella of leadership along with six other components: (1) dreaming, (2) visioning, (3) boundary management, (4) risk taking, and (6) mastery. Dreaming is the antecedent to having a vision. It may be night or day dreaming,

P

conscious and unconscious associations with parts and pieces of ideas, experiences, and feelings. Vision is the result of dreaming and the intentional framing of pictures in the mind that portray the possible and the impossible becoming a reality. A vision has a destination requiring action, even if the pathway and the required resources are in question. However, it is with the use of boundary management that visions are shared with others, the colleagues and the followers. Leaders need to know the extent of their influence and where and when to build a bridge of collaboration, authority, or guidance with the others or simply when to lead and when to follow. Bridge building may not always be timely or effective and the leader may find one's self in a situation where there is a need to move forward without the safety of a bridge. This is the risk taking component of leadership. Mastery is the owning and acknowledgment by others of one's expertise, knowledge, skills, abilities, and experiences. These six components of leadership provide useful resources for the journey, but without power they tend to dissipate quickly.

Montana and Charnov (2008, p. 253) claim that power "enables leadership to influence subordinates and peers by controlling organizational (system) resources." This is accomplished through the following types of power originally described by French and Raven in 1960.

INFORMATIONAL POWER

Nurses in hospitals or communities possess more information than any other provider about the patient/consumer of services. This information is critical to the organizational functioning of any health care system. The nurse leader stands at the front of the line in terms of informational power.

LEGITIMATE POWER

This type refers to positional or earned power legitimized by the organizational system or an outside body. The nurse's license is a clear example of legitimate power. The nurse is authorized by the appropriate state(s) to practice and provide care to the citizens of that state.

CHARISMATIC POWER

This is displayed and maintained by the nurse showing the joy or passion for what one does. In nursing, there at times seems to be a greater emphasis on the difficult or painful aspects of the profession which limits the expression of one's passion for nursing. This type of power is easily accessible with rebalancing the equation to emphasize one's passion for the opportunity to serve and make a difference. Passion is an essential incentive in attracting followers and colleagues.

COERCIVE POWER

A simple definition of this challenging type of power is being in a position to offer two alternatives: one being more attractive than the other (e.g., getting a bonus if you do something versus not getting it if you do not). It involves a narrowing of the choices someone else has, but can be managed in a positive, less punitive manner if the nurse leader chooses.

REFERENT POWER

Interestingly, this is power gained by association. The most useful exemplar of this type of power is mentoring. The protégés gain status or use of resources due to their association with their mentors. For additional information on mentoring, see the entry "Leadership Development" in this volume,

Encourage Mentors (www.encourage-mentors.com), Leaders Mentoring (www.leadermentoring.com), and the National Mentoring Partnership (www.mentoring.org).

Maraldo (2008) states that "The relationship of power to leadership is unmistakable. It is a key component of leadership." Leadership must have an ongoing power generator. For nursing, the power generator is developed and sustained by the people we serve.

French, J. P. R. Jr., & Raven, B. (1960). The bases of social power. In D. Cartwright & A. Zander (Eds.), *Group dynamics* (pp. 607–623). New York, NY: Harper and Row.

Grace, M. (2003). *Origins of leadership: The etymology of leadership.* Paper presented at the International Leadership Association Conference, November 6–8, 2003, in Guadalajara, Jalisco, Mexico. Retrieved from http:www.ila-net.org/Publications/Proceedings/2003/mgrace.pdf

Maraldo, P. (2008). Leadership and power. In H. R. Feldman (editor-in-chief), *Nursing leadership: A concise encyclopedia.* New York, NY: Springer Publishing.

Montana, P. J., & Charnov, B. H. (2008). *Management.* Hauppauge, NY: Barron's Educational Series, Inc.

Beverly Louise Malone

PRECEPTORSHIP: PATHWAY TO SAFE PRACTICE AND CLINICAL REASONING

Clinical preceptors fulfill vital roles both in the development of new staff and in collecting evidence of competent practice (Boyer, 2008). They protect patients, staff, students, and the agency by observing the practice of the learner/orientee to ensure safe, effective care that adheres to

protocols. The preceptor also serves as coach, role model, and mentor as the new nurse endeavors to understand the practice environment and adapt to the responsibilities associated with being a nurse. Preceptors serve these roles for students, new graduates, experienced hires, temporary staff, and allied health care colleagues. In fact, throughout their professional careers, nurses vividly remember their first preceptor as well as their first work experience as a nurse. This fact alone tells us that the preceptor role is a critical variable in the development of a nurse's perception of the profession. The importance of the preceptor's role grows as past and current research validates the core educational challenges involved in developing nurses (Benner, 1984; Benner, Sutphen, Victoria, & Day, 2010) and updates the transition shock, crisis, and role development issues experienced during that first year of nursing practice (Benner, 1984; Duchscher, 2009; National Council for State Boards of Nursing, 2010).

The National Council for State Boards of Nursing (2010) has established a transition to practice model that is intended for collaborative implementation by education and practice. The delivery of this model calls for 6 months of clinical preceptor support. During this period, the preceptor maintains a safe care, safe practice, and safe learning environment, while fostering the development of clinical reasoning in the new care provider. This is the clinical reasoning that makes possible the "life or death" decision making that is core to both nursing and medical care. "The quality of the new nurse/preceptor partnership had a direct relationship with how competent a new RN felt about his/her nursing practice. Of equal importance was the finding that a higher competency score reported by a new RN correlated with fewer practice errors at both four

P

and six months" (Foundation for Nursing Excellence, 2009, p. 2).

The development of a preceptor program in a health care institution is a "best practice strategy" that allows experiential learning to occur while protecting the safety of both patient (Hickey, 2009; Luhanga, 2008) and learner. Most nurses are not inherently successful preceptors. Unique knowledge and skills need to be introduced, role modeled, assessed, and supported for success to be achieved in this role. Consequently, a fully developed nurse preceptor training program is vital for a safe and effective patient care and for achieving successful recruitment/retention outcomes (Lee, Tzeng, Lin, & Yeh, 2009; Porter-O'Grady, 2009). The preceptor role must be operationally defined, recognition and reward determined, selection criteria specified, and distinct responsibilities outlined. Some basic prerequisites for the selection of preceptors include (1) completion of a predetermined amount of time as a registered nurse within an institution, (2) effective communication and interpersonal skills with colleagues and patients, (3) applies nursing process to adapt the plan of care to patient's changing needs, (4) role models positive professional attributes, and (5) completes preceptor development course. The protocol also delineates the "when and how" for completing the assigned task or role. A reduction in patient assignment is generally required to fulfill the core roles in a safe, effective manner.

With role expectations clear, the preceptor course curriculum must be developed (Vermont Nurses in Partnership, 2008). The teaching methodology needs to include content delivery that integrates role playing, case-based learning exercises, and interactive strategies for resolving conflicts and giving feedback. The teaching plan used by the Vermont evidence-based internship program (Boyer, 2010) includes a transition from traditional learning objectives to performance outcomes expectations that connect with clinical performance as a preceptor. Content areas address the core communication, interpersonal, and teaching/learning theory that enables the preceptor to fulfill their defined roles. Thus, the instruction that is needed is shaped by the expected roles, responsibilities, challenges, and resources within the system.

Delivery of this education and support has a twofold purpose. The first is to improve capability related to teaching, coaching, mentoring, leadership, communication, and evaluation. Second, the program supports a transition from the current crisis-driven, intimidating, and isolating work place to a more supportive environment designed to assist the transition of a novice into successful practice. Effective preceptor development and support is established with the addition of annual updates for these clinical instructors. The fields of effective, experiential, and reflective learning grow with the same complexity and intensity as our highly technical clinical practice. Both of these fields require continuing education to ensure that both knowledge and skills remain current. Content for advanced preceptor development might explore a core topic in greater depth or delve into new interpersonal, teaching/learning, or leadership content such as emotional intelligence, appreciative inquiry, crucial conversations, and so forth. Links to possible options and further resources can be found as you scroll down through the topics and links at www.vnip.org/links.html.

The effective preceptor program is designed to build capacity both in individuals and in the environment. This learning fosters effective work with students, orientees, and interns to help them gain capability and meet competencies expected within orientation or student experiences.

It fosters the development of leadership skills and professionalism at a "grassroots" level. Most importantly, it sets the stage for safe, effective, experiential learning that is crucial to the development of effective nursing judgment and clinical reasoning.

See also Coaching Nurses; Conflict Management; Constructive Feedback; Cultural Diversity; Dedicated Education Unit; Delegation; Emotional Intelligence; Externships; Generational Differences in Leadership and Mentoring; Human Resource Management; Internships; Leadership Development; Managing Anger/ Emotions; Mentoring; Nurse Residency; Orientation and Staff Development; Teamwork

Benner, P. (1984). *From novice to expert: Excellence and practice power in clinical nursing*. Menlo Park, CA: Addison Wesley.

Benner, P., Sutphen, Victoria, M. L., & Day, L. (2010). *Educating nurses: A call for radical transformation*. San Fransico, CA: Jossey-Bass.

Boyer, S. (2010, June 15). *Vermont Nurses in Partnership*. Retrieved July 14, 2010, from http://www.vnip.org

Boyer, S. A. (2008). Competence and innovation in preceptor development—Updating our programs. *Journal for Nurses in Staff Development, 24*(2), E1–E6.

Duchscher, J. B. (2009). Transition shock: The initial stage of role adaptation for newly graduated registered nurses. *Journal of Advanced Nursing, 65*(5), 1103.

Foundation for Nursing Excellence. (2009). *Evidence-based transition to nursing practice initiative in North Carolina: Summary of Phase 1 findings*. Raleigh, NC: NC Center for Nursing Excellance. Retrieved from http://www.ffne.org

Hickey, M. (2009). Preceptor perceptions of new graduate nurse readiness for practice. *Journal for Nurses in Staff Developmen. 25*(1), 35–41.

Lee, T.-Y., Tzeng, W.-C., Lin, C.-H., & Yeh, M.-L. (2009). Effects of a preceptorship programme on turnover rate, cost, quality and professional development. *Journal of Clinical Nursing, 18,*1217–1225.

Luhanga, F. Y. (2008). Hallmarks of unsafe practice: What preceptors know. *Journal for Nurses in Staff Development, 24*(6), 257–264.

National Council for State Boards of Nursing. (2010). *Transition initiatives*. Retrieved July 13, 2010, from https://www.ncsbn.org/363.htm

Porter-O'Grady, T. (2009). Commentary on Lee T-Y, Tzeng W-C, Lin C-H., & Yeh M-L (2009). Effects of a preceptorship programme on turnover rate, cost, quality and professional development. *Journal of Continuing Education in Nursing*, 3207–3209.

Susan A. Boyer

PROFESSIONAL PRACTICE MODEL

The importance of working in a professional practice environment has been well known since the first Magnet Hospital Study (McClure, Poulin, Sovie, & Wandelt, 1983). From this landmark study, the essential components of professional practice were identified, including autonomy, control over practice, and collaborative relationships with physicians. Professional practice models are generally based on theory, are not stagnant, are designed to evolve over time, and are a basis for guiding ways nurses can clearly articulate belief systems (Ives Erickson, 1996; McEwen & Willis, 2002). Professional practice models describe the relationships of important organizational concepts and can support organizational activities designed to advance nursing practice. One of the most effective strategies for aligning nurses and clinicians across the disciplines is the articulation of a professional practice model. When a team becomes aligned, a commonality of direction emerges, and individual energies harmonize. There is a shared purpose and understanding of how to complement one another's efforts (Senge, 1995). In the white paper *Hallmarks of the Professional Nurse Practice Environment*, the American Association of Colleges of Nursing (2002) cites the following as characteristics of the practice setting that best support professional nursing practice:

- Manifest a philosophy of clinical care emphasizing quality, safety, interdisciplinary collaboration, continuity of care, and professional accountability.
- Recognize contributions of nurses' knowledge and expertise to clinical care quality and patient outcomes.
- Promote executive level nursing leadership.
- Empower nurses' participating in clinical decision making and organization of clinical care systems.
- Maintain clinical advancement programs based on education, certification, and advanced preparation.
- Demonstrate professional development support for nurses.
- Create collaborative relationships among members of the health care provider team.
- Utilize technological advances in clinical care and information systems.

The operational challenge in articulating a professional practice model is in defining concepts in such a way that brings significance to daily practice. Each component is critical to practice and care delivery. If a model is to work, each clinician needs to understand, embrace, and master the skills involved and be willing to learn—continuously learn—because the environment in which care is delivered is rapidly changing. This is a journey that the health care team takes together.

An example of a professional practice model is the interdisciplinary model utilized at Massachusetts General Hospital, which provides a comprehensive view of professional practice (Picard & Jones, 2005). This professional practice model consists of nine essential elements including vision and values, standards of practice, narrative culture, professional development, patient centeredness, clinical recognition and advancement, collaborative decision making, research and innovation, and entrepreneurial teamwork. The professional practice model is a framework for achieving clinical outcomes, for assuring the identity, integrity, and development of each discipline, and for working collaboratively in the care of patients and families. Because each component is inherently related to all others, an "interlocking" puzzle was chosen to represent the model. Each is connected to the need to truly understand the patient experience and ways to improve the patient care process (Figure 4).

The creation of a professional practice model serves many purposes, including the following:

- articulates the work of clinicians across a variety of settings;
- provides a framework to guide clinical practice, education, administration, and research;
- promotes communication among disciplines and between clinicians and the organization;
- provides a framework for setting a strategic direction and achieving goals and clinical outcomes;
- guides the allocation of resources;
- serves as a framework for the evaluation of practice; and
- functions as a marketing tool to visually describe clinical practice both internally and externally.

The model gathers the components of nurses' contributions and fits them

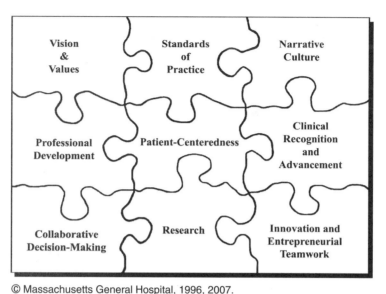

© Massachusetts General Hospital, 1996, 2007.

FIGURE 4. Massachusetts General Hospital professional practice model.

together to reveal the whole or essence of nursing practice. In addition, it takes the often-invisible work of nurses and other members of the health care team and makes it visible.

See also American Association of Colleges of Nursing; Magnet Hospitals

American Association of Colleges of Nursing. (2002). *Hallmarks of the professional nurse practice environment*. White paper. Washington, DC: Author.

Ives Erickson, J. (1996). *Caring headlines*. Boston, MA: Massachusetts General Hospital.

McClure, M. L., Poulin, M. A., Sovie, M. D., & Wandelt, M. (1983). *Magnet hospitals: Attraction and retention of professional nurses*. Washington, DC: American Nurses Publishing.

McEwen, M., & Willis, E. M. (2002). *Theoretical basis for nursing*. Philadelphia, PA: Lippincott Williams & Wilkins.

Picard, C., & Jones, D. (2005). *Giving voice to what we know: Margaret Neuman's theory of health as expanding consciousness in practice, research and education*. Sudbury, MA: Jones and Bartlett Publishers.

Senge, P. (1995). *The fifth discipline*. New York, NY: Doubleday/Currency.

Jeanette Ives Erickson
Marianne Ditomassi

PROFESSIONAL PRESENCE

Professional presence or presentation of self helps to establish an aura of competence and authority. How one presents oneself controls the impression one makes on others, especially those with whom we interact. It is a subject that some nurse leaders are reluctant to discuss. Attitudes often include notions that "I want to be me, just the way I am." A common thought is, "I've come this far, why change now?" Still others say, "I don't have time for make-up and hair styling." Despite attitudes such as these, impressions are important. One has limited time to establish a first impression; first impressions become lasting impressions. These impressions influence professional relationships and communications among people. In fact, Lavington (1997, p. 1) makes clear that "it only takes people three seconds to know where you're coming from." Like it or not, the way we dress, how we look, and how we act conveys credibility, competence, and authority.

Look only to the major TV newscasters to see role models of impeccable dress: Diane Sawyer, Katie Couric, and Brian Williams. As nurse leaders, we serve as role models to others with whom we work. We can all improve how we look and dress by working with needed changes and emphasizing our strengths. For women and men, dark tailored suits with white blouses or shirts provide a basic wardrobe design which can be changed with colored blouses or shirts and conservative scarves and ties. One current fashion trend of wearing sleeveless dresses in the work place is out of place despite its prominence; sleeveless dresses or tops belong in social settings. Timeless, tailored dressing projects good taste and confidence.

Other aspects of dressing should be considered also. Shoes and hair styles reveal much about one's status (Lavington, 1997, p. 96). Shoes should be in good condition, of high quality, in conservative colors, and well shined. Hair should be styled to suit one's face and cut to appropriate length. Women's hair should be no longer than shoulder length, or if longer, should be pulled back from the face. Otherwise hair becomes a distraction rather than a frame for the face. For women, jewelry is best when it is tasteful and conservative rather than trendy where too-big necklaces or earrings not only detract from one's face, but detract from what one is saying and the message being delivered. Makeup

illuminates the face and should be so subtle that it is difficult to detect. Women's handbags look best when appropriate in size, and backpacks are never considered professional for men or women. Ties for men should end no more than two inches below the waist-line and socks always match the trousers (Smith, 2006a, 2006b). By creating our own image, we make a positive impression on others which helps to establish a sense of position and power.

How we look and act over all, in addition to how we dress, also conveys confidence. Observe the behaviors of those who appear self-confident. A firm handshake is essential for a good first impression. Notice also the leader who enters a room full of people, ready to provide the keynote address. The speaker walks briskly to the microphone, smiles at the audience while being introduced, then stands with erect posture, both feet on the floor, makes eye contact with a few in the audience, uses gestures from the shoulder to punctuate the air at certain times to make a specific point. The speaker is poised, dignified, and confident. It is said that we hear only approximately 7% of the content of a presentation but that a large percentage of what we take in is visual. Body language sends signals of attitude, values, and emotions. For example, crossing one's arms across the body suggests withdrawal and does not project openness to relationships or discussion. Constantly looking down rather than making eye contact with others suggests shyness and even lack of understanding. We must watch for incongruence between what we say and what our body language says because the latter is so powerful. Voice is another determinant of perceived authority. Men have an advantage of having a deep voice that can be heard across the room, suggesting power and authority. Women's voices tend to be higher pitched and often soft. A woman can deliberately lower her voice to make communication more powerful. It is worth noting that some women nurse leaders speak too tentatively to be taken seriously. We tend to "ise" words like, "I wonder if..." when presenting a new idea. Or we might say, "Do you think we..." when an action is suggested. Sometimes we begin a sentence with, "I think maybe...," rather than stating a more positive self-owned idea. It is wise to be aggressive in speech, not aggressive to the point of abusive, but aggressive enough to own the point and show confidence in our competence.

As nurse leaders, we benefit from enhancing and projecting professional presence to our peers, colleagues, employers, employees, patients, and communities. We enter our leadership positions having had extraordinary nursing curricula of skills that include observation, assessment, interpersonal relationships, planning, communication, and evaluation. We are experienced, determined, persuasive, and passionate about our profession. We remain at the top of the list of health professionals most trusted by the public. Yet the public image of nursing and nurses suggests that only *we* know the myriad responsibilities and accomplishments that we perform each day. Of the many ways to change the perception of our profession, one is certainly to promote our individual and collective professional presence. Mitchell (2002, p. 109) suggests that we make every effort to create the most positive impression possible and to ask ourselves, "How do I want to be perceived?" and "Am I showing the people with whom I'm associating, the respect they deserve." After all, the point of striving for professional presence is to convey confidence, credibility, authority, and power and to use those dynamics to promote and improve health and health care for all people and communities.

Lavington, C. (1997). *You've only got three seconds.* New York, NY: Broadway Books.

Mitchell, M. (2002). *Class acts: How good manners create good relationships and good business.* New York, NY: M Evans and Company, Inc.

Smith, J. R. (2006a). *From clueless to class act: Manners for the modern man.* New York, NY: Sterling Publishing Inc.

Smith, J. R. (2006b). *From clueless to class act: Manners for the modern woman.* New York, NY: Sterling Publishing Inc.

Shirley S. Chater

Quality and Safety Education for Nurses

At the turn of the century, the Institute of Medicine (IOM) produced a series of reports on the quality of health care in America, documenting that quality, safety, and patient-centered care were *not* key features of the lived experiences of a high percentage of patients and families (Aspden, Corrigan, Wolcott, & Erickson, 2004; Committee on the Quality of Health Care in America, 2001). In 2003, the IOM report *Health Professions Education: A Bridge to Quality* issued a call for change, specifically, to alter learning experiences that form the basis for professional identity formation so that graduates of health professional educational programs would be educated to deliver *patient-centered care* as members of an *interdisciplinary team*, emphasizing *evidence-based practice, quality improvement approaches*, and *informatics* (IOM, 2003).

Nursing educators who were members of an interprofessional learning community (the Institute for Healthcare Improvement–sponsored Dartmouth Summer Symposium for Teaching Healthcare Improvement with leader Paul Batalden) conceived the *Quality and Safety Education for Nurses* (QSEN) project, which has been funded by the Robert Wood Johnson Foundation (RWJF) since 2005. With the leadership of a principal investigator 10 quality and safety thought leaders in nursing and representatives of professional organizations involved in nursing licensure, certification, and accreditation of nursing programs worked on behalf of nursing to answer the questions: What does this challenge mean for nursing education? What quality and safety competencies describe what it means to be a respected nurse? What teaching strategies will prepare graduates with the knowledge, skills, and attitudes to continuously improve the quality and safety of the health care systems in which they work?

Six competency definitions were developed: patient-centered care, teamwork and collaboration, evidence-based practice, quality improvement, safety, and informatics. Nurse educators were engaged in focus groups, surveys, and organizational feedback to assist QSEN leaders as they generated statements about the knowledge, skills, and attitudes that should be developed for each competency during prelicensure and advanced practice educational programs (Cronenwett et al., 2007; Cronenwett, Sherwood, Pohl, et al., 2009). These products served as guides for curricular development in formal academic programs, transition to practice and continuing education programs, and as frameworks for use by professional regulatory bodies that set standards for licensure, certification, and accreditation of nursing education programs.

As QSEN leaders engaged in conversations with faculty at multiple schools and meetings, the consistent plea was to "tell us how to teach" the knowledge, skills, and attitudes that are not embedded in current curricula. By March 2007, the QSEN Web site (www.qsen.org) began serving as a vehicle for sharing annotated references and strategies for classroom, skills/simulation laboratory, and clinical site teaching. In July 2007, 15 schools from ADN, diploma, and BSN prelicensure programs were selected through a competitive process to receive RWJF funding in support of their work to generate curricular change and teaching strategies. Over the subsequent 18 months, faculty responsible for classroom, simulation, and clinical teaching from each school participated in the QSEN Learning Collaborative, generating and sharing ideas with each other and through the QSEN Web site (Cronenwett, Sherwood, & Gelmon, 2009).

By 2009, the American Association of Colleges of Nursing (AACN) had incorporated quality and safety competency development in documents that set standards for accreditation of BSN and DNP programs, and the National Council of State Boards of Nursing was advocating that QSEN competencies be included in their framework for new graduate residency programs. A phase of widespread faculty development began under two RWJF grants, one to University of North Carolina–Chapel Hill (Dr. Linda Cronenwett) and one to AACN (Dr. Geraldine Bednash).

The AACN faculty (Barnsteiner from the University of Pennsylvania, Disch from the University of Minnesota, and Johnson from George Washington University) currently lead regional train-the-trainer conferences, where schools send two faculty members who receive in-depth training and materials to support curricular change. The University of North Carolina faculty lead additional approaches to securing the desired changes in nursing education. The first annual QSEN National Forum was held in June 2010 in Denver, Colorado, with a sold-out attendance of 324 participants, including multiple textbook authors and publishers. Faculty development is supported on the Web site by a series of self-guided faculty learning modules, developed under the leadership of Pamela Ironside. Shirley Moore leads the interprofessional VA Quality Scholars program, and QSEN provides support for the faculty mentors of the pre- and postdoctoral medical and nursing VAQS scholars selected in six sites to receive training in quality improvement science. Gwen Sherwood and Jane Barnsteiner are co-editing a textbook *Quality and Safety in Nursing: A Competency Based Approach to Improved Outcomes*, and QSEN faculty consult with other textbook authors who wish to incorporate content to support quality and safety education.

With 6 years of generous funding from the RWJF, the impact of QSEN-led work has stimulated fundamental changes in nursing education. It will take more time to accomplish the paradigm shift required of faculty and students in every nursing program in the country, but with regulatory and textbook changes that provide added impetus to change, the outlook is positive.

Nurse executives and staff educators are concerned with QSEN as well. The opportunities for academic-practice partnerships that develop role models among faculty and clinicians for the competencies we seek in all health professionals will be the next frontier. The end goal is for nurses and all health professionals to value identities that describe a "good, respected health professional" as one who can care for individual patients in an excellent manner but also improve the quality and safety of health care systems as part of their daily work.

Aspden, P., Corrigan, J. M., Wolcott, J., & Erickson, S. M. (Eds.). (2004). *Patient safety: Achieving a new standard for care.* Washington, DC: National Academies Press.

Committee on the Quality of Health Care in America. (2001). *Crossing the quality chasm: A new health system for the 21st century.* Washington, DC: National Academies Press.

Cronenwett, L., Sherwood, G., Barnsteiner, J., Disch, J., Johnson, J., Mitchell, P., et al. (2007). Quality and safety education for nurses. *Nursing Outlook, 55*(3), 122–131.

Cronenwett, L., Sherwood, G., & Gelmon, S.B. (2009). Improving quality and safety education: The QSEN Learning Collaborative. *Nursing Outlook, 57*(6), 304–312.

Cronenwett, L., Sherwood, G., Pohl, J., Barnsteiner, J., Moore, S., Sullivan, D.T., et al. (2009). Quality and safety education for advanced nursing practice. *Nursing Outlook, 57*(6), 338–348.

Institute of Medicine. (2003). Health professions education: A bridge to quality. Washington, DC: National Academies Press.

Linda Cronenwett

R

RAISE THE VOICE!

Raise the Voice! is a campaign launched by the American Academy of Nursing (AAN) in 2007 to identify and promote the work of nurses, specifically those who have created new models of care delivery that are accessible, cost effective, replicable, and holistic. This initiative, conceived by the authors while members of the AAN Board, highlights the work of Edge Runners—nurses who are practical innovators in creating new ways to deliver health care that improves quality, reduces costs, and provides a personalized experience. The intended audience for the campaign includes the public, the policymakers, the administration, the health care leaders, and all committed to progressive change.

The goal of the campaign is to ensure that Americans hear and understand the exciting possibilities for transforming the health care system—and that nurses are leading the way in developing solutions that achieve significant clinical and financial outcomes. According to the AAN Web site (www.aannet.org), this is a call for "not just reformation but transformation—moving American health care away from its current hospital-based, acuity-oriented, physician-dependent paradigm toward a patient-centered, convenient, helpful, and affordable system. America needs a system that keeps people as healthy as possible, treats the patient promptly, comprehensively and effectively."

At present, the AAN has recognized 46 Edge Runner programs. Two examples illustrate the innovative thinking and impact of all of the programs found on the AAN Web site:

- 11th Street Family Health Services (Patricia Gerrity, PhD, RN, FAAN)—a trans-disciplinary health center managed by nurses that serves residents in four public housing developments. The program provides a range of primary care, dental services, behavioral health services, and health promotion and disease prevention to a population where 57% of patients are covered by the state Medicaid plan and 33% are uninsured. Outcomes include improved control of hypertension (68% of clients versus 50% for African Americans), increased immunization rates, decreased depression rates, reduced number of low birth weight infants, and a 20% reduction in hemoglobin A1C.

- Nurse–Family Partnership (Harriet Kitzman, PhD, RN, FAAN)—an evidence-based nurse home visitation program, from pregnancy through the child's first two years of life—to improve pregnancy outcomes, child health and development, and the economic self-sufficiency of low-income, first-time parents and their children. Outcomes include 79% reduction in preterm delivery for women who smoke, 35% fewer hypertensive disorders of pregnancy, a decrease in smoking, a 28-month greater interval between the birth of first and second child, a 23% reduction in subsequent pregnancies by child age 2 years, and 39% fewer injuries among children.

The campaign has been well supported by a diverse coalition of individuals and organizations. A Raise the Voice! Advisory Board of national leaders is chaired by Edward G. Rendell, former Governor of Pennsylvania; the initial chair was Dr. Donna Shalala. This impressive group advises the current co-chairs and AAN staff on issues related to promotion, networking, fundraising, and taking these programs to scale. A grant from the Robert Wood Johnson Foundation has also provided support for the campaign.

Joanne Disch
Karlene Kerfoot

RAPID RESPONSE TEAMS

Rapid response teams (RRT), also known as medical emergency teams, bring teams of clinicians with critical care experience to the patient's bedside. The RRT was part of Institute for Healthcare Improvement's 100,000 lives campaign, an initiative to protect patients from harm. Although protocols and membership of RRTs are structured differently in each setting and no two teams seemingly operate alike, most have some combination of the following: the process is initiated by the nurse caring for the patient and the RRT is comprised of a critical care nurse, a respiratory therapist, a senior resident, and/or a hospitalist. The

criteria established for initiating the RRT vary but generally include acute changes in the following: respiratory status, blood pressure and heart rate, level of consciousness, and decreased urine output without a history of renal dysfunction. In the evolution of RRTs, the level of discomfort of the nurse caring for the patient has been added to the criteria for calling the RRT (Scholle & Mininni, 2006). The RRT is expected to arrive at the patient's bedside within 10 minutes of a call initiating the team response. Communication is critical in this process, and the use of situation, background, assessment, and recommendation techniques has assisted in the effective use of the RRTs (Simmonds, 2005).

RRTs have been widely implemented across the United States and gained further acceptance after the Institute for Healthcare Improvement encouraged their implementation as a strategy to decrease preventable deaths. The implementation of RRTs has grown to more than 1,600 hospitals in the United States, and in multiple nations there is little consensus on its effect in decreasing preventable deaths or other outcome measures such as intensive care unit admission rates. There is increasing discussion not only on the outcome measures but also on the effect of the RRT from the perspective of the nurse who generally initiates the RRT. Several hospitals have expanded the RRT to allow family members to initiate the RRT, analogous to a 911 when patients seem to be experiencing an emergency. These teams function by bringing consultation from critical care experts directly to the bedside no matter the location. The development of the RRT was thought to result in better support to patients and the staff caring for them. In addition, improved patient outcomes, decreased untoward events that may require a higher level of care, improved survival rates, and altered patterns of transfers into critical care areas were expected with the initiation of these teams.

Studies of the effectiveness of RRTs varied, and although the RRT provides a systems approach in dealing with critically ill patients, the benefits are not yet well defined in measuring outcomes (Cretikos & Hillman, 2003). Recent studies (Hillman et al., 2005) suggest that the use of the RRT has increased but that the negative outcomes such as unplanned admission to critical care, reduced mortality rates, or reduced cardiac arrest rates have not occurred (Chan, Renuka, Nallmothu, Berg, & Sasson, 2010). Qualitative data are emerging (Shapiro, Donaldson, & Scott, 2010) not only on the clinical outcomes mentioned earlier but also on the nurses' ability to recognize the deteriorating signs of patients, the nurses' work environment, empowering nurses to take control of their work environment, and the effect on job satisfaction. Clearly, this debate persists and new questions continue to emerge. Nursing leaders need to evaluate the potential effectiveness of the RRT in their own organizations and settings to determine its value in affecting the lives of patients we serve and our collective responsibility to reduce harm to patients under our care.

See also Institute for Healthcare Improvement

Chan, P., Renuka, J., Nallmothu, B., Berg, R., & Sasson, C. (2010). Rapid response teams: A systematic review and meta-analysis. *Archives of Internal Medicine, 170*(1), 18–26.

Cretikos, M., & Hillman, K. (2003). The medical emergency team: Does it really make a difference? *Journal of Internal Medicine, 33*(11), 511–514.

Hillman, K., Chen, J., Cretikos, M., Bellomo, R., Brown, D., Doig, G., et al. (2005). Introduction of the medical emergency team (MET) system: A cluster randomised controlled trial. *Lancet, 365*(9477), 2091–2097.

Scholle, C., & Mininni, N. (2006). How a rapid response team saves lives. *Nursing, 36*(1), 36–40.

Shapiro, S., Donaldson, N., & Scott, M. (2010). Rapid response teams seen through the eyes of the nurse. *American Journal of Nursing, 110*(6), 28–34.

Simmonds, T. C. (2005). Best-practice protocols: Implementing a rapid response system of care. *Nursing Management, 36*(7), 41–59.

Ingrid E. Brodin

REGULATORY BOARDS

The 10th Amendment to the U.S. Constitution reserves to the states, as part of their police powers, the right to regulate professions to protect the health, safety, and welfare of the public. Regulatory boards are created when state legislators are convinced that the practice of a profession requires regulation to protect the public. The resulting laws that are passed are referred to as *practice acts*. For nursing, the first such practice acts were passed in 1903. Practice acts distinguish the practice of nursing from that of other health care providers and define and differentiate the scope of practice and professional responsibilities for registered professional nurses (RNs), licensed practical nurses (LPNs), and advanced practice nurses (APNs). Generally, practice acts are written in broad terms to permit the acquisition of new knowledge, technological advances, and the gradual evolution of the profession. Practice acts designate the creation of a regulatory board and grant authority to the board to enforce the provisions of the law. The regulatory board serves as the administrative body to assure that provisions of the practice act are met. A list of nursing regulatory boards can be found at www.ncsbn.org by clicking on the link labeled *Boards of Nursing*. There is at least one nursing regulatory body in each of the 50 states and the District of Columbia. Although some states have more than one such body, for example, a separate board for LPNs, another for RNs, and a distinct board for APNs, the most common configuration is that of a single board that manages regulatory issues of RNs, LPNs, and APNs. Regulatory boards, based on the authority provided in the practice act, generally function to establish criteria for licensure, including education, experience, examination, age, and citizenship; determine grounds for removal of a license; establish policies to conduct disciplinary proceedings; determine licensure renewal requirements, including continuing competence or continuing education; and arbitrate scope of practice issues, that is, make legal opinions on those activities that can and cannot be provided by the licensed professionals within the board's purview. Requirements for membership on regulatory boards are specified in the nursing practice act. In the early history of nursing, regulatory boards included only RNs as members. LPNs began to be added in the 1940s and in the 1970s jurisdictions began to include public members as board members with full voting rights and privileges. The structure of regulatory boards across states and jurisdictions is marked by considerable diversity. Some boards are essentially independent and operate autonomously on licensure revenues. Such boards have the authority to promulgate regulations, initiate new legislation, and make declarative statements regarding scope of practice issues. Other boards function within an umbrella organization in a department, such as health, education, or labor, which regulates numerous other disciplines. This hierarchical structure strongly affects the authority of the regulatory board and its ability to control its budget, to determine the outcome of licensure for applicants, and to make decisions on scope of practice issues. Regulatory boards also have gathered to form associations of regulatory boards. Voting membership in such associations is usually limited to the regulatory board or body within each individual state authorized to regulate the specific profession. The National Council of State Boards of Nursing serves as an example of an association of regulatory nursing boards. Further information about the National Council of State Boards of Nursing can be obtained by accessing their Web site at www.ncsbn.org.

See also Continuing Professional Education; National Council of State Boards of Nursing, Inc.

Barbara Zittel

RESEARCH INTEGRITY

Facilitating public trust in the scientific endeavors of the numerous investigators, especially in the field of health, is critical. Research integrity is not easily defined because it involves both individuals and research institutions that provide an environment for integrity and excellence in the science. From an individual perspective, the Institute of Medicine (IOM) suggests that integrity refers to commitment to "intellectual honesty and personal responsibility" for the studies that one conducts and a special emphasis on the responsible conduct of research, including protection of one's subjects (IOM, 2002, p. 5). Individual research integrity is characterized by a set of behaviors:

• intellectual honesty and analysis of study protocols;

- scrutinizing data-based contributions for accuracy;
- rigorous, systematic, and fair review of peer's intellectual work;
- sharing scientific theory and research results with colleagues for critique and consideration of accuracy and rigor;
- transparency regarding conflicts of interest.
- high priority given to the protection of human and animal subjects.

Most research is conducted by teams of senior and junior investigators and their staff. Each of these individuals needs to understand their responsibility for preventing research misconduct. The principal investigator is ultimately responsible for the integrity of the study, the actions of the research team members, and the accuracy of the data.

Institutional commitment entails "creating an environment that promotes responsible conduct" and encourages integrity through the provision of structures, policies, procedures, and senior mentors with integrity (IOM, 2002, p. 5). Institutional research integrity is characterized by the following:

- developing leadership structures for support of individual scientists to conduct responsible research;
- promoting constructive, consistent interaction between mentors/mentees and among the research team members;
- advocating knowing, understanding, and adhering to the policies and procedures for the responsible conduct of research;
- monitoring and managing when necessary, conflicts of interest involved with research programs;
- providing opportunities for educational workshops and modules on research integrity; and

- following up on any allegations of misconduct in research programs of the institution's scientists.

A common practice flowing from the recommendations of the IOM report is the implementation of a self-assessment plan and protocol for research institutions. This is a "police ones' self" type of strategic that has been strongly adopted by the institutions although resources are required for such assessments.

Many of the individual scientist and institutional standards for research integrity have been developed by the Department of Health and Human Services, Office of Research Integrity (ORI). Because of past abuses and misconduct of research from around the 1930s to the 1970s, a number of Codes of Conduct for Research were produced, for example, the Nuremberg Code, the Declaration of Helsinki, and the National Commission for the Protection of Human Subjects in Biomedical and Behavioral Research (The Belmont Report). A series of laws resulted that led to the establishment of the ORI and similar offices in other federal agencies that systematically monitor the federal government's investment in science, especially biomedical and behavioral research. The ORI oversees the conduct of research within approximately 4,000 institutions worldwide, which are expected to monitor their individual scientists.

In the ORI, research integrity is operationalized as the misconduct of research. The definition of misconduct includes several areas:

- Fabrication refers to altering or making up data in some manner and reporting or recording them.
- Falsification involves "manipulating" the data, equipment, data protocols, or

omitting data in some manner to achieve a specific research outcome.

- Plagiarism is the use of other people's words, ideas, protocols, and so forth, without giving credit to those colleagues.

The ORI is clear that honest errors or misinterpretation of data do not constitute research misconduct. Having a difference of opinion with a colleague or reporting systematically analyzed data that differs from prior research studies also does not indicate misconduct of research. There is concern in the literature that the three categories of fabrication, falsification, and plagiarism do not constitute the entire realm of misconduct of research and that this concept needs to be expanded.

Research integrity also involves scientific ethics. This factor refers to the morals and values guiding an investigators decisions and actions while in the process of conducting and disseminating research as well as the ethics of how other professionals implement the research in practice and policy. Scientists' ethics guide their adoption and commitment to the individual characteristics of research integrity, that is, intellectual honesty, safeguarding accuracy of data, rigorous peer review, transparent conflicts of interest, and especially a strong focus on the protection of human and animal subjects. These factors are paramount in all stages of the research process, from conducting to disseminating to implementing the findings.

There are major pressures to enter into misconduct of research from enhancing a reputation to obtaining resources that scientists must manage and control. The pressures are particularly difficult for junior investigators who are in the process of building their reputations and are being pushed to obtain extramural funding in order to be promoted and tenured in academic institutions. Senior mentors, who both support and sponsor the young investigators, are critical in promoting the conduct of responsible research and facilitating careers. Education programs outlining strategies for the responsible conduct of research are required from institutions receiving federal funds and are major factors in socializing young scientists and raising awareness for all researchers.

In summary, research integrity encompasses and is required of both individual scientists and the institutions in which research is conducted. Education for learning how to safeguard the integrity of a study and the presence of senior mentors for young scientists is interactive with the research environment of the institution in ensuring research integrity.

Institute of Medicine & National Research Council. (2002). *Integrity in scientific research: Creating an environment that promotes responsible conduct.* Washington, DC: National Academies Press.

Ada Sue Hinshaw

RESOURCE DEVELOPMENT

Resources are the foundation of any organization and the tools by which administrators execute their role. They are the source of our ability to achieve organizational goals and the manner in which they are allocated communicates the priorities of the organization. Organizational resources are most commonly thought of as money or funds but they can also be people, space, services, or any other valuable commodity that can be used to accomplish organizational goals. One of the primary responsibilities of a nurse leader is the acquisition of resources to meet the strategic priorities of the organization.

There are several areas that drive the development of resources in organizations and should be of primary concern to nurse leaders. First, resource development should be consistent with the mission and vision of the organization. For example, an organization whose primary mission is the education of nursing students should examine all dimensions of that mission to determine if there are opportunities to develop new services for the existing population or to expand the existing services to new markets. It is critical to avoid the temptation to move outside the boundaries of the mission to begin services or programs that confound the core work of the organization.

The strategic plan of the organization is a driver for resource development and a business plan is the map used to determine how resources will be allocated. A focused and thoughtful strategic plan will illuminate the areas in which new or supplemental resources are needed. A defined strategic initiative aligned with the priorities of the organization provides the nurse leader with an opportunity to secure resources from donors, administration, and others who share a passion for that initiative. The business plan will give direction on how resources are deployed and the mechanism for evaluating the effectiveness of the new initiative. Partnerships and consortia can extend the impact of the organization's resources by sharing the cost and work of developing new initiatives.

Organizations are often faced with the challenge of acquiring sufficient resources to accomplish their defined goals. In times of scarce resources, organizational goals are often forfeited. Scarce resources may negatively affect morale, influence the perception of the organization in the community, and make it impossible to compete for new staff, clients, or students. As such, resource development is a skill that is critical to the success of a nurse leader. Many organizations are allocated resources based on past performance, and the nurse leader is constrained from innovation because of a lack of funds. Taking an entrepreneurial approach to the development of resources will allow for the possibility of new revenue streams, which will seed innovative approaches to practice and organizational development.

Resources can also be realized through the elimination of existing programs or services which frees up revenue to fund new initiatives. The elimination of ineffective or out-of-date programs or services is critical to a well-functioning organization, but it often comes with staff challenges, especially if staff feels that their employment is in jeopardy because of this organizational change. The elimination of programs or services to free up resources must be executed in line with the organization's strategic plan, keeping members of the organization informed of the necessary changes to the current structure of programs or services. Using data in decision making is critical to the effective implementation of change in organizations.

Resource development is a critical skill of the nurse leader. There are challenges to resource development in both times of prosperity and scarcity. A thoughtful approach to fiscal management, coupled with creativity and entrepreneurship, will provide the foundation for the development of the necessary resources for organizational effectiveness.

Additional information is available from the following sources:

American Association of Colleges of Nursing. (2005). *Academic leadership in nursing: Making the journey.* Washington, DC: Author.

Buller, J. L. (2007). Setting budgetary priorities. In *The essential academic dean: A practical guide to college leadership* (pp. 174–181). San Francisco, CA: Jossey-Bass.

Donnelly, G. (2005). A budget model to determine the financial health of nursing education programs in academic institutions. *Nursing Leadership Forum, 9* (4), 143–147.

Stuart, G. W., Erkel, E. A., & Shull, L. H. Allocating resources in a data-driven college of nursing. *Nursing Outlook, 58*(4), 200–206.

Paula Milone-Nuzzo

RISK MANAGEMENT IN THE HEALTH CARE SETTING

The Joint Commission (2007) defines risk management as "clinical and administrative activities undertaken to identify, evaluate, and reduce the risk of injury to patients, staff, and visitors, and the risk of loss to the organization itself." Risk management was practiced in the insurance industry for many years before becoming a specific competency within health care organizations. The initial function of risk management was to help mitigate the escalating costs of health care premiums, which had been rising as a result of an increasing number of claims and lawsuits. As expenses rose in the 1970s, a need developed to examine the liability concerns that affected patient care and the outcomes of these situations. In addition, the risk manager's role was focused on proactively managing activities within the health care system that could broaden the knowledge and behaviors of providers in response to negative outcomes of care. Risk managers were initially seen as the guardians of the information chest of adverse events and their effect on patients and staff.

In many institutions today, risk managers collect and analyze occurrence reports, participate in the defense of malpractice cases, offer guidance and education dealing with difficult patients and situations, and initiate sentinel event case review. It is through the risk manager's assessment and interaction with providers that liability concerns are identified. In addition, the risk manager helps to identify system weaknesses or vulnerabilities within hospital settings that may allow adverse events to occur. During the interview and investigative process, the risk manager also has the opportunity to assess not only the safety of patients, but also the emotional well-being of providers involved in an adverse event, who are often referred to as the *second victim*. According to Wu (2000), "Many errors are built into existing routines and devices, setting up the unwitting physician and patient for disaster. And, although patients are the first and obvious victims of medical mistakes, doctors are wounded by the same errors: they are the second victims." Nurses also hold the same vulnerability as physicians and assessing their response to an event and assuring support will foster a just culture within your environment. As nurse leaders, ensuring identification and education of potential risks is key to a reliable risk management program.

Since the release of the 2001 Institute of Medicine publication *To Err Is Human*, the world of risk management and patient safety has begun to coalesce and move to new prominence in health care. Identification of risk, development of corrective action plans, event disclosure, and providing apology to patients and their families are some of the responsibilities that risk managers undertake.

There are many ways that risk managers can help to analyze concerns. Communication is the number one tool of an effective risk manager (Carroll, 2006). Understanding the causes of errors is crucial to preventing their recurrence as well as litigation in the future. Risk managers look for ways to make improvements in work processes to prevent harm from reaching others. Nurses are key to the process of a case analysis or root cause analysis; however, it is often challenging to create an environment free from blame that allows people to speak freely about their fears and concerns. Reviewers have moved away from the process of asking, "Who did it?" to asking "What happened and why?"

Risk identification and reporting is a major tool used in risk management. "The values of reporting events, to learn what factors contribute to their occurrence, and to take actions to reduce or eliminate those factors is now recognized as key to improving patient safety" (Shostek & Pronovost, 2006). Assuring a nonpunitive culture for risk reporting will foster an increase in risk identification.

Creating a *fair and just culture* is one way that nurse leaders can collaborate with risk managers to prevent errors and identify system vulnerabilities. According to Frankel (2004), "A fair and just culture means giving constructive feedback and critical analysis in skillful ways, doing assessments that are based on facts, and having respect for the complexity of the situation. It also means providing fair-minded treatment, having productive conversations, and creating effective structures that help people to reveal their errors and help the organization learn from them."

As nurse leaders work to create transparencies in health care and patient care delivery systems, it is important to involve patients in the prevention and management of risk. At times, the fear of litigation prevents health care providers from acknowledging to the patient that something has gone wrong. The provider often feels unable to offer an apology. According to cancer specialist, Dr. Robert Buckman (1992), who has written extensively about disclosure and apology of medical error,

"Patients were significantly more likely to either report or sue the physician when he or she failed to acknowledge the mistake. From this, one may hypothesize that if clinicians disclose all pertinent information, patients will be less likely to sue" (Federico, 2003).

"In a survey conducted by the National Patient Safety Foundation (NPSF) as many as 95% of the respondents wanted to know about even the most insignificant error" (Federico, 2003, p. 2). By receiving open and honest communication from their providers, patients have the potential to be knowledgeable about their health care and feel safer. Open and direct communication is crucial for a patient to understand what has happened when there is an error, and it is essential to remaining in control of health care decisions. This in turn will lead to a more satisfied patient relationship and also may lead to a decrease in malpractice litigation (Atkins, 1995).

For too long, health care providers have not been accountable to their patients and society for errors that have occurred. The public now demands more. The core competencies of risk managers are focused on supporting providers with information about risk avoidance as well as the management of adverse events when they occur. Their contributions help to foster and create a patient care culture of transparency, safety, and performance improvement and will expect no less from the hands they place their lives in. This is not unlike teaching our children the importance of owning up to a mistake.

See also Accreditation in Nursing Practice; Sentinel Events

Atkins, P. M. (1995). Reducing risks through quality improvements, infection control, and risk management. *Critical Care Nursing Clinics of North America, 7*(4), 733–741.

R

Buckman, R. (1992). *How to break bad news: A guide for health care professionals*. Baltimore, MD: Johns Hopkins University Press.

Carroll, R. (2006). *Risk management handbook*. Chicago, IL: American Hospital Publishing.

Federico, F. (2003). Disclosure of medical error. *Forum, 23*(2), 2–3.

Frankel, A. (2004). *Dana-Farber Cancer Institute: Principles of a fair and just culture*. Retrieved August 24, 2007, from http://www.maco-alition.org/Initiatives/docs/Dana-Farber_PrinciplesJustCulture.pdf

Institute of Medicine. (2001). *To err is human*. Washington, DC: National Academies Press.

Shostek, K., & Provonost, P. (2006). Managing Risks and Improving Safety in the Intensive Care Unit. In *Risk management handbook*. Chicago, IL: American Hospital Publishing.

The Joint Commission. (2007). *Sentinel event glossary of terms*. Retrieved August 24, 2007, from http://www.jointcommission.org/SentinelEvents/se_glossary.htm

Denise Peterson

ROBERT WOOD JOHNSON FOUNDATION EXECUTIVE NURSE FELLOWS PROGRAM

The Executive Nurse Fellows Program, supported by the Robert Wood Johnson Foundation, is a national three-year fellowship opportunity for nurses in advanced leadership positions, who aspire to lead and shape the health care delivery system in their organizations or communities. Commencing on 2011, the program is administered by the Center for Creative Leadership (CCL) in Greensboro, NC, and the University of North Carolina, Chapel Hill, School of Nursing (UNCCH). David Altman, PhD, Executive Vice President, Research, Innovation and Product Development at CCL and Linda Cronenwett, PhD, RN, FAAN, Dean Emerita, School of Nursing at UNCCH, serve as Co-Program Directors. The National Program Office to which inquiries may be sent is located at CCL in Greensboro. The fellowship program admits up to 20 fellows every year from all aspects of nursing including health services, academic and research organizations, public-, health-, and community-based organizations or systems, and national professional, governmental, and policy organizations. It allows participants to remain in their current positions while they enhance their knowledge and skills necessary to address the unprecedented changes in health and health care delivery.

The curriculum provides learning experiences that expand concepts of leadership including, but not limited to, self-awareness, communication and interpersonal skills, strategic thinking and implementation, creativity, and innovation and change agent skills. The program consists of seminars, webinars, individual coaching sessions, group work, and personal mentoring. Each fellow completes a leadership project during the fellowship. The project addresses an issue important to the home organization and often can be applied to a broader health care system (Morjikian & Bellack, 2005).

HISTORY

Terrance Keenan, a senior vice president and program officer of the Robert Wood Johnson Foundation, was the visionary who dedicated much of his professional life to supporting nursing initiatives. One such initiative was the development of the Executive Nurse Fellows Program that would focus not on management, but on advanced leadership skills, intended for nurses who hold senior level positions. The Center for the Health Professions at the University of California, San Francisco, was chosen in 1997 as the initial site of the program. Edward H. O'Neil, PhD, FAAN, Director of the Center for the Health Professions, was named Project Director and Marilyn Chow, DNSc, RN, FAAN, Vice President, Patient Care Services, Kaiser Permanente, served as the Program Director. The Robert Wood Johnson Foundation appointed a sixteen member National Advisory Committee, chaired by Shirley S. Chater, PhD, RN, FAAN, whose major responsibilities included reviewing applications and interviewing candidates for recommendation to the program. In 1998, the first cohort of 15 fellows was accepted, and 20 fellows per year were admitted thereafter. The program soon achieved national prominence and continued to be administered by the Center for the Health Professions until 2011.

ALUMNI

By 2011, more than 250 executive nurse leaders completed the program. An active alumni association assures continuous contact among fellows, some continuing to work together on initiatives of mutual interest, often consulting with each other to expand existing projects. Many fellows extend the projects completed during the program into the future, bringing innovation and change to their organizations and communities. A description of selected fellows' executive level work since graduating from the program appears in the book titled, *Nurse Executive*, edited by Linda Thompson Adams, former fellow, and Edward H. O'Neil, Director, Center for the Health Professions, University of California, San Francisco (Adams & O'Neil, 2009). Alumni meetings are held annually in conjunction with a regular program seminar to encourage the inclusion of new fellows and to guarantee social and professional networking among cohorts.

Adams, L. T. & O'Neil, E. (Eds.). (2009). *Nurse executive.* New York, NY: Springer Publishing Co.

Bellack, J. & Morjikian, R. (2005). The RWJ executive nurse fellows program, Part 2. *Journal of Nursing Administration, 35*(12), 533–540.

Fralic, M. F. & Morjikian, R. (2006). The RWJ executive nurse fellows program, Part 3. *Journal of Nursing Administration, 36* (2), 96–102.

Morjikian, R. & Bellack, J. (2005).The RWJ executive nurse fellows program, Part 1. *Journal of Nursing Administration, 35*(10), 431–438.

www.executive nursefellows.org

Shirley Chater

ROBERT WOOD JOHNSON FOUNDATION NURSE FACULTY SCHOLARS PROGRAM

In 2008, the Robert Wood Johnson Foundation (RWJF) created the Nurse Faculty Scholars Program to address the long-term structural nursing shortage by lessening the nursing faculty shortage (www.nursefacultyscholars.org). The purpose of the program is to develop the next generation of national leaders in academic nursing through career development awards for outstanding junior nursing faculty and also to strengthen the academic productivity and overall excellence of nursing schools by providing mentorship, leadership training, salary, and research support to young faculty. The program is administered by a national program office located at Johns Hopkins University School of Nursing. Personnel includes National Program Director, Dr. Jacquelyn Campbell, a deputy director and administrative staff,

R

with leadership provided by the RWJF Program Officer, Dr. MaryJoan Ladden, under the Human Capital Program Area of RWJF, and the National Advisory Committee (NAC) chaired by Dr. Angela Barron McBride.

Between 12 and 15 scholars are chosen each year through a call for proposals, and review is according to well-publicized selection criteria by the NAC with an interview of the top applicants to make final selections. Eligible candidates are between 2 and 5 years of their first appointment as full time faculty after PhD or post doctoral training. Scholars receive substantial (60% time) salary support and research funding to complete in 3 years the research project they proposed as well as to participate in leadership training provided by the program.

Major content areas of the leadership training include personal development, research and scholarship, management skills, policy formation, teaching excellence, and university/community leadership. In addition, participants receive mentorship from three senior scholars, first their primary mentor from their own school of nursing, who provides mentoring in advancing their nursing career at their own institution and becoming an academic nursing leader and supports their application. Second, an interdisciplinary research mentor from their own university provides mentorship to the scholar in developing an interdisciplinary research career and the science in their field as well as becoming known for that expertise in their university. Finally, the program assigns participants to a national nursing mentor who facilitates their development as a national nursing leader.

Evaluation of the program is based on the following criteria: scholars' achievements in research and scholarship, national stature in the discipline, leadership in their school, university, and community, and achievement of teaching excellence. In addition, the program is evaluated on criteria of diversity of the scholars (ethnic, gender, and research intensity and type of baccalaureate schools of nursing) and its contribution to the academic productivity and overall excellence of the nursing schools where the scholars are located. To assure diversity in schools of nursing, a school can have no more than two active scholars at a time. The Nurse Faculty Scholars Program demonstrates the support of the RWJF for the profession of nursing as well as its commitment to investing in preparing health professionals for leadership.

Jacquelyn Campbell
MaryJoan Ladden
Angela Barron McBride

ROBERT WOOD JOHNSON FOUNDATION'S INITIATIVE ON THE FUTURE OF NURSING

Nursing is a critical component of the Robert Wood Johnson Foundation (RWJF)'s mission to improve the health and health care of all Americans. Over the years, the Foundation has made a significant investment in nursing because fundamental to the Foundation's role is that it is not possible to address the challenges faced by our nation's health care system without also addressing the challenges faced by nursing. The initiative on the future of nursing (IFN) has provided an opportunity to further this investment and to work in partnership with the Institute of Medicine to find solutions to the challenges confronting nursing and health care.

Some of the nation's top minds were brought together for fresh thinking about these challenges. The results of this initiative released in October 2010 in a landmark Institute of Medicine (IOM) report, *The Future of Nursing: Leading Change, Advancing Health*, represents the finest kind of collaboration with experts and health professionals from a wide range of fields, crossing over boundaries and working outside of traditional silos to develop solutions that are grounded in evidence-based research.

The report contains recommendations for an action-oriented blueprint on the future of nursing. It is a call to action for everyone who considers health and health care a priority for our nation. The message is clear: we must address the challenges faced by nursing if we are to improve health and health care.

Nursing leadership repeatedly came to the forefront of the IOM committee's deliberations. They felt that leadership is crucial to advancing the profession. Nurses need to be full partners with physicians and other health professionals in redesigning health care in the United States. Nurses must see policy as something they shape, rather than something that happens to them.

To ensure that nurses are ready to assume leadership roles, the committee felt that leadership-related competencies need to be embedded throughout nursing education; leadership development and mentoring programs need to be made available for nurses at all levels; and a culture that promotes and values leadership needs to be fostered. Equally important is that all nurses—from students, to bedside and community nurses, to chief nursing officers and members of nursing organizations, to researchers—must take responsibility for their personal and professional growth by developing leadership competencies. They must exercise these competencies in a collaborative environment in all settings, including hospitals, communities, schools, boards, and political and business arenas, both within nursing and across the health care professions.

Two of the eight IOM recommendations focus specifically on leadership: expanding opportunities for nurses to lead and preparing and enabling nurses to lead change to advance health. The other recommendations seek to remove scope of practice barriers, improve education, and create an infrastructure for interprofessional health care workforce data collection. Overall, the recommendations call for significant improvements in public and institutional policies at the national, state, and local levels.

Implementing these recommendations must happen to achieve the vision of a reformed health care system where all Americans have access to high-quality patient-centered care. RWJF is committed to leading the implementation of these recommendations, but cannot do it alone. Addressing the challenges faced by nursing must be seen as a societal issue. To that end, the Foundation has joined forces with AARP on the Future of Nursing: Campaign for Action. RWJF and AARP are leading a broad-based coalition of organizations that represent hospitals and health systems, insurance companies and other payers, higher education, state and federal governments, consumers and other health professionals and nurses. The National Summit on Advancing Health through Nursing was also held to mark the launch of the IFN implementation phase, where over 500 leaders from nursing, government, insurance industry, advocacy organizations, philanthropy and others pledged to take action to make the recommendations a reality.

It is a fantastic start, but all nursing leaders are needed to join in this effort. Visit www.thefutureofnursing.org to

R

R

decide how to get involved. Details are provided about the recommendations, research, and data behind them; examples of local programs that exemplify the promise of the recommendations; personal stories that bring to life the principles behind the recommendations; ongoing blog posts and opportunities for readers to provide feedback; ideas, action steps and resources on how organizations can become involved; and toolkits and template materials for those working on the ground to advance the recommendations in their communities.

All nursing leaders must join to address the challenges faced by nurses and the overall health care workforce. The nursing profession has the potential to effect wide-reaching improvements in the health care system to directly improve patient care. Nurses must seize this opportunity.

Florence Nightingale said, "May we hope that when we are all dead and gone, leaders will arise who have been personally experienced in the hard, practical work, the difficulties and the joys of organizing nursing reforms, and who will lead far beyond anything we have done." We have got an opportunity to follow her footsteps. Let us get to work to transform our field and improve patient care.

Susan Hassmiller

ROBERT WOOD JOHNSON HEALTH POLICY FELLOWSHIP PROGRAM

The Robert Wood Johnson (RWJ) Health Policy Fellowship Program offers a unique opportunity for nurses to increase their expertise and influence in the health policy arena, while bringing the special knowledge and skills of nursing to the debate. The program was created in 1973 and remains the second longest running program of the Robert Wood Johnson Foundation. Over the course of almost 40 years of placing mid-career health-related professionals/scientists in policy positions in Washington, DC, the Fellowship experience has prepared over 200 leaders who have contributed to the development and implementation of health-related legislation and policy. More than 20 nurses have participated in the program, and they continue to influence health policy in significant ways (Derksen & Whelan, 2010; Ridenour & Trautman, 2009; http://www.rwjf.org/files/research/HPF.final.pdf; Sharp, 2003).

Designed to provide the Fellows with expertise and access to policy leaders at the national level, the Fellows contribute professional health care expertise to the policy debate while learning the insider's view of the workings of health policy and legislation. As an added professional bonus, the Fellowship alumni program provides a network that is invaluable throughout one's career. The program, funded by the Robert Wood Johnson Foundation and conducted by the Institute of Medicine (IOM) of the National Academy of Sciences, provides exceptional opportunities for outstanding mid-career professionals who exhibit the following characteristics: (1) possess the skills and commitment to use the fellowship experience to provide leadership in improving health, health care, and health policy at the national, state, or local level; (2) bring a depth of expertise and knowledge about health and health care to the policy-making process; and (3) can offer an informed perspective on important and complex challenges facing health policymakers. Competitive mid-career professional applicants demonstrate a record of publication and expertise in a specified area, community and policy engagement, and commitment to post-fellowship policy engagement (http://www.healthpolicyfellows.org/fellowship.php).

The 3-year fellowship requires a minimum of 12 months in residence in Washington, DC, with full-time commitment to the Fellowship in the first year, with an option to extend the Washington, DC, experience beyond the first 12 months. Years 2 and 3 of the Fellowship are dedicated to individually directed policy initiatives in each Fellow's home institution/community. After the first year, Fellows become members of the alumni association with opportunities to continue to network with policymakers and issues beyond the Washington, DC placement.

The first 3 months include a comprehensive orientation to the health policy arena. Fellows interact with leadership at the IOM and other leading policy experts in think tanks, nonprofit organizations, advocacy groups, lobbyists, and federal agencies including a trip to the Centers for Disease Control and Prevention (CDC) in Atlanta. The orientation also includes 4 weeks with the Congressional Fellows of the American Political Science Association (http://www.apsanet.org/content_3031.cfm). The Congressional Fellows are journalists, political scientists, international governmental representatives, and federal agency employees. This interdisciplinary orientation provides an invaluable foundation and network that enhances the field placement and supports future work after the fellowship.

During the orientation process, Fellows begin negotiating for placements. Most Fellows find opportunities in either the Senate or House in Congressional Offices or with Committee staff on Committees with jurisdiction over health issues. Opportunities exist to work in federal agencies and in the White House. During the course of the 12-month residency, Fellows make fact-finding trips as a group to select state governments and individually to meet with constituents relative to their field placement. Additional opportunities exist to work with the Canadian Parliament in Ottawa and collaborate with Canadian Congressional Fellows visiting in Washington, DC.

Work assignments include activities such as drafting legislation, arranging and staffing Congressional hearings, briefing legislators for committee sessions and floor debates, responding to constituent requests, and serving as the liaison between elected officials and the executive branch, interest groups, trade associations, think tanks, and the health care community. During the course of the year, Fellows have opportunities for media training, individual executive coaching, and briefings on topics such as health economics, health care finance, the Congressional budget process, international health perspectives, science and technology, and health information technology (http://healthpolicyfellows.org/pdfs/rwjf_brochure_final.pdf).

This resource-rich Washington experience prepares Fellows with expertise and networks to influence the future of public health and health care and accelerate their own career development while bringing the Fellows health care expertise to the policy debate. Alumni of the Fellowship become part of a robust alumni network. Alumni opportunities include invitation to IOM annual meetings and involvement in Fellowship activities.

In 2011, up to six grants of up to $165,000 each will be made. Nurses possess the skills and expertise to enhance health policy development, implementation, and evaluation. It is very important for more

R

nurses to apply for this very important and prestigious fellowship (http://www. healthpolicyfellows.org/home.php).

Congressional Fellowship Program. Retrieved May 4, 2011, from http://www.apsanet.org/content_3031.cfm

Derksen, D. & Whelan, M. (2010). Closing the health care workforce gap. Retrieved May 4, 2011, from http://www.americanprogress.org/issues/2010/01/health_workforce.html

Health Policy Fellows. Retrieved May 4, 2011, from http://www.healthpolicyfellows.org/fellowship.php

Ridenour, N. & Trautman, D. (2009). A primer for nurses on advancing health policy. *Journal of Professional Nursing, 25*(6), 358–362.

Robert Wood Johnson Health Policy Fellowships Program. Retrieved May 4, 2011, from http://healthpolicyfellows.org/pdfs/rwjf_brochure_final.pdf

Robert Wood Johnson Health Policy Fellows Program. Retrieved May 4, 2011, from http://www.rwjf.org/files/research/HPF.final.pdf

Robert Wood Johnson Health Policy Fellows Program. Retrieved May 4, 2011, from http://www.healthpolicyfellows.org/home.php

Sharp, N. (2003). Health policy internships and fellowships in Washington, DC. *Newborn and Infant Nursing Review, 3*(1), 32–35.

Nancy Ridenour

Self-Renewal

When the joy of service turns into work distress and career discontent, it is time to take stock and be intentional about personal and professional renewal efforts. Renewal involves balancing your personal needs with the demands of work and caring for others, so that you have fresh energy for yourself and your activities (Kurth & Schmidt, 2003). Renewal is accomplished by clarifying one's strengths, values, gifts, and talents and using those gifts with intention. A strengths-based approach to renewal involves helping people understand their individual differences, signature themes, and natural talents. Nurse leaders need to engage inner work in order to more effectively provide outer service (Pesut, 2001).

Dr. Frederick Hudson (1999) is a pioneer in the psychology of adult development and renewal. The Hudson Institute (http://www.hudsoninstitute.com) has been investigating and supporting people in professional renewal efforts since 1986. On the basis of his theory of the adult developmental life cyle and his theory about the renewal cycle, he observes that personal or professional regeneration consists of four phases: (1) the go-for-it phase, (2) the doldrums, (3) the cocooning, and (4) the renewal. The go-for-it phase supports dreams related to work, purpose, goals, and achievements. As experience plateaus, management of the doldrums is necessary. If disenchantment of self persists, inner work and cocooning are advised to heal wounds, make discoveries, and renew purpose and passion. Successful cocooning leads to a life transition that supports a new purpose and new beginnings. This cycle seems to repeat itself every decade in an adult's developmental life. Hudson's research suggests that people who have mastered the art of professional renewal had the following characteristics in common:

- Self-renewing adults are value driven—committed to values, purposes, and preferences, and they possess a personal self-authority, which inspires them to live their beliefs.

- Self-renewing adults are connected to the world around them. They actively seek friends, contacts, and take care in their communications and build networks of information, resources, and causes to which they commit. They need solitude and quiet and honor inner life and outer boundaries. They plan time for introspection, interaction, and decision making. They refill their own cups before they get emptied.

- Self-renewing adults pace themselves—scheduling episodic breaks from routines

S

for travel, holidays, vacations, retreats, seminars, and sabbaticals. They are more interested in quality than busyness, effectiveness over efficiency, and integrity and style rather than short term results.

- Self-renewing adults enjoy contact with nature and all the elements—wind, rain, sun, stars, and mountains, panoramic views, earth, seas, and seashore are dependable sources of renewal for them. They are creative and playful; they are active not passive. They explore, exercise, experiment, laugh, and enjoy art, life, and creative forms of expression.

- Self-renewing adults adapt to change and pursue best options. They feel life and loss. They evaluate life with care. They are competent at entering, sustaining, and letting go of emotional attachments. They learn from down times. They live through the down times of their lives and embrace conflict as a means to produce clarity and renewal in relationships.

- Self-renewing adults trust the process of self-renewal and realize renewal is often found at the end of a grieving process. They are always in training.

- Self-renewing adults never stop learning. Self-renewing adults realize learning leads to new competencies and possibilities and self-mastery. They are future oriented. They focus on "what if" and the "not yet." They consciously live today with intentions for tomorrow.

- Self-renewing adults manage the necessary, entertain the possible, and develop foresight about desired future states.

When Pesut (2004) served as president of the Honor Society of Nursing, Sigma Theta Tau International, his presidential call was to "Create the Future Through Renewal." In his remarks he provided the following logic:

As self is renewed; commitments to service come forward more easily. Renewed commitments to

service require attention to mindfulness and reflective practice. Mindful reflective practice begets questions that support inquiry. Such inquiry guides knowledge work and evidence-based care giving. Care giving supports society as knowledge, values and service intersect. Knowledgeable people and especially knowledgeable nurses provide care that society needs. Creating a caring society is the spirit work of nursing. In order to continue the spirit work of nursing personal and professional renewal is a vital consideration for nurse leaders.

Hudson, F. (1999). *The adult years: Mastering the art of self-renewal*. San Francisco, CA: Jossey-Bass.

Kurth, K., & Schmidt, S. (2003). *Running on plenty at work: Renewal strategies for individuals*. Potomac, MD: Renewal Resources Press.

Pesut, D. J. (2001). Healing into the future: Recreating the profession of nursing through inner work. In N. Chaska (Ed.), *The nursing profession: Tomorrow and beyond* (chap. 70, pp. 853–867). Thousand Oaks, CA: Sage.

Pesut, D. J. (2004). Create the future through renewal. *Reflections on Nursing Leadership*, *30*(1), 24–25, 56.

Daniel J. Pesut

SENTINEL EVENTS

In the mid-1990s, the Joint Commission on Accreditation of Healthcare Organization Accreditation (now renamed The Joint Commission [TJC]) used the term "sentinel events." A sentinel event is an unexpected occurrence involving death or serious physical or psychological injury, or the risk thereof. Serious injury specifically includes loss of limb or function. The phrase "or the risk thereof" includes any process variation for which a recurrence would carry a significant chance of a serious adverse outcome. Such events are called "sentinel" because they signal the need for immediate investigation and response (The Joint Commission

Policy and Procedures on Reviewable Sentinel Events, 2008). Organizations using TJC accreditation process are strongly encouraged to report any sentinel event identified in the following list. TJC may also request a report if it becomes aware of a sentinel event by some other means such as communication from a patient, a family member, or an employee or the hospital, a JC surveyor, or through the media. In those organizations using TJC accreditation process, TJC may review a patient care event that has resulted in an unanticipated death or major permanent loss of function, not related to the natural course of the patient's illness or underlying condition, or a specific event occurring during the hospitalization may also be reviewed. The subset of sentinel events that is subject to review by TJC includes any occurrence that meets any of the following criteria:

- Event has resulted in an unanticipated death or major permanent loss of function, not related to the natural course of the patient's illness or underlying condition.
- Event is one of the following (even if the outcome was not death or major permanent loss of function unrelated to the natural course of the patient's illness or underlying condition):
  ○ Suicide of any patient receiving care, treatment, and services in a staffed around-the-clock care setting or within 72 hours of discharge
  ○ Unanticipated death of a full-term infant
  ○ Abduction of any patient receiving care, treatment and services
  ○ Discharge of any infant to the wrong family
  ○ Rape (see details in policy)
  ○ Hemolytic transfusion reaction involving administration of blood or blood product having major blood group incompatibilities
  ○ Surgery on the wrong patient or wrong body part
  ○ Unintended retention of a foreign object in a patient after surgery or other procedure
  ○ Severe neonatal hyperbilirubinemia (bilirubin >30 mg/dl)
  ○ Prolonged fluoroscopy with cumulative dose >1500 rads to a single field or any delivery of radiotherapy to the wrong body region or >255 above the planned radiotherapy dose (The Joint Commission Policy and Procedures on Reviewable Sentinel Events, 2008).

Sentinel events are voluntarily reported to TJC and these data are used to identify trends. In addition, TJC uses the sentinel event data to formulate TJC National Patient Safety Goals.

On a quarterly basis, TJC releases sentinel event statistics for all facilities accredited by the TJC. These data provide critical information in the prevention of sentinel events to accredited health care organizations and the public. From these data, the TJC issues "sentinel event alerts" designed to assist organizations in identifying, mitigating and eliminating health care patient safety issues. Sentinel event statistics that organizations may use as comparative data are available on the TJC Web site.

TJC requires review of sentinel events using the root cause analysis format. The root cause analysis methodology focuses primarily on systems and processes and not on individual performance. TJC further requires an action plan for any issues identified as a result of the analysis. The plan should address responsibility for implementation, oversight, pilot testing (as appropriate), time lines, and strategies for measuring the effectiveness of the actions (The Joint Commission Policy and Procedures on Reviewable Sentinel Events, 2008).

Although other industries, such as airlines, have used a similar reporting format with success for many years, the concept of sentinel events was controversial when first introduced. Because sentinel events also may be litigated events, many organizations feared that peer review information reported to TJC could lose privilege and become admissible in a lawsuit. Over time, however, the sentinel event concept has successfully identified and provided an evidence base and methodology for the prevention and mitigation of health care error. Please refer to TJC Web site for a complete and current description of the sentinel event policy.

See also Accreditation in Nursing Practice; Risk Management in the Health Care Setting

The Joint Commission. (2008). *Sentinel event policies and procedures.* Retrieved November 29, 2010, from http://www.jointcommission.org/ Sentinel_Event_Policy_and_Procedures

Jo Ann Brooks

Shared Governance Is Structure Not Process

Shared governance is a structure, not a program or a process (Simplicio, 2006). This is an important distinction as it informs both thinking and acting with regard to making it a sustainable reality. Too many leaders have seen shared governance as another contemporary process that reflects the current landscape of health care and, therefore, something that must be considered and implemented. More organizations say they have shared governance than actually demonstrate it.

What is shared governance exactly? There are any number of definitions, but most converge around the notion that shared governance is an organizational frame for configuring accountable professional decision making that fully engages the stakeholders by placing right decisions made by the right people in the right place at the right time for the right purpose (Gaguski & Begym, 2009). The simplicity of this definition belies the complexity of its construction. The mechanics of shared governance require an organizational construct that makes shared decision making the way of doing business within an accountable, professional work setting.

Shared governance is an accountability-based concept insofar as it builds on the notion of legitimate accountability and ownership for the outcomes of particular work (Pinkerton, 2008). The system approaches accountability from its defining elements and constructs the organization frame around the locus of control for the exercise of particular accountabilities. Construction depends on the articulation of the definers of accountability, autonomy, authority, and competence, and the specific enumeration of just what accountabilities exist in the organization and where best they are placed to assure their appropriate and sustainable exercise (Porter-O'Grady, 2010).

Once accountability for decisions has been clearly numerated and role and performance expectations outlined, decisions that relate to the expression of those accountabilities are allocated and distributed throughout the organization. An infrastructure for advancing their legitimacy and its exercise is constructed to define, link, and integrate decisions and activities through an intersecting and seamless dynamic that assures organizational integrity and the achievement of related outcomes. Normally, decision capacity is identified within the context of management or organizational decisions and clinical or professional decisions. Traditionally, shared governance structures build on the delineation of the five management accountabilities of human, fiscal, material, support, and systems processes and the professional alignment of accountability for practice, quality, and competence (Porter-O'Grady, 2010). The general rule of engagement for a shared governance system is the clear (exclusive or reserved) delineation of these functional alignments, demonstrating the partnership necessary to make each demarcation work effectively and intersect safely and productively. In shared governance systems, managers do not make clinical decisions and clinicians do not make management decisions.

This distinction between organizational and management accountability (often called resource accountability or contextual accountability) and professional accountability (also called content accountability) is a critical distinction within a shared governance system (Porter-O'Grady, 2010). Accountability does assume some exclusivity or reserved powers on the basis of the rule and performance expectations related to them. Within this logic, it is essential that the accountability specific or distinct to managers be articulated and allocated, and just as vital is the need to clearly state the accountabilities that belong to the professional. In the case of nursing shared governance, the professional accountabilities that are unique to the discipline are practice, quality, competence, and knowledge creation and generation (research) as would be delineated within the context of any professional discipline. Within the shared governance rubric, these

would be reserved to the profession, and all decisions, activities, and processes related to them would fall within the performance expectations of the professional. The obligation of the system, managers, and support structures would be evidenced in their responsiveness to these decisions made exclusively by the professional staff. The shared elements in the decisional process are exercised in the strategic integration between organizational goals and professional obligations. The organizational and work infrastructure of shared governance is designed to support and advance these intersecting accountabilities and unique role capacities.

Finally, there is the notion of partnership: one of the critical elements related to implementation and exercise of shared governance principles. Here, organizational infrastructure and systems support must be constructed within the context of horizontal linkages between the parties accountable and the partnerships among them as necessary to sustain the mutual goals of all stakeholders. In these partnership arrangements, all members have specific and unique obligations to the partnership and roles to play in advancing its purposes. Professionals at the point of service, consultants, experts, and clinical specialists (or advanced practitioners) all play a role and make a unique contribution to the clinical concert that is nursing practice. Managers, too, play a significant role in creating a context and advancing the effective decisions of the organization regardless of their locus of control. Each party to this mosaic of interactions and intersections must fully engage his or her role and play that part that maintains and sustains the collaboration necessary to achieve the outcomes that cannot be obtained without it. This mutuality and collateral set of relationships is pivotal to both the structuring and expression of shared governance in the clinical system.

Shared governance represents the consonance of necessary forces to ensure that both professional and collaborative practices converge and by converging sustain their positive impact on purpose and patient care. Built on the foundations of accountability, reflecting the fundamental characteristics of professional obligation, constructed on an appropriately conceived organizational infrastructure, representing the characteristics of professional partnership, and exhibiting the elements of a clearly articulated locus of control, shared governance reflects the best in supporting organizational architecture for the practice of professionals (Malloch & Porter-O'Grady, 2009). In an increasingly complex and horizontally linked clinical environment, the prerequisites of accountability partnership and discipline-specific integrity are accelerated. The shared governance organizational infrastructure creates a frame for the behaviors and relationships necessary to truly advance an evidence-driven patient-centered clinical environment necessary to build the future of professional, quality-based health care.

Gaguski, M., & Begyn, P. (2009). A unique model of shared governance. *Ocology Nursing Forum, 36*(4), 385–389.

Malloch, K., & Porter-O'Grady, T. (2009). *Introduction to evidence-based practice in nursing and healthcare.* Boston, MA: Jones & Bartlett.

Pinkerton, S. (2008). The unit practice council: The center of professional practice. *Nursing Economics, 26*(6), 401–407.

Porter-O'Grady, T. (2010). *Interdisciplinary shared governance.* Boston, MA: Jones & Bartlett.

Simplicio, J. (2006). Shared governance: An analysis of power on the modern university campus. *Education 126*(4), 763–770.

Tim Porter-O'Grady

SHORTAGE OF NURSING FACULTY

Professional nurses are well-established as essential partners in the provision of safe, high-quality health care to members of our society. As such, the assurance of a strong workforce in nursing is an important health care requirement, one in which nurses should take an active leadership role. To provide that workforce, it is essential that nursing have a strong cadre of well-prepared and committed faculty. Unfortunately, despite increases in numbers of faculty, and significant increases in graduate education in nursing, the faculty shortage is, in fact, worsening.

A number of factors have come into play in recent years to address the faculty shortage that became a national issue more than 5 years ago and was projected to increase due to the increased numbers of nursing faculty approaching retirement age. Chief among these has been the increase in federal support for nurses pursuing graduate study to prepare them for faculty roles. The Nurse Faculty Loan Program was specifically designed to provide financial support to this group of students. Essentially, this program enables students who served as nurse faculty after graduation from such a program to have up to 85% of their loan cancelled. Table 2 reflects a tripling in enrollment in master's programs in nursing focused on the development of nurse educators, leading to a 300% increase in graduations in that specialty.

Table 2 merely reports on the growth and expansion of programs of study at the master's level, specifically designed to foster development of academic teachers in nursing education. In addition, there has been a very significant expansion in most master's-level programs in nursing.

Table 2
ENROLLMENT DATA IN MASTER'S PROGRAMS
WITH A MAJOR IN NURSING EDUCATION

Year	No. of Schools	Students	Graduates
2006–2007	193	4,966	890
2007–2008	233	8,916	1,160
2008–2009	243	10,474	2,227
2009–2010	258	12,111	2,816
2010–2011	304	15,243	3,864

The National Sample Survey estimates a 68% increase in enrollments in master's programs from 257,812 in 2000 to 375,794 in 2008. While most of these individuals study some aspect of advanced clinical practice, they nonetheless meet the minimum requirement in most states for faculty appointment, that is, the master's degree.

The growth in master's preparation has been accompanied by a similar expansion of doctoral education. The National Sample Survey reports a 60% increase in nurses achieving the doctorate, from 17,256 in 2000 to 28,369 in 2008. In a summary of enrollment and graduation changes in the last 5 years in doctoral programs, the American Association of Colleges of Nursing (AACN) reports an average annual increase of 157 students enrolled in research-focused doctoral programs. At the same time, the enrollment in Doctor of Nursing Practice (DNP) programs has doubled. In 2009, AACN reported a total of 3,415 students enrolled in such programs, whereas in 2011 that number had risen to 7,034. Career aspirations of the graduates of these doctoral programs are diverse, yet 48% of the PhD graduates and 21% of the DNP graduates express a commitment to faculty positions.

These expansions in enrollment suggest that the pool for qualified faculty has increased, even though many of these individuals holding advanced degrees in nursing have not been prepared to function as nurse faculty. Despite this drawback, the fact that the potential has grown so much provides hope for more successful recruitment of legally qualified faculty, who could then profit from faculty development programs.

NUMBERS OF FACULTY

The actual number of nurses employed as faculty reflect a marked growth. In 2005, the total number of full-time faculty employed in all schools of nursing was estimated to be approximately 23,000. This figure was derived from combining data from the AACN and the National League for Nursing (NLN), which each identified between 11,416 to 11,635 faculty employed full time in baccalaureate or higher degree programs, and the NLN database that included faculty from associate degree and diploma programs, which number 11,166 and 919, respectively. At the same, time the NLN identified a total of 18,654 nurses who worked part time as faculty. The grand total of faculty in all programs of study in nursing was 41,654.

Recent data from the U.S. Department of Health Resources and Services Administration (HRSA) in the 2008 National Sample Survey of Registered Nurses report a highly expanded workforce base. The HRSA report of numbers of faculty includes individuals who work in programs of study leading to licensure as an LPN/LVN. Notwithstanding this additional element, the totals in 2011 are 65,193 nurse faculty. This total was fairly equally distributed between full- and part-time faculty with 30,527 filling full-time positions and 34,666 occupying part-time positions. Data available from the AACN provides information related to full-time faculty, identifying a total of 15,726 full-time faculty employed in programs of study in nursing and another 15,711 part-time for a

S

S

total of 31,437 in baccalaureate and higher degree programs. A personal communication from Dr. Kathleen Kaufman, senior researcher, reflects that NLN faculty data for 2009 estimates a total of 59,951 individuals employed in nursing education. This figure includes full- and part-time employment and all programs of study. Given this substantial increase in personnel employed by schools of nursing, how can we document that a shortage continues to exist and threatens to worsen?

DEMAND FOR NURSE FACULTY

As documented earlier, the last 5 years have witnessed a very substantial increase in numbers of faculty in the nation's schools of nursing. Yet at the same time, there has been a marked increase in the demand for education in nursing in all academic programs. Furthermore, in all of the data noted previously, the only attempt to specially prepare nurses to function effectively in faculty roles is found in the data related to individuals achieving masters in nursing education. Research-focused doctoral programs leading to the PhD pay minimal attention to the teaching role, emphasizing the functions related to the generation and dissemination of new knowledge, whereas the focus of DNP programs emphasizes advanced *clinical* practice and not the advanced practice in nursing found in disseminating knowledge and preparing neophytes.

FACTORS IN THE FACULTY SHORTAGE

Both the NLN and AACN report that their constituents continue to leave faculty positions unfilled and turn away a significant number of qualified applicants to the nation's schools of nursing. In a news release, the AACN reported that 67,563 qualified applicants were not accepted at

schools of nursing during 2010 due to the shortage of faculty. Concomitantly, the vacancy rate among faculty in schools of nursing continues to grow. Nationally, there were almost 2,000 unfilled faculty positions in 2007, which was distributed among one third of the nation's schools of nursing.

In 2010, the NLN developed a Nurse Educator Shortage Fact Sheet, which summarized the issues in faculty recruitment to include workload and compensation. Respondents to national surveys regarding faculty consistently report inability to offer competitive salaries as an obstacle to recruitment and retention of nursing faculty. In fact, the 2010 NLN Fact Sheet (2011) reports that the primary reasons for the continued shortage of faculty relate to: "an aging and overworked faculty who earn less than nurses entering clinical practice, and less than holders of advanced degrees in other academic disciplines." Anecdotal reports among colleagues confirm high levels of recruitment difficulties and limited array of potential candidates from which to select compatible additions to a school's workforce. Workload issues are rampant as well with faculty reporting consistent workweeks in excess of 52 hours, during the regular school year, and 8 to 10 hours per week on weekends and holidays. Thus, validating frequently made references to faculty burnout and overload.

In an AACN study completed in 2009–2010, schools of nursing reported on reasons additional full-time faculty were not hired. Chief among these was insufficient funds to hire new faculty. This may have been due to inadequate funding from the institution to the nursing division or that funds allocated were not competitive to attract qualified applicants. Additional reasons, however, related to the inability to compete for qualified applicants and limitations on numbers of qualified applicants available in the region. The net result from unsuccessful recruiting is all too often increased workload for remaining faculty, which may lead to retention issues with the faculty currently employed. One point worth noting from the National Sample Survey is that nurse faculty seemed more satisfied with their work, than many nurses serving in other sectors of practice. This may be a perspective that should have more attention and celebration.

WORRIES FOR THE FUTURE

Among the chief concerns as nursing attempts to plan for the future is the high volume of nurse faculty in the upper age brackets. According to 2009 NLN annual Faculty Census Data, 30% of all faulty are over 60 years of age. In addition, 63% are between the ages of 46 and 60. The most dramatic increase among faculty in terms of age was the 7% increase in numbers of faculty over 60. These data moved from 9% in 2006 to nearly 16% in 2009. Essentially, 48% of nurse faculty is 55 or over, and fully one half of all faculty report that they expect to retire within the next 10 years. This would require a dramatic increase in the number of faculty prepared annually.

SUMMARY

Despite strong developments in the graduate preparation of nurses, positions in clinical settings carry substantially more compensation and offer more opportunities for advancement than do positions in the academy. Furthermore, due to limited attention to the preparation of faculty in the full academic role, it may be that as a profession we do not strive to excite neophytes about a career as an educator. Based on the age margin of currently employed nurse faculty and employment trends among nurses holding advanced degrees, nursing education is on the cusp of a dire shortage in faculty, not to mention faculty in leadership positions. The profession needs to find ways to advocate more for careers in nursing education and nurses in leadership positions can be these strong advocates.

See also Faculty Recruitment to Academic Settings; Faculty Retention

Fang, D., Tracey, C., & Bednash, G. D. (2011). 2010–2011 *Salaries of instructional and administrative nursing faculty in baccalaureate and graduate programs in nursing.* Washington, DC: American Association of Colleges of Nursing.

Health Resources and Services Administration. (2010). *2008 National sample survey of registered nurses.* Washington, DC: Health and Human Services, Division of Nursing.

National League for Nursing. (2010). *NLN Nurse Educator Fact Sheet.* Retrieved April 3, 2011, from www.nln.org/governmentalaffairs/pdf/Nurse Faculty Shortage.pdf

Eileen H. Zungolo

SIGMA THETA TAU INTERNATIONAL

The Honor Society of Nursing, Sigma Theta Tau International (STTI; www.nursingsociety.org), provides leadership and scholarship in practice, education, and research to enhance the health of all people. STTI supports the learning and professional development of members striving to improve nursing care worldwide. Membership is by invitation to baccalaureate and graduate nursing students who demonstrate excellence in scholarship and to nurse leaders exhibiting exceptional

S

achievements in nursing. Founded in 1922 by six nurses, the name is derived from the Greek words *Storgé*, *Tharos*, and *Timé*, meaning "love," "courage," and "honor." The honor society was incorporated in 1985 as Sigma Theta Tau International, Inc., a not-for-profit organization with a 501(c)(3) tax status in the United States. With 130,000 active members in 86 countries, the STTI has 470 chapters on college campuses in Australia, Botswana, Brazil, Canada, Colombia, Ghana, Hong Kong, Japan, Kenya, Malawi, Mexico, the Netherlands, Pakistan, Singapore, South Africa, South Korea, Swaziland, Sweden, Taiwan, Tanzania, Wales, the United Kingdom, and the United States.

From its inception, the honor society has recognized the value of scholarship and excellence in nursing practice. In 1936, the honor society became the first U.S. organization to fund nursing research. Today, the honor society supports these values through numerous professional development products and services that focus on the core areas of education, leadership, career development, evidence-based nursing, research, and scholarship. These products and services advance learning and professional development of members and all nurses who strive to improve the health of the world's people. STTI also produces publications including books, journals, and Web-based documents that support the learning and professional development of nurses and houses in its Indianapolis headquarters the Virginia Henderson International Nursing Library; a premier, online library offering a collection of more than 37,000 nursing research studies; and also researchers' demographic information and study abstracts. The library also contains abstracts from major nursing research conferences, including research events sponsored by the honor society.

A Biennial Convention brings together colleagues from around the world to participate in continuing education, leadership, and career development as well as to conduct the business of the association in its House of Delegates. Research conferences and leadership summits also offer members opportunities to learn, to explore, and to develop leadership, scholarship, and research skills.

Diane Mancino

STAFF RECRUITMENT

Staff recruitment for a health care organization can be defined as the search for the "best candidate using a swift, outcome-oriented approach" (National Association for Health Care Recruitment, 2005). The "best candidate" is one who meets basic competency for the position and is aligned with the mission and values of the organization. The search is composed of a number of strategies, processes, and procedures that when combined and evaluated will contribute to the success of the health care organization. A successful recruitment program begins with knowledge of appropriate employment laws and regulations governing the process and the development of a recruitment plan that is based on information gathered from a variety of sources.

The recruitment plan should start with a review of the organization's strategic plan for health care program creation or growth. Questions to be answered in defining the scope of a recruitment plan include the following: What will the personnel needs for new programs look like? Will there be corresponding redesign of existing services that may require redeployment of current staff with needs for additional education and training? Does the organization have educational resources in place to support program change and staff training? What is the available labor market for the specific categories of staff needed? What is the hiring competition with that market? What is the organization's reputation within the community and does the workforce reflect the cultures of the communities it serves? Understanding these internal and external influences that impact recruitment of staff is critical to the success of a recruitment plan.

Other data necessary for the planning process include measures of vacancy and turnover rates for various health care positions, the number of days on average it takes to fill a vacant position, and the average cost per hire. These figures should be tracked and trended on a regular basis to determine appropriate allocation of recruitment staff and financial resources. By using the projected numbers of staff needed and the cost per hire, a budget can be determined to support various sourcing and marketing strategies. Vacancy information can also be used to determine how budgeted monies should be allocated.

A successful recruitment plan begins with the recruiter. The recruiter represents the organization not only to external customers but to internal customers as well. Building a positive and productive relationship with managers is critical to successful recruiting. In addition to traditional sourcing mechanisms—such as the use of targeted health care employment and niche Web sites, local and national print advertisement, onsite hiring events, and outside career fairs—utilization of social media has become an effective method to reach both active and passive candidates. The use of Facebook, LinkedIn, and blogs can drive candidates to an organization's Web site. According to Forken (2011), the first online destination for a prospective employee when conducting a job search is the employer Web site, followed by niche sites, job boards, search engines, and social networking. The organization's Web site should be easy to navigate, engaging, and appealing to a multigenerational and diverse workforce. A successful recruitment plan also acknowledges the efforts of current employees in attracting candidates to the organization through an employee referral program. The message conveyed to prospective candidates through each of these venues should reflect the mission, vision, and values of the health care organization and how it aligns with an applicant's own personal philosophy.

The dual impact of health care reform and the economy as well as the expected retirements of employees from the baby boomer generation will also influence an organization's recruitment plan. In times of uncertainty and change, health care organizations may be required to reduce positions or delay hiring. The advent of health care reform may also require health care organizations to redesign services and position requirements to attract a workforce that will best meet the changing business requirements of their organization. By creating and implementing a focused workforce planning strategy, organizations can identify high potential candidates, develop and mentor them, and cultivate future leaders to address the requirements of reform and other components of the health care environment (Holm, 2011).

To determine the success of the various sourcing strategies, it is necessary to maintain statistics, such as the number of completed applications from qualified applicants, what venues are identified by the applicants, and how long it took to fill the vacancy. Another aspect of recruitment planning involves how applicants will be screened, interviewed, and selected. "Applicants become candidates when they [are screened] and interviewed for a specific position" (National Association for Health Care Recruitment, 2005). The completed application provides contact information, educational preparation, a detailed outline of the applicant's work experience and history, and the applicant's dated signature acknowledging the accuracy of the information provided. The interview and selection procedures use questions that allow the hiring manager to determine the applicant's specific qualifications for the position and assess the basic competencies needed to carry out the associated responsibilities of the job. The questions should be open ended and focus on the applicant's work experiences and behaviors. By using "behavioral-based" questions that seek examples of past experience, the hiring manager can assess future professional or technical competency in a related situation.

The interview is also a time when the applicant is assessed for "fit" or how professional conduct and work behaviors in previous positions or roles will translate into the prospective work unit or organizational culture. The goal in this part of the plan is to select the "best candidate" for a position using an outcome-oriented approach. Follow-up and the offer should be done quickly, with the offer of employment contingent upon completion of the post-offer screening process (background/reference information, license and credential verification, health and drug screening, and any other verification of employment documentation). A continuous review of the recruitment plan and the associated information collected and trended provides the opportunity to evaluate the overall success of the organization's staff recruitment program and how it contributes to organizational success.

Forken, M. (2011, January). *Harvey Research National Study of RNS*. New York, NY: Harvey Research, Inc.

Holm, A. (2010, November–December). *Why is work force planning important to us* (Vol. 46, pp. 16–17). Orlando, FL: Directions, National Association for Health Care Recruitment, XVX.

National Association for Health Care Recruitment. (2005). *Recruiter's handbook*. Orlando, FL: Author.

Mary Ann Radioli

STAFF RETENTION

The cost of replacing a registered nurse (RN) is between 75% and 125% of the RN's annual salary (Pine & Tart, 2007), making it essential that nurse leaders develop effective techniques for retaining each RN on their staff. Experienced nurses are being lost because of burnout, physical exhaustion, and dissatisfaction with the work environment. The RN shortage will reach 285,000 by 2020 (Donelan, Buerhaus, DesRoches, Dittus, & Dutwin, 2008). Consequently, the profession has intensified efforts to produce more graduates to address the shortage, but disillusioned new graduates often leave hospital work within 1 year after graduation (Pellico, Brewer, & Kovner, 2009). In a survey by Bowles and Candela (2005), 30% of respondents left nursing in their first year of practice and 57% by their second year. The most frequently cited reason was unsafe nurse-to-patient ratios, followed by management issues such as lack of support and guidance. Pellico et al. (2009) found that new RNs experienced "colliding expectations" between their personal ideals and the reality of practice, analogous to the "reality shock" identified by Kramer (1974) long ago. In addition to issues of work overload, the study participants bemoaned mistreatment by physicians and colleagues, which was often ignored by management (Pellico et al., 2009).

What most nurses look for in a job is socioemotional compensation (Censullo, 2008). When the work environment does not provide fulfillment of a nurse's ideology, leaving may be the only tenable option (Censullo, 2008). Fortunately, there are a number of proactive strategies that a nurse leader can use to promote job satisfaction: (1) convey support and appreciation to staff, especially during stressful periods; (2) promote staff autonomy; (3) create team camaraderie and cohesion by socializing outside the workplace (picnics, potlucks) and by celebrating promotions, certifications, and advanced degrees; and (4) listen carefully to staff concerns and take prompt action, especially if conflict or bullying is occurring (Thomas, 2009). When a unit culture condones bullying behavior, nurses may not only leave that particular unit but also leave the profession (Stevens, 2002). Definitive steps can be taken to change a bullying culture. Nursing turnover, which had reached 28% at one hospital, was significantly reduced after workshops were held and clear anti-bullying practices were instituted (Stevens, 2002).

Coaching and mentoring are essential for socialization of new nurses and assimilation into existing work teams (Anthony et al., 2005). Steps that managers can take to welcome new graduates include (1) developing a plan to promote team acceptance of the new grads, (2) monitoring new grads for reality shock or alienation, (3) encouraging individualism rather than mandating conformity to unit norms, (4) providing supportive preceptors and mentors, and (5) promoting membership in professional organizations and workplace committees (Duchscher & Cowin, 2004).

Research provides useful information on the factors that contribute to nurses' job satisfaction. Predictors of job satisfaction in a meta-analysis of 31 studies, representing 14,567 study participants, were (1) greater autonomy, (2) greater collaboration with physicians, and (3) lower job stress (Zangaro & Soeken, 2007). Team performance effectiveness is another significant predictor of RN job satisfaction; conflict among the team has direct negative effects on job satisfaction (Cox, 2003). It is time for nurse managers to apply these research findings. Although reduction of job stress is not always within a manager's control, a collegial and mutually respectful climate can be created and maintained. The nurse manager must serve as the "chief retention officer" (Nursing Executive Center, 2000).

Anthony, M. K., Standing, T. S., Glick, J., Duffy, M., Paschall, F., Sauer, M., et al. (2005). Leadership and nurse retention: The pivotal role of nurse managers. *Journal of Nursing Administration, 35*, 146–155.

Bowles, C., & Candela, L. (2005). First job experiences of recent RN graduates. *Journal of Nursing Administration, 35*, 130–137.

Censullo, J. L. (2008). The nursing shortage: Breach of ideology as an unexplored cause. *Advances in Nursing Science, 31*(4), E11–E18.

Cox, K. B. (2003). The effects of intrapersonal, intragroup, and intergroup conflict on team performance effectiveness and work satisfaction. *Nursing Administration Quarterly, 27*, 153–163.

Donelan, K., Buerhaus, P., DesRoches, C., Dittus, R., & Dutwin, D. (2008). Public perceptions of nursing careers: The influence of media and nursing shortages. *Nursing Economics, 26*, 143–150, 165.

Duchscher, J. E., & Cowin, L. S. (2004). The experience of marginalization in new nursing graduates. *Nursing Outlook, 52*, 289–296.

Kramer, M. (1974). *Reality shock*. St. Louis, MO: C.V. Mosby.

Nursing Executive Center. (2000). *Reversing the flight of talent*. Washington, DC: The Advisory Board Company.

Pellico, L., Brewer, C., & Kovner, C. (2009). What newly licensed registered nurses have to say about their first experiences. *Nursing Outlook, 57*, 194–203.

Pine, R., & Tart, K. (2007). Return on investment: Benefits and challenges of a baccalaureate nurse residency program. *Nursing Economics, 25*, 13–18, 39.

Stevens, S. (2002). Nursing workforce retention: Challenging a bullying culture. *Health Affairs, 21*, 189–193.

Thomas, S. P. (2009). *Transforming nurses' stress and anger: Steps toward healing.* New York, NY: Springer Publishing.

Zangaro, G., & Soeken, K. (2007). A meta-analysis of nurses' job satisfaction. *Research in Nursing and Health, 30*, 445–458.

Sandra P. Thomas

STAFFING EFFECTIVENESS

An important component of executive nursing practice is the appropriate allocation and utilization of human resources. Whether it is through an annual budgeting process or day-to-day staffing, providing the right number of nurses to meet the care requirements of patients is an art and a science. Accurate definition and quantification of the work of nursing is critical to the identification of appropriate nursing resource requirements. In acute care settings, the most common definition of nursing work is the patient day, and nursing resource requirements are expressed as hours per patient day or, in more recent discussions, as nurse–patient ratios (Graf, Millar, Feilteau, Coakley, & Ives Erickson, 2003). There does not exist, however, a single methodology that is the answer for every health care organization.

Providing the optimal number of nursing personnel with the appropriate mix of registered nurses to unlicensed assistive personnel to meet the needs of patients is based on numerous factors including patient acuity, experience of the nurse, environment of care, and technology and other staff support systems (Ives Erickson, 2002). The identification of required direct care staffing occurs at three levels: long-term projections for the fiscal year, near-term scheduling for successive time-plan cycles, and daily staffing for shift-to-shift requirements. Commonly, staffing levels are based on volume and acuity of patients (nursing workload) and factored for distribution of workload over various time periods, experience, and mix of staff as well as logistical and support issues (Curtin, 2003; Ives Erickson, 2002). Each organization must look at structure and process to determine the right approach to nurse staffing to effectively meet the patient's requirements for nursing care. Staffing effectiveness involves "defining competencies and expectations for all staff. Staffing includes assessing those defined competencies and allocating the human resources necessary for patient safety and improved patient outcomes" (The Joint Commission, 2010). Staffing projections and total budgeted full-time equivalent requirements are developed in conjunction with the overall organizational budgeting process. The budgeting process is based on anticipated volume, admissions, length of stay and procedure volume, and patient acuity. These data are then used to develop unit-specific staffing budgets. Key target ratios, such as hours per unit of work, staff mix, and nonproductive factors, are identified using current and historical data.

One approach to staffing is the implementation of a system that identifies the patient's needs for nursing care. Patient acuity systems or nursing workload measurement systems provide an indication of staffing requirements. Graf et al. (2003)

explain that "in addition to assisting in day-to-day staffing decisions acuity systems provide an opportunity for storing the raw data from the system at their most basic level provides and opportunities for more extensive analyses and informed, data-driven decision-making related to resource allocation, performance improvement and productivity enhancement" (p. 76).

At a time when many states in the country are considering enacting nurse staffing legislation to establish staffing ratios for hospitals (Aiken et al., 2010), it is important that everyone understand the issues and challenges of staffing to meet the care requirements of the patient and keep practice safe. Nurse staffing ratio advocates point to the need to mandate minimum staffing. The rationale is that the rates of poor patient outcomes are well known when staffing levels are poor. Several research studies have found significant associations between lower levels of nurse staffing and higher rates of pneumonia, failure to rescue, upper gastrointestinal bleeding, and urinary tract infections (Aiken et al., 2010; Hickman et al., 2003; Needleman, Buerhaus, Mattke, Stewart, & Zelevinsky, 2002). Other studies found associations between lower staffing levels and pneumonia, lung collapse, falls, pressure ulcers, thrombosis after major surgery, pulmonary compromise after surgery, longer hospital stays, and 30-day mortality rates. Researchers caution, however, that the research does not advocate for mandated staffing levels. Instead, research indicates that those patient outcomes that are driven primarily by the interventions of the nurse (nursing-sensitive indicators) should be viewed as poor outcomes rather than as measures of the impact of nurse staffing on patient outcomes. Opponents of ratio legislation point out that with staffing ratios, health care organizations run the

risk of replacing critical nursing judgment and assessment with fixed numbers. The debate needs to be informed by considering the patient population in need of nursing care. Not all patients are the same. Care needs vary from patient to patient and for the same patient over time (Ives Erickson, 2002). Patient outcomes depend not only on the kind and severity of patients' illnesses but also on human resources factors such as the mix of nurses, doctors, and auxiliary personnel, and on the work environment or culture of the hospital. The key tenet is that no matter what the pressures may be, it is absolutely essential that we be able to provide the right clinician to the right patient at the right time, every time.

Aiken, L., Sloane, D., Cimiotti, J., Clarke, S., Flynn, L., Seago, J., et al. (2010). Implications of the California nurse staffing mandate for other states. *Health Services Research, 45*(4), 904–921.

Curtin, L. L. (2003). An integrated analysis of nurse staffing and related variables: Effects on patient outcomes. *Online Journal of Issues in Nursing, 9*(3). Retrieved from www.nursing world.org/MainMenuCategories/ANAMarketplace/ANAPeriodicals/OJIN/KeynotesofNote/StaffandVariablesAnalysis.aspx

Graf, C., Millar, S., Feilteau, C., Coakley, P., & Ives Erickson, J. (2003). Patients' needs for nursing care, beyond staffing ratios. *Journal of Nursing Administration, 33*(2), 76–81.

Hickman, D. H., Severance, S., Feldstein, A., Ray, L., Gorman, P., Schuldheis, S., et al. (2003, May). *The effect of health care working conditions on patient safety.* Evidence Report/Technology Assessment Number74. (Prepared by Oregon Health & Science University under Contract No. 290–97-0018). AHRQ Publication No. 03-E031. Rockville, MD: Agency for Healthcare Research and Quality.

Ives Erickson, J. (2002, March 7). In the debate over arbitrary staffing ratios, we must be the voice of reason, *Caring Headlines*, 2–3.

Joint Commission, Department of Publications, Joint Commission Resources. (2010). *2010 hospital accreditation standards.* Oakbrook Terrace, IL: Author.

S

Needleman, J., Buerhaus, P., Mattke, S., Stewart, M., & Zelevinsky, K. (2002). *Nurse-staffing levels and patient outcomes in hospitals.* Final report for Health Resources and Services Administration. Contract No. 230–99-0021. Harvard.

Jeanette Ives Erickson

STRATEGIC PLANNING

Strategic planning is the process of identifying directions and facilitating the alignment of purpose, people, plans, and actions with the aim of serving a cocreated, value-driven, desired outcome. Strategic planning is supported by strategic learning. Schwartz (1991) makes a useful distinction between "strategic" and "tactical" planning. Strategic planning includes attention to the "big picture" of a situation whereas "tactical" planning focuses on detailed local activities. Horwath (2009) suggests that the essentials to strategic planning and learning include the following: (1) acumen—the ability to generate critical insights through a step-by-step evaluation of a business and its environment; (2) allocation—focusing on limited resources through strategic trade-offs; and (3) action—implementing a system to guarantee effective execution of strategy at all levels of your organization (Strategic Thinking Institute, 2010). The essential components of strategic planning involve core leadership competencies of anticipation, alignment, and action (Deering, Dilts, & Russell, 2002).

Pietersen (2002) proposes a four-stage strategy for strategic planning: learning, focusing, aligning, and executing. Strategic planning requires an organization and its leadership to ask and answer three key questions (Pietersen, 2002): (1) What is the environment in which our organization must compete and win? (2) What are those few things our organization must do outstandingly well to win and go on winning in this environment? (3) How will we mobilize our organization to implement these things faster and better than our competitors? The strategic learning cycle involves generating insight into changing environments, making strategic choices, aligning an organization behind a chosen strategic focus, and implementing and experimenting with an executed strategy while concurrently learning throughout the process. Robert Dilts (1996) also defines strategic thinking as the ability to identify a relevant desired state, assess the starting state, and then establish and navigate the appropriate path of transition states required to reach the desired state.

A key element of effective strategic thinking is related to discerning which people and processes will most efficiently and effectively influence and change the present state in the direction of the desired state. Dilts (1996, 1998) offers a logical-level model for thinking and acting in terms of learning and planning (Alpha Leadership, 2010). There are three levels to consider in the Dilts Model: meta, macro, and micro. Meta-level planning involves attention and mindfulness to organizational issues of spirit, vision, and identity. Macro-level planning involves attention to path finding, culture building, beliefs, and values that support organizational identity and role-performance configurations. Micro-level planning involves attention to environmental variables related to efficiency, task, relationship, and capabilities as well as behaviors that support or inhibit strategic alignment of purpose, people, plans, and actions that serve a greater good or desired outcome. At each level of learning and planning, a specific leadership skill is called forth. For example, at the meta leadership level, one needs leadership influence that involves the development of a charismatic leadership skill set. This also requires attention to the learning from changes taking place in the environment and developing some insight into the environmental changes. At the level of identity, one needs to craft leadership influence with some consideration for individual talents and strengths within an organization and a focus on strategic choices related to the special mission of the organization and its contribution to the environment. At the level of values and beliefs, one needs to influence and inspire people in the organization, serve as cheerleader and coach, and challenge people to consider how they might rethink their own ideas in light of organizational aspirations and goals.

Leadership for strategic planning is about helping people think through old problems in new ways with intelligence, rationality, and careful outcome specification. As leadership attends to issues of behavior, action, and execution, clear representation of desired goals and evidence for achievement of those goals is essential. Implementing and experimenting with the execution of a strategic plan involves reliance on the capabilities and resources of individuals and the organization to engage in reflective learning processes that contribute to insights and ongoing organizational learning. As the leader's attention turns to specific behaviors, leadership concerns turn attention to contracting rewards for effort and being clear about expectations in exchange for effort and special commendations associated with promotions for good work. Most strategic plans fail because of failure

to define end state objectives clearly or because of a poor implementation strategy (Borgesson, 2007).

Alpha Leadership. Retrieved September 10, 2010, from http://www.alphaleaders.com

Borgesson, M. (2007). *Scenario planning resources.* Retrieved September 10, 2010, from http://www.well.com/~mb/scenario_planning

Deering, A., Dilts, R., & Russell, J. (2002). *Alpha leadership.* Hoboken, NJ: John Wiley.

Dilts, R. (1996). *The new leadership paradigm.* Retrieved September 10, 2006, from http://www.nlpu.com/Articles/article8.htm

Dilts, R. (1998). Moving from vision to action. Retrieved September 10, 2010, http://www.nlpu.com/Patterns/pattern8.htm

Horwath, R. (2009). *Deep dive: The proven method for building strategy, focusing your resources and taking smart action.* Austin, TX: Greenleaf Book Press.

Pietersen, W. (2002). *Reinventing strategy: Using strategic learning to create and sustain breakthrough performance.* Hoboken, NJ: John Wiley.

Schwartz, P. (1991). *The art of the long view.* New York, NY: Doubleday Currency.

Strategic Thinking Institute. Retrieved September 10, 2010, from http://www.strategyskills.com/strategy_facilitation.asp

Daniel J. Pesut

STUDENT RECRUITMENT

According to the U.S. Department of Labor, Bureau of Labor Statistics (2011), the employment of registered nurses is expected to grow by 22% from 2008 to 2018, with more than 581,500 new RN positions being created. Although the American Association of Colleges of Nursing (AACN) reported a 3.6% enrollment increase in entry level baccalaureate programs in nursing in 2009, this

S

increase is not sufficient to meet the projected job growth. Recruitment strategies, whereas varied and innovative, need to start at the academic level to interest both potential students in the profession and nursing school graduates in the need to further their education to facilitate career advancement. To prepare for an influx of students, academic leaders will need to plan for additional educational opportunities. This presents its own challenges in terms of sites for clinical education and an ongoing faculty shortage (AACN, 2010a). In communicating the annual enrollment survey results, for example, AACN notes that there were 54,000 prospective undergraduate nursing students and 9,500 prospective graduate students turned away in fall 2009 (AACN, 2010b, 2010c).

Many recruitment strategies can be used at both the undergraduate and graduate level. An example of these strategies is participation in organizational career fairs such as those sponsored by the state nurses' association, student nurse associations, and professional journals. Membership in local, state, and national health care recruiter organizations such as the National Association for Healthcare Recruitment (nahcr.com), Greater New York Association of Nurse Recruiters (gnyanr.org), and Hudson Valley Healthcare Recruitment Association (hvhra.com) enables a school to network and affiliate with area hospitals and health care organizations to collaborate on recruitment incentives, such as salary ranges, sign on bonuses, and senior year tuition remission, and participation in mentorship programs that pair new nurses with experienced staff nurses.

At the undergraduate level, recruitment can start at an early age, by reaching out to middle and high school students to increase their awareness of the benefits of a career in nursing. With the help of school guidance counselors, information can be

disseminated regarding: participating in a summer scholars camp for students to spend a week at a school of nursing with faculty counselors, visits to a school of nursing to tour and learn and perform hands on skills such as assessing vital signs and working with simulation in the school's learning resource lab, and pairing a high school and a nursing school students for a shadowing experience. Nursing school recruiters should be a presence at the local middle and high schools by participating in career day sessions to represent the profession with information about health care career options and demonstrations of basic skills. There are also collaborating health care facilities that are affiliated with local high schools, funded via grants, to introduce students to the world of nursing via classes at the high school and mentorships at the facility, with summer employment at the affiliating site.

At the high school level, University Enrollment Management builds a pool of prospective students by buying lists from organizations such as SAT, ACT, and the *Princeton Review*. Once a potential student is contacted, invitations to open houses and school tours and meetings with the nurse recruiter help convert the "contacts" to "applicants." Various school-based "conversion events," such as "phonathons" where nursing faculty and recruiters contact accepted/undecided students, "preview weekends" where potential students are paired with nursing students, mock classes and overnights on campus, and scholarship dinners, help convert applicants to accepted and deposit paid students.

Another group of potential nursing students is the "second career" group. These are people who have baccalaureate degrees and are interested in a nursing career. They may have heard about second career opportunities from a colleague or family member or decided to come into nursing because of a difficult health experience of a family member or close friend. Traditional undergraduate open house programs are not the appropriate venue for this group, but evening information sessions provide an opportunity for individuals that work or have other daytime obligations to learn about a program or nursing in general.

There needs to be a great deal of creativity when recruiting graduate nursing students. Because they are already registered nurses, their place of work is an excellent opportunity for recruitment. This can be done by collaborating with the nursing education or human resources departments of the health care agency to arrange a mutually convenient time and location to conduct recruitment sessions. Electronic media and social networking provide other venues to recruit this population. One example is delivering e-mail blasts to potential students, informing them of upcoming information sessions and announcements regarding new programs. Another use would be participation in online chats, where prospective students are invited to participate in a virtual "chat" with nursing school faculty and representatives from enrollment management. Yet another use of the Internet would be using social networking to further explore nursing programs and communicate with prospective students. Further, prospective students can communicate with each other and with students currently in the program. Examples of these sites are as follows:

- Allnursingschools.com
- Nurse.com
- Advanceweb.com
- Minoritynurse.com
- Aboutnursing.com
- Jnj.com
- NAHCR.com
- Facebook.com
- Twitter.com
- Myspace.com
- LinkedIn.com

Despite the fact that we are in challenging economic times, we are still facing a nursing shortage that must be addressed now and in the next several years. These strategies and others can place colleges and universities in a prime position to expand the nursing workforce by preparing qualified graduates to alleviate the disparity between projected need and actual enrollment of nursing students.

American Association of Colleges of Nursing. (2010a, September). *Nursing faculty shortage*. Retrieved March 24, 2011, from http://www.aacn.nche.edu/Media/FactSheets/FacultyShortage.htm

American Association of Colleges of Nursing. (2010b, September). *Nursing shortage*. Retrieved February 3, 2011, from http://www.aacn.nche.edu/media/factsheets/nursingshortage.htm

American Association of Colleges of Nursing. (2010c, March). *Final data from AACN's 2009 survey indicate ninth year of enrollment and admissions increases in entry-level baccalaureate nursing programs*. Retrieved March 24, 2011, from http://www.aacn.nche.edu/media/newsreleases/2010/enrollchanges.html

Additional information is available from these Web sites:

Bureau of Labor Statistics, U.S. Department of Labor. (2011). *Occupational outlook handbook, 2010–2011 edition: Registered nurses*. Retrieved February 3, 2011, from http://www.bls.gov/oco/ocos083.htm

DiscoverNursing.com. (2006, September). *Job opportunities*. Retrieved February 3, 2011, from http://www.discovernursing.com/job-opportunites

Mintzer Herlihy, S. (2010, April). *The best practices for recruitment for nursing schools*. Retrieved February 3, 2011, from http://www.ehow.co.uk/list_6165717_practices-recruitment-nursing-schools.html

Judi DeBlasio
Jane Dolan

S

STUDENT RETENTION

Many factors contribute to the retention of students in nursing programs: student-program fit; program progression policies, opportunities for remediation; financial issues; and cultural and student support issues. Retention strategies need to be planned and implemented long before students are admitted to nursing programs. At the same time, retention strategies need to be consistent not only with the type of program, philosophy of enrollment, diversity of the student population, and the human and fiscal resources that underpin a successful retention program but also with what factors students believe matter most in their staying the course. Noel-Levitz (2008) conducted the 2008 National Student Satisfaction and Priorities survey between 2005 and 2008, surveying 279,575 students and 13,451 faculty, staff, and administrators. Overall, students ranked instructional effectiveness, academic advising, and safety and security as the top three most important factors influencing satisfaction. At the same time, campus personnel surveyed ranked concern for the individual, recruitment and financial aid, and instructional effectiveness as the most important determinants of satisfaction and ultimately retention. Results indicate that instructional effectiveness (i.e., instructional and program quality) is the key factor in student retention and success. The entire report can be read at www.noellevitz.com. Evidence is also emerging that social networking sites may play a role in increasing student retention rates. Two British colleges are using social networking sites to connect students to teachers, to interpret assignment requirements, and to remind students of deadlines. These strategies are having positive effect on motivation and achievement of this cyber generation (Coughlan, 2009).

RETENTION AND ADMISSION

There is a strong relationship between admission criteria and retention rates; the better the student's admission profile (Scholastic Aptitude Test scores, high school quintile, and high school grade point average [GPA]), the more likelihood of student success. If the admission of academically disadvantaged students is part of the program's mission, there needs to be a well-designed, formal retention plan and program that tracks student progress and provides the necessary supports, such as tutoring, counseling, and programming for study, organizational, cultural adaptation, and stress management skills. A successful retention program cannot be left entirely to full-time nursing faculty carrying full teaching loads. Staff or specially designated faculty support for remediation need the time and tools to conduct a successful retention program.

RETENTION AND PROGRESSION

Every accredited nursing program publishes progression criteria so that students understand the performance level they must achieve to move through the program. Because of the clinical nature of nursing programs, nursing progression criteria may be set higher than the overall university policy. It is useful for programs to develop a database that tracks the following: (1) the number of "F" and "D" grades that nursing students earn throughout the course of their program; (2) the number and demographic profile of students that successfully repeat "F" and "D" grade courses and progress on;

and (3) the number and demographic profile of students that drop out of the nursing program. The demographic profile can include faculty-selected variables such as overall GPA and Scholastic Aptitude Test on admission; GPA in selected science courses; and admission status, for example, transfer or freshman standing. These cumulative data can provide a predictive success model for faculty to use in their admission process and in improving retention programs and in improving student retention and success.

RETENTION AND NCLEX-RN SUCCESS

Success on the National Council Licensure Examination for Registered Nurses (NCLEX-RN) needs to be part of nursing program retention strategies. It is the responsibility of every nursing program to ensure that the graduate is prepared to attain licensure to practice. The inability to secure a registered nurse license after the successful completion of any nursing program can be devastating to the student and to the family's investment in an education. There are a variety of strategies that include periodic testing across the nursing curriculum as well as a summative, comprehensive test with predictive values. Any testing program selected or designed by faculty or by a standardized testing service should be accompanied by a systematic remediation policy and program for those students who fall below the passing standard.

SUMMARY

Retention programs in schools of nursing should be derived not only from the admission and progression philosophy and policies of the nursing program but also from data provided by students on those factors that contribute most highly

to their success. Faculty who design retention programs should be sensitive to students' generational needs and to the ongoing collection and analysis of retention data that will point the way to improvement.

See also Licensure

Arizona State University. (n.d.). *College of nursing exemplary programs for retention.* Retrieved October 7, 2006, from http://www.asu.edu/retention/exemplary/pdf/KA_Nursing.pdf

Coughlan, S. (2009). Facebook "cuts student drop-outs." *BBC News.* Retrieved September 18, 2010, from http://news.bbc.co.uk/go/pr/fr/-/2/hi/uk_news/education8299050.stm

Noel-Levitz, Inc. (2008). *The 2008 National Student Satisfaction and Priorities Report— Four Year Private Colleges and Universities.* Retrieved September 18, 2010, from http://www.noellevitz.com

Gloria F. Donnelly

SWOT ANALYSIS

Strategic management is the process through which an organization analyzes the competitive environment to understand organizational strengths, weaknesses, opportunities, and threats (SWOT). On the basis of that understanding, strategies are devised and implemented to neutralize threats and take advantage of opportunities. A SWOT analysis involves evaluation of internal organizational resources and capabilities and an evaluation of the external environment to identify market opportunities and competitive forces. It is helpful in identifying how internal and external factors might interact to create a market advantage, or increase competitive pressures. The analysis will highlight areas where an organization is vulnerable, where it is constrained, and

S

where it can leverage strengths to increase market share. A SWOT analysis is a key tool in the strategic management process.

STRENGTHS AND WEAKNESSES

Effective strategic management requires an understanding of internal organizational competencies, capabilities, and resources that lead to a competitive advantage. An internal analysis (strengths and weaknesses) should consider the following:

- What is the fit between the external environment and the present internal characteristics of the organization?
- Which services meet the key preferences and selection criteria of customers (i.e., patients, physicians and staff) in the target market?
- What is the value of the services provided by the organization versus that of competitors in the minds customers?
- Can the organization anticipate the future and respond to changing conditions?
- Do management information systems support business and clinical operations and inform decisions?
- How are the organization's financial resources, including debt position, financial returns, working capital, liquidity, and cash management?

Several strengths and weaknesses will be identified as a result of an internal analysis. Strengths might include a cost advantage, customer loyalty, attractive physical or service characteristics of the facility, company culture, exclusive contracts, clinical quality outcomes, and high satisfaction levels for patients, physicians, and staff. Weaknesses may include a narrow product line, lack of management depth, high-cost operations, poor clinical outcomes, or a weak market image.

OPPORTUNITIES AND THREATS

The external environment has increasingly become a factor in the success of health care organizations, and organizations must anticipate and respond to significant shifts taking place within that environment. External factors include technological, social, regulatory, political, economic, and competitive forces. External factors also include demographic shifts, changes in motivation for workers, and changes in the values, preferences, and expectations of customers. Organizations must understand and anticipate the impact of these external forces to stay in touch with the needs of the market. An external environmental analysis (opportunities and threats) should consider the following:

- What current and emerging issues, regulations, and governmental policies affect the organization's existing position in the market?
- How do industry structures, changing economics, and general trends impact key success factors?
- What is the competition's size, growth rate, service quality, and profitability?
- What kinds of future issues will have a significant impact on the organization's mission, vision, values, objectives, and strategy?

Several opportunities and threats will be identified as part of the external analysis. Opportunities might include the opportunity to add to existing product lines, to enter new markets, or to acquire new technologies. Threats might include new competition, unfavorable government policies, shifting customer loyalties, or innovations that will radically change care delivery.

EFFICIENCY VERSUS EFFECTIVENESS

SWOT analysis is an effective method within the strategic management process to help organizations become more efficient and effective in their market. Organizational effectiveness can only occur when an organization is well positioned to accomplish its mission, with economies in the use of capital, personnel, and the physical plant. Creating and sustaining a competitive advantage requires a balance between the ability to work skillfully with controllable internal factors (strengths and weaknesses) while adapting to factors outside of the organization's direct control (opportunities and threats).

Additional information is available from the following sources:

Barney, J. B. (2010). *Gaining and sustaining competitive advantage* (4th ed.). Reading, MA: Addison-Wesley Publishing Company.

Ginter, P. M., Swayne, L. M., & Duncan, W. J. (2006). *Strategic management of health care organizations* (5th ed.). Malden, MA: Blackwell Publishers.

Kalisch, B., & Curley, C. (2008, February). Transforming a nursing organization. *Journal of Nursing Administration, 38*(2), 76–83.

Pearce, C. (2007, May). Ten steps to carrying out a SWOT analysis. *Nursing Management, 14*(2), 25.

Nancy Hollingsworth

T

TEAMWORK

Professional nurses have many roles, but all require the skill of working with others. Teamwork involves working collaboratively rather than individually. The nature of nursing work directs us to work collaboratively with other professionals, unlicensed health care workers, and most importantly our patients. Working together with others toward a common goal is a broad definition of teamwork. A team is usually a small group of people with complementary skills who are committed to a common purpose. There is a set of performance goals for which team members hold themselves mutually accountable. The work product of the team is produced through the joint contributions of its members. The work produced by the team is greater than the work that could be produced by each individual. In other words, a team is more than a sum of its parts (Katzenbach & Smith, 2005).

In health care, the nurse might be a member of multiple teams. There are patient care teams responsible for the care of individual patients and families. There are work teams established for a given task that are dismembered when the goal is achieved. There are ongoing teams established to manage and monitor specific outcomes such as patient safety, length of patient hospital stay, or skin care. Regardless of the type of team or its goal, there are fundamental underpinnings of all successful teams. They include competent leadership, open communication, clear purpose and goals, and measurable outcomes.

Leadership of a team is crucial to the team's success. Team leaders motivate and manage members. In health care, the membership of the care giving team is usually made up of several different specialists that are collectively responsible for the care of a patient. The leader is responsible to ensure that members understand their roles and have the opportunity and ability to communicate and participate in the decision making and care planning. The leader must manage the flow of communication and the complementary effect of the individual professional work.

Effective communication is also crucial to success. The leader is responsible for ensuring that all members are heard, remembering that silence may not indicate acceptance. Because health care teams have become more culturally diverse, leaders must to be open to the cultural expectations of the members. Through effective open communication, ideas, opinions, and dialogue are valued and encouraged. This reinforces the value of each team member and requires active listening, verbally checking your perception of what you heard (Chinn, 2004). Effective communication between team members, especially nurse–physician communication, has been linked to better patient outcomes (Institute of Medicine, 2010; Page, 2004)

Conflict and disagreement are germane to team building. With a diverse group of caregivers and professionals from different cultural and educational backgrounds, conflicts sometimes arise. An important leadership skill is the ability to deal with conflict and facilitate turning conflict into something positive. Conflict avoidance will result in anxiety and friction and hinder the team process; however, addressing conflict, while at the same time acknowledging its presence, is a first step in leading to resolution.

Team members need to have clear goals with set expectations and definitive timeframes. Whether it's a patient care team or a task team, identifying measurable goals is the first step for a team trying to shape a purpose meaningful to its members. When goals are clear, discussions focus on how to pursue them and are more productive than when goals are ambiguous. Performance goals are symbols of accomplishment that motivate and energize the team (Katzenbach & Smith, 2005). These goals need to be measurable and each member needs to fully understand her or his responsibility in working toward the team's success. To keep members engaged in the work of the team, it is helpful to identify critical measurement points as the team works toward goals. In this way, team members can feel positive about their progress toward reaching the goal. At the end of every success, the team should celebrate its accomplishment. Enthusiasm for the work to be done and accomplished are important aspects of maintaining team spirit.

Not all team work has successful outcomes. This does not mean the work of the team was a failure. For task teams, time for objective evaluation and reflection needs to be built into the team's schedule. Regardless of the outcomes, opportunities for improvement should be addressed. For patient care teams and ongoing work teams there should be time set aside for team evaluation. Such evaluation needs to focus on the team building process as well as specific outcome measures. Team building is an ongoing effort and the responsibility of all members.

The Institute of Medicine calls for nurses to practice to the full extent of their education and training and be full partners with physicians and other health care professionals to redesign health care in the United States (Institute of Medicine, 2010). This goal challenges nurses to take professional responsibility and participate with colleagues as an active member of the team.

Chinn, P. (2004). *Peace and power: Creative leadership for building community* (6th ed.). Boston, MA: Jones & Bartlett Publishers.

Institute of Medicine. (2010). *The future of nursing leading change, advancing health report brief.* Retrieved on November 20, 2010, from http://www.nap.edu/catalog/12894.html

Katzenbach, J., & Smith, D. (2005). The discipline of teams. *Harvard Business Review, 83*(7/8), 162–171.

Page, A. (2004). Keeping patients safe: Transforming the work environment of nurses. *Committee on the work environment for nurses and patient safety, Institute of Medicine.* Washington, DC: National Academies Press.

Christine Coughlin

TECHNOLOGY

Technology abounds in nursing and has been "inexorably linked" since the late 19th century (Honey, 2011; Sandelowski, 2000, p. 1). Technology serves to define nursing (the IV nurse) and be defined by nursing. Patient care areas have been defined by the technologies used, for example, hemodialysis units, critical care units, operating rooms. Hoffman (2011, para 1) states "Nurses must increasingly master a host of complex technologies, from 'smart' medical devices to tablet PCs."

Technology is used in patient care to assess patients, track and monitor aspects of nursing care and clinical responses (central venous catheters, cardiac monitors, laboratory results), or assist with medication administration, documentation and patient information. Technology is used in nursing administration for staffing, tracking patient acuity, assuring patient safety, and managing quality improvement initiatives. In nursing education, technology is used to present information, measure attainment of skills and knowledge, and validate knowledge and skills. In nursing research it is used to obtain, analyze, and disseminate information and evidence for practice.

Clinical information systems integrate information of the patient's medical records, including physician/primary care provider order entry, patient allergies, medical diagnoses, laboratory results, radiology reports, medication administration, and for provider documentation. Clinical information systems can provide checks and balances that help prevent repetition of tests and alert caregivers about medication interactions, or duplication and patient allergies. Electronic medical records are used to assure patient safety and prevent errors in practice such as medication errors. Computerized patient records allow easy access to vital patient information at point of care instead of having to wade through a myriad of papers in a patient chart.

Technologies used by nurses in the care of patients vary in complexity and are used wherever nursing care is realized. Devices include medical devices such as beds, thermometers, stethoscopes, sphygmomanometers, bedside monitors, IV pumps, and invasive catheters. In addition, nurses use information technologies, such as personal digital assistants and computer databases, to help them keep abreast of the latest changes impacting patient care. The expanding use of wireless technology can enhance communication among nursing staff and improve response time to patient calls, improving patient safety. Personal digital assistants are used to assist nurses with the myriad of information needed to provide safe care such as information on medications, diagnostic tests, and calculations (Courtney, Demiris, & Alexander, 2005; Guarascio-Howard, 2011; Wälivaara, Andersson, & Axelsson, 2010).

New technologies are constantly being introduced into patient care. Technologies such as bar code scanning may help to reduce or prevent medication errors but also increase the time needed to provide patient care. Computerized documentation systems provide timely recording of activities provided to the patient and communication with all health care providers. Handheld computers are being evaluated as point-of-care information systems to enhance or change workflow. Computer decision support systems are being used to gather large amounts of data to identify trends and group data and to summarize data to be translated by the user to intervene appropriately in patient care (Mann & Salinas, 2009). Telemedicine with videoconferencing has been implemented for palliative and hospice care, cardiac rehabilitation monitoring, patient education and patient monitoring (Courtney et al., 2005).

The scope of technology used in nursing education is also changing at a rapid pace. Educators use technology to help students and nurses increase their knowledge base and maintain competence via videos, online courses. Online courses are offered both for basic nursing education and for continuing education, offering nurses the ability to attain degrees especially if they live a distance from an educational facility. Online courses are taught in real time and asynchronously and classroom discussion takes place through the use of virtual chat rooms and blogs. Technology also helps to track the competency of nurses, keeping record of courses the nurse has completed or needs to complete, and sending reminders of courses needing to be completed (Courtney et al., 2005; Wälivaara et al., 2010).

Computerized patient classification systems and scheduling systems assist nursing management in assigning the appropriate level of personnel to provide safe, effective patient care. The patient classification system indicators such as nursing time for teaching, intravenous medications and fluids, suctioning, or frequent turning and assessment, are defined by each institution because each institution's patient population is unique. The number of nursing hours needed to care for each client is then defined. The scheduling systems assign the appropriate number of staff for daily unit coverage based on the number of nursing care hours needed each day. Although the classification systems help identify the level of nursing care needed and the scheduling systems assure an appropriate number of personnel, the manager must consider staff competency, staffing levels, and skill mix (Marquis & Huston, 2009).

Information technology skills are used to examine patient records to discover trends in patient care, quality improvement issues, risk management, staffing, and patient acuity.

Although technology assists nurses to provide safe effective patient care both directly and indirectly, the nurse must remain vigilant of the information provided by the technology, the impact it has on patient care and develop new techniques of communication. Nurses must be educated on the technologies used, technical skills and cognitive skills needed. Technology does not replace good judgment; nurses must rely on their assessment skills to assure accuracy of information provided by the technology. Technology can and does malfunction. Processes and support systems must be in place to provide staff with the resources necessary to address the situation when technology malfunctions (Haghenbeck, 2005).

See also Electronic Health Record

Courtney, K. L., Demiris, G., & Alexander, G. L. (2005). Information technology. *Nursing Administration Quarterly, 29*(4), 315–322.

Guarascio-Howard, L. (2011, Winter). Examination of wireless technology to improve nurse communication, response time to bed alarms, and patient safety. *HERD, 4*(2), 109–120.

Haghenbeck, K. T. (2005, Spring/Summer). Critical Care Nurses' Experience when Technology Malfunctions. *Journal of New York State Nurses Association 36*(1), 13–19.

Hoffman, A. (2011). Technology in Nursing. Retrieved April 19, 2011, from http://career-advice.monster.com/in-the-office/workplace-issues/technology-in-nursing/article.aspx

Mann, E. A., & Salinas, J. (2009). The use of computer decision support systems for the critical care environment. *AACN Advanced Critical Care, 20*(3), 216–219.

Marquis, B., & Huston, C. J. (2009) *Leadership roles and management functions in nursing: Theory and application* (6th ed.). Philadelphia, PA: Lippincott, Williams & Wilkins

Sandelowski, M. (2000). *Devices & desires: Gender, technology, and American nursing.* Chapel Hill, NC: University of North Carolina Press.

Wälivaara, B., Andersson, S., & Axelsson, K. (2010). General practitioners' reasoning about using mobile distance-spanning technology in home care and in nursing home care. *Scandinavian Journal of Caring Science, 25,* 117–125.

Karen Toby Haghenbeck

TELEHEALTH

The Health Resources and Services Administration (HRSA, 2001) defined *telehealth* as "the use of electronic information and telecommunications technologies to support long-distance clinical health care, patient and professional health-related education, public health and health administration." The use of telehealth can increase the quality of health services by removing the barriers of space and time and make health resources accessible, affordable, and convenient to many consumers and providers who feel empowered by these tools (Hebda & Czar, 2009). In rural and underserved areas, telehealth can decrease isolation and distance barriers; in school health, off-site clinicians can provide needed physical exams; in correctional health, the risk of escape in patient transfer can be decreased; in emergency care, evaluation and treatment can begin in ambulance transport; in critical care, access to specialists can improve patient outcomes; and in home care, aging immobile patients can be monitored to decrease emergency visits. Some of the technologies used in telehealth include telephone and faxes paired with an integrated data exchange, computers, interactive video transmissions, direct links to health care instruments, transmission of images, and telecommunications that use audio and video (American Telemedicine Association, 2010).

KEY ISSUES

The potential benefits of telehealth, however, bring challenges related to reimbursement, cross-state licensure, standards, privacy, and the need for guiding principles to direct its use. There is evidence to support the usability and cost savings for telehealth (HRSA, 2001) but reimbursement for these services can be complex. Medicare coverage for telehealth services includes a limited number of medical or other health services, like office visits and consultations provided using an interactive two-way telecommunications system (like real-time audio and video) by an eligible provider who is at a location different from that of the patient. Medicare coverage applies only if the patient is located at a doctor's office, hospital, rural health clinic, federally qualified health center, hospital-based dialysis facility, skilled nursing facility, or community mental health center (Centers for Medicare and Medicaid Services, 2010).

In addition to reimbursement issues, some states restrict interstate telemedicine practice . With challenges regarding cross-state licensure, many states have adopted the Interstate Nurses Licensure Compact, a licensure model based on mutual recognition of licensure for nurses. Despite this progress, many clinicians are reluctant to use telehealth citing the technology is intrusive both personally and professionally. Nurses often get caught up in "fixing" the technology, which disrupts routine care. Some fear this technology could impact their relationship with patients (Thomas et al., 2009).

Safety, standards, and privacy are increasingly important. Safety may be compromised if there is equipment failure or malfunction or when the use of telehealth does not provide the patient with the same level of service as direct "hands-on" care (Hebda & Czar, 2009). Without widely adopted standards and guidelines, interoperability and interconnection are not possible. Older and newer equipment need to interconnect and different brands of the same equipment must operate with one another. In addition, clinical protocols and guidelines such as telecommunications transmission specifications are needed. For example, the clinical technical standard for image quality in a video transmission should specify what is required to correctly diagnose a patient. Regarding privacy, the general principles for the use and disclosure of personally identifiable health information are applicable regardless of the format of the information, methods of transmission, time sequence of its creation and use, or the way it is communicated. Differences between federal and individual state privacy laws, however, make this a challenge for teleheath participants (HRSA, 2001). Regulations and guidelines for privacy, security, and certification of health information technology are defined by the federal government (Office of the National Coordinator).

TELEHEALTH PRINCIPLES

In 1999, the American Nurses Association (ANA) defined 12 core principles to guide the development and use of telehealth. The principles assert that the basic standards of professional conduct and the practitioner's responsibility to provide high-quality and ethical care must not be compromised by telehealth technologies (ANA, 1999). Telehealth applications should only be used for services that are legally or professionally authorized. Although additional licensure should not be required to use telehealth, these services must adhere to basic assurances of quality. Nurses have a responsibility to examine how telehealth changes the patterns of care delivery and what modifications to standards may be

required. The development of guidelines for telehealth needs to be based on empirical evidence; competencies for using such technologies must be ensured. It is important to protect the confidentiality and the integrity of data when using telehealth applications, and documentation requirements for recording telehealth services received need to be developed. When embracing the power of this technology, it is essential that the integrity and therapeutic value of the client/health care practitioner relationship be preserved. To this end, clients must be informed about the process, risks and benefits, and their rights and responsibilities when using telehealth. Patient safety needs to be assured through the appropriate use of hardware and software. Finally, the ANA calls for a systematic and comprehensive research agenda for the ongoing assessment and evaluation of telehealth services.

THE FUTURE

In an era of increased health costs, an aging population for which chronic conditions call for continuous monitoring, and access to providers that is sometimes limited, telehealth has the capacity to provide a vehicle for creative delivery, administration, and education for health care. Nurses are challenged to harness this capacity to create the future of health.

See also American Nurses Association; Technology

American Nurses Association. (1999). *Core principles on telehealth*. Retrieved July 14, 2006, fromhttp://www.nurse.org/acnp/telehealth/th.ana.core.shtml

American Telemedicine Association. (2010). *Telemedicine defined*. Retrieved August 20, 2010, from http://www.americantelemed.org/i4a/pages/index.cfm?pageid=3333

Centers for Medicare and Medicaid Services. (2010). *Medicare & you 2010*. Retrieved August

10, 2010, from http://www.medicare.gov/publications/pubs/pdf/10050.pdf

Health Resources and Services Administration. (2001). *Report to Congress on telemedicine.* Retrieved July 14, 2006, from http://www.hrsa.gov/telehealth/pubs/report2001.htm

Hebda, T., & Czar, P. (2009). *Handbook of informatics for nurses and health care professionals* (4th ed.). Upper Saddle River, NJ: Prentice Hall.

Office of the National Coordinator for Health Information Technology. (n.d.). Homepage. Retrieved August 25, 2006, from http://www.hhs.gov/healthit

Thomas, E. J., Lucke, J. F., Wueste, L., Weavind, L., & Patel, B. (2009). Association of telemedicine for remote monitoring of intensive care patients with mortality, complications, and length of stay. *JAMA, 302*(24), 2671–2678. Retrieved August 20, 2010, from http://jama.ama-assn.org/cgi/content/short/302/24/2671?rss=1

Carol A. Romano
Charlotte A. Seckman

TRANSFORMATIONAL LEADERSHIP

The Great Man theory of leadership was the primary concept guiding all leadership literature before the 1900s and introduced the thought that the masses were led by a superior few leaders (Dowd, 1993). These leaders shaped the institutions and organizations they led, and they thought that only through their high degree of intelligence, energy, and moral force that the masses were led. Covey (2004) divides the approaches to leadership theories into five categories…"trait, behavioral, power-influence, situational, and integrative" (p. 352). As a response to Great Man theories, trait and behavioral theories began to emerge, followed by theorists analyzing situational and environmental factors in leadership. More recently in the latter half of the 1900s, integrative theories that include goal attainment, change theory, contingency theories, and people and situations have been developed. This entry focuses on one theory of leadership, an integrative theory that is transformational and value based. Both Burns (1978) and later Bass and Avolio (1990) are considered the seminal theorists of transformational leadership. Burns (1978, p. 19) defined transformational leadership as a "process whereby leaders and followers raise one another to higher levels of morality and motivation."

James M. Burns (1978) was the first to introduce the concept of leadership in relation to both the leader and the follower. "The genius of leadership lies in the manner in which leaders see and act on their own and their followers' values and motivations" (Burns, 1978, p. 19). The evolution of transformational leadership emerged from an understanding of leadership based on transactions, where an exchange of incentives occurs for desired accomplishments (Bass, 1990). This movement from transactional leadership to transformational leadership is based on an exploration of characteristics that move beyond the transactional mode of relationship. Transactional leadership was defined by Burns as having an emphasis on work standards, assignments, task orientation, and task completion. Transactional leadership style included rewards and punishments based on this compliance-based form of working. Although Burns proposed that leadership is both a transactional and transformational process, it was Bass (1990) followed by other researchers (Avolio, Waldman, & Yammarino, 1991) who identified the characteristics of transformational leadership. The qualities include:

1. Individualized consideration—the ability of a leader to treat each person equally,

but differently, to give personal attention, functioning as a coach or mentor (Atwater & Yammarino, 1993).

2. Intellectual stimulation—the ability of the leader to ask questions and find ways to problem solve, to encourage followers to create solutions and try new ideas; questioning assumptions, reframing problems, and approaching old situations in new ways (Avolio et al., 1991); including the followers in the generation of solutions.

3. Charisma—a leader's ability to generate excitement and provide vision and a sense of direction

4. Inspiration—the communication of the shared vision on the part of the leader to the follower, motivating and inspiring others by providing meaning and challenge to followers' tasks (Howell & Avolio, 1993).

5. Idealized influence—a leader's ability to behave as a role model and emulate high ethical standards.

Burns's (1978) transformational leadership theory described the emergence of leaders who raise the awareness of followers by appealing to their elevated ideals and values. Early attempts to measure these characteristics were described in Bass's (1985) work, and pilot study survey questions began to differentiate the concepts of transactional and transformational leadership qualities. The components and definitions of transactional and transformational leadership behaviors are included in Table 3. These studies were replicated through multiple businesses, government, and industry, with similar results (Bass, 1985, p. 32).

Many social scientists have studied transformational leadership and its application to business (Atwater & Yammarino, 1993; Bass & Avolio, 1990). These applications include leadership development in the ranks of the military (Atwater & Yammarino,

Table 3
DEFINITION OF TRANSFORMATIONAL LEADERSHIP BEHAVIORS (BASS, 1990)

Leadership behavior	Definition
Idealized influence (attributed and behavioral)	Provides vision and sense of mission, instills pride, and gains respect and trust
Inspirational motivation	Communicates high expectations, uses symbols to focus efforts, and expresses important purposes in simple ways
Intellectual stimulation	Promotes intelligence, rationality, and careful problem solving
Individualized consideration	Gives personal attention, treats each employee individually, coaches, and advises

1993) and leveraging leadership characteristics to increase global competitiveness (Tichy & Devanna, 1990). Management behaviors and traits also have implications for creating cultures of innovation, where business problems can be solved (Kanter, 1982), group potency and effectiveness can be increased (Sosik et al., 1997), and change management strategies can be used (Pearce & Sims, 2002).

TRANSFORMATIONAL LEADERSHIP AND NURSING

One of the first studies in nursing examining transformational leadership was completed by Dunham and Klafehn (1990). This descriptive study with cross-sectional survey methods was conducted in one moderate sized hospital to explore transformational leadership characteristics and skills in nurse executives. The use of the multifactorial leadership questionnaire (Avolio & Bass, 1999) was used to reveal that nurse executives were transformational as perceived by themselves and their staff. Meighan (1990) furthered the study of characteristics of transformational

T

leadership and investigated individual consideration and charisma. By identifying characteristics of a strong leader, staff nurses expected managers to demonstrate transformational leadership characteristics. This was reinforced by the nurse executives studied by Murphy and DeBack (1991), who recognized transformational qualities as important for the nurse executive role. Nurses demonstrating transformational leadership qualities have also been studied, and the emergence of courage development was identified by Aprigliano (2000). The different levels of leadership in nursing that have been explored include the executive role, the middle manager role, and the staff nurse role as a leader and follower. McDaniel and Wolf (1992) tested the theory of transformational leadership in nursing and found that higher level transformational leadership qualities were found in the nurse executive than in the middle manager. In addition, work satisfaction was above average correlated to the higher scoring transformational leadership qualities in the nurse executive. McDaniel and Stumpf (1993) furthered this work by suggesting that there may be a relationship between work satisfaction and transformational leadership scores of nurse managers. Nurse managers had moderate transformational leadership scores compared with nurse executives.

The application of leadership theory to nursing practice is evident in the Magnet Recognition Program®, and there are requirements for transformational leadership through the sources of evidence (Magnet Application Manual, p. 25). The areas of transformational leadership that the Magnet program requires include evidence of strategic planning, advocacy and influence, visibility, accessibility, and communication. Through these transformational leadership requirements, the chief nurse in a Magnet organization leads both planned and unplanned change and is a leader for patient care.

American Nurses Credentialing Center. (2005). *Magnet recognition program recognizing excellence in nursing services: Application manual 2005.* Silver Spring, MD: Author.

Aprigliano, T. (2000). The experience of courage development in transformational leaders. *Journal of Emergency Nursing, 26*(2), 104.

Atwater, L. E., & Yammarino, F. J. (1993). Personal attributes as predictors of superiors' and subordinates' perceptions of military academy leadership. *Human Relations, 46*(5), 645–668.

Avolio, B. J., & Bass, B. M. (1999). Re-examining the components of transformational and transactional leadership using the multifactor leadership questionnaire. *Journal of Occupational and Organizational Psychology, 72,* 441–462.

Avolio, B. J., Waldman, D. A., & Yammarino, F. J. (1991). Leading in the 1990's: The four I's of transformational leadership. *Journal of European Industrial Training, 15*(4), 9–16.

Bass, B. M. (1985). *Leadership and performance beyond expectations.* New York, NY: The Free Press.

Bass, B. M. (1990). *Bass and Stogdill's handbook of leadership: Theory, research, and managerial applications: third edition.* New York, NY: The Free Press.

Bass, B. M., & Avolio, B. J. (1990*). Transformational leadership development: Manual for Multifactor Leadership Questionnaire.* Palo Alto, CA: Consulting Psychologist Press, Inc.

Burns, J. M. (1978). *Leadership.* New York, NY: Harper & Row Publishers.

Covey, S. R. (2004). *The eighth habit: From effectiveness to greatness.* New York, NY: Free Press.

Dowd, J. (1993). *Control in human societies.* New York, NY: Appleton-Century.

Dunham, J., & Klafehn, K. A. (1990). Transformational leadership and the nurse executive. *Journal of Nursing Administration, 29*(4), 28–34.

Howell, J. M., & Avolio, B. (1993). Transformational leadership, transactional leadership, locus of control, and support for innovation: Key predictors of consolidated business-unit performance. *Journal of Applied Psychology, 78*(6), 891–902.

McDaniel, C., & Stumpf, L. (1993). The organizational culture: Implications for nursing service. *Journal of Nursing Administration, 23* (4), 54–60.

McDaniel, C., & Wolf, G. A. (1992). Transformational leadership in nursing service: A test of theory. *Journal of Nursing Administration, 22*(2), 60–65.

Meighan, M. M. (1990). The most important characteristics of nursing leaders. *Nursing Administration Quarterly, 15*(1), 63–69.

Murphy, M. M., & DeBack, V. (1991). Today's nursing leaders: Creating the vision. *Nursing Administration Quarterly, 16*(1), 71–90.

Karen Drenkard

TRANSFORMING CARE
AT THE BEDSIDE

In 2003, the Institute for Healthcare Improvement and the Robert Wood Johnson Foundation launched Transforming Care at the Bedside (TCAB) nationwide, in part to answer the call to action from the Institute of Medicine to improve care in hospitals and clinic settings. Although many improvement strategies center on critical care units and emergency rooms, TCAB targets medical/surgical units where it is estimated that 35% to 40% of unexpected deaths occur (Rutherford, Lee, & Greiner, 2004). TCAB calls for extensive redesign of the care models and processes in medical/surgical units. The intent is "to transform the elements that affect care on medical/surgical units: care delivery processes, nursing care models, physical environments, organizational cultures and norms, and care team collaboration and performance" (Rutherford et al., 2004). Three innovative hospitals initially were selected as prototypes for conceptual framework development: Seton Northwest Hospital, Austin,

TX; UMPC Shadyside, part of University of Pittsburgh Medical Center (UMPC), Pittsburgh, PA; and Kaiser Foundation Hospital, Roseville, CA. These hospitals developed and tested ideas and project viability. Early work assisted in the further development of the current conceptual framework. Five main themes are addressed in the TCAB framework for improvement:

- Safety and reliable care: Care for moderately sick patients who are hospitalized is safe, reliable, effective and equitable.

- Vitality and teamwork: Care is provided in a joyful and supportive environment that nurtures professional formation and career development; effective teams strive for excellence.

- Patient-centered care: Honors the whole person and family, respects the individual values and choices, and ensures continuity of care. Patients will say, "They gave me exactly the help I want (and need), exactly when I want (and need) it."

- Value-added care processes: All care processes are free of waste and promote continuous flow (Martin et al., 2007).

- Transformational leadership: Leaders at all levels of the organization make the commitment to the resources necessary to support and sustain the innovations and empower the frontline leaders and staff who are identifying and testing new processes to improve patient care (Rutherford, Moen, & Taylor, 2009).

TCAB work later expanded to 10 hospitals in the second and third phases. In 2007, a Robert Wood Johnson Foundation grant to the American Organization of Nurse Executives helped spread the initiative, and two additional components were added to the TCAB framework: caring and nurse ownership of practice.

T

TCAB is different from other quality improvement initiatives because it relies on the engagement and empowerment of first-line managers and frontline staff who spend the most time providing care to patients and families. Second, TCAB is transformative change and requires unit managers and frontline staff to challenge old paradigms and past experience. Finally, TCAB is grounded in continuous learning and continuous improvement as teams test new ideas and processes. Fundamental to TCAB is the Model for Improvement (Langley et al., 2009), which includes the use of three questions: What are we trying to accomplish? How will we know that a change is an improvement? What changes can we make that will result in improvement?

The experience at UPMC Shadyside is a good example of the how this initiative was launched using the initial four-point framework and six core values of work redesign to empower frontline staff.

- Work redesign is done with staff that does the work in the place where the work happens and as it happens.
- Improvement efforts are centered on a patient's or employee's need.
- Support from executive leadership is critical.
- First test with a small sample, learn, and then spread to a larger scope.
- Teach as you go because once done, the approach will need to apply to other problems.
- Make it happen tomorrow (Martin et al., 2007).

The use of methodologies such as brainstorming and nominal group technique is essential to engage staff in identifying areas for improvement. Staff is encouraged to vision what the perfect patient or staff experience would look like in each of the four themes. Interviews with patients and families also are essential to gain insight into their needs, desires, and priorities to ensure that a patient-centered focus is maintained (Martin et al., 2007). It is not unusual that a large number of ideas will be generated. The experience at Shadyside suggests that staff be encouraged to select a few easy or quick wins in one or more of the focus areas. This serves to motivate staff with early accomplishments and quick positive impact to the quality of care. The teams are then moved to a small number of ideas that were mentioned most often to reinforce a sense of urgency and universality. In later phases, teams are asked to identify one problem area in each of the themes (Martin et al., 2007).

At the end of Phase 3 of the pilot, and based on the results from 10 of the TCAB hospitals, a number of "high-leverage changes" were identified for each of the themes. High leverage changes are defined as those most likely to result in improved outcomes (Rutherford et al., 2009). Some examples under each theme include the following:

Safe and reliable care

- Rapid response teams—using trigger criteria for early detection and quick response to a change in the patient's condition
- Family-initiated rapid response team calls such as "Condition H"

Vitality and teamwork

- Build competencies of frontline staff for leading innovation and process improvement using the PDSA model and lean engineering methods
- Empower staff with shared leadership models

Patient-centered care

- Patient and family involvement in rounds at the bedside and bedside nursing change-of-shift reports
- Include patients and families on all quality improvement teams

Value-added care processes

- Acuity adaptable rooms
- Eliminate waste and improve work flow for the admission process, medication administration process, handoffs, and discharge process

There is a growing business case for TCAB initiatives. Quality improvement and cost containment have been persistent health care imperatives for some time but few programs to date have focused on nursing care and even fewer on nursing care in medical-surgical units. TCAB has been the exception (Unruh, Agrawal, & Hassmiller, 2011). In a study based on data from the original "TCAB 10," the analysis indicates that on average the TCAB units had fewer patient falls with harm and less RN turnover and overtime compared with to national averages (Unruh et al., 2011). The study goes on to state that although a cost of implementation per unit was $222,258 per unit, the outcomes resulted in financial benefits of $847,861 per unit from 2004 to 2007 (Unruh et al., 2011).

Costs to implement a TCAB program include reorganization of staff, redesign of units, staff education, and time off the unit to participate in meetings (Unruh et al., 2011). A second study cited that after TCAB strategies were implemented, between February 2005 and December 2007, the proportion of reported medication errors, falls that resulted in harm and pressure ulcers as reported in clinical incidents reports were reduced from 46.3% to 17.1%, from 97.0% to 51.0%, and from 91.3% to 46.6%, respectively, representing an absolute reduction

by about one half. Additional benefits can include a reduction in the number of patient codes on medical-surgical units, fewer medication administration errors of all types, improved patient, family and staff satisfaction, and increased time in direct nursing care at the bedside (Martin et al., 2007; Unruh et al., 2011).

Hundreds of hospitals have adopted the program or many of the practice innovations generated through TCAB program. However, there needs to be more work quantifying the return on investment for patient quality outcomes, operating efficiencies, and patient and staff satisfaction. There are only a few American publications regarding this topic (Chaboyer, Johnson, Hardy, Gehrke, & Panuwatwanich, 2010).

Chaboyer, W., Johnson, J., Hardy, L., Gehrke, T., & Panuwatwanich, K. (2007, May). Transforming care strategies and nursing-sensitive patient outcomes. *Journal of Advanced Nursing, 66*(5), 1111–1119.

Langley, G. J., Nolan, K. M., Norman, C. L., Provost, L. P., & Nolan, T. W. (2009). *The improvement guide: a practical approach to enhancing organizational performance* (2nd ed.). San Francisco: Jossey-Bass.

Martin, S. C., Greenhouse, P. K., Merryman, T., Shovel, J., Liberi, C. A., & Konzier, J. (2007, October). Transforming care at the bedside: Implementation and spread model for single-hospital and multihospital systems. *Journal of Nursing Administration, 37*(10), 444–451.

Rutherford, P., Lee, B., & Greiner, A. (2004). *Transforming care at the bedside*. Cambridge, MA: Institute for Healthcare Improvement. IHI Innovation series white paper. Retrieved from http://www.ihi.org

Rutherford, P., Moen, R., & Taylor, J. (2009). TCAB: The "how" and the "what": Developing an initiative to involve nursing in transforming change. *AJN, 109*(11), 5–17.

Unruh, L., Agrawal, M., & Hassmiller, S. (2011, April–June). The business case for transforming care at the bedside among the "TCAB 10" and lessons learned. *Nursing Administration Quarterly, 35*(2), 97–109.

Marilyn Cox

T

TRANSITIONAL CARE MODEL

The transitional care model (TCM) is an evidence-based, nurse-led, team-based model of care that was designed by a multidisciplinary team of researchers at the University of Pennsylvania (Penn) in 1980 and originally referred to as "Quality Cost Model of Advanced Practice Nurse (APN) Transitional Care." Initially, the model was developed to promote safe, earlier discharge of high risk women and infants by substituting a portion of the hospitalization with home follow-up by nurse specialists (Brooten et al., 1986). This approach to care has since been adapted to address the needs of chronically ill, older adults who experience frequent transitions among providers and across settings and who are at high risk for negative outcomes (AARP, 2009).

The term "transitional care" refers to a range of time limited services and environments that complement primary care and are designed to ensure health care continuity and avoid preventable poor outcomes among at risk populations as they move from one level of care to another, among multiple providers, and across settings (Coleman & Boult, 2003; Naylor, 2000). TCM is a multidimensional approach to transitional care designed not only to avoid breakdowns in care that are commonly experienced during transitions but also to interrupt the cycle of repeated hospitalizations with the goal of promoting long-term positive outcomes.

Specifically, TCM provides comprehensive in-hospital planning and home follow-up for chronically ill high-risk older adults hospitalized for common medical and surgical conditions. Transitional care nurses (TCNs) with master's degrees in nursing and additional preparation in the care of people with multiple chronic conditions serve as the primary coordinator of care for patients receiving TCM. A TCN begins to interact with a patient, family caregivers, and involved health professionals at hospital admission. The same TCN continues to address the patient's individual needs and preferences throughout the hospitalization and for an average of two months after hospital discharge, providing an evidence-based protocol that includes regular home visits, ongoing, accessible telephone support, and personal communication with each patient's primary care physician during his or her first follow-up medical appointment to assure effective communication between providers.

TCM emphasizes coordination and continuity of care, prevention and avoidance of complications, and close clinical treatment and management to facilitate patients' transitions and their abilities to manage their care at home. Patients and family caregivers are actively engaged in the provision of care through the identification of health goals and education and community support. By developing streamlined, rational plans of care and by identifying and responding to health care risks and symptoms earlier, patterns of frequent acute hospital and emergency department use are interrupted, health status decline is prevented, and longer term positive outcomes are achieved.

In the three National Institute of Nursing (NINR)–funded randomized controlled clinical trials completed to date (Naylor et al., 1994, 1999, 2004), patients in the TCM intervention groups have consistently demonstrated significant improvements in clinical and economic outcomes when compared with control groups. Patients receiving TCM in the most recently completed multisite trial, for example, experienced significant improvements in physical function and quality of life in the short term, enhanced satisfaction with care, increased time to first readmission or death, and fewer total rehospitalizations through 52 weeks postdischarge (Naylor et al., 2004). After accounting for the cost of the intervention, the mean savings in total health care costs were $5,000 per patient.

Ongoing funding from the National Institute of Aging (NIA) and NINR as well as a number of foundations (the Commonwealth Fund, the Jacob and Valeria Langeloth Foundation, the John A. Hartford Foundation, Inc., the Gordon & Betty Moore Foundation, the California HealthCare Foundation, the Marian S. Ware Alzheimer's Program, and the Alzheimer's Association) has enabled University of Pennsylvania School of Nursing researchers to compare the effects of TCM to lower intensity interventions among cognitively impaired hospitalized older adults (NIA, R01-AG023116-06) (Naylor, 2004), examine changes in the trajectory of health and quality of life among frail elders who are newly transitioning to long term care (NIA and NINR, R01-AG025524-05) (Naylor, 2005), and establish partnerships with payers (e.g., Aetna Corporation, Kaiser Permanente Health Plan) to translate TCM into "real-world" clinical practice and to determine if the clinical and economic outcomes achieved in the randomized controlled clinical trials can be replicated.

In response to the aging of the population, the prevalence of chronic illness, and escalating health care costs, the demand for high value transitional care services has grown. Under the Affordable Care Act (ACA) (2010), for example, a community-based care transitions program has been enacted (Sec. 3026). Through ACA, $500 million in funding has been made available to implement transitional care programs targeting high-risk Medicare beneficiaries. TCM, as an effective, evidence-based approach, offers an innovative nurse-led, team-based solution that is responsive to the growing demand for high value transitional care services.

AARP. (2009). *Chronic Care: A Call to Action for Health Reform*. Washington, DC: Author.

Affordable Care Act, Pub. L. No. 111-148, § Sec. 3026. (2010).

Brooten, D., Kumar, S., Brown, L P., Butts, P., Finkler, S A., Bakewell-Sachs, S., et al. (Oct 9, 1986). A randomized clinical trial of early hospital discharge and home follow-up of very-low-birth-weight infants. *New England Journal of Medicine, 315*(15): 934–939.

Coleman, E. A., & Boult, C. (2003). Improving the quality of transitional care for persons with complex care needs. *Journal of the American Geriatrics Society, 51,* 556–557

Naylor, M. D. (2000). A decade of transitional care research with vulnerable elders. *Journal of Cardiovascular Nursing, 14*(3), 1–14.

Naylor, M. D. (2004). *Hospital to home: Cognitively impaired elders and their caregivers*. Sponsored by the National Institute on Aging, R01-AG023116-06, and the University of Pennsylvania Marian S. Ware Alzheimer's Program.

Naylor, M. D. (2005). Health related quality of life: Elders in long-term care. Sponsored by the National Institute on Aging, the National Institute of Nursing Research, R01-AG025524–05, and the University of Pennsylvania Marian S. Ware Alzheimer's Program.

Naylor, M. D., Brooten, D., Campbell, R., Jacobsen, B.S., Mezey, M.D., Pauley, M.V., et al. (1999). Comprehensive discharge planning and home follow-up of hospitalized elders: A randomized clinical trial. *Journal of the American Medical Association, 281,* 613–620.

Naylor, M. D., Brooten, D. A., Campell, R. L., Maislin, G., McCauley, K.M., & Schwartz, J.S. (2004). Transitional care of older adults hospitalized with heart failure: a randomized, controlled trial. *Journal of the American Geriatrics Society, 52,* 675–684.

Naylor, M., Brooten, D., Jones, R., Lavizzo-Mourey, R., Mezey, M., & Pauley, M. (1994). Comprehensive discharge planning for the hospitalized elderly. *Annals of Internal Medicine, 120,* 999–1006. Retrieved from http://www.transitionalcare.info

Mary D. Naylor

TRANSLATIONAL SCIENCE

Translational science is the bridge between laboratory discoveries and the applied sciences of health care disciplines. It ultimately develops knowledge about approaches that are both successful (efficacious) and useful (effective) in improving health care diagnosis, treatment, prevention, and health care delivery systems. While there is lack of consensus that translation is a "science," there is agreement that it is a significant paradigm shift, connecting previously siloed basic laboratory discoveries to human trials and then to point-of-care implementation. The shift also underscores that this must be accomplished through cross disciplinary collaboration and engagement of provider communities and consumer communities.

In the translational science continuum of research, connections between basic science and clinical care are specified during early community engagement. The first stage of translational science emphasizes the meaningfulness of bench research in human clinical trials. The latter portion of the translational science continuum focuses on health care service redesign that enhances rapid adoption of practices shown to be effective.

Translational science is considered essential for improving health care and outcomes. Those in the field investigate concepts about the individual patient and provider, the healthcare organization and system, and healthcare policies. Translational science is important to health care in that what works under controlled conditions is tested to see if it works in real-life situations: Does bench science translate into an efficacious treatment that can then shape bedside care and population health? Nurse scientists contribute research to each

stage along this continuum of translational science. Nurse leaders play essential roles in applying the findings for best practice, particularly in the latter stage of translational research.

Translational science and translational research are new terms in health care and both the scientific field and the definitions are still evolving. The term *translational science* became widely known in 2006, when the National Institutes of Health (NIH) launched the Clinical and Translational Science Award program (Zerhouni, 2005). Although today's literature contains a plethora of definitions for the term (Westfall, Mold, & Fagnan, 2007), the following description is cited in the recent NIH announcement for Clinical and Translational Science Awards: "Translational research includes two areas of translation. One is the process of applying discoveries generated during research in the laboratory, and in preclinical studies, to the development of trials and studies in humans. The second area of translation concerns research aimed at enhancing the adoption of best practices in the community. The comparative effectiveness of prevention and treatment strategies are [sic] also an important part of translational science" (NIH, 2010).

Accordingly, two translational blocks are referred to in translational science: T1 and T2. T1 refers to transferring laboratory discoveries about disease mechanisms into new methods for diagnosis, therapy, and prevention by first testing them in humans. T2 focuses on the translation of clinical studies results into clinical practice and health decision making (Sung et al., 2003). T1 is well developed as the enterprise that moves basic science into new drugs, devices, and treatment options for patients and is vital to advancing care. However, U.S. patients receive only half of recommended services (McGlynn et al.,

2003) because a second set of barriers exist in moving the evidence about effective treatment into widely practiced care; these barriers are the target of T2 research. The study of T2 processes is less developed than T1. However, it is an area of research of importance to nurses because it is concerned with closing the quality gap and improving access, refining systems of care, supporting informed choices of patient and clinicians, and providing point of care decision support tools (Woolf, 2008).

The focus of T2 translational research is to discover effective strategies to redesign care to be safe, efficient, and effective and to implement change and spread and sustain improvement. According to some experts (Dougherty & Conway, 2008), the translation continuum should extend to T3 activities that address the "how" of improving health care delivery. An example of this is discovering ways that health care can be delivered reliably to all patients in all settings of care and contribute to improving the health of individuals and populations. T3 activities include the development policy changes necessary to foster attempts to foster improve health outcomes. The paradigm shift heralded by translational science offers an unprecedented opportunity for productive collaboration between nurse leaders and academic scientists. Nurse leaders play essential roles in the investigation of T2-T3 questions, such as (1) identifying factors that speed adoption of best practices and (2) changing the context of the health care agency to spread and sustain best practices. As nurse leaders actively engage in translational science, it is likely that we will see rapid adoption of improvement changes by providers, patients, and the public.

Dougherty, D., & Conway, P. H. (2008). The "3T's" road map to transform US health care: The "How of high-quality care." *Journal of*
the American Medical Association, 299(19), 2319–2321.

McGlynn, E. A., Asch, S. M., Adams. J., Adams, J., Keesey, J,. Hicks, J., et al. (2003). The quality of health care delivered to adults in the United States. *New England Journal of Medicine, 348*(26), 2635–2645.

National Institutes of Health. (2010). Request for Applications (RFA) Number: FA-RM-10-001. Retrieved from http://grants.nih.gov/grants/guide/rfa-files/RFA-RM-10-001.html#SectionI

Sung, N. S., Crowley, W. F. Jr., Genel, M., Salber, P., Sandy, L., Sherwood, L. M., et al. (2003). Central challenges facing the national clinical research enterprise. *Journal of the American Medical Association, 289*(10), 1278–1287.

Westfall, J. M., Mold, J., & Fagnan, L. (2007). Practice-based research—"Blue highways" on the NIH roadmap. *Journal of the American Medical Association, 297,* 403–406.

Woolf, S. H. (2008). The meaning of translational research and why it matters. *Journal of the American Medical Association, 299*(2), 211–213.

Zerhouni, E. A. (2005). Translational and clinical science—Time for a new vision. *New England Journal of Medicine, 353*(15), 1621–1623.

Kathleen R. Stevens

TRUTH ABOUT NURSING

In 2001, the Center for Nursing Advocacy was established by seven graduate nursing students at Johns Hopkins University School of Nursing who came together to help address the nursing shortage. In 2008, the Center for Nursing Advocacy announced the dissolution of the Center as a corporation and re-branded itself as the Truth About Nursing, which continued to pursue its previous, original mission. The founders hoped that using informal, alternative, or hybrid approaches to media analysis would help to dispel myths and commonly held beliefs about the nursing

T

profession that made it less attractive to pursue for employment. This mission—to increase public understanding of the central, front-line role that nurses play is health care—is accomplished by attempting to promote positive portrayals of nurses in the media and encouraging the media to consult with expert nurses. Using comic or irreverent elements to critique the media, the Truth About Nursing seeks to capture the attention and interest of those who create media. Some of their activities include ranking best and worst media portrayals of nursing, the use of letter-writing campaigns to make nurses' voices heard, reviewing and analyzing media, discussion forums for exchange of ideas, encouraging nurses to create nurse-friendly media, and monitoring the media. In addition, the Web site has links for frequently asked questions, general information on nurses and nursing, an archive of news about nurses and nursing in the media, individual media reviews, literature supporting the work of the organization, a press room for information available to the media, and an opportunity to contact the organization and use their search function. The Truth About Nursing hosted its first conference, Empowering Nurses and Improving Care through Better Understanding of Nursing, in the spring of 2011, to create a national opportunity to participate with experts to develop and hone abilities to gain respect for the profession of nursing. Information about success stories about a number of large and small corporations that have modified their advertising to be more sensitive to how nurses is portrayed and their image exploited for financial gain is also found on the website. Donations are welcome because the Truth About Nursing is nonprofit and needs donations to sustain its mission of advocacy. Ultimately, the Truth About Nursing seeks to improve the image of nursing, which, in turn, will attract people to the nursing profession, thereby providing a long-term solution to the fluctuating global nursing shortage.

Paule V. Joseph
Harriet R. Feldman

W–Z

World Health Organization (WHO)

The World Health Organization (WHO) was founded April 7, 1948, a day that is celebrated annually as World Health Day. WHO (www.who.int) is a component of the United Nations and is an international agency with a variety of purposes including: providing leadership on an international view of health issues, creating research efforts focused on health issues, establishing policy standards, and monitoring the health issues across the world (WHO, 2010a). The World Health Assembly governs this organization and meets in Geneva, Switzerland, on a yearly basis. This meeting is attended by delegates representing the 193 member states. The Executive Board is made up of 34 members who agree to serve for 3-year terms; the Executive Board meets semiannually. The primary functions of the Executive Board are to advise and assist the inner workings of the World Health Assembly. WHO has a primary Director-General who is appointed by the World Health Assembly upon the recommendation of the Executive Board. This position is a 5-year term (www.who.int/mediacentre/events/governance/eb/en/index.html). A major priority of WHO continues to be the control and prevention of three deadly infectious diseases: HIV/AIDS, tuberculosis, and malaria. Six million people die of these diseases every year, and 2.7 million people were newly infected with HIV in 2008 alone. It is estimated that 33.4 million people were living with HIV in 2008. Unfortunately, only 37% will have access to prevention or transmission information and tragically, millions are without antiretroviral medications (WHO, 2010b). A second goal current goal is to decrease deaths of children under the age of 5 years, as close to 11 million young children die each year with the largest numbers located in sub-Saharan Africa and south Asia. Ninety percent of these deaths are a result of six medical causes, including diarrhea, HIV/AIDS, malaria, measles, neonatal difficulties, and pneumonia (WHO, 2010a). A third priority of WHO in 2006 was to improve the health of all women, with focus on new mothers as more than 500,000 women die each year in either pregnancy or childbirth. Unfortunately, these deaths are not disease related but rather caused by severe lack of prenatal and birthing care. Recent studies confirm that the health care needs of women from adolescence through older age are severely lacking and urgent action has been requested to address this surprising, new development (WHO, 2010c).

World Health Organization. (2010a). *About WHO*. Retrieved November 18, 2010, from http://www.who.int/about/en

World Health Organization. (2010b). *HIV/AIDS: Data and statistics*. Retrieved November 18, 2010, from http://www.who.int/hiv/data/en

World Health Organization. (2010c). *Women and health: Today's evidence tomorrow's agenda*. Retrieved November 19, 2010, from http://www.who.int/gender/women_health_report/en/index.html

Ronda Mintz-Binder

WRITING FOR PUBLICATION

Writing for publication is a form of expression that allows the nurse leader to communicate to a wide audience. A nurse leader's thoughts published in an academic journal, clinical magazine, or even the local paper have a potential audience of thousands of interested readers. Those readers may be peers in the field of health care, members of other disciplines, or the general public. Nurse leaders who publish need not be possessed of advanced degrees nor have extensive writing experience. In fact, nurses who lead change at any level of their organization or community will find that they can contribute in a way that will be of interest and benefit to others. Several compelling arguments exist for why nurse leaders should write for publication. By engaging in this process, nurses can advance nursing knowledge, advance the nursing profession, and advance themselves personally.

Nurses disseminate specialized nursing knowledge to their colleagues when they share the results of targeted literature reviews, evidence-based practice projects, local research, or even successful change efforts in their organization. Nurse leaders are active problem solvers and are thus constantly looking for ways to improve the quality of care received by patients. By publishing the results of their efforts, they not only provide a foundation for others with similar problems but open a dialogue between nurses that may lead to enhanced solutions. Peers from multiple locations and organizations can work together to refine new ideas and innovations as well as suggest creative alternatives. Ultimately, by advancing nursing knowledge through publication, nurse leaders can lead widespread change in patient care.

Nurse leaders also contribute to the advancement of the nursing profession when they generate and disseminate nursing knowledge. Publication of this knowledge allows nurses to regulate their profession through the testing of others' ideas, thus maintaining nursing as a unique discipline among the health care professions. In addition, publishing is one method of advancing the profession to the public. Nurse leaders can write letters to the editor or commentaries for newspapers and magazines about a wide range of topics, increasing nursing's voice in the development of public policy. These public forums can also be used to educate the community about clinical and practice issues. When nurse leaders use their expertise to write about common health problems, such as managing heart failure or diabetes, it increases the visibility and credibility of the nursing profession while providing a valuable service to the community.

Personal advancement is another compelling reason for nurse leaders to write for publication. The process of constructing an argument and polishing it for publication often provides new insights into the process, problem, or solution under consideration, enhancing the nurse leader's practice in that area. The skills developed while writing for publication also lend themselves to improvement in other leadership activities, such as developing project proposals or evidence-based practice protocols. Writing for publication can not only contribute to enhanced job performance but also benefit one's career as well. Publications are impressive entries on curriculum vitae and may be necessary for career advancement, consultative positions, and awards and honors. An article published in a professional journal often brings feedback from previously untapped sources, which provides networking opportunities that may prove beneficial for both learning and career advancement. Finally, seeing one's efforts published in a permanently archived forum is extremely satisfying, and provides a sense of lasting accomplishment.

Given the many reasons to write for publication, nurse leaders may be excited to get started but unsure where to begin. Fortunately, there are many resources available to assist nurse leaders in their writing endeavors. Several books and articles provide guidance for style, grammar, and formatting of references, as well as "how-to" instructions for the creation and submission of papers to professional journals. Beginning writers should invest in texts such as *The Elements of Style* (Strunk & White, 2000) and the *Publication Manual of the American Psychological Association* (American Psychological Association, 2010), as these will be useful throughout their career. However, most importantly, nurse leaders should realize they already possess the basic skills to communicate with and educate others; using and expanding those skills to write for publication will benefit nursing knowledge, the profession, and the nurse.

American Psychological Association. (2010). *Publication manual of the American Psychological Association* (6th ed.). Washington, DC: Author.

Strunk, W., & White, E.B. (2000). *The elements of style* (4th ed.). Needham Heights, MA: Allyn & Bacon.

Patricia S. Groves
Vicki S. Conn

W–Z

HISTORICAL LEADERSHIP FIGURES

Gina M. Myers

INTRODUCTION

The nurses included in this section embodied leadership skills that continue to be relevant to current practice. While there are many nurses in history who are admired for their accomplishments, those included speak directly to nurse leaders in administration, academia, research, and practice. Their successes and struggles provide useful lessons for obtaining equity in the profession, maintaining the integrity of nursing practice, and the adoption of innovative programs and practices in the face of resistance. Their endeavors inspire our continued work in advancing the profession.

Leaders in academia include Rachel Louise McManus who is celebrated as one of the first nurses to obtain a doctoral degree. Her achievement encouraged others to do the same by making the PhD a possibility for nurses at a time when the necessity of the degree was not well understood. By opening this door, she provided the profession an access to the training needed to establish and grow our knowledge base. Annie Warburton Goodrich and Mary Adelaide Nutting were among those who used their expertise to open schools, allowing nurses better access to opportunities to advance their education at the baccalaureate and master's level.

Isabel Hampton Robb first advocated for standardization of nurse training when there were no guidelines in place, and Veronica M. Driscoll carried out this difficult task more recently in her role in creating the blueprint for higher education in nursing. Their efforts have helped to create the culture in which anyone who is called a registered nurse is known to be held to consistently high standards. Others developed specialized programs to address gaps in nursing, such as the associate degree nursing program by Mildred L. Montag, which continues to educate a large part of our nursing workforce today.

These leaders also had a hand in advancing nursing specialty practice, including the development of psychiatric nursing by Hildegard Peplau and the progression of public health nursing by Lillian Wald. Both were forerunners in setting their practice arenas apart as specialties and developed lasting programs to help nurses learn and refine the skills required to meet unique patient needs. More recently, Karen Buhler-Wilkerson focused her talents on developing a university-based home care program, showing that nurse leaders can make old ideas new again by using their resources and connections in innovative ways. Nursing was also impacted by the creation of the clinical nurse specialist role by Laura L. Simms and the contribution of the concept of team nursing by Eleanor C. Lambertson; both concepts are still widely used in health care organizations.

Alongside the advancement in specialty practice was the growth in status of ethnically diverse nurses. Leaders in the movement to bring about equality for all nurses included Mabel Keaton Staupers, Estelle Massey Osborne, Mary Elizabeth Carnegie, and most recently Ildaura Murillo-Rohde. Without their courageous efforts and willingness to put themselves in controversial positions, the advancement of African American and Hispanic nurses would not have made the leaps and bounds as it did. An environment has been created in which diversity is embraced and equality expected by tackling issues of discrimination in the profession, including the need for minority nurses to organize so that their voices could be heard.

Other leaders, including Lucille Elizabeth Notter and Harriet Werley advanced nursing science by pioneering and leading the efforts of some of the most esteemed nursing research journals and books. From Florence Nightingale's efforts in the Crimean War early on to Notter's work in establishing the credibility and prestige of the journal *Nursing Research* in more recent times, these leaders kept the focus on advancing nursing scholarship by generating new knowledge through research, disseminating findings to those in practice, and providing the resources for nurses to learn more about the research process.

This section inspires nurses at all levels to take on leadership roles, whether they be formal or informal. The past leaders presented in this encyclopedia have demonstrated that it does not take an army of nurses to make great changes. Many of their accomplishments did not happen quickly or easily; the necessary ingredients for success were the ability to persevere, skill in presenting nursing's needs clearly and with conviction, and an unrelenting vision of a better profession. Most of these individuals did not have access to funding or technology, but used what they had wisely, relied on their network of nurse colleagues, and employed remarkable problem-solving and program-planning skills in completing their goals. Their examples inspire us to push past our own limits to move the profession forward in meaningful ways that will create better-prepared nurses, stronger organizations, and optimal patient outcomes.

M. Janice Nelson is acknowledged as the original contributor to a number of the Historical Leadership Figures written about in this section.

CLARISSA HARLOWE BARTON
(1821–1912)

Clarrisa [Clara] Harlowe Barton is most notably remembered as the founder of the American Red Cross (1881), holding the position of president for 22 years. She is regarded as a truly dedicated American patriot for her work in the Civil War and her devotion in bringing quality health care practices to the United States (Halamandaris, n.d.). Clara was an energetic leader who did not hesitate to roll up her sleeves and role model professional nursing behaviors by acting as a health care advocate and philanthropist. She frequently organized efforts to collect donations of supplies for soldiers and was also instrumental in locating missing soldiers after the war (Faust, 1986). Barton was extremely influential in global politics and health care abroad as well as domestically, fueling the movement of public health nurses locally and internationally. Barton was a recipient of the Iron Cross of Merit and authored a number of books about the initiation of the Red Cross and the Red Cross Movement in general (American Red Cross Museum, n.d.; Halamandaris, n.d.). She also wrote the American amendment to the Red Cross constitution and founded the National First Aid Society in 1904. She was inducted into the National Women's Hall of Fame in 1973 in recognition of her commitment to the well-being of society (National Women's Hall of Fame, n.d.).

American Red Cross Museum. (n.d.). *Clara Barton: Founder of the American Red Cross.* Retrieved November 6, 2010, from http://www.redcross.org/museum/history/claraBarton.asp

Faust, P. I. (Ed.). (1986). *Historical times illustrated encyclopedia of the Civil War.* Retrieved November 6, 2010, from http://www.civilwarhome.com/bartonbio.htm

Halamandaris, V.J. (n.d.). *Profiles in caring* (Column 101). Retrieved November 6, 2010, from http://www.nahc.org/NAHC/Val/Columns/SC10.html

National Women's Hall of Fame. (n.d.). *Women of the hall: Clara Barton.* Retrieved November 6, 2010, from http://greatwomen.org/women.php?action=viewone&id=17

KAREN BUHLER-WILKERSON
(1944–2010)

Karen Buhler-Wilkerson was an innovative leader in the field of home care and also a passionate nurse historian. She received both her bachelor's degree (1966) and master's degree (1969) from Emory University, going on to complete a PhD from the University of Pennsylvania in Health Care History and Policy (University of Pennsylvania, 2010). One of her most remarkable achievements includes being a founder of Penn Nursing Living Independently for Elders program. This program provides home care to residents of West Philadelphia who are considered poor and frail. It has been in existence since 1999 and is the only university-based program of its type in the country (Milone-Nuzzo, 2010). Buhler-Wilkerson's scholarship activities have contributed to approximately 40 publications and three books in nursing. Her best-known work is *No Place Like Home: A History of Nursing and Home Care in the United States* (2001). She also wrote *The Call to the Nurse: Healing at Home: Visiting Nurse Service of New York, 1893–1993* (Milone-Nuzzo, 2010; University of Pennsylvania, 2008).

Buhler-Wilkerson was also the director of the Barbara Bates Center for the Study of the History of Nursing and has twice received the Lavinia Dock Award for Exemplary Historical Research and Writing from the American Association for the History of Nursing as well as the Agnes Dillon Randolph Award for Significant Contributions to the Field of Nursing History from the Center for Nursing Inquiry at the University of Virginia School of Nursing. She was invited to be a fellow of the American Academy of Nurses in 1989 (University of Pennsylvania, 2008, 2010).

Milone-Nuzzo, P. (2010). In Memoriam: Dr. Karen Buhler-Wilkerson. *Home Healthcare Nurse, 28*(6), 325–326.

University of Pennsylvania. (2008). *Karen Buhler-Wilkerson, PhD, FAAN, RN: Professor of Community Health Nursing*. Retrieved December 29, 2010, from http://www.nursing.upenn.edu/faculty/profile.asp?pid=125

University of Pennsylvania. (2010). A tribute to Karen Buhler Wilkerson. *The Chronicle, 22*(1), 1–7. Retrieved December 29, 2010, from http://www.nursing.upenn.edu/history/Documents/spring10.pdf

MARY ELIZABETH CARNEGIE
(1916–2008)

Mary Elizabeth Carnegie was a courageous and committed nurse who was devoted to removing the barriers that stood in the way of the advancement of Black nurses. She graduated from Lincoln Hospital School for Nurses (1937) and went on to receive a bachelor's degree from West Virginia State College, a master's degree from Syracuse University, and a doctorate in public administration from New York University (American Nurses Association [ANA], 2008; New York Nurse, 2008). In 1948, she became president of the Florida State Chapter of the National Association of Colored Graduate Nurses; at the same time, she was appointed a "courtesy member" of the Florida State Nurses Association but was not given the privilege of speaking or voting. However, Carnegie ignored the rules and spoke freely at the meetings and was elected to the Florida State Nurses Association Board the following year. Her victory started a domino effect that ended the period of all-White state nurses associations in the South (New York Nurse, 2008). She served as the first dean of the Florida A&M University School of Nursing and initiated the baccalaureate nursing program at Hampton University in Virginia (ANA, 2008; Foundation of the New York State Nurses Association, 2010). Dr. Carnegie mentored many young nurses, encouraging them to advance their education. She worked for the *American Journal of Nursing* (1953–1978), was an editor emeritus of *Nursing Research*, and wrote *The Path We Tread: Blacks in Nursing Worldwide, 1854–1994*. Her awards include the George Arens Pioneer Medal from Syracuse University, the President's Award from Sigma Theta Tau International, and the Living Legend Award from the Association of Black Nurse Faculty in Higher Education. She was inducted into the ANA Hall of Fame in 2000 (ANA, 2008).

American Nurses Association. (2008). *Mary Elizabeth Carnegie (1916–2008) 2000 Inductee.* Retrieved January 6, 2011, from http://www.nursingworld.org/MaryElizabethCarnegie

Foundation of the New York State Nurses Association. (2010). *In memoriam: Dr. Mary Elizabeth Carnegie.* Retrieved January 3, 2011, from http://foundationnysnurses.org/inmemoriam/index.php

New York Nurse. (2008). *Mary Elizabeth Carnegie—The pathfinder.* Retrieved January 6, 2011, from http://www.nysna.org/publications/newyorknurse/2008/feb/carnegie.htm

LAVINIA LLOYD DOCK
(1858–1956)

Lavinia Lloyd Dock, the ardent suffragette, political activist, and author graduated from the Bellevue Training School for Nurses in 1886. Dock held a number of positions, including Assistant Superintendent of Nurses under the leadership of Isabel Hampton Robb at the Johns Hopkins Training School for Nurses in Baltimore. For a short time, she was Superintendent of Nurses at the Illinois Training School and worked with Lillian Wald at the Henry Street Settlement for some 20 years (American Association of the History of Nursing, 2006). Dock authored one of the first nursing text books, *Materia Medica for Nurses*, served as the foreign editor for the *American Journal of Nursing*, and authored the four volumes of *History of Nursing*; the first two volumes of which were co-authored with Mary Adelaide Nutting. This well-connected early leader insisted that nursing would never be accepted as a respectable profession until women "get the vote!" (Christy, 1969). This was her vision and passion for women and nurses. After the age of 50, she devoted most of her time to women's suffrage and political action.

In an autobiographical sketch, Dock wrote that she was most satisfied with two events in her life, "…doing the history with Miss Nutting and going to jail with the Women's Party" (Dock, 1930). Dock was inducted into the American Nurses Association Hall of Fame in 1976 (American Nurses Association, 2008).

American Association of the History of Nursing. (n.d.). *Gravesites of prominent nurses.* Retrieved November 7, 2010, from http://www.aahn.org/gravesites/dock.html

American Nurses Association. (2008). *1976 Inductee. Lavinia Lloyd Dock. 1858–1956.* Retrieved November 7, 2010, from http://www.nursing world.org/FunctionalMenuCategories/About ANA/Honoring-Nurses/HallofFame/ 19761982/dockll5531.aspx

Christy, T. E. (1969). *Cornerstone for nursing education. A history of the division of nursing education of Teachers College, Columbia University, 1899–1947.* New York, NY: Teachers College Press.

Dock, L. L. (1930). Autobiographical Sketch. *Lavinia L. Dock by Lavinia Lloyd Dock.* Typewritten manuscript. Archives of the Alumnae Association of the Bellevue School of Nursing, Inc. Veronica M. Driscoll Center for Nursing, Albany, NY.

Veronica M. Driscoll
(1926–1994)

Veronica M. Driscoll spent much of her career advancing the nursing profession and advocating for the economic security of nurses through better pay, better benefits, and an acceptable work environment. She was a graduate of St. Catherine's Hospital School of Nursing in Brooklyn (1948). She went on to receive her bachelor's degree from St. John's University (1953), her master's degree from New York University (1958), and her doctorate degree from Teachers College, Columbia University (Birnbach, 2000). She held positions in nursing education and administration before she joined the New York State Nurses Association (NYSNA) as deputy executive director in 1960; she served as executive director from 1969 to 1979 (*New York Times*, 1994). As executive director, she worked to double the organization's membership and streamline operations and established NYSNA as the largest RN collective bargaining unit nationwide (American Nurses Association [ANA], 2007). While she was in this position, the NYSNA publications *Report* and *Journal* were introduced and the Foundation of NYSNA was established; she served as the first executive director (Birnbach, 2000). In addition, Driscoll was active in the 1972 revision of New York State's Nurse Practice Act, which is still in place today. She also had a hand in developing *A Blueprint for the Education of Nurses in New York State*, which supported higher education for nurses, specifically the bachelor's degree (Birnbach, 2000; Foundation of NYSNA, 2010). Driscoll was active nationally with the ANA, serving as the chairperson of the Commission on Economic and General Welfare. She was inducted into the ANA's Hall of Fame in 2002 (ANA, 2007). The foundation's corporate headquarters was designated in her name when she resigned in 1979 (Foundation of NYSNA, 2010).

American Nurses Association. (2007). *Veronica Margaret Driscoll (1926–1994): 2002 Inductee.* Retrieved from http://www.nursingworld.org/VeronicaMargaretDriscoll

Birnbach, N. (2000). Veronica Margaret Driscoll 1926–1994. In V. Bullough & L. Sentz (Eds.), *American Nursing: A Biographical Dictionary* (Vol. 3). New York: Springer Publishing Company.

Foundation of New York State Nurses Association. (2010). Retrieved January 5, 2011, from http://foundationnysnurses.org/aboutus/VeronicaDriscollCenter.php

New York Times. (1994). Veronica Driscoll, 67, Head of Nurses' Group. Retrieved January 5, 2011, from http://www.nytimes.com/1994/02/02/obituaries/veronica-driscoll-67-head-of-nurses-group.html

ANNIE WARBURTON GOODRICH
(1866–1954)

Annie Warburton Goodrich held a variety of administrative positions in acute care, home care, and education; her last being the Dean of the nursing program at Yale University. While in that role, she spoke about the need for ethics in nursing and the importance of education, not just training, highlighting the need for nursing to move forward in knowledge rather than relying on past practice (Smith, 1980). She obtained her nursing education at New York Hospital in 1892. She was awarded the honorary degree of Doctor of Science from Mount Holyoke College (1921), the honorary degree of Master of Arts from Yale University (1923), and the honorary degree of Doctor of Laws from Russell Sage College (1936) (Burst, 1998). In 1924, Goodrich developed and became dean of the first nursing program at Yale University; it was the first university in the United States to grant the Bachelors degree to nurses (Tomes, 1980). Ten years later, she put the graduate program into place (American Nurses Association [ANA], 2007). She served the profession as president of the ANA, president of the Association of Collegiate Schools of Nursing, president of the American Society of Superintendents of Training Schools for Nurses, and president of the International Council of Nurses (ANA, 2007; Burst, 1998). Her numerous honors include Fellow of the American College of Hospital Administrators, Medal of National Institute of Social Science, Distinguished Service Medal of the United States, Walter Burns Saunders Medal, Adelaide Nutting Medal, and the Yale Medal "for outstanding service to Yale" (Burst, 1998). She was inducted into the ANA Hall of Fame in 1976 (ANA, 2007).

American Nurses Association. (2007). *Annie Warburton Goodrich (1866–1954) 1976 Inductee.* Retrieved January 3, 2011, from http://www.nursingworld.org/Functional MenuCategories/AboutANA/Honoring-Nurses/HallofFame/19761982/goodaw5541. aspx

Burst, H. V. (1998). *Yale University School of Nursing: A brief history.* Retrieved January 5, 2011, from http://www.med.yale.edu/library/nursing/historical/deans/goodrich.html

Smith, J. P. (1980). Dean Annie Warburton Goodrich: A nurse of our time. *Journal of Advanced Nursing, 5,* 347–348.

Tomes, N. (1980). Goodrich, Annie Warburton. In B. Sicherman & C. Green (Eds.). *Notable American women: The modern period (Vol. 4).* United States: Radcliffe College. Retrieved January 5, 2011, from http://books.google.com/books?id=CfGHM9K U7aEC&pg=PA288&lpg=PA288&dq=An nie+Warburton+Goodrich&source=bl& ots=Oq4Gqco8es&sig=94w9_sSgW9avh-QPom3p0xffiPQ&hl=en&ei=xQp0TKG_ AoP78AbAt5n2CA&sa=X&oi=book_result& ct=result&resnum=9&ved=0CC4Q6AEwCD gU#v=onepage&q=Annie%20Warburton%20 Goodrich&f=false

VIRGINIA A. HENDERSON
(1897–1996)

Virginia Avenel Henderson was a multi-faceted, forward-thinking leader in nursing whose national and international endeavors are often compared to those of Florence Nightingale (American Nurses Association, 2007). She held many accomplished positions including a faculty member for 14 years at Teachers College, Columbia University, a cofounder of the Interagency Council on Information Resources in Nursing, a cofounder of the New England Regional Council on Library Resources for Nursing, the first chairperson of the *International Index* Editorial Advisory Committee, and a member of the International Nurses Council. Henderson produced the first *Annotated Index of Nursing Research* while on faculty at Yale University, inciting a research movement in the field that led to the recognition of nursing as a professional and respected occupation. She was one of the first nurses to elucidate that nursing was not just merely following physicians' orders but could be used as a therapeutic mechanism in and of itself. Henderson was an innovator in identifying key concepts such as continuity of care, patient advocacy, multidisciplinary scholarship, outcomes orientation, and health promotion. She created a definition of nursing that was internationally accepted and clearly delineated the field of nursing from the field of medicine (Allen, n.d.). Further, she has been called the "greatest nurse advocate for libraries" (Allen, n.d.). The Sigma Theta Tau International Library is named to honor her (Sigma Theta Tau International, 2010). Henderson was inducted posthumously into the American Nurses Association Hall of Fame in 1996 (American Nurses Association, 2007).

Allen, M. (n.d.). *Interagency Council on Information Resources for Nursing (ICIRN) Tribute to Virginia Avernal Henderson 1897–1996.* Retrieved November 7, 2010, from http://www.sandiego.edu/academics/nursing/theory/henderson.htm

American Nurses Association. (2007). *Virginia A. Henderson (1897–1996): 1996 inductee.* Retrieved November 7, 2010, from http://www.nursingworld.org/VirginiaAHenderson

Sigma Theta Tau International. (2010). *Virginia Henderson International Library: About the library.* Retrieved November 7, 2010, from http://www.nursinglibrary.org/portal/Main.aspx?PageID=4002

ELEANOR C. LAMBERTSEN
(1915–1998)

Eleanor C. Lambertsen was a leader at the bedside and in the education arena. She earned her bachelor's, master's, and doctoral degrees at Teachers College, Columbia University (Foundation of New York State Nurses, 2010). Her dissertation spearheaded the concept of team nursing as a model for nursing practice. Her work was carried out in a demonstration project at Francis Delafield Hospital and attracted the attention of administrators all over the country (Saxton, 1998). In her career, she served the profession as a president of the American Nurses Foundation, as a director of the Division of Nursing of the American Hospital Association, as a dean of the Cornell University/New York Hospital School of Nursing, as a senior associate director of Nursing at New York Hospital, and as a director of the Division of Health Services, Sciences, and Education while concomitantly serving as a Helen Hartley Professor of Nursing Education and Chair of the Department of Nursing at Teachers College. Lambertsen was also a member of the Surgeon General's Consulting Group that initiated the first Nurse Training Act, which provided a significant source of federal funding for nursing education (New York Times, 1998), and her work strongly contributed to the revised legal definition of nursing in the New York State Practice Act (Foundation of New York State Nurses, 2010). Her experiences in education and service enabled her to educate the public on the value of nursing education and on the need to change the structure of hospital nursing services (University of Pennsylvania, 2010).

Foundation of New York State Nurses. (2010). *Bellevue Alumnae Center for Nursing History: Eleanor Lambertsen Papers.* Retrieved November 7, 2010, from http://foundation-nysnurses.org/bellevue/guidetoarchivalrecords/collections/collections_abs02.php

New York Times. (1998). *Lambertsen, Eleanor C., ED.D, R.N. New York Times Paid Notice: Deaths.* Retrieved November 7, 2010, from http://www.nytimes.com/1998/04/01/classified/paid-notice-deaths-lambertsen-eleanor-c-edd-rn.html

Saxton. W. (1998). *Eleanor C. Lambertsen, 82; Introduced Use of Nurse Teams. New York Times Obituaries.* Retrieved November 7, 2010, from http://www.nytimes.com/1998/04/10/nyregion/eleanor-c-lambertsen-82-introduced-use-of-nurse-teams.html

University of Pennsylvania. (2010). *Lambertsen, Eleanor C., Papers, 1915–1977, BC2.* Retrieved November 7, 2010, from http://www.nursing.upenn.edu/history/Documents/Eleanor%20C%20Lambertsen.pdf

Rachel Louise McManus
(1896–1993)

Rachel Louise McManus was a leader who was committed to advancing the nursing profession through education and ensuring quality nursing care through the standardization of knowledge necessary for licensure. She earned her nursing diploma at the Massachusetts General Hospital School of Nursing and went on to complete her baccalaureate, master's, and doctoral degrees at Teachers College, Columbia University. She remained connected with Teachers College for 36 years, serving in the roles of faculty and dean. McManus was the first nurse to earn a PhD and was a vital part of the effort to establish schools of nursing in colleges and universities (National Women's Hall of Fame, n.d.). In collaboration with the Committee on Measurements and Educational Guidance of the National League for Nursing Education, she was instrumental in the development of prenursing tests, pre-tests for clinical nursing courses, achievement tests in the sciences, and tests in clinical nursing. The application of these batteries of tests brought about national standardization of nurse licensing exams (Christy, 1969). In recognition of her contributions, the National Council of State Boards of Nursing established the R. Louise McManus Award and the Meritorious Service Award in her honor (Rothwell, 2006). The R. Louise McManus Medal was established by the Teachers College Nursing Education Alumni Association to recognize longstanding contributions of a distinguished nature to the nursing profession (Nursing Education Alumni Association, n.d.). R. Louise McManus was inducted into the National Women's Hall of Fame in 1994 for her accomplishments (National Women's Hall of Fame, n.d.).

Christy, T.E. (1969). *Cornerstone for nursing education. A History of the division of nursing education of teachers college, Columbia University, 1899–1947.* New York: Teachers College Press.

National Women's Hall of Fame. (n.d.). *Women of the hall: R. Louise McManus.* Retrieved November 8, 2010, from http://www.greatwomen.org/women.php?action=viewone&id=108

Nursing Education Alumni Association. (n.d.). *Achievement awards. Criteria for specific NEAA achievement awards.* Retrieved November 8, 2010, from http://www.tcneaa.org/awards/achievementawards.html

Rothwell, K. (2001). *National women's history month: Honoring nurses' courage and vision.* Retrieved November 8, 2010, from http://www.nursezone.com/Nursing-News-Events/more-features/National-Women%E2%80%99s-History-Month-Honoring-Nurses%E2%80%99-Courage-and-Vision_21014.aspx

MILDRED L. MONTAG
(1908–2004)

Mildred Louise Montag earned a baccalaureate degree in history from Hamline University, St. Paul, Minnesota, in 1930, a baccalaureate in nursing from the University of Minnesota, and a master's and doctorate in Nursing Education (EdD) at Teachers College, Columbia University. She is most widely known for her doctoral dissertation, *The Education of Nursing Technicians*, completed at Teachers College. This work ignited the associate degree movement in nursing and helped it evolve from an idea into hundreds of programs held at community and junior colleges across the nation. Montag was instrumental in increasing the number of nurses in this country and changing the nursing population by providing greater access for minorities, males, adult learners, married students, and other diverse populations of students who were interested in becoming nurses (Klainberg, n.d.; Teachers College, 2004). Throughout her career, Montag held a number of professional positions, which include a faculty member at the University of Minnesota School of Nursing and an instructor at St. Luke's Hospital School of Nursing (New York). She is credited with developing and growing the School of Nursing at Adelphi University. She served as its director from 1943 until she left to do her doctoral work at Teachers College in 1948 (Klainberg, n.d.).

Klainberg. M. (n.d.). *History of the school: Dr. Mildred Montag.* Retrieved November 8, 2010, from http://nursing.adelphi.edu/about/history.php

Teachers College, Columbia University News. (2004). *News and Publications: Mildred Montag, 95, dies.* Retrieved November 8, 2010, from http://www.tc.columbia.edu/news/article.htm?id=4717

ILDAURA MURILLO-ROHDE
(1920–2010)

Ildaura Murillo-Rohde, PhD, RN, FAAN, was born in Panama on September 6, 1920, and arrived in the United States in 1945. She died in 2010. One of her greatest accomplishments was founding the National Association of Hispanic Nurses (NAHN; nahnnet.org/NAHNFounder. html) in 1975 and serving as its first president (NAHN, 2011). She realized the pressing need for this group early in her career; very few Hispanic nurses were working in academia, conducting research, or providing information to policymakers regarding the health care needs of the Hispanic people. Her goal was to provide an organization in which Hispanic nurses could have a more formal and collective voice to enhance their professionalism and practice. She also felt strongly that part of the role of the NAHN was to strongly encourage and support members in pursuing advanced nursing education (Chwedyk, 2001). Murillo-Rohde can claim a few other "firsts." She was the first Hispanic nurse to earn a PhD from New York University (1971), the first Hispanic Associate Dean at the University of Washington, and the first Hispanic Dean at the School of Nursing at New York University (Millan, 2010). Her practice background was in psychiatric nursing and she offered her nursing expertise internationally while working with UNICEF (New York University, 2010). The NAHN has established an award and scholarship in her name. The award honors members who have outstanding accomplishments in education, research, or practice, and the scholarship supports students enrolled in nursing school (NAHN, 2011). Murillo-Rohde has received the Hildegard Peplau Lifetime Achievement Award and was named a Living Legend of the American Academy of Nursing in 1994. Both honors recognize her continuous commitment and professional contributions to the Hispanic nursing community (American Academy of Nursing, 2010; Millan, 2010).

American Academy of Nursing. (2010). *AAN living legend, Ildaura Murillo-Rohde, passes away.* Retrieved from http://www.aan-net.org/i4a/headlines/headlinedetails.cfm?id=280

Chwedyk, P. (2001). 25 and counting: The National Association of Hispanic Nurses marks its first quarter century of advancing the agenda for Hispanic health care needs. *Minority Nurse.* Retrieved from http://www.minoritynurse.com/associations-and-organizations/25-and-counting

Millan, A. (2010). President's message. *National Association of Hispanic Nurses at a Glance, 4*(1), 1. Retrieved from http://www.thehispanic-nurses.org/newsletter/2010ANovemberNAHNataGlance.pdf

National Association of Hispanic Nurses. (2011). *History.* Retrieved from http://nahnnet.org/AboutNAHN.html#History

New York University. (2010). NYU College of Nursing creates a legacy of deans. *NYU Nursing, 6*(1), 8. Retrieved from http://www.thehispanicnurses.org/newsletter/2010ANovemberNAHNataGlance.pdf

FLORENCE NIGHTINGALE
(1820–1910)

Florence Nightingale has been described as brilliant, inspiring, witty, and dedicated yet has also been called stubborn and meddling by some (Vicinus & Nergaard, 1987). These characteristics contribute to her versatility as a leader and her tireless passion to provide quality care for patients using research evidence. She was a staunch hospital reformer and a brilliant statistician whose organizational skills revolutionized hospital environments when she introduced ventilation and sanitation. Her early research efforts brought about great changes for the military. Nightingale's accomplishments during the Crimean War are legendary. Her attention to the environment and application of basic hygiene principles reduced the death rate from nearly 43% to 2.5% among the wounded soldiers (Cook, 1913). Nightingale pioneered the use of graphics in statistical analysis; she originated the use of pie graphs and tables to illustrate her points—a tactic which was previously unknown in nursing (Palmer, 1977). In 1860, she established the *Nightingale Training School for Nurses* in London (Baly, 1998). Despite her incapacitation in later years, Nightingale published books and pamphlets, and she wrote more than 10,000 letters—most of which are housed in the Library of the British Museum and the Greater London Record Office (Vicinus & Nergaard, 1989).

Baly, M. E. (1998). *Florence Nightingale and the nursing legacy*. Bainbridge Books: Philadelphia.

Cook, Sir E. (1913). *The life of Florence Nightingale* (Vol. 1). London: Macmillan.

Palmer, I. S. (1977). Florence Nightingale: Reformer, reactionary, researcher. *Nursing Research, 26*(2), 84–89.

Vicinus, M., & Nergaard, B. (Eds.). (1989). *Ever yours, Florence Nightingale. Selected Letters.* London: Billings & Sons, Ltd.

LUCILLE ELIZABETH NOTTER
(1907–1993)

Lucille Elizabeth Notter was a visionary nurse educator and researcher who was committed to the conduction and dissemination of nursing research during a time when research was thought of as separate from the role of nursing and nursing practice itself (Downs, 1993). She graduated from Saints Mary and Elizabeth Hospital School of Nursing in Kentucky (1931), going on to complete her bachelor's (1941), master's (1946), and doctorate degrees (1956), all from Teachers College, Columbia University (Foundation of New York State Nurses Association [NYSNA], 2010). Notter was the first editor of the journal *Nursing Research*; under her leadership, it became the first nursing journal to be included in MEDLINE. Her work included assisting the American Nurses Association (ANA) in securing funding for a series of research conferences in which she was the main organizer. She was also the first editor of the International Nursing Index and served as a mentor to many novice nurse researcher (Downs, 1993). Notter authored *Essentials of Nursing Research* and coauthored with Eugenia K. Spalding *Professional Nursing: Foundations, Perspectives, and Relationships* (ANA, 2007). In addition, she served as a nurse advisor to the New York State Education Department and New York City Committee on Prison Health Services, a secretary and president of NYSNA, and a president and Treasurer of Nurses House. Her awards and honors include the Distinguished Service to Public Health Nursing Award from the American Public Health Association, the R. Louise McManus Medal from Teachers College Nursing Education Alumni Association, Honorary Recognition for Distinguished Service to the Nursing Profession from NYSNA, and induction into the ANA Hall of Fame (ANA, 2007; Foundation of NYSNA, 2010).

American Nurses Association. (2007). *Lucille Elizabeth Notter (1907–1993) 1996 Inductee.* Retrieved January 3, 2011, from http://www.nursingworld.org/FunctionalMenu Categories/AboutANA/Honoring-Nurses/HallofFame/19962000Inductees/nottle5555.aspx

Downs, F.S. (1993). An editor for all seasons. *Nursing Research, 42*(3), 131.

Foundation of New York State Nurses Association. (2010). *Bellevue Alumnae Center for Nursing History Limited Edition Nursing Pins: Lucille Elizabeth Notter—2008.* Retrieved January 4, 2011, from http://foundationnys-nurses.org/giftshop/Notter.php

MARY ADELAIDE NUTTING
(1858–1948)

Mary Adelaide Nutting was a leader who promoted education for nurses. She graduated from the Johns Hopkins Hospital Training School for Nurses in 1991 and within 2 years became the assistant Superintendent of Nurses and Principal of the Training School. She held the position until 1907 when she assumed charge of the course in Hospital Economics at Teachers College, Columbia University. Nutting was the director of the first university-connected department of nursing and the first nurse ever to be appointed to a professorship in a university (Christy, 1969). Eventually, the nursing program at Teachers College became a hub for international nursing education. Nutting laid the foundation for graduate education in nursing when she insisted that only those nurses with a high school diploma who had completed a 2- or 3-year nurse training program would be eligible for admission. In addition, Nutting laid the groundwork to create an accelerated nursing curriculum for college graduates. Through her work with the American Society of Superintendents of Training Schools for Nurses (later to become the National League for Nursing Education), Nutting worked ardently to establish a universal standardized nursing curriculum (Christy, 1969). She was also a versatile writer who coauthored the first two volumes of the *History of Nursing* with Lavinia Dock and also wrote *A Sound Economic Basis for Nursing*, which was a collection of her articles (Alan Mason Chesney Medical Archives of the Johns Hopkins Medical Institutions, n.d.). Nutting was posthumously inducted into the American Nurses Association Hall of Fame in 1976 (American Nurses Association, 2007).

Alan Mason Chesney Medical Archives of The Johns Hopkins Medical Institutions. (n.d.). *Personal paper collections: Mary Adelaide Nutting Collection.* Retrieved November 8, 2010, from http://www.medicalarchives.jhmi.edu/papers/nutting.html

American Nurses Association. (2007). *1976 Inductee. Mary Adelaide Nutting: 1858–1948.* Retrieved November 8, 2010, from http://www.nursingworld.org/MaryAdelaide Nutting

Christy, T. E. (1969). *Cornerstone for nursing education. A history of the division of nursing education of Teachers College, Columbia University, 1899–1947.* New York, NY: Teachers College Press.

Estelle Massey Osborne
(1901–1981)

Estelle Massey Osborne fought tirelessly to eradicate discrimination for Black nurses, especially in the military and professional nursing organizations, so they would have the same opportunities for education and professional advancement as White nurses. Osborne's nursing education began at the segregated St. Louis City Hospital School (Fondiller, 2001). She obtained both her bachelor's (1929) and master's (1931) degrees from Teachers College, Columbia University; she was the first Black nurse with a master's degree. She was appointed to the National Nursing Council for War Service during a time when Black nurses were not allowed in military service. Under her influence, the number of schools admitting both Black and White students rose from 14 to 38, and the Army and Navy no longer refused Black nurses for service. She was elected president of the National Association of Colored Graduate Nurses (1934) and in her role fostered relationships with the American Nurses Association (ANA), the National League for Nursing, and the National Organization for Public Health Nursing (ANA, 2007; Fondiller, 2001). In 1946, she was the first Black nurse to become faculty at New York University. Her numerous awards and honors include the Mary Mahoney Award (1946), the establishment of the Estelle Massey Scholarship at Fisk University, Nashville, Nurse of the Year by the New York University Division of Nurse Education (1959), the Honorary Life Membership Award from Teachers College Nursing Education Alumni Association (1976), the Honorary Life Membership Chi Eta Phi, Omicron Chapter, and an honorary membership in the American Academy of Nursing in 1978 (New York University, n.d.; Pitts-Mosley, 2002). She was inducted into the ANA Hall of Fame in 1984 (ANA, 2007).

American Nurses Association. (2007). *Estelle Massey Osborne (1901–1981): 1984 Inductee.* Retrieved January 7, 2011, from http://www.nursingworld.org/EstelleMassey Osborne

Fondiller, S. H. (2001). Pioneers in the forefront of integration. *Nursing and Health Care Perspectives, 22*(2), 64–66.

New York University. (n.d.). A Brief History of the College. Retrieved January 7, 2011, from http://www.nyu.edu/nursing/thecollege/history.html

Pitts-Mosley, M. O. (2002). Great Black nurses series: Estelle Massey Riddle Osborne. *Association of Black Nursing Faculty Journal.* Retrieved January 7, 2011, from http://find-articles.com/p/articles/mi_m0MJT/is_5_13/ai_93610984/ ?tag= content;col1

SOPHIA PALMER
(1853–1920)

Sophia French Palmer was a born administrator who used her leadership skills to restructure hospitals, to develop schools of nursing, and to establish professional nursing organizations. She also expended great effort to obtain legislation requiring registration for nurses (American Nurses Association, 2008; Death of the Journal Editor, 1920). Palmer graduated from the Boston Training School for Nurses in 1876. In her career, she is noted to have reorganized Garfield Memorial Hospital in Washington and City Hospital in Rochester, New York. She also established St. Luke's Hospital and Training School in Massachusetts and the Garfield School in Washington (Death of the Journal Editor, 1920). Sophia Palmer was one of the early nursing leaders involved in establishing the Associated Alumnae of United States and Canada (later to be renamed the American Nurses Association) and the Society for Superintendents of Training Schools for Nurses (later to become the National League for Nursing Education; American Nurses Association, 2008). She was also influential in the establishment of the New York State Nurses Association (Pavri, 2000) and the Genesee Valley Nurses Association in Rochester, New York (Rochester General Hospital, n.d.). Palmer was the first President of the New York Board of Examiners and the first editor of the *American Journal of Nursing*, a position which she held until her death (Death of the Journal Editor, 1920). She was inducted into the American Nurses Association Hall of Fame in 1976 (American Nurses Association, 2008).

American Nurses Association. (2008). *The hall of fame inductees: Sophia French Palmer.* Retrieved November 9, 2010, from http://www.nursing world.org/FunctionalMenuCategories/AboutANA/Honoring-Nurses/HallofFame/19761982/palmsf5561.aspx

Death of the journal editor. (1920). *American Journal of Nursing, 20*(7). Retrieved November 9, 2010, from http://www.jstor.org/stable/3406946

Pavri, J. M. (2000). *Honoring our past: Building our future, a history of the New York State Nurses Association, NYSNA.* Franklin, VA: Q Publishing.

Rochester General Hospital. (n.d.). Sophia French Palmer. Retrieved November 9, 2010, from http://www.rochestergeneral.org/rochester-general-hospital/about-us/rochester-medical-museum-and-archives/Baker-Cederberg-Museum-and-Archives/biographies/sophia-french-palmer

HILDEGARD PEPLAU
(1909–1999)

Hildegard Peplau was a leader in the field of psychiatric nursing and is often referred to as the "mother of psychiatric nursing" (American Nurses Association, 2007). She graduated from Pennsylvania Hospital School of Nursing (1931), received a Bachelor of Arts degree from Bennington College (1943), went on to earn a master's degree at Teachers College, Columbia University (1947), and a Doctor of Education degree (EdD) in Curriculum Development from Teachers College (1953) (Forchuk, 2007). Peplau was a committed figurehead in nursing education and an advocate of higher education in nursing. She spearheaded the first clinical Nurse Specialist program at Rutgers University in 1954. This graduate program had a focus in psychiatric/mental health nursing (Rust, 2004). Peplau was the only nurse to serve as the Executive Director and then President of the American Nurses Association. She served on the International Council of Nurses and received the Christiane Reimann Prize from that organization (Anonymous, 1999). Peplau contributed revolutionary and pivotal ideas to the field of nursing and health care, such as patient–nurse relationship, mental health nursing constructs, inciting patients to more actively participate in their health care, and interpersonal relationships between health care providers and their clients (Gregg, 1999). Peplau was posthumously inducted into the American Nurses Association Hall of Fame in 1998 (American Nurses Association, 2007).

American Nurses Association. (2007). *The 1998 Hall of Fame Inductees: Hildegard Peplau.* Retrieved December 9, 2010, from http://www.nursingworld.org/Functional MenuCategories/AboutANA/Honoring-Nurses/HallofFame/19962000Inductees/peplauh5563.aspx

Anonymous. (1999). In memoriam: Hildegard E Peplau, 1909–1999. *Journal of Child and Adolescent Psychiatric Nursing, 12*(2), 51–51.

Forchuk, C. (2007). *Hidegard Peplau nursing theorist homepage.* Retrieved December 9, 2010, from http://publish.uwo.ca/~cforchuk/peplau

Gregg, D. E. (1999). Hildegard E. Peplau: Her contributions. *Perspectives in Psychiatric Care, 35*(3), 10–12. Retrieved December 9, 2010, from http://findarticles.com/p/articles/mi_qa3804/is_199907/ai_n8870487/pg_5/?tag=content;col1

Rust, J. E. (2004). Dr. Hildegard Peplau. *Clinical Nurse Specialist, 18*(5), 262–263.

ISABEL HAMPTON ROBB
(1860–1910)

Isabel Hampton Robb was a graduate of the Collegiate Institute of St. Catherine's (Ontario, Canada) and was subsequently admitted to the Bellevue Hospital Training School for Nurses in 1883. Robb was passionate about establishing and maintaining standardized training for nurses during a time when many hospitals were opening schools to gain access to student nurses for staffing (Christy, 1969). During her career, she served as Superintendent of the Illinois Training School in Chicago (1886–1889), Superintendent of Nurses and Principal of the Training School at John Hopkins Training School for Nurses (1889–1894) (American Association for the History of Nursing, Inc., n.d.). Robb was also responsible for establishing the course in Hospital Economics at Teachers College, Columbia University (1899). It was designed for graduate nurses serving in administrative or teaching roles across the country (Christy, 1969). Robb's leadership activities reached national proportions in the formation of the American Society of Superintendents of Training Schools for Nurses, which was later renamed the National League for Nursing Education. She also took the lead in forming the Nurses' Associated Alumnae of United States and Canada, which later became the American Nurses Association; she served as the first president of the Associated Alumnae (1896–1897). Robb was also among the original members of the committee to establish the *American Journal of Nursing*. In addition, she wrote three books during her career: *Nursing: Its Principles and Practices* (1893), *Nursing Ethics* (1900), and *Educational Standards for Nurses* (1907) (Alan Mason Chesney Medical Archives of Johns Hopkins Medical Institutions, n.d.), and was posthumously inducted into the ANA Hall of Fame in 1976 (American Nurses Association, 2008).

American Association for the History of Nursing, Inc. (n.d.). Isabel Adams Hampton Robb (1860–1910). Retrieved December 28, 2010, from http://www.aahn.org/gravesites/robb.html

American Nurses Association. (2008). *1976 Inductee: Isabel Adams Hampton Robb (1860–1910)*. Retrieved December 28, 2010, from http://www.nursingworld.org/Functional MenuCategories/AboutANA/Honoring-Nurses/HallofFame/19761982/robbia5575.aspx

Christy, T. E. (1969). *Cornerstone for nursing education. A history of nursing education of Teachers College, Columbia University, 1899–1947*. New York, NY: Teachers College Press.

The Alan Mason Chesney Medical Archives of The Johns Hopkins Medical Institutions. (n.d.). *The Isabel Hampton Robb Collection*. Retrieved December 28, 2010, from http://www.medica-larchives.jhmi.edu/papers/robb.html

Jessie M. Scott
(1915–2009)

Jessie M. Scott was a retired assistant surgeon general in the U.S. Public Health Service who made her mark on nursing education with her involvement in the 1964 Nurse Training Act. She was a strong advocate for improved nurse training and testified before congress on numerous occasions. She graduated from Wilkes–Barre General Hospital School of Nursing (1936) and went on to receive her bachelor's degree from the University of Pennsylvania. She received her master's degree in personnel administration from Columbia University (1949) and developed a program of field training in counseling for graduate students. She joined the U.S. Public Health Service in 1957 and became the director of the Division of Nursing in 1964; during this time, she worked to address the nursing shortage nationally and also spent time traveling internationally to observe and advise nursing education programs. Her honors include a distinguished service medal from the U.S. Public Health Service, the National League for Nursing's honor for national and international leadership, and the Spirit of Nursing Award on the 100th anniversary of the Visiting Nurse Service of New York City (Sullivan, 2010). She was also named a "Living Legend" in 1994 (American Academy of Nursing, 2010). In 1979, the Jessie M. Scott Award was established in her name by the American Association of Nursing and is presented to a registered nurse whose accomplishments in a field of practice, education, or research demonstrate the interdependence of these elements and their significance for the improvement of nursing and health care (American Nurses Association, 2010).

American Academy of Nursing. (2010). *1994 living legends*. Retrieved January 3, 2011, from http://www.aannet.org/i4a/pages/index.cfm?pageid=3463

American Nurses Association. (2010). *ANA National Awards Program*. Retrieved from http://www.nursingworld.org/FunctionalMenuCategories/AboutANA/Honoring-Nurses/NationalAwardsProgram/CriteriaApplications/JessieMScott_1.aspx

Sullivan, P. (2010). Public health official promoted nurse training. *The Washington Post*. Retrieved January 3, 2011, from http://www.washingtonpost.com/wp-dyn/content/article/2009/10/29/AR2009102904545.html

Laura L. Simms
(1919–2009)

Laura Simms was a valuable nurse leader in New York State whose contributions had a lasting impact on professional practice. She earned her nursing degree at Parkland Hospital School of Nursing in Texas, her Masters at Southern Methodist University in Texas, and her doctorate at Teachers College, Columbia University. Her doctoral dissertation focused on the significance of the role of the Clinical Nursing Specialist, a role which she pioneered during her time in practice. Simms's work as chairperson of the New York State Nurses Association (NYSNA) Special Committee to Study the Nurse Practice Act in 1969 paved the way for the revised legal definition of professional nursing practice in 1972. This new definition identified the diagnostic privilege and autonomous nature of nurses; other states used this definition as their model (Driscoll, 1976; Foundation of NYSNA, 2010). In addition, she played an important role of an Incorporator of the Foundation of New York State Nurses and was instrumental in the construction of the Veronica M. Driscoll Center for Nursing. She also guided the creation of the Foundation's centers for nursing history, public education, and research. Further, she served as the Foundation's first president and then trustee at large. Simms earned the Honorary Recognition Award from NYSNA, the Driscoll Award from the Foundation, and The R. Louise McManus Medal from Teachers College, Columbia University; all deemed the highest honor by each organization. She was also a member of the National League for Nursing and president and director at large of NYSNA (Foundation of NYSNA, 2010).

Driscoll, V. M. (1976). *Legitimizing the profession of nursing: The distinct mission of the New York State Nurses Association.* Schenectady, New York: The Foundation of the New York State Nurses Association.

Foundation of New York State Nurses Association. (2010). *In memoriam: Laura Simms EdD, RN.* Retrieved January 2, 2011, from http://foundationnysnurses.org/inmemoriam/index.php

Mabel Keaton Staupers
(1890–1989)

Mabel Keaton Staupers was a courageous nursing leader and Black activist who fought for the rights of Black nurses and for better care of Black patients (American Nurses Association [ANA], 2007). She graduated with honors from the Freedmen's Hospital School of Nursing in Washington, DC, in 1917. Observant of segregated schools of nursing, segregated hospital beds, and rank segregation in organizations, which included the National League for Nursing Education and the ANA, Staupers was resolved to initiate change that would generate and guarantee equal rights for Black nurses that would alert the public to disparities in treatment of Blacks and which would ultimately result in improved access to health care services for Black Americans everywhere (Carnegie, 1995). She was the first executive secretary of the National Association of Colored Graduate Nurses and led the fight to integrate Black nurses into the armed forces and professional nursing organizations. Because of her tireless efforts, the recognition and the acceptance of Black nurses into the institutional structures of American nursing were greatly improved (Foundation of New York State Nurses Association, 2010). Staupers was a recipient of numerous awards, including the Mary Mahoney Medal in 1914, the prestigious Springarn Medal from the NAACP in 1931, the Sojourner Truth Medal in 1947, the National Urban League Team Work Award, 1967, and the Medgar Evers Human Rights Award in 1965 (Carnegie, 1995). She authored the book *No Time for Prejudice* and was inducted into the ANA Hall of Fame in 1996 (ANA, 2007).

American Nurses Association. (2007). *1996 Inductee: Mabel Keaton Staupers, 1890–1989.* Retrieved January 4, 2011, from http://www.nursingworld.org/FunctionalMenu Categories/AboutANA/Honoring-Nurses/HallofFame/19962000Inductees/stauperm5584.aspx

Carnegie, M. E. (1995). *The path we tread. Blacks in nursing worldwide* (3rd ed.). New York: National League for Nursing Press.

Foundation of New York State Nurses Association. (2010). *Bellevue Alumnae Center for Nursing History: Mabel Keaton Staupers—1994.* Retrieved January 4, 2011, from http://foundationnysnurses.org/giftshop/Staupers.php

LILLIAN WALD
(1867–1940)

Lillian Wald was a born leader and innovator who showed unending determination by putting her time, energy, and program planning skills into assisting those lacking access to healthcare. Through her work, she coined the term "public health nurse" (Jewish Women's Archive, 2010). Wald juggled many roles at one time including nurse, social worker, reformer, teacher, activist, philanthropist, and humanitarian. When confronted with the poverty and untenable living conditions among the sick poor and immigrants in the lower east side of Manhattan, she turned her attention toward their needs (Christy, 1969). Wald's administrative skills enabled her to plan and execute a city wide visiting nurse program and establish the Henry Street Settlement—the forerunner of the Visiting Nurse Service of New York. This program became the national model and eventually a worldwide model for public health nursing (Visiting Nurse Service of New York, 2010). She was also the founder and first president of the National Organization of Public Health Nurses and is notably responsible for the initiation of the Federal Children's Bureau under President Theodore Roosevelt. Before her death, she was named in the *New York Times* (1922) as one of the twelve greatest living American women (National Women's History Museum, n.d.). Wald was inducted into the American Nurses Association Hall of Fame in 1976 (American Nurses Association, 2008) and the National Women's Hall of Fame in 1993.

American Nurses Association. (2008). *Hall of fame inductee: Lillian Wald (1867–1940).* Retrieved from http://www.nursingworld.org/LillianDWald

Christy, T. E. (1969). *Cornerstone for nursing education. A history of the division of nursing education of Teachers College, Columbia University. 1899–1947.* New York: Teachers College Press.

Jewish Women's Archive. (2010). *History makers: Lillian Wald: Public health nursing.* Retrieved from http://jwa.org/historymakers/wald/public-health-nursing

National Women's Hall of Fame. (n.d.). *Women of the hall: Lillian Wald.* Retrieved from http://www.greatwomen.org/women.php?action=viewone&id=162

National Women's History Museum. (n.d.). *Lillian D. Wald (1867–1940).* Retrieved from http://www.nwhm.org/education-resources/biography/biographies/lillian-wald

Visiting Nurse Service of New York. (2010). *Lillian Wald.* Retrieved from http://www.vnsny.org/community/our-history/lillian-wald

HARRIET WERLEY
(1914–2002)

Harriet H. Werley received her nursing diploma from the Jefferson Medical College Hospital School of Nursing in Philadelphia, going on to obtain her bachelor's degree from the University of California, Berkeley (1948), and her master's degree in Nursing Administration from the Teachers College at Columbia University (1951). Before earning her PhD in psychology from the University of Utah (1969), she served in a variety of positions in the United States Army, one being the first chief of the Department of Nursing Research at the Walter Reed Army Institute of Research (Lewis, 2007; University of Illinois at Chicago, n.d.). Werley is best known for her pioneering work in nursing informatics, advocating for the use of clinical data for research and patient management; she led the way in the development of the science of nursing informatics. One of her big achievements was collaborating with Norma Lang in the creation of Nursing Minimum Data Sets that included nursing diagnoses, interventions, outcomes, and nursing intensity (Lewis, 2007; Ozbolt, 2003). Further, she was a founding editor of the journals *Research in Nursing and Health* and the *Annual Review of Nursing Research*. Werley was the first nurse to be given the Award for Outstanding Contribution to Nursing and Psychology from the American Psychological Association (University of Illinois at Chicago, n.d.). In 1996, she was presented with a distinguished service award from the University of Illinois-Chicago and given the President's Award from the American Medical Informatics Association (Lewis, 2007). In 1973, Werley became a Charter Fellow of the American Academy of Nursing. In 1991, the American College of Medical Informatics elected her to fellowship, and in 1994, the American Academy of Nursing designated her a "Living Legend" (Ozbolt, 2003).

Lewis, D. (2007). Editorial: A tribute to Harriet Helen Werley. *CIN: Computers, Informatics, Nursing, 25*(2), 59–60.

Ozbolt, J. G. (2003). Harriet Helen Werley, PhD, RN, FAAN, FACMI. *Journal of the American Medical Informatics Association, 10*(2), 224–225.

University of Illinois at Chicago. (n.d.). Harriet H. Werley Papers, 1959–2002. Retrieved January 1, 2001, from http://www.uic.edu/depts/lib/specialcoll/services/lhsc/ead/017–20-04f.html

INDEX